SLEEP AND THE MATURING NERVOUS SYSTEM

Based on a symposium, "The Maturation of Brain Mechanisms Related to Sleep Behavior," held at Boiling Springs, Pennsylvania, June 21–24, 1970, sponsored by The National Institute of Child Health and Human Development, National Institutes of Health.

Sleep and the Maturing Nervous System

Edited by

CARMINE D. CLEMENTE

Department of Anatomy
School of Medicine
University of California at Los Angeles
Los Angeles, California

DOMINICK P. PURPURA

Department of Anatomy and the Rose F. Kennedy
Center for Research in Mental Retardation and
Human Development
Albert Einstein College of Medicine
Bronx, New York

FLORENCE E. MAYER

Growth and Development Branch
National Institute of Child Health and Human
Development
Department of Health, Education and Welfare
National Institutes of Health
Bethesda, Maryland

ACADEMIC PRESS   New York and London   1972

ACADEMIC PRESS, INC.
111 Fifth Avenue, New York, New York 10003

United Kingdom Edition published by
ACADEMIC PRESS, INC. (LONDON) LTD.
24/28 Oval Road, London NW1

LIBRARY OF CONGRESS CATALOG CARD NUMBER: 72-84277

PRINTED IN THE UNITED STATES OF AMERICA

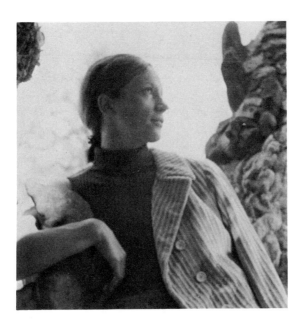

To the memory of Dr. Danièle Jouvet-Mounier (1935–1970). Her research on the maturation of sleep patterns in different species will remain forever a cornerstone in the building of our knowledge of sleep-wakefulness behavior. Its importance was amply illustrated by the frequent references to her work throughout the conference and in the pages that follow.

Contents

3 **Maturing Neuronal Subsystems: The Dendrites of Spinal Motorneurons**

Madge E. Scheibel and Arnold B. Scheibel

NEUROCHEMICAL FACTORS IN THE MATURATION OF SLEEP BEHAVIOR

4 **Coordination between Excitation and Inhibition: Development of the GABA System**

Eugene Roberts

5 **Contributions of Differential Housing to Brain Development: Some Implications for Sleep Behavior**

Walter B. Essman

6 **The Role of Biogenic Amines in Sleep**

Oscar Resnick

7 Developmental Changes in Neurochemistry during the Maturation of Sleep Behavior

Williamina A. Himwich

8 Maturation of Neurobiochemical Systems Related to the Ontogeny of Sleep Behavior

Peter J. Morgane

DEVELOPMENT OF EEG AND ACTIVITY PATTERNS IN RELATION TO SLEEP

9 Development of Wakefulness-Sleep Cycles and Associated EEG Patterns in Mammals

Robert J. Ellingson

10 The Basic Rest-Activity Cycle and Sleep: Developmental Considerations in Man and Cats

M. B. Sterman

11 Development of States in Infants

Arthur H. Parmelee, Jr., and Evelyn Stern

DEVELOPMENT OF REFLEX PATTERNS IN SLEEP

12 The Somatosensory Cerebral Evoked Potentials of the Sleeping Human Newborn

John E. Desmedt

13 Patterns of Reflex Excitability during the Ontogenesis of Sleep and Wakefulness

Michael H. Chase

14 Patterns of Reflex Behavior Related to Sleep in the Human Infant

H. F. R. Prechtl

Contents

DEVELOPMENTAL ASPECTS OF NORMAL
AND ABNORMAL SLEEP BEHAVIOR

15 Sleep Deprivation and the Organization of the Behavioral States

William C. Dement

16 Development of Sleep Patterns in Autistic Children

Edward M. Ornitz

17 Sleep in Mental Retardation

Olga Petre-Quadens

18   Maternal Toxemia, Fetal Malnutrition, and Bioelectric Brain Activity of the Newborn

F. J. Schulte, Gabriele Hinze, and Gerlind Schrempf

19   Summary and Concluding Remarks

Donald B. Lindsley

List of Participants

YOSHIO AKIYAMA, Department of Developmental Neurology, University of Gröningen, The Netherlands

THOMAS F. ANDERS, Department of Psychiatry, Albert Einstein College of Medicine at Montefiore Hospital, Bronx, New York

FLOYD E. BLOOM, Laboratory of Neuropharmacology, Division of Special Mental Health Research, National Institute of Mental Health, Saint Elizabeth Hospital, Washington, D.C.

DAVID BODIAN, Department of Anatomy, Johns Hopkins University School of Medicine, Baltimore, Maryland

MICHAEL H. CHASE, Departments of Anatomy and Physiology, University of California, School of Medicine, Los Angeles, California

CARMINE D. CLEMENTE, Department of Anatomy, University of California, School of Medicine, Los Angeles, California

PAUL D. COLEMAN, Department of Anatomy, University of Rochester School of Medicine and Dentistry, Rochester, New York

WILLIAM C. DEMENT, Department of Psychiatry, Stanford University, School of Medicine, Stanford, California

JOHN E. DESMEDT, Brain Research Unit, University of Brussels, Brussels, Belgium

ROBERT J. ELLINGSON, Nebraska Psychiatric Institute, University of Nebraska, Medical Center, Omaha, Nebraska

WALTER B. ESSMAN, Department of Psychology, Queens College, C.U.N.Y., Flushing, New York

HARRY H. GORDON, Rose Fitzgerald Kennedy Center for Research in Mental Retardation and Human Development, Albert Einstein College of Medicine, Bronx, New York

WILLIAMINA A. HIMWICH, Thudichum Psychiatric Research Laboratory, Galesburg State Research Hospital, Galesburg, Illinois

GABRIELE HINZE, Department of Pediatrics, University of Gottingen, Göttingen, Germany

BARRY J. HOFFER, Laboratory of Neuropharmacology, Division of Special Mental Health Research, Saint Elizabeth Hospital, Washington, D.C.

NATHANIEL KLEITMAN, 222 Washington Avenue, Santa Monica, California

DONALD B. LINDSLEY, Departments of Psychology, Physiology, and Psychiatry, and Brain Research Institute, University of California, Los Angeles, California

DENNIS J. McGINTY, Neuropsychology Research, Veterans Administration Hospital, Sepulveda, California

DAVID R. METCALF, Department of Psychiatry, University of Colorado Medical Center, Denver, Colorado

PETER J. MORGANE, Laboratory of Neurophysiology, Worchester Foundation for Experimental Biology, Shrewsbury, Massachusetts

EDWARD M. ORNITZ, Department of Psychiatry, University of California, School of Medicine, Los Angeles, California

ARTHUR H. PARMELEE, JR., Department of Pediatrics, University of California, School of Medicine, Los Angeles, California

H. F. R. PRECHTL, Department of Developmental Neurology, University of Gröningen, The Netherlands

JAMES W. PRESCOTT, National Institute of Child Health and Human Development, Bethesda, Maryland

DOMINICK P. PURPURA, Department of Anatomy and the Rose F. Kennedy Center for Research in Mental Retardation and Human Development, Albert Einstein College of Medicine, Bronx, New York

OLGA PETRE-QUADENS, Department of Developmental Neurology, Born-Bunge Research Foundation, Berchem-Antwerp, Belgium

OSCAR RESNICK, Worchester Foundation for Experimental Biology, Shrewsbury, Massachusetts

EUGENE ROBERTS, Division of Neurosciences, City of Hope National Medical Center, Duarte, California

HOWARD ROFFWARG, Department of Psychiatry, Albert Einstein College of Medicine at Montefiore Hospital, Bronx, New York

GUENTER H. ROSE, Laboratories of Developmental Psychobiology, University of Nebraska Medical School, Omaha, Nebraska

MORTIMER G. ROSEN, Department of Obstetrics-Gynecology, University of Rochester School of Medicine and Dentistry, Rochester, New York

ARONOLD B. SCHEIBEL, Departments of Anatomy and Psychiatry, University of California, School of Medicine, Los Angeles, California

MADGE E. SCHEIBEL, Departments of Anatomy and Psychiatry, University of California, School of Medicine, Los Angeles, California

GERLIND SCHREMPF, Department of Pediatrics, University of Göttingen, Göttingen, Germany

F. J. SCHULTE, Department of Pediatrics, University of Göttingen, Göttingen, Germany

ROBERT J. SHOFER, Department of Anatomy and the Rose F. Kennedy Center for Research in Mental Retardation and Human Development, Albert Einstein College of Medicine, Bronx, New York

GEORGE R. SIGGINS, Laboratory of Neuropharmacology, Division of Special Mental Health Research, National Institute of Mental Health, Saint Elizabeth Hospital, Washington, D.C.

M. B. STERMAN, Neuropsychology Research, Veterans Administration Hospital, Sepulveda, California

EVELYN STERN, Department of Pediatrics, University of California, Center for Health Sciences, Los Angeles, California

ELLIOT D. WEITZMAN, Department of Neurology, Albert Einstein College of Medicine, Bronx, New York

DONALD J. WOODWARD, Department of Physiology, School of Medicine and Dentistry, University of Rochester, Rochester, New York

Preface

It is now well established that both genetic and environmental factors play important roles in determining the morphological and electrophysiological maturation of the brain. What is not known, however, is how such maturational features contribute to the progressive elaboration of complex neural interactions that characterize the development of sleep-wakefulness activities in the maturing organism. There can be little doubt that this problem is central to the issue of the development of complex behaviors in general. This follows from the fact that such behaviors are expressed upon a background of variable wakefulness which requires the integrative activity of many different neuronal organizations. But equally impressive is the fact that transitions from sleep to wakefulness and vice versa bring into operation perhaps more complex neural and biochemical mechanisms. Thus the understanding of how maturational processes are related to the development of sleep-wakefulness behavior should provide information essential for the adequate appreciation of the biological basis of behavior in the broadest sense.

The conference, held at the Allenberry Inn in Boiling Springs, Pennsylvania from June 21-24, 1970, was organized to explore the extent to which basic data on brain maturation and data on the ontogeny of sleep-wakefulness behavior might be discussed from the standpoint of their mutual relevancy. Additional aspects of the conference focused on the developmental implications of conditions, experimental or otherwise, which might lead to the establishment of normal and abnormal sleep behavior in maturing organisms. The program was divided into five sessions: (1) The Maturation of Neural Elements, (2) Neurochemical Factors in Maturation of Sleep Behavior, (3) Development of EEG and Activity Patterns in Relation to Sleep, (4) Development of Reflex Patterns in

Sleep, and (5) Developmental Aspects of Normal and Abnormal Sleep Behavior. The proceedings were summarized by Dr. Donald B. Lindsley.

The editors of this symposium volume were joined in the planning stages of the conference by Dr. Robert J. Ellingson, Dr. Donald B. Lindsley, and Dr. Merrill S. Read. Grateful acknowledgment is also made to Miss Wanda Burnett for editorial assistance in the preparation of the final manuscript and to the Growth and Development Program of the National Institute of Child Health and Human Development whose enthusiastic support and sponsorship of the conference made this volume possible.

Carmine D. Clemente
Dominick P. Purpura
Florence E. Mayer

THE MATURATION OF NEURAL ELEMENTS

1

Principles of Synaptogenesis and Their Application to Ontogenetic Studies of Mammalian Cerebral Cortex*

Dominick P. Purpura and Robert J. Shofer

Newborn altricial mammals exhibit relatively little awake behavior (crying, crawling, sucking, etc.) and quiet sleep in contrast to the large proportion of time they spend in "active" or rapid eye movements sleep (REMS). Maturation of sleep-wakefulness cycles results in an increasing capacity for wakefulness, as Kleitman has correctly insisted, and a reorganization of temporospatial patterns of various sleep states. Although the neurobiological processes underlying these developmental events are poorly understood, maturation of sleep-wakefulness behavior is evidently as much a consequence of the reorganization of early established patterns of activity as it is the elaboration of new modes of operation in developing neuronal subsystems. Considering the prominence of the physiological mechanisms subserving active sleep in the altricial neonate, it is difficult

*Supported in part by grants from NINDS (NS-07512) and The Given Foundation.

3

to imagine any further maturation of these mechanisms during the postnatal period. Indeed, the real "paradox" in paradoxical sleep (PS) in the immature born animal is that it expresses the operation of brain stem neuronal organizations that are as functionally mature at birth as they will ever be. Viewed in this fashion, it could be argued that the maturation of sleep-wakefulness behavior involves the development of control systems for effective and purposeful utilization of the intervals between periods of REMS. Whether these control systems reside in brain stem organizations or at both diencephalic and cortical levels is unimportant for present purposes. (Available evidence, reviewed elsewhere in this volume, suggests their representation at virtually all neuraxial levels.) The key problem is not *where* these control systems reside, but how their functions are expressed at different postnatal developmental stages.

Central to this problem is the prickly issue of the meaning and significance of "maturation" as applied to such complex activities as sleep and wakefulness. Analyses of maturation in terms of overt sensorimotor and autonomic activities or electrographic, biochemical, and neuroendocrinological events suffice to provide conceptual definitions of the concatenation of processes implicated in brain development. But just as the most complex behaviors must ultimately yield to analytical approaches capable of dissecting individual elements of the behavior, however hazardous this may seem, so is it necessary that the processes of brain maturation be similarly comprehended. It is no longer sufficient to specify parameters of brain development exclusively in terms of gray/white coefficients, cell size, shape and location, cortical electrical activity, or myelination of central pathways. What must be understood is the nature and functional significance of dynamic interactions in developing neuronal subsystems. No less important is the problem of defining maturational changes in the physiological properties of immature neurons and their synaptic relations. For it is the authors' prejudice that elucidation of fundamental principles of synaptogenesis and electrogenesis in developing neuronal organizations will greatly facilitate future analysis of control mechanisms implicated in sleep-wakefulness behavior in the immature animal.

This report considers several types of ontogenetic studies ranging from analyses of excitability properties and synaptic processes in single immature cortical neurons to structure-function correlations in developing cortical neuronal subsystems. The complex processes involved in cortical maturation represent decisive events in the elaboration of control systems regulating sleep-wakefulness activity. Hence, studies of elementary operations of immature cortical neurons and their synaptic connections can be expected to provide a basis for assessing the development of these forebrain mechanisms and their influence on manifestations of sleep states at different developmental stages.

COMPARATIVE NEURONAL MORPHOGENESIS AND
SYNAPTOGENESIS IN IMMATURE CEREBRAL
CORTEX: FUNCTIONAL IMPLICATIONS

Morphological studies at the light and electron microscope level have provided a consistent picture of the pattern of postnatal development of neurons and synapses in feline cerebral cortex (Noback and Purpura, 1961; Voeller *et al.*, 1963; Purpura and Pappas, 1968; Schwartz *et al.*, 1968; Scheibel and Scheibel, 1964). It has been established that in newborn kittens pyramidal neurons exhibit relatively well-developed apical dendrites in both neocortex and hippocampus, but only the latter cortical structure contains pyramidal neurons with well-developed basilar dendritic systems in the neonatal period. Utilizing the criteria of basilar dendritic growth as a rough index of cortical neuronal maturation, it is evident that hippocampal neuronal development in the kitten is approximately 2 weeks in advance of neocortical development in respect to the elaboration of total dendritic surface area available for synaptic inputs on trunks or spines.

The existence of well-developed apical dendrites in neocortex and both apical and basilar dendrites in hippocampus of newborn kittens has permitted definitive analysis of the mode of synaptogenesis in cortex as revealed in electron microscopic studies. Although axodendritic synapses in cerebral cortex are clearly evident at birth (Voeller *et al.*, 1963) in the kitten, these synapses are far more abundant in hippocampus than in neocortex (Schwartz *et al.*, 1968). In neocortex axodendritic synapses exhibiting all the fine structural features characteristic of mature synapses are related largely to dendritic trunks and dendritic branches in the immediate neonatal period. Spines are not present on apical dendrites of neocortical pyramidal neurons in the newborn kitten, but these become prominent during the second postnatal week (Noback and Purpura, 1961; Scheibel and Scheibel, 1964). In contrast to this, both apical and basilar dendrites of hippocampal pyramidal neurons exhibit well-developed spines in the neonatal period (Fig. 1), which is consistent with the more advanced maturational state of hippocampal neurons. This is further reflected in the extraordinary development of axodendritic synapses of the hippocampal neuropil in the neonatal kitten. These synapses are related to a variety of dendritic processes, including dendritic spines (Fig. 2).

The major postnatal morphogenetic event in neocortical pyramidal neurons in the kitten is the elaboration of basilar dendrites which proceeds to completion during the first postnatal month. During this period apical dendrites increase in volume, develop many branches and finer processes and, as noted above, acquire their complement of spines as do the basilar dendrites. Axon-collateral

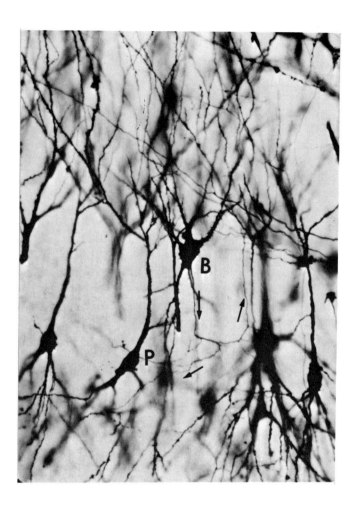

Fig. 1. Golgi-Cox preparation showing pyramidal and nonpyramidal neuron relations in hippocampus of a 3-day-old kitten. P, pyramidal neurons in superficial parts of stratum pyramidale; basilar dendrites and spines on apical and basilar dendrites are detectable. B, a modified basket-pyramid neuron of the stratum radiatum. Dendrites arising from the superior pole of this neuron are thick, covered with prominent spines, and are distributed in the stratum moleculare. Dendrites from the inferior pole course downward. The cell body of this neuron also exhibits prominent spines. The main stem axon, clearly visible, descends to the stratum pyramidale and bifurcates. One branch ascends along the apical dendritic shafts of pyramidal neurons, the other descends along basilar dendrites of these cells. × 250. (From Purpura and Pappas, 1968.)

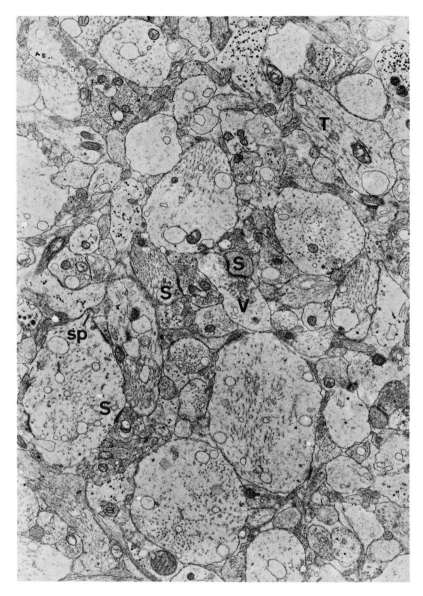

Fig. 2. Electron micrograph of neuropil of the hippocampus in a 1-day-old kitten. Large numbers of very fine processes are discernible, as well as many axodendritic synapses (S). Presynaptic elements of these synapses contain numerous vesicles (V). Note that axodendritic synapses are related to large as well as to very small dendritic processes. Sp, dendrite spine; T, microtubules. × 8500. (From Schwartz *et al.*, 1968.)

proliferation and increase in axon diameter are additional morphogenetic events in the postnatal period. For the most part these events precede the onset of myelination of pyramidal neuron axons (Purpura *et al.*, 1964a), which is a relatively prolonged maturational process in the kitten.

It is particularly noteworthy that the development of axodendritic synapses in cerebral cortex proceeds well in advance of the initial proliferation of axosomatic synapses (Voeller *et al.*, 1963). The same holds for the immature hippocampus despite the more mature appearance of its pyramidal neurons (Schwartz *et al.*, 1968). The fact that axodendritic systems related to trunks and spines are already well organized prior to the maturation of axosomatic synapses is especially relevant to the mode of synaptic engagement of cortical neurons by excitatory and inhibitory pathways in the early postnatal period (see below).

Axosomatic synaptogenesis is completed by the end of the first postnatal month in both neocortex and hippocampus. It has not been possible to detect obvious differences in the fine structure of neuropil in feline neocortex or hippocampus after the first month at which time cortical neuropil is similar to that found in the adult cat (Pappas and Purpura, 1961). These observations on the fine structure of neuropil should not be taken to indicate that no further morphogenesis occurs in kitten cerebral cortex beyond the first postnatal month. Subtle alterations in dendritic fine processes, the progressive elaboration of spine synapses and axon-terminal proliferation represent continuing developmental events which could readily escape detection unless more quantitative light and electron microscopic correlation techniques are employed. A step in this direction has been taken in studies of synaptogenesis in rat cerebral cortex (Aghajanian and Bloom, 1967).

Electrophysiological studies of immature neurons in neocortex and hippocampus have provided considerable information on the properties of these elements and their synaptic relations. Despite the "fragility" of immature neurons, in comparison to mature neurons, intracellular recording and stimulation techniques have been applied to the study of spike generation and synaptic processes in cortical neurons at different developmental stages. Because of the "fragility" of immature neurons a somewhat confused picture has emerged in regard to the question of resting membrane potentials in neurons of immature cortex. Studies carried out in the young rat (Deza and Eidelberg, 1967; Mareš, 1964) have suggested very low membrane resting potentials (10-30 mV) during the first 2 postnatal weeks. These results are most likely attributable to failures by these workers to secure satisfactory intracellular recordings from immature rat cortex neurons. When attempts are made to obtain stable recordings, it is clear that resting membrane potentials of cortical neurons in the young kitten, even in the immediate neonatal period, are in the range of 40-60 mV (Purpura *et al.*, 1965, 1968).

One of the major characteristics of intracellularly recorded postsynaptic

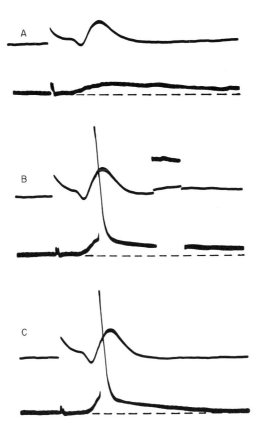

Fig. 3. Prolonged EPSP's (80-100 msec) evoked by ventrolateral thalamic stimulation in a sensorimotor cortex neuron from a 6-day-old kitten. Upper channel records indicate cortical surface activity, negativity upward. Amplitude of cortical surface responses, 200 μV. A, weak stimulation elicits an 18-20 msec latency EPSP with slow rise time and prolonged declining phase. B and C, stronger stimulation decreases rise time and increases amplitude of EPSP. Cell discharge secured at crest of EPSP. Note duration of spike potential, lack of repetitive responsiveness and failure of spike discharge to alter time course of the EPSP. Calibration in B, 50 mV; 20 msec. (From Purpura *et al.*, 1965.)

potentials (PSP's) in immature cortical neurons is their relatively long duration. This holds for both excitatory and inhibitory postsynaptic potentials (EPSP's and IPSP's) but is far more evident in IPSP's. Significant also is the slow rise time and peak amplitude of EPSP's evoked in immature neocortical neurons by stimulation of specific thalamocortical projections (Fig. 3). Such slowly evolving EPSP's are generally not observed in mature neocortical neurons responding to specific thalamic stimulation (Creutzfeldt *et al.*, 1966; Purpura and Shofer, 1964; Purpura *et al.* 1964b). It should also be noted (Fig. 3) that an unusually long latency intervenes between a stimulus to the thalamic relay nucleus and the onset of the EPSP. This long latency is referable to conduction delay in poorly myelinated or unmyelinated thalamocortical afferents. Temporal dispersion in such axons may also account for the slow rise time of the EPSP, but this is also related to dendritic location of the synapses on immature neurons (Purpura, 1967; Rall, 1967).

Despite the magnitude and duration of specific evoked EPSP's in immature neurons such synaptically induced depolarizations are rarely effective in triggering repetitive spike potentials, especially in very young kittens. This lack of repetitive responsiveness of immature cortical neurons has been repeatedly observed in intracellular studies of the authors and extracellular unit studies of others (Armstrong-James, 1970; Huttenlocher, 1967). Intracellular recording has also disclosed that spike potentials are longer in duration in immature neurons than in mature neurons, thereby suggesting fundamental differences in the kinetics of ionic processes underlying spike electrogenesis in immature and mature elements (Purpura, 1969a).

Although EPSP's are well developed in immature cortical neurons they do not exhibit the potency that is evident in neurons of older kittens. In part this is explicable by the limited excitability of immature neurons and probably the paucity of excitatory synapses and their remote location on dendritic trunks. It should be recalled that EPSP's evoked by thalamic stimulation are detectable in neocortical neurons prior to the development of axodendritic spine synapses (Fig. 3). If spine synapses are largely excitatory in function, as a number of workers have suggested (cf. Jones and Powell, 1970), their absence in immature neurons could account for the relative ineffectiveness of EPSP's elicited by afferent pathways with synaptic terminals distributed largely in relation to dendritic trunks. As pointed out by Rall (1967) EPSP's generated at adjacent sites on the same dendrite can be expected to exhibit nonlinear summation. Spine synapses, on the other hand, could serve to restrict the conductance change that underlies the EPSP by virtue of the high longitudinal resistance of the neck of the spine (Llinás and Hillman, 1969). This would allow for linear summation of electrotonically propagating EPSP's in dendritic branches and trunks.

A remarkable finding in intracellular studies of immature cortical neurons has been the prominence of IPSP's elicited by various modes of synaptic activation. Prolonged IPSP's have been observed in the neonatal period in neocortical neurons (Fig. 4) and both spontaneous and evoked IPSP's have been particularly prominent in immature hippocampal neurons (Fig. 5). In the latter elements such IPSP's have all the characteristics of IPSP's observed in adult animals (Kandel *et al.*, 1961; Andersen *et al.*, 1964). This is evident in regard to the duration of IPSP's and their distribution in hippocampal pyramidal neurons following particular modes of stimulation (Fig. 6). Prolonged (>500 msec)

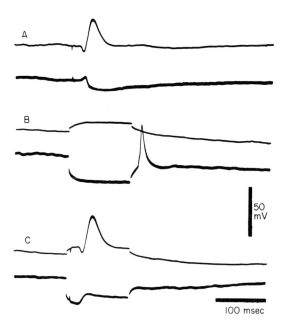

Fig. 4. Prolonged depressant effect of residual IPSP on directly evoked response of a neuron from a 5-day-old kitten. A, ventrolateral thalamic stimulation elicits a cortical evoked response predominantly surface-negative in configuration. The partially depolarized neuron exhibits an early EPSP and succeeding long duration IPSP. B, membrane hyperpolarization and succeeding anode-break response produced by an inward current pulse of about 120 msec duration. Note inflection on rising phase of anode-break response. C, thalamic stimulation during induced membrane hyperpolarization. Early phase of IPSP is inverted to depolarizing response which summates with the initial EPSP. Anode-break response is suppressed by residual hyperpolarization of the IPSP, whose time course is unaltered by inversion of early phase during current injection. (From Purpura *et al.*, 1965.)

IPSP's in neocortical neurons have commonly been observed in older kittens following thalamic relay nucleus stimulation. It is the authors' experience that similar single-shock specific thalamic stimulation in adult animals does not result in the production of such long-duration IPSP's in neocortical neurons (Purpura and Shofer, 1964; Purpura *et al.*, 1964b). Since synaptic events elicited in cortical neurons by thalamic stimulation are composites of EPSP's and IPSP's generated at different somadendritic membrane sites, it is likely that the long duration of IPSP's in immature neocortical neurons reflects, in part, the relative paucity of EPSP's which might ordinarily "attenuate" prolonged hyperpolarizing potentials by algebraic summation. The extent to which the development of axodendritic spine synapses might contribute countervailing EPSP's to limit the effectiveness of prolonged IPSP's is not known. However, it should be recalled

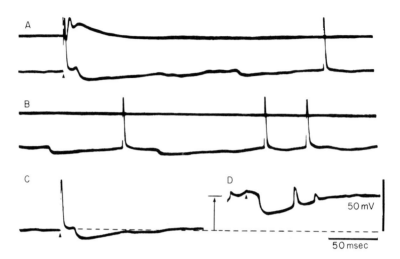

Fig. 5. Spontaneous and fimbrial-evoked IPSP's in a hippocampal neuron from a 3-day-old kitten. Upper channel: Monopolar recording from the ventricular surface of the hippocampus at the fimbrial-hippocampal junction. A, fimbrial stimulation at arrowhead. A directly evoked spike is elicited due to coupling between stimulating and recording electrodes; this spike is followed by a small EPSP which is terminated by a prolonged IPSP. Note recurring IPSP's and spontaneous spikes in this and record B. C and D, comparisons of IPSP characteristics when cell has satisfactory resting potential (C) and when partial depolarization occurs (D); partial spikes are evident in (D). IPSP duration in partially depolarized cell exhibits only a small decrease in duration and a minimal decrease in rise time. Arrow between C and D indicates approximate loss of membrane potential. (From Purpura *et al.*, 1968.)

that prolonged IPSP's in response to single thalamic stimuli have been observed in neocortical neurons of kittens 3-4 weeks of age (Fig. 7), i.e., well after the phase of peak axodendritic spine synapse proliferation.

The demonstration that prolonged IPSP's exhibiting all the electrographic features of IPSP's in adult animals can be recorded intracellularly in cortical neurons of neonatal kittens prior to the development of axosomatic synapses indicates that at least in early postnatal periods inhibition of cortical neurons is effected by axodendritic synapses (Purpura *et al.*, 1965). The morphophysiological data in support of this conclusion have been particularly compelling in regard to inhibitory activities generated in immature hippocampal pyramidal neurons by fornix or fimbria stimulation (Figs. 5 and 6) (Purpura *et al.*, 1968). Examination of many profiles of hippocampal pyramidal neuron cell bodies in the electron microscope has failed to reveal axosomatic synapses despite the presence of axon terminals in close apposition to cell bodies. It is indeed remarkable that, despite this relationship, such terminals are generally in synaptic contact with dendrites and not cell bodies (Fig. 8) (Schwartz *et al.*,

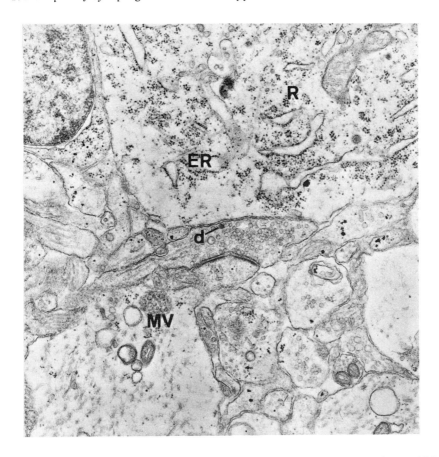

Fig. 8. A well-developed synapse adjacent to the cell body of a hippocampal pyramidal neuron in a newborn kitten. The presynaptic terminal contains a large number of vesicles including a dense core granule (d). The terminal is clearly in synaptic relation to a dendritic process which exhibits a prominent postsynaptic density. Note 'clusters of ribosomes (R) and the rough endoplasmic reticulum (ER) in the cell body. A multivesicular body (MV) is seen in a large dendritic process. × 21,100. (From Schwartz *et al.*, 1968.)

the soma. There can be little doubt that when primary impulse trigger sites in the soma-initial segment region are suppressed by IPSP's impulse initiation and spike generation in dendrites occur in accordance with the data and schema of Fig. 11 (Purpura *et al.*, 1965). While these observations have required a critical reexamination of the functional activity of dendrites and have established criteria for evaluating dendritic spike generation and conduction (Purpura, 1967, 1971), they have also revealed a developmental process in cortical neurons which could not have been predicted from previous evoked potential studies. From the large number of intracellular investigations of *mature* neocortical neurons it is

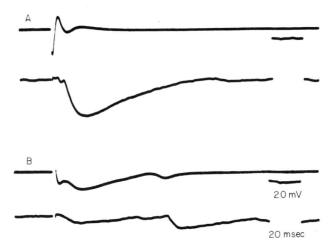

Fig. 9. Characteristics of IPSP's evoked in a hippocampal pyramidal neuron by different modes of stimulation in a 2-day-old kitten. Upper channel: Monopolar recordings from ventricular surface of hippocampus. A, fimbrial stimulation evokes a short-latency antidromic field potential which is recorded intracellularly. This is succeeded by a prominent and prolonged IPSP. B, stimulation of the perforant pathway in the subiculum elicits a multiphasic short and long-latency IPSP in the same neuron. (From Purpura, Prelevic, and Santini, unpublished data.)

evident that spike generation and propagation rarely, if ever, occur in these cells under ordinary conditions. Inasmuch as *immature* cortical neurons may exhibit dendritic spikes, it follows that the absence of spike-generating properties in mature neurons reflects a developmental alteration, perhaps linked in some obscure fashion to dendritic and synaptic morphogenesis. The implication in this is that cortical neuronal maturation must include a component of change in the physiological properties of dendrites in addition to more obvious changes associated with morphogenetic events.

The hypothesis has been proposed that partial spikes in dendrites of mature neurons may serve to increase the efficacy of remote axodendritic excitatory synapses (Spencer and Kandel, 1961). Since the afferent input to immature cortical neurons is exclusively dendritic in distribution, the capacity for partial and full spike generation in dendrites may reflect a mechanism for increasing the synaptic security of these inputs with a paucity of terminals on dendritic trunks (Purpura, 1969a). Additionally, spike generation in distal dendrites may compensate for suppression of primary impulse initiation sites by IPSP's that exert their effects largely on soma and proximal dendritic segments. Paradoxically, inhibition in this instance could become an effective mechanism for activating sites in dendrites potentially capable of exhibiting partial or full spike generation and propagation. The records shown in Fig. 11 illustrate this in immature cortical neurons, and other examples of this have been found in

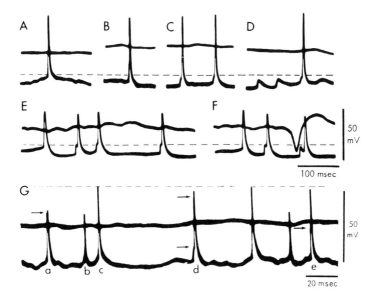

Fig. 10. Various types of spontaneous discharges recorded in immature neocortical neurons. A-D, from a 5-day-old kitten. A, spike potential triggered on a slow depolarizing prepotential. B and C, transition stages with development of fast prepotentials seen in isolation and in association with cell discharge. E and F, from a neuron in a 13-day-old kitten. Various dissociations between spikes and fast prepotentials seen during increases in membrane polarization. G, different varieties of spikes recorded during a 250-msec period of spontaneous activity of a neuron in an 18-day-old kitten. The different types of spikes are labeled a-e for purposes of identification. Arrows indicate points of inflections. Broken horizontal line in G indicates maximum amplitude of spikes such as those labeled c, which lack discontinuities. Note in particular differences in amplitude, duration, and points of inflections. Calibrations in F apply to records A-F. (From Purpura *et al.*, 1965.)

mature hippocampal pyramidal neurons (Purpura, 1966). Thus, the potentiality for multiple sites of impulse initiation and spike propagation in dendrites implies far more complex integrative functions than can be inferred on the basis of the spinal motoneuron model (Purpura, 1971). To the extent that plasticity of function is adequately reflected in heterogeneous excitability properties of developing dendritic systems, the integrative capacities of immature cortical neurons may be more impressive than has been suspected previously.

CORRELATION OF SYNAPTOGENESIS AND EVOKED POTENTIALS OF IMMATURE CEREBRAL CORTEX

It has long been established that primary cortical evoked potentials in newborn altricial mammals and the human premature neonate are initially surface-negative in configuration. Maturation of these responses results in the appear-

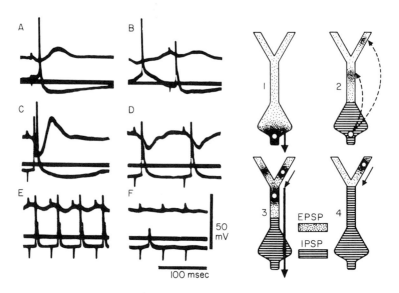

Fig. 11. Impulse initiation and propagation in dendrites of a neuron from a 21-day-old kitten. Upper channel record: cortical surface-evoked response to ventrolateral thalamic stimulation. Third beam of oscilloscope was placed at resting membrane potential level established in absence of stimulation. A, single shock thalamic stimulus evokes small EPSP which triggers "normal" spike potential. Latter is succeeded by an IPSP. B, spontaneous discharge initiated by slow EPSP precedes stimulus. When stimulus occurs on small succeeding IPSP, evoked spike is smaller in amplitude and arises from a lower firing level. C, early phase of 5-Hz thalamic stimulation during which IPSP-summation leads to sustained membrane hyperpolarization. Spike potential is evoked with shorter latency than in A. Spike arises directly from baseline and exhibits rapid rise time. Note second component on shoulder of first spike. D and E, increase in stimulus frequency results in reduction of second component. F, failure of all-or-none spikes and appearance of partial response whose latency is similar to second component of spikes in E. 1, Original conditions similar to those in A when EPSP's trigger impulse at normal spike initiation sites (white dot). 2, IPSP's produce transitory shift in impulse trigger sites in dendrites. 3, Repetitive stimulation as in C through E leads to depression of primary impulse trigger site by IPSP's and activation of dendritic loci by axodendritic EPSP's. Large arrow indicates all-or-none propagating spike. Small arrow represents partial spike. 4, Conditions such as those in F, at a stage when partial response arising in distal dendritic site is incapable of initiating conducted dendritic spike. (Modified from Purpura *et al.*, 1965.)

ance of typical initially surface-positive responses of specific projection cortex (cf. reviews in Himwich, 1970; and elsewhere in this volume). Surface-negative responses are also prominent in a variety of evoked cortical potentials of immature neocortex, including the locally evoked superficial negative responses (Purpura *et al.*, 1960) (Fig. 12). The presence of well-developed axodendritic synaptic pathways in superficial regions of cortex in the newborn kitten has

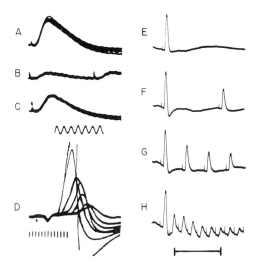

Fig. 12. Composite of different varieties of potentials evoked in the neocortex of neonatal kittens. Negativity upward in all records. A, superficial cortical response to local surface stimulation consists in long-duration negativity. Stimulus frequency in A, 0.5 Hz. B, increase in stimulus frequency (12 Hz) produces marked depression of response which persists for many seconds after return to 0.5 Hz stimulus frequency. C, calibration, 100 Hz. D, superimposed responses recorded from the anterior suprasylvian gyrus during 0.5-Hz stimulation in medial pontomesencephalic reticular regions in a 2-day-old kitten. Early low amplitude surface-positive component is unaltered, whereas late prominent negativity rapidly attenuates at this stimulus frequency. Cal. 100 Hz. E-H, Predominantly surface-negative specific responses evoked in posterior sigmoid gyrus following stimulation of ventrolateral thalamic nuclei and their projections in a newborn kitten. Stimulus frequency as follows: E, 0.5; F, 2 Hz; G, 5; and H, 10 Hz. Depression of response is evident during 2-Hz stimulation and profound during 10-Hz stimulation. Time calibration 0.5 sec. (From Purpura, 1964.)

suggested that surface-negative potentials prominent in neonatal preparations reflect the precocious and differential development of such pathways (Purpura, 1961a,b). This hypothesis initially supported by observations on normal patterns of neuronal morphogenesis (Noback and Purpura, 1961) and synaptogenesis (Voeller *et al.*, 1963) has been examined further in recent preliminary studies aimed at defining the laminar distribution of geniculocortical afferents in immature cortex at a developmental stage in which primary visual evoked responses (VER) consist largely of long-latency surface-negative potentials. The initial results of this exploratory study may be summarized in the morphological data illustrated in Figs. 13-16 (Laemle *et al.*, 1971).

Application of the Fink-Heimer (1967) technique for degenerating axons and axon terminals has revealed that several days following an electrolytic lesion of the geniculocortical radiations in a 6-day-old kitten superficial laminae of striate

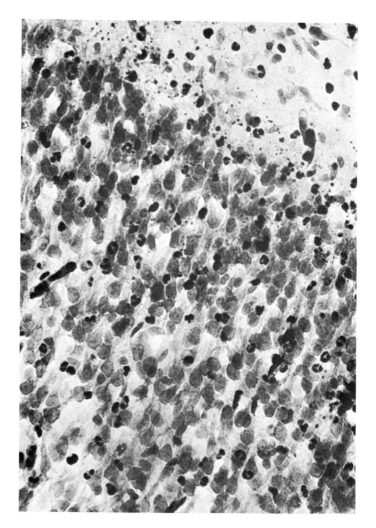

Fig. 13. Demonstration of deposits of silver spherules characteristic of degenerating axons as revealed in a Fink-Heimer preparation of visual cortex in an 8-day-old kitten 2 days following an electrolytic lesion of the geniculocortical radiations. The molecular layer is to the upper right. Note relative density of spherules at base of molecular layer and upper laminae II and III. × 640. (From Laemle *et al.*, 1971.)

cortex exhibit silver spherules characteristic of degenerating processes (Fig. 13). What is particularly striking is that the deposits are largely restricted to the molecular layer, subjacent lamina II and superficial lamina III. The relatively sharp demarcation of silver spherules is suggestive of a predominant distribution of degenerating geniculocortical axons in superficial regions of striate cortex in the very young kitten.

Confirmation of the foregoing observations has been obtained in parallel electron microscope studies of degenerating axons and axon terminals from the same lesioned kittens employed in the light microscope studies (Laemle *et al.*, 1971). It should be pointed out that although axodendritic synapses are well developed in superficial cortex of young mammals, the number of these in the neonatal animal is considerably less than in the adult (Aghajanian and Bloom, 1967). Furthermore, it can be expected that the number of terminal processes associated with a single afferent fiber is likely to be smaller in the immature than in the adult animal. These factors have combined to make detection of degenerating presynaptic terminals in immature cortex a difficult task. On the other hand, no difficulty has been encountered in finding degenerating axons in superficial layers of striate cortex following lesions of the geniculocortical pathway.

Examples of the appearance of early degeneration in axons of the molecular layer in an 8-day-old kitten, 2 days following a lesion of the radiations, are shown in Fig. 14A, B. The cytoplasm of these degenerating axons contains electron-opaque amorphous material with variable condensation characteristics. The relatively large amount of this amorphous material in degenerating axons is consistent with the size of silver spherules observed in the Fink-Heimer preparations (Fig. 13), assuming that such spherules represent the coalescence of many silver particles that have been deposited on the argyrophilic condensation material in the degenerating axon (Heimer and Peters, 1968). In some instances the condensed material inside a degenerating axon has been extremely electron-opaque as in the axons shown in Fig. 15A, B from layers III and I, respectively. More typical appearing degenerating axons, one exhibiting the features of a degenerating presynaptic terminal, are illustrated in Fib. 16A, B.

These preliminary findings of degenerative changes in axons of the molecular layer and subjacent superficial regions of striate cortex a few days following geniculocortical radiation lesions in 4-6-day-old kittens are entirely consistent with the hypothesis (Purpura, 1961b) that the initial surface negativity of the primary VER in immature neocortex is generated by geniculocortical pathways that effect synaptic relations with dendritic elements in the superficial neuropil. Although considerably more work is required in evaluating the significance of experimentally induced degenerative changes in immature axons, the data at hand strongly suggest that geniculocortical radiations have a fundamentally different intracortical distribution in immature than in mature visual cortex. Further, it is clear from the paucity of axodendritic spine synapses and basilar dendrites in immature visual cortex that such radiation axons synaptically engage dendrites of immature cortical neurons differently from mature neurons. Despite obvious differences in intracortical afferent distribution, synaptic development, and excitability of neurons in immature visual cortex, it has been shown that "before a kitten opens its eyes, and long before the eyes are used in visual exploration, single cells of the primary cortex respond to natural

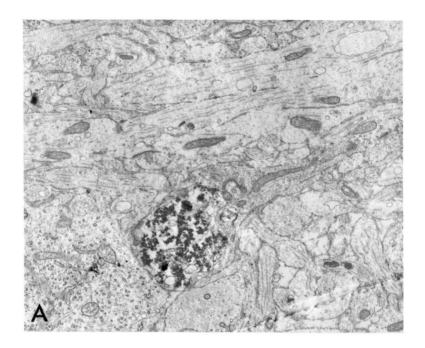

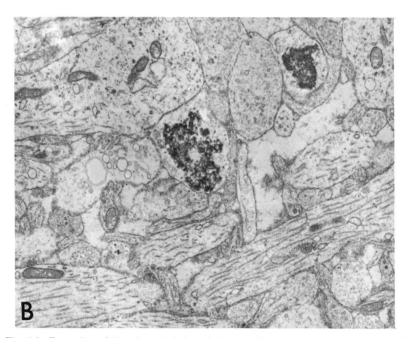

Fig. 14. Examples of the characteristics of degenerating axon processes as revealed in electron micrographs of visual cortex from an 8-day-old kitten, 2 days following an electrolytic lesion of the geniculocortical radiations. (A) Large degenerating process in the molecular layer. (B) Two axons similarly located in the molecular layer. Note variable appearance of electron-dense amorphous condensation material in degenerating process. × 14,200. (From Laemle *et al.*, 1971.)

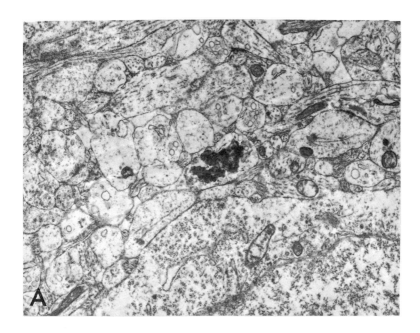

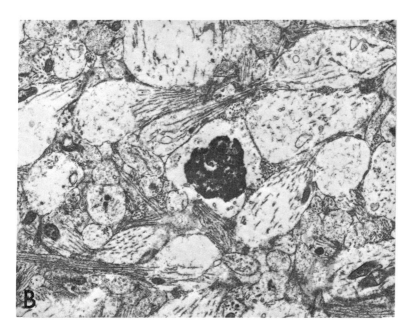

Fig. 15. Further examples of degenerating axonal processes in visual cortex of an 8-day-old kitten, 2 days following an electrolytic lesion of the geniculocortical radiations. (A) Degenerating axonal process located in superficial region of lamina IV. (B) Lamina I, degenerating axon. × 14,200. (From Laemle et al., 1971.)

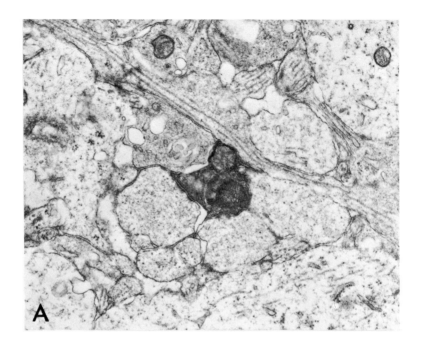

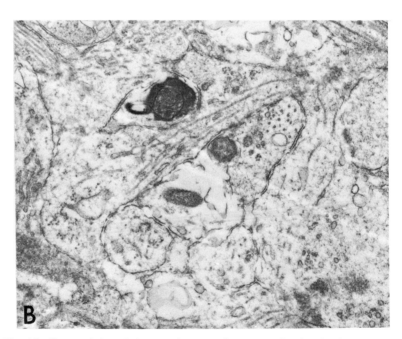

Fig. 16. Characteristics of degenerating axonal processes in the visual cortex from a 6-day-old kitten, 2 days following a lesion of the geniculocortical radiations. (A) Degenerating axon terminal in lamina IV. Note preservation of postsynaptic dense material and marked opacity and condensation of axoplasm of the presynaptic process. (B) Degenerating axonal process in lamina II. × 23,300. (From Laemle *et al.*, 1971.)

stimulation with the same specificity as is found in the adult" (Hubel and Wiesel, 1965, p. 1041). While it is clear from this that the initial synaptic relations formed in immature visual cortex reflect an extraordinary degree of innate specificity in early developing retinogeniculocortical connections (Hubel and Wiesel, 1963), more dynamic properties of these relations, as defined by various statistical parameters of spike train discharges etc., are undoubtedly postnatal acquisitions (Bergström, 1968). The problem of elucidating the significance of these dynamic aspects of information-processing in developing neuronal subsystems has only recently been explored (Hyvärinen, 1966; Shofer *et al.*, 1969; Stenberg, 1967; Woodward *et al.*, 1969). These data promise to provide heuristically valuable hypotheses for correlating structure and functional alterations at different neuraxial sites with the information-carrying capacity of developing neuronal networks (Bergström, 1969). In the case of visual cortex, preliminary studies of the statistical relations of primary evoked potentials and unit discharges have revealed differences in the preferred firing times of units responding to flash in young kittens as compared with adult animals. It is well known that unit discharges are characteristically associated with the initial surface-positive component of the primary evoked response in adult animals (Purpura, 1959). In contrast to this, such preferred firing occurs in relation to the long-latency initial negative wave in young kittens (Fig. 17). Other features of unit discharges in immature visual cortex including the paucity of spontaneous discharges and lack of repetitive responsiveness, as noted above, are also indicative of the functional immaturity of early established anatomically specified neuronal relations in primary projection cortex.

A characteristic finding in studies of evoked potentials in immature animals and the human neonate has been the observation of rapid "fatigability" of repetitively evoked responses (cf. elsewhere in this volume). In many instances relatively low-frequency stimulation of corticopetal projections that would ordinarily sustain high-frequency activation in the mature animal may result in marked depression of evoked activity. In the newborn kitten, specific as well as nonspecific projection pathways to neocortex may exhibit profound fatigability even at stimulus frequencies below 0.5 Hz (Fig. 12) (Purpura, 1964). One explanation for the singular susceptibility to depression exhibited by afferent projection pathways in the immature brain following repetitive activation may be sought in the low-level excitability and lack of repetitive responsiveness of immature neurons as discussed above. Differences in the properties of presynaptic terminals as well as unusual postsynaptic receptor desensitization may be cited as possible additional contributory mechanisms for response depression in the immature brain. It should also be recognized that the activation of well-developed inhibitory synaptic pathways in immature cerebral cortex, and perhaps at other sites in the immature brain, could play a major role in limiting the responsiveness of neurons driven by repetitive afferent volleys (Purpura, 1969a).

The easy fatigability of cortical evoked potentials in the immature animal must

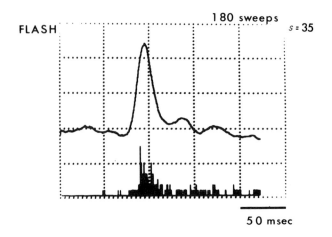

Fig. 17. Poststimulus time histogram and averaged evoked response from visual cortex of a 10-day-old kitten. Negativity upward. Primary response to flash stimulation is of long latency and predominantly surface-negative. PST histogram indicates similar time of occurrence for the modal latency of evoked single unit activity recorded with a microelectrode inserted in cortex close to the site of registration of the surface response. Stimulus for each sweep occurs 25 msec before the abscissal origin. *s* indicates number of spikes represented at maximal height. (From Shofer and Purpura, unpublished data.)

be clearly distinguished from another more complex process underlying response decrement. This process has all the overt features of "habituation" in that the depression succeeding low-frequency repetition of a stimulus may be reversed ("dishabituation") by a brief change in stimulus frequency (Purpura, 1961a). It is noteworthy that these events in the neocortex of the neonatal kitten have been demonstrated only in respect to cortical evoked responses elicited by stimulation of pontomesencephalic reticular regions. Such stimulation evokes long-latency surface-negative responses in anterior suprasylvian gyrus as shown in Fig. 12D. Repetition of the stimulus at 0.5 Hz results in rapid attenuation of the evoked negativity (Fig. 12D) as is clear in the first few responses of Fig. 18A. It is further shown in Fig. 18 that continuation of the 0.5 Hz stimulation results in complete "habituation" of the evoked response. However, it is only necessary to increase the stimulus frequency to 25 Hz for a few seconds to induce a marked augmentation of the response as in Fig. 18B. Cycles of "habituation and dishabituation" may be induced by similar changes in stimulus frequency for long periods of observation (Fig. 19) (Purpura, 1961a).

The results illustrated in Figs. 18 and 19 provide evidence suggesting the potential operation of rather complex transactions involving axodendritic synapses. Additionally, the data indicate a functional capability of nonspecific projection systems in the immature brain that is not evident in specific projections. If the cyclic alterations in evoked potentials produced by transient

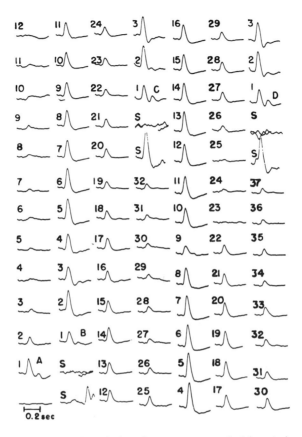

Fig. 18. Continuous series of cortical surface responses evoked in anterior suprasylvian gyrus of a 2-day-old kitten by stimulation of medial pontomesencephalic reticular regions. The figure is to be read from lower left to upper right. Each record shows the response to single-shock stimulation once every 2 sec (0.5 Hz). First series (A1-12) was initiated after a 30-min rest period. The first stimulus (A1) elicits a prominent surface-negative response which rapidly attenuates during successive stimulation (A2-12). Thereafter, second column, bottom, a 4-sec period of 25 Hz stimulation was applied through the same stimulating electrodes (S-S) and the 0.5 Hz stimulation continued in series B1-32. Note progressive enhancement then attenuation of response. Additional series C1-37 and D1-3 were interrupted by similar brief periods of 25 Hz stimulation. (From Purpura, 1961a. Reprinted by permission of the New York Academy of Sciences.)

variations in stimulus frequency are confined to axodendritic synapses in nonspecific cortex, it follows that the functional properties of these synapses may be different from axodendritic synapses involved in specific evoked responses of primary projection cortex in the immature animal. Such differences may be reflected in their capacity for transmitter mobilization and release,

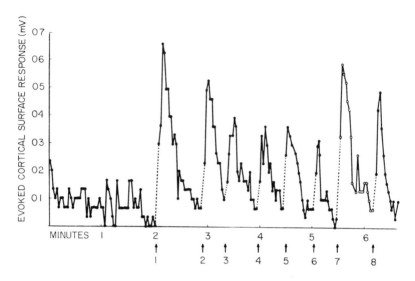

Fig. 19. Graphical representation of data similar to that shown in Fig. 18, but from another continuous series lasting more than 6 min. Amplitude of response evoked every 2 sec in anterior suprasylvian gyrus rapidly decreases over a 2-min period. At first arrow, stimulus frequency is abruptly changed to 25 Hz for 4 sec (dotted portion of curve). Postactivation facilitation of 0.5 Hz evoked response is profound initially, but during brief presentation of 25 Hz stimulation (arrows 2-6) the latter stimulus becomes less effective. The magnitude of the postactivation facilitation is partially restored after 50 Hz stimulation (arrow 7, series with open circles) and again with 25 Hz stimulation (arrow 8). (From Purpura, 1961a. Reprinted by permission of the New York Academy of Sciences.)

persisting changes in excitability of presynaptic terminals and other factors implicated in response decrement and postactivation facilitation (Eccles, 1964). These differences may not be confined to excitatory axodendritic synapses but may be evident as well in inhibitory synapses linked to nonspecific projection systems. Intracellular studies of events, such as those illustrated in Figs. 18 and 19, will be required to determine the validity of these suggestions. For present purposes it suffices to emphasize that the functional immaturity observed in one class of early specified synaptic connections (e.g. primary visual cortex) may not be observed in other types of synaptic relations in immature cortex.

COMMENTS

The complexity of maturational processes in the mammalian brain has been amply illustrated in the foregoing survey devoted to the analysis of several major features of synaptogenesis and the properties of immature cortical neurons. This complexity is evident in the demonstration that any one maturational event is shown to consist of a variety of interrelated processes each of which has a unique significance. Thus, a morphological change in dendrites implies developmental alterations in the type, number, and distribution of axodendritic synapses. Concomitant maturational alterations in dendritic spike electrogenesis also occur, but these changes are not reflected in obvious gross or fine structural characteristics. Assessment of the "immaturity" of cortical neurons is further complicated by differential features of synaptogenesis. It seems appropriate to consider neurons "immature" until they have acquired their full complement of synapses, however this may be evaluated. Yet synaptic inhibition is well expressed in immature cortical neurons and cannot be viewed as a functionally immature process. The same cannot be said for excitatory synaptic activities. It will be of considerable interest to determine whether the precocious development of inhibitory synaptic pathways in immature cerebral cortex is paralleled by a similar differential development of inhibition at other neuraxial sites. The demonstration of "habituation and dishabituation" phenomena in certain nonspecific reticulocortical projection systems in the neonatal kitten is strongly suggestive of the operation of such complex inhibitory activities within these systems.

The maturational events examined here have little direct bearing on more classical parameters of development such as myelination of central pathways. This is not to minimize the important contribution of myelination to the optimal operation of input-output transactions in cerebral cortex and elsewhere (Purpura *et al.*, 1964a). But myelination has been overemphasized as a milestone of maturation at the expense of more dynamic processes which underlie the capacity for effecting such transactions. The fact that maturation of sleep-wakefulness behavior precedes myelination of most forebrain pathways further indicates the tenuous relevancy of myelination to the *early* establishment of complex synaptic interrelations in neuronal subsystems mediating this behavior.

No attempt has been made in this report to extend findings on the properties of immature cortical neurons and their synaptic organizations to the analysis of mechanisms subserving sleep states in the immature animal. It goes without saying that many of the developmental features examined above are likely to be encountered in neurons located in brain stem and diencephalic structures implicated in various aspects of sleep-wakefulness activity. The question of the relationship of sleep behavior in the neonate to the functional capacity of the immature brain may be far more intriguing but certainly no less important. Any answers to this question must of necessity be limited by the paucity of information on elementary morphophysiological processes subserving sleep-wakefulness states in the immature brain, or for that matter, in the mature brain. There can be little doubt that the lack of organized sleep spindles or EEG patterns of "active" sleep in the newborn animal reflects the functional immaturity of thalamocortical synchronizing mechanisms (Purpura, 1969b) as well as other subcortical-cortical and brain stem integrative activities. But analysis of these immature neuronal subsystems awaits the application of quantitative techniques for elucidating their elementary properties.

It may be argued, perhaps not without justification, that the microdissection of elementary processes in sleep-wakefulness behavior may be irrelevant, if not ill-advised. The same might have been argued in the early period of the analysis of movement control mechanisms in terms of simple reflex actions. For as Sherrington (1906) cautioned: "A simple reflex is probably a purely abstract conception, because all parts of the nervous system are connected together and no part of it is probably ever capable of variation without affecting and being affected by various other parts, and it is a system certainly never absolutely at rest. But the simple reflex is a convenient, if not probable, fiction." What is required at this stage in the analysis of the developmental neurobiology of sleep-wakefulness behavior is a "convenient fiction" as powerful as the concept of the "simple reflex" has been in the study of motor control systems. Implicit in the approach described here is the "fiction" that detailed studies of the properties of immature neurons and their synaptic relations will eventually permit an adequate understanding of the maturation of sleep-wakefulness mechanisms. To this end we have sacrificed "relevancy" in the hope of acquiring quantitative morphophysiological data on elementary developmental processes.

REFERENCES

Aghajanian, G. K., and Bloom, F. E. (1967). The formation of synaptic junctions in developing rat brain: a quantitative electron microscopic study. *Brain Res.* 6, 716-727.

Andersen, P., Eccles, J. C., and Løyning, Y. (1964). Pathway of postsynaptic inhibition in the hippocampus. *J. Neurophysiol.* 27, 608-619.

Armstrong-James, M. A. (1970). Spontaneous and evoked single unit activity in 7-day rat cerebral cortex. *J. Physiol. (London)* 208, 10P.

Bergström, R. M. (1968). Development of EEG and unit electrical activity of the brain during ontogeny (with special reference to the development of entropy relations of the brain). *In* "Ontogenesis of the Brain" (L. Jílek and S. Trojan, eds.), pp. 61-71, Universita Karlova, Praha.

Bergström, R. M. (1969). An entropy model of the developing brain. *Develop. Psychobiol.* 2, 139-152.

Creutzfeldt, O. D., Lux, H. D., and Watanabe, S. (1966). Electrophysiology of cortical nerve cells. *In* "The Thalamus" (D. P. Purpura and M. D. Yahr, eds.), pp. 209-235, Columbia Univ. Press, New York.

Deza, L., and Eidelberg, E. (1967). Development of cortical electrical activity in the rat. *Exp. Neurol.* 17, 425-438.

Eccles, J. C. (1964). "The Physiology of Synapses." Springer Verlag, Berlin and New York.

Eccles, J. C. (1969). "The Inhibitory Pathways of the Central Nervous System." Thomas, Springfield, Illinois.

Eccles, J. C., Libet, B., and Young, R. R. (1958). The behavior of chromatolyzed motoneurones studied by intracellular recording. *J. Physiol (London)* 143, 11-40.

Fink, R. P. and Heimer, L. (1967). Two methods for selective silver impregnation of degenerating axons and their synaptic endings in the central nervous system. *Brain Res.* **4**, 369-374.

Heimer, L. and Peters, A. (1968). An electron microscope study of a silver stain for degenerating boutons. *Brain Res.* **8**, 337-346.

Himwich, W. A., ed. (1970). "Developmental Neurobiology." Thomas, Springfield, Illinois.

Hubel, D. H., and Wiesel, T. N. (1963). Receptive fields of cells in striate cortex of very young, visually inexperienced kittens. *J. Neurophysiol.* **26**, 994-1002.

Hubel, D. H. and Wiesel, T. N. (1965). Binocular interaction in striate cortex of kittens reared with artificial squint. *J. Neurophysiol.* **27**, 1041-1059.

Huttenlocher, P. R. (1967). Development of cortical neuronal activity in the neonatal cat. *Exp. Neurol.* **17**, 247-262.

Hyvärinen, J. (1966). Analysis of spontaneous spike potential activity in developing rabbit diencephalon. *Acta Physiol. Scand.* **68**, Suppl. 278, 1-67.

Jones, E. G. and Powell, T. P. S. (1970). An electron microscopic study of terminal degeneration in the neocortex of the cat. *Phil. Trans. Roy. Soc. London, Ser. B.* **257**, 45-62.

Kandel, E. R., Spencer, W. A., and Brinley, F. J., Jr. (1961). Electrophysiology of hippocampal neurons. I. Sequential invasion and synaptic organization. *J. Neurophysiol.* **24**, 225-242.

Laemle, L., Benhamida, C., and Purpura, D. P. (1972). *Brain Res.* In press.

Llinás, R. and Hillman, D. E. (1969). Physiological and morphological organization of the cerebellar circuits in various vertebrates. *In* "Neurobiology of Cerebellar Evolution and Development" (R. Llinás, ed.) pp. 43-74. Amer. Med. Ass. Press, Chicago, Illinois

Mareš, P. (1964). Ontogenetic development of membrane potentials in telencephalic structures in the rat. *Physiol. Bohemoslov.* **13**, 256-262.

Noback, C. R. and Purpura, D. P. (1961). Postnatal ontogenesis of neurons in cat neocortex. *J. Comp. Neurol.* **117**, 291-307.

Pappas, G. D. and Purpura, D. P. (1961). Fine structure of dendrites in the superficial neocortical neuropil. *Exp. Neurol.* **4**, 507-530.

Purpura, D. P. (1959). Nature of electrocortical potentials and synaptic organizations in cerebral and cerebellar cortex. *Int. Rev. Neurobiol.* **1**, 47-163.

Purpura, D. P. (1961a). Morphophysiological basis of elementary evoked response patterns in the neocortex of the newborn cat. *Ann. N. Y. Acad. Sci.* **92**, 840-859.

Purpura, D. P. (1961b). Analysis of axodendritic synaptic organizations in immature cerebral cortex. *Ann. N. Y. Acad. Sci.* **94**, 604-654.

Purpura, D. P. (1964). Relationship of seizure susceptibility to morphologic and physiologic properties of normal and abnormal immature cortex. *In* "Neurological and Electro-encephalographic Correlative Studies in Infancy" (P. Kellaway and I. Peterson, eds.), pp. 117-154. Grune and Stratton, New York.

Purpura, D. P. (1966). Activation of "secondary" impulse trigger sites in hippocampal neurons. *Nature (London)* **211**, 1317-1318.

Purpura, D. P. (1967). Comparative physiology of dendrites. *In* "The Neurosciences: A Study Program" (G. C. Quarton, T. Melnechuk, and F. O. Schmitt, eds.), pp. 372-393. Rockefeller Univ. Press, New York.

Purpura, D. P. (1969a). Stability and seizure susceptibility of immature brain. *In* "Basic Mechanisms of the Epilepsies" (H. Jasper, A. A. Ward and A. Pope, eds.), pp. 481-505. Little, Brown, Boston, Massachusetts.

Purpura, D. P. (1969b). Interneuronal mechanisms in thalamically induced synchronizing and desynchronizing activities. *In* "The Interneuron" (M. A. B. Brazier, ed.), pp.

467-496. U.C.L.A. Forum in Medical Sciences, Los Angeles, California.

Purpura, D. P. (1971). Dendrites: heterogeneity in form and function. *Proc. Int. EEG Cong.* (in press).

Purpura, D. P., and Pappas, G. D. (1968). Structural characteristics of neurons in the feline hippocampus during postnatal ontogenesis. *Exp. Neurol.* **22**, 379-393.

Purpura, D. P., and Shofer, R. J. (1964). Cortical intracellular potentials during augmenting and recruiting responses. I. Effects of injected hyperpolarizing currents on evoked membrane potential changes. *J. Neurophysiol.* **27**, 117-132.

Purpura, D. P., Carmichael, M. W., and Housepian, E. M. (1960). Physiological and anatomical studies of development of superficial axodendritic synaptic pathways in neocortex. *Exp. Neurol.* **2**, 324-347.

Purpura, D. P., Shofer, R. J., Housepian, E. M., and Noback, C. R. (1964a). Comparative ontogenesis of structure-function relations in cerebral and cerebellar cortex. *Progr. Brain Res.* **4**, 187-221.

Purpura, D. P., Shofer, R. J., and Musgrave, F. S. (1964b). Cortical intracellular potentials during augmenting and recruiting responses. II. Patterns of synaptic activities in pyramidal and nonpyramidal tract neurons. *J. Neurophysiol.* **27**, 133-151.

Purpura, D. P., Shofer, R. J., and Scarff, T. (1965). Properties of synaptic activities and spike potentials of neurons in immature neocortex. *J. Neurophysiol.* **28**, 925-942.

Purpura, D. P., Prelevic, S., and Santini, M. (1968). Postsynaptic potentials and spike variations in the feline hippocampus during postnatal ontogenesis. *Exp. Neurol.* **22**, 408-422.

Rall, W. (1967). Distinguishing theoretical synaptic potentials computed for different soma-dendritic distributions of synaptic input. *J. Neurophysiol.* **30**, 1138-1168.

Scheibel, M., and Scheibel, A. (1964). Some structural and functional substrates of development in young cats. *Progr. Brain Res.* **9**, 6-25.

Schwartz, I. R., Pappas, G. D., and Purpura, D. P. (1968). Fine structure of neurons and synapses in the feline hippocampus during postnatal ontogenesis. *Exp. Neurol.* **22**, 394-407.

Sherrington, C. S. (1906). "The Integrative Action of the Nervous System." Yale Univ. Press, New Haven, Connecticut.

Shofer, R. J., Sax, D. S., and Strom, M. G. (1969). Analysis of auditory and cerebro-cortically evoked activity in the immature and adult cat cerebellum. *In* "Neurobiology of Cerebellar Evolution and Development" (R. Llinás, ed.), pp. 703-717. Amer. Med. Ass. Press, Chicago, Illinois.

Shofer, R. J., and Purpura, D. P. (1971) In preparation.

Spencer, W. A., and Kandel, E. R. (1961). Electrophysiology of hippocampal neurons. IV. Fast prepotentials. *J. Neurophysiol.* **24**, 272-285.

Stenberg, D. (1967). The ontogenesis of the spontaneous electrical activity of the lower brain stem. *Acta Neurol. Scand.* **43**, Suppl. 31, 162.

Voeller, K., Pappas, G. D., and Purpura, D. P. (1963). Electron microscope study of development of cat superficial neocortex. *Exp. Neurol.* **7**, 107-130.

Woodward, D. J., Hoffer, B. J., and Lapham, L. V. (1969). Correlative survey of electrophysiological, neuropharmacological, and histochemical aspects of cerebellar maturation in rat. *In* "Neurobiology of Cerebellar Evolution and Development" (R. Llinás, ed.), pp. 725-738. Amer. Med. Ass. Press, Chicago, Illinois.

2

The Development of Synapses
in the Rat Cerebellar Cortex

Barry J. Hoffer, Floyd E. Bloom,
George R. Siggins, and Donald J. Woodward

Clearly, sleep is an active function involving the integration of many central nervous loci. Since such interactions in mammals occur by chemically transmitting synapses, it is germane to consider the maturation of synaptic function at a conference of this nature. Moreover, since there is a great deal of evidence implicating the monoamines, norepinephrine (NE) and serotonin (5-HT), in the production of sleep (Jouvet, 1969), the maturation of monoaminergic synapses is particularly significant in terms of development of sleep mechanisms.

We have studied the maturation of synapses onto rat cerebellar Purkinje cells, especially the maturation of the newly described NE-containing afferent pathway (Bloom *et al.*, 1971). There are a number of important reasons for choosing the rat cerebellum. First, the animal is extremely immature at birth. Indeed, all major elements of the cerebellar cortex are either in the neuroblast

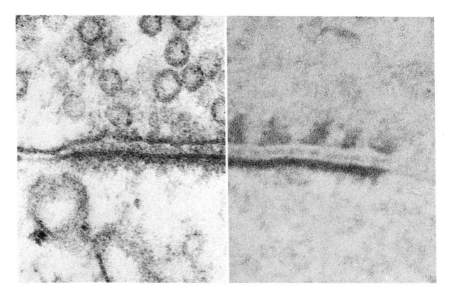

Fig. 1. Comparison of electron micrographs of adult synapses stained with osmium (left) and E-PTA (right). In osmium-stained sections, pre- and postsynaptic membranes and synaptic vesicles are apparent. In E-PTA-stained sections, the presynaptic dense projections, postsynaptic band, and intersynaptic line are seen. The presynaptic and postsynaptic membranes are electronlucent. × 108,000.

stage or the process of migration at the time of birth. Second, the cerebellar cortex of adult mammals has been extensively studied, both anatomically and physiologically (Eccles *et al.*, 1967); well-defined excitatory and inhibitory pathways synapse on the Purkinje cell soma and dendritic tree. Furthermore, the various excitatory and inhibitory pathways each possess characteristic well-defined actions on Purkinje cell discharge.

In order to quantitate synaptic development, it is necessary to employ a multidisciplinary approach. In this chapter, I should like to present morphological studies showing development of synaptic structure, physiological experiments indicating maturation of synaptic function, and pharmacological investigations showing the development of receptivity to neurotransmitters. All studies were carried out on midline vermis just behind the primary fissure (Larsells' lobules, VI and VII). Autoradiographic evidence has indicated that these are the areas of cerebellar cortex which are the slowest to mature (Altman, 1969).

Using ethanolic phosphotungstic acid (E-PTA) without osmication, it is possible to selectively stain the synaptic complex (Bloom and Aghajanian, 1966) (Fig. 1). Central junctions stained with this technique show characteristic presynaptic dense projections and postsynaptic bands; an intersynaptic line is

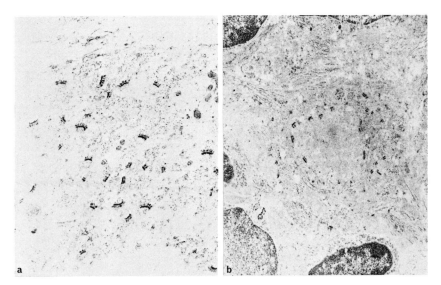

Fig. 2. (a) Electron micrograph of contacts between axons and dendrites in the molecular layer of the cerebellar cortex from a 6-day-old animal as stained by the E-PTA technique. Note the adult-like morphology. × 30,000. (b) Electron micrograph of contacts in presumed mossy fiber terminals of 12-day-old cerebellum stained by E-PTA technique. Multiple specialized contacts can be seen. × 30,000.

TABLE I   *Rat Cerebellar Cortical Synapse Development: Number of E-PTA Stained Synaptic Contacts of the Molecular Layer in Folium VII*

No. of contacts per 100 μ^2 [a]	Postnatal day
0	1
0	2
0.5	3
3.2	5
4.5	6
6.1	7
8.7	8
9.6	9
10.3	11
10.7	12
16.9	14
26.8	20
36.5	70

[a]Each value is the mean of 10-14 samples of 100 μ^2.

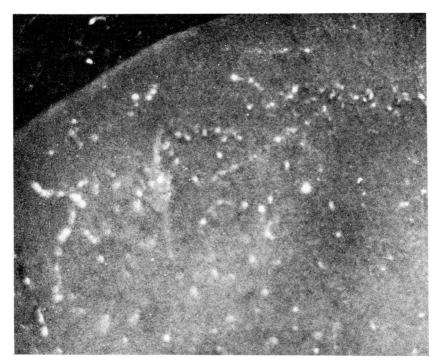

Fig. 3. Norepinephrine-containing axons in the molecular layer of the cerebellar cortex of a 14-day-old animal demonstrated by fluorescence microscopy after condensation of freeze-dried tissue with formaldehyde vapor. Note characteristic varicosities. × 350.

also visible. If one compares the adult and neonatal (Fig. 2) cerebellar cortices, one finds that the E-PTA morphology of individual junctions is quite similar. In other words, as early as synapses stain, they possess a near-adult morphological appearance. What changes markedly is the density (i.e., the number/unit area) of synapses (Table I). Prior to 3 days of age, no E-PTA stained synapses are detectable, but synaptogenesis increases rapidly thereafter. The major increments are between days 3 and 9, and days 12 and 26. Since all samples were taken from the nascent molecular layer, it is assumed that most of the synapses are from parallel fibers to Purkinje cell dendrites.

In order to study the morphological development of the NE-containing afferents to the Purkinje cells, the fluorescence technique of Falck and Hillarp was used (Falck *et al.*, 1962). Fluorescent fibers with characteristic varicosities were seen as early as 5 days of age (Fig. 3).

The onset of parallel fiber and climbing fiber excitation of the Purkinje cell has also been studied with electrophysiological techniques. Activation of Purkinje cells by parallel fiber stimulation and spontaneous climbing fiber bursts both

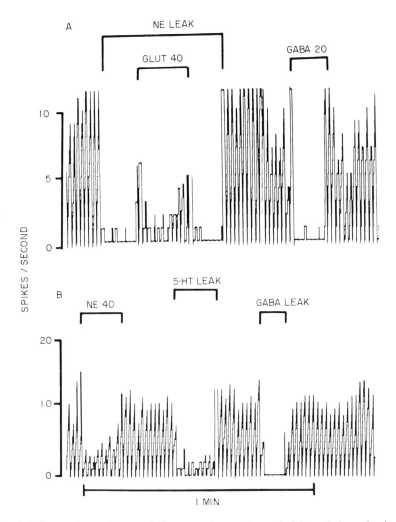

Fig. 4. Effects of putative cerebellar neurotransmitters administered by microion-tophoresis on spontaneous neonatal Purkinje cell discharge. Numbers after each drug indicate ejection current in nanoamperes ("leak" indicates removal of the retaining current, thus allowing the drug to simply diffuse from the pipette tip). Duration of drug application indicated by brackets. (a) 1 day of age. (b) 2 days of age. NE, norepinephrine; Glut, glutamate; GABA, γ-aminobutyric acid; 5-HT, serotonin.

appear only after 3½-4 days of age, and are reasonably similar to such excitation in the adult.

Since there is little or no morphological synapse development prior to day 5, responses of Purkinje cells to putative neurotransmitters prior to this age should

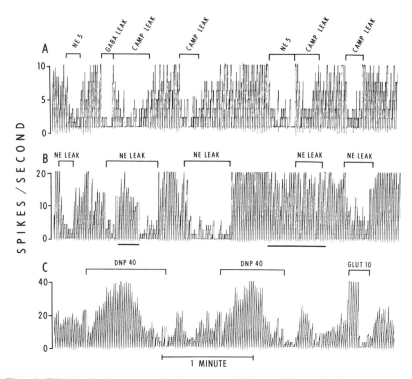

Fig. 5. Effects of pharmacological agents, administered by microiontophoresis on spontaneous neonatal Purkinje cell discharge. Numbers after each drug indicate ejection current in nanoamperes. Duration of drug application indicated by brackets. NE, norepinephrine; PGE, prostaglandin; GABA, γ-aminobutyric acid; cAMP, cyclic $3',5'$-adenosine monophosphate; DNP, dinitrophenol; Glut, glutamate. (A) cAMP mimicry of NE-induced depression of discharge in a 2-day-old animal. (B) PGE blockade of NE-induced depression of discharge in a 3-day-old animal. The black bars beneath the integrated spike record indicate duration of microiontophoresis of PGE, 5nA. (C) Acceleration of discharge produced by DNP and Glut in a 4-day-old animal. (Spontaneous discharge in records (B) and (C) was augmented by the continuous leak of glutamate from one barrel of the micropipette throughout the time of recording.)

be determined solely by postsynaptic receptivity. The effect of various potential transmitter agents has been studied by administering them to spontaneously active Purkinje cells by the technique of microiontophoresis. Purkinje cells of 1- and 2-day-old rats respond to virtually all putative neurotransmitters (Fig. 4). They are excited by glutamate (Glut) and are inhibited by NE, 5-HT, and γ-aminobutyric acid (GABA). Indeed, the immature Purkinje cells are considerably more sensitive to these agents than their adult counterparts (Woodward *et al.*, 1971). This is especially relevant in terms of Dr. Purpura's findings of pronounced and prolonged IPSP's in immature cells. There may be both increased postsynaptic receptivity as well as persistence of transmitter.

In the adult cerebellum, there is evidence that the effects of NE on Purkinje cells are mediated by cyclic $3',5'$-adenosine monophosphate (cAMP) and that NE responses are blocked by prostaglandins (Siggins *et al.*, 1971). This cAMP mimicry and prostaglandin blockade of NE is also evident in 2- and 3-day-old animals (Fig. 5); hence, this very sophisticated "metabolic" inhibitory mechanism also develops prior to the formation of specific synaptic connections.

In summary, postsynaptic receptivity of the Purkinje cell antedates significant synaptogenesis. The morphological appearance of the individual synapse appears quite mature as early as it can be detected, and the major developmental change is in terms of number of synapses. This correlates well with the electrophysiological data, which indicates that the synapses function in a nearly adult fashion almost as soon as they are formed. Finally, I would like to emphasize that the cerebellar cortex is used here as a model. We must now apply these types of multidisciplinary analyses to particular brain structures like the raphe nuclei and locus coeruleous before we can determine the neuronal basis of the maturation of sleep in the central nervous system.

REFERENCES

Altman, J. (1969). Autoradiographic and histological studies of postnatal neurogenesis. *J. Comp. Neurol.* **136**, 269-294.

Bloom, F. E., and Aghajanian, G. (1966). Cytochemistry of synapses: selective staining for electron microscopy. *Science* **154**, 1575-1577.

Bloom, F. E., Hoffer, B. J., and Siggins, G. R. (1971). Studies on norepinephrine-containing afferents to Purkinje cells of rat cerebellum. I. Localization of the fibers and their synapses, *Brain Res.* **25**, 501-522.

Eccles, J. C., Ito, M., and Szentagothai, J. (1967). "The Cerebellum as a Neuronal Machine." Springer Publ., New York.

Falck, B., Hillarp, N. A., Thieme, G., and Thorp, A. (1962). Fluroescence of catecholamines and related compounds condensed with formaldehyde. *J. Histochem. Cytochem.* **10**, 348-354.

Jouvet, M. Biogenic amines and the states of sleep. *Science* **163**, 32-41.

Siggins, G. R., Hoffer, B. J., and Bloom, F. E. (1971). Studies on norepinephrine-containing afferents to Purkinje cells of the rat cerebellum. III. Evidence for mediation of norepinephrine effects by cyclic $3',5'$-adenosine monophosphate. *Brain Res.* **25**, 535-554.

Woodward, D. J., Hoffer, B. J., Bloom, F. E., and Siggins, G. R. (1971). The ontogenetic development of synaptic junctions, synaptic activation and responsiveness to neurotransmitters in rat cerebellar Purkinje cells. *Brain Res.* **34**, 73-98.

INVITED DISCUSSION (CHAPTER 1 AND 2):
GUENTER H. ROSE

I would like to comment on two of Dr. Purpura's basic points: 1) the precocious development of synaptic inhibition in cerebral cortex, and 2) the early development of axodendritic synapses in the molecular cortical layer in contrast to later developing axosomatic synapses.

If Dr. Purpura is correct concerning early synaptic inhibition in the cerebral cortex, one can speculate on the utility of such a process to act as a brake against overstimulation or overexcitation before appropriate sensorimotor systems are mature, thereby inducing stability in the immediate postnatal period. In support of this, as recently reviewed by Ellingson and Rose (1970) and Purpura (1969), various species of animals in the immediate postnatal period are less susceptible to topical or systemic administration of CNS excitants, such as Metrazol, both in seizure production and EEG reactivity. The threshold of seizure induction generally decreases with age.

In spite of this, one would expect that extreme hyperstimulation of a particular sensory system would overtax stability in the neonatal period thus producing prolonged effects. In this regard we found (Fig. 6) that exposing kittens to continuous light, 24 hr/day, from birth to 8 months of age, resulted in considerable increase in amplitude of visual electrocortical responses (VER) over that obtained from normal age controls and in the adult mother kept with the kittens. The relative involvement of subcortical and peripheral changes awaits future assessment.

Turning to neurophysiological studies, we have been interested in the past several years (Rose and Lindsley, 1965, 1968; Rose, 1971) in the development of the VER in kittens to brief controlled flashes. These studies have been undertaken in anesthetized as well as unanesthetized preparations, and it is the contrast between these two preparations during development upon which I wish to focus.

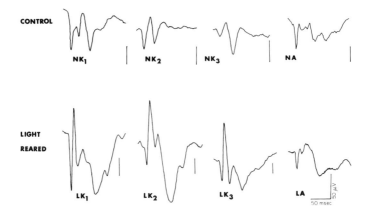

Fig. 6. Visual evoked potentials from light-reared and control animals. Tracings are monopolar recordings obtained from awake, unanesthetized animals with skull screws and represent the algebraic summation of 50 responses. Pupils dilated with homatropine; LK, light-reared kittens; LA, light-reared adult (mother); NK, normal kittens; NA, normal adult. Kittens are 8 months of age. Vertical lines: 50 μV. (Rose, Gruenau, and Spencer, 1972.)

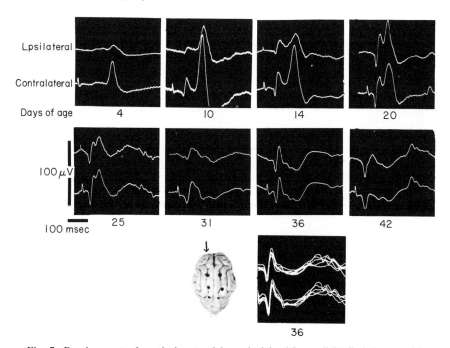

Fig. 7. Development of cortical potentials evoked by 15-μsec light flash in same kitten studied at successive age levels; monocular stimulation by collimated light beam brought to a focus near cornea of animal's right eye; pupil dilated with homatropine. Monopolar recordings from ipsilateral (R6) and contralateral (L5) visual cortex. Arrow indicates eye stimulated. Initial upward deflection indicates light flash. Superimposed tracings at day 36 show consistency of response (flash at onset of trace). In this and all figures, upward deflection indicates negativity at the active electrode. Calibration: 100 msec; 100 μV. (Adapted from Rose and Lindsley, 1965, 1968.)

Figure 7 illustrates the sequence of electrocortical changes during development in the anesthetized kitten (Nembutal) to brief single light flashes. The initial long-latency response between 2 and 4 days of age correlates with the precocious development of the apical dendrites and axodendritic connections. By 10 days of age, the amplitude of response increases markedly, and its latency decreases. Concurrently, this component is preceded by a shorter-latency positive-negative complex, coincident with the later maturation of the deeper basilar dendrites and axosomatic synapses (Purpura, Chapter 1, this volume). The resultant waveform by the end of the second postnatal week is a clearly definable positive-negative-negative response. As the animal matures, this later developing complex continues to increase in amplitude. At the same time, the original long-latency negative wave decreases in amplitude and latency until, at approximately 30 days of age, either the two negative waves coalesce or there is a disappearance, under Nembutal, of the original long-latency wave, resulting in a positive-negative VER typical of that recorded from the adult preparation.

Figure 8 illustrates the sequence recorded either in an awake preparation with implanted electrodes or from an unanesthetized but paralyzed preparation. One of the striking results obtained in these studies is that the sequence of development in the anesthetized as well as in the unanesthetized preparation is identical within the first 2 postnatal weeks. The sequence obtained under chloralose is likewise identical. It is only beginning with the third postnatal week, that is, beginning at about 14 days of age, that a divergence in waveform configuration between the anesthetized and the unanesthetized preparations occurs. This consists of the temporary appearance of a small negative component between the original negative waves, as well as an increase in positivity preceding the original long-latency negative wave and the maintenance of this latter component which evolves into a W-shaped VER typical of the adult unanesthetized preparations.

Stated otherwise, as illustrated in Figure 9, Nembutal (B) introduced in the unanesthetized preparations (A) causes no changes in waveform in the first 2 weeks. This is in contrast to the older preparations where Nembutal removes the later components.

One final point needs to be stressed regarding the period after 2 weeks of age. Not only is there a divergence in waveform as a function of lack of anesthesia, but, as illustrated in Figure 10, there are differences within a recording session as a function of the behavioral states of the animal, i.e., whether in aroused, drowsy, or sleeping condition. Such states, if present in the animal under 2 weeks of age have no effect on the waveform of the VER.

REFERENCES

Ellingson, R. J., and Rose, G. H. (1970). Ontogenesis of the electroencephalogram. *In* "Developmental Neurobiology" (W. A. Himwich, ed.), pp. 441-474. Thomas, Springfield, Illinois.

Purpura, D. P. (1969). Stability and seizure susceptibility of immature brain. *In* "Basic Mechanisms of the Epilepsies" (H. H. Jasper, A. A. Ward, and A. Pope, eds.), pp. 481-505. Little, Brown, Boston, Massachusetts.

Rose, G. H. (1971). The relationship of electrophysiological and behavioral indices of visual development in mammals. *In* "Brain Development and Behavior" (M. B. Sterman, D. J. McGinty, and A. M. Adinolfi, eds.). p. 145-183. Academic Press, New York.

Rose, G. H., Gruenau, S. P., and Spencer, J. W. (1972). Maturation of visual electrocortical responses in unanesthetized kittens: Effects of barbiturate anesthesia. *Electroencephalogr. Clin. Neurophysiol.* (in press).

Rose, G. H., and Lindsley, D. B. (1965). Longitudinal development of evoked potentials in kittens. *Electroencephalogr. Clin. Neurophysiol.* 18, 525 (abstr.).

Rose, G. H., and Lindsley, D. B. (1968). Development of visually evoked potentials in kittens: Specific and non-specific responses. *J. Neurophysiol.* 31, 607-623.

GENERAL DISCUSSION (CHAPTER 1 AND 2)

Dr. Clemente: Dr. Purpura, you emphasized strongly that cortical neurons in very young animals appear not to be mature in respect to their properties for excitation and inhibition. Your work refers principally to the maturation of the intrinsic inhibitory and excitatory mechanisms of cortical neurons, but these same immature cortical neurons, as yet, do not express their influences on lower centers such as the hypothalamus, brain stem, and spinal cord. Another point which I wish to bring up with regard to your paper is whether you would like to extend your concept on the maturation of neuronal membranes. You mentioned that cortical units were difficult to record in the early period. Do you see any differences in the morphology of the membranes of cortical neurons in the immature animal in comparison to the mature animal?

Dr. Purpura: We have not observed any changes in the morphological appearance of unit membranes with development. That is precisely one of the points I was trying to make. The fact is that there are a variety of developmental alterations in the physiological properties of

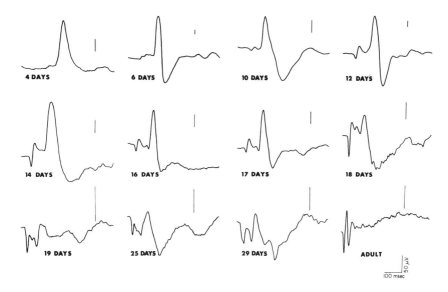

Fig. 8. Computer-averaged visually evoked potentials from contralateral visual cortex of unanesthetized (Flaxedilized) kittens at ages indicated. Focused monocular stimulation occurs at onset of trace. Monopolar recordings; neck reference (with ear reference check). Traces are algebraic summation of 25 responses. (Rose, Gruenau, and Spencer, 1972.)

excitable membranes of cortical neurons that are not reflected in obvious fine structural characteristics. That is one of the problems.

There is something quite interesting about the development of unit discharges in immature cortex as has been observed by many workers, some of whom I have cited in my report. In general, spontaneous activity is virtually absent in the immediate neonatal period and units are difficult to "drive" with peripheral stimulation. It is of interest that when discharge frequency increases and patterns of unit activity become more consistently mature in appearance, there is an increase in activity of the Na-K activated ATPase system (Huttenlocher and Rawson, 1968). What is not known is whether the increase in unit firing precedes the increase in enzyme activity or vice versa.

Several factors undoubtedly contribute to the increase in repetitive responsiveness of neurons during postnatal ontogenesis. There is, of course, the increase in the number of excitatory synapses that will lead to augmented excitatory drives. But this must be associated with a parallel change in the capability of neurons to exhibit repetitive firing and this is essentially a problem of spike electrogenesis and its sequelae. Perhaps immature neurons have prominent delayed rectification and rapid Na-inactivation coupled with a low level operation of pump mechanisms for rapidly restoring ionic distributions to predischarge levels. These factors indicate a relationship of the discharge properties of immature cortical neurons to intracellular metabolic events occurring in the early postnatal period.

The increase in potency of excitatory synaptic drives does have a correlation in the morphological development of synapses. Evidently if a synapse looks morphologically "mature" it is probably capable of adequate functional activity. However, there is no question but that synapses may form and "look" perfectly mature in the electron microscope before such synapses have participated in any organized functional activity. Dr.

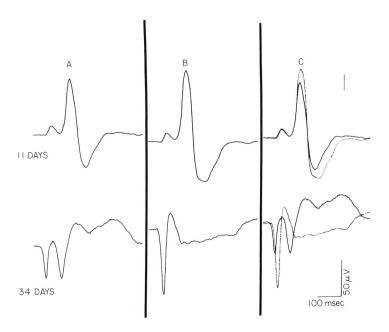

Fig. 9. Effect of pentobarbital anesthesia on visual electrocortical response recorded in unanesthetized (Flaxedilized) preparation at two different age levels. A = Flaxedil, B = Flaxedil plus pentobarbital (Nembutal), C = superimposition of A and B. Tracings are algebraic summation of 25 responses. (Rose, 1971.)

Stanley Crain, together with Dr. Pat Model, Dr. Murray Bornstein, and Dr. George D. Pappas, who are all investigators in the Kennedy Center at the Albert Einstein College of Medicine, have shown that cultures of fetal mouse cerebrum that are allowed to differentiate in xylocaine and Mg^{2+} (which block impulse conduction and synaptic transmission) will continue to elaborate all varieties of synapses. The obvious conclusion from these preliminary studies is that early phases of synaptogenesis are programmed by innate processes which are not at all dependent upon functional activity.

There are two phases in the postnatal development of cortical neuronal interactions. One phase is dependent on information transcribed from "genetic tapes" and is deterministic in operation, such as early patterns of dendritic growth and synaptogenesis. A second phase, perhaps sequentially overlapping the first, involves feedback from the external and internal milieu. Once a certain pattern of connectivity has developed, it would appear to require some degree of appropriate function to maintain these connections, at least for some types of neuronal interaction, as shown in the work of Hubel and Wiesel (1963, 1965). It remains an open question as to whether the early synaptogenetic processes can be "influenced" by environmental perturbations, even at the microsynaptogenetic level. Certainly, by the time new dendritic spines develop on cortical neurons in the second week, as the Scheibels have also shown, this is quite late from the standpoint of cortical synaptogenesis. It must be recalled that the primary afferent pathways are already distributed onto dendrites in superficial laminae in the early postnatal period, before spines are prominent. This would appear to be a relatively ineffective mode of activating immature cortical neurons in the neonatal period.

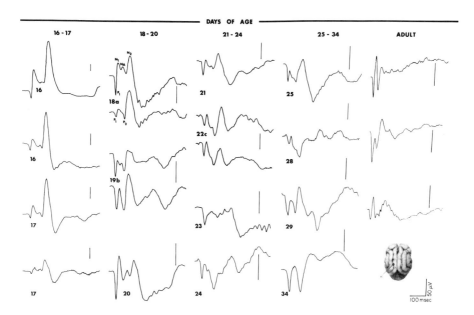

Fig. 10. Computer-averaged visual evoked potentials from contralateral visual cortex of unanesthetized (Flaxedilized) kittens at older ages indicated. Focused monocular stimulation occurs at onset of trace. Monopolar recordings: neck reference. Letters after age indicate two recordings from same animal. Tracings are algebraic summation of 25 responses. (Rose, Gruenau, and Spencer, 1972.)

But insofar as the visual cortex is concerned, kittens are not highly visual animals in the first 2 weeks. The same cannot be said for somesthetic functions.

In regard to your question concerning the maturation of inhibition in cortex, our data have shown that inhibitory synapses are functionally quite mature and that inhibition is well developed in contrast to excitation. Obviously, other aspects of inhibitory systems, such as the spread of inhibition in cortex, the activity of recurrent inhibitory mechanisms, etc. may not show the same degree of maturation as is reflected in the registration of IPSP's from single neurons.

Dr. Roberts: I am a little worried about the interpretation of inhibition being present before excitation in a really functional way. One can elicit the kinds of results you have by artificial stimulation, but behaviorally one gets the feeling that excitation occurs sometime before its real coordination is achieved. The latter is what I would expect inhibition to be doing; and I am just wondering whether, with the type of stimulation you use, there is just a big release of GABA which would give a long-lasting IPSP.

The mechanisms during early stages may not be very effective for binding GABA and transporting it away from the synaptic cleft, which is the way of inactivating it. It is questionable whether functionally in the animal inhibition is really effective at these early times of development, even though the machinery for liberating an inhibitory transmitter might be available if one gives it a big electrical boost.

Dr. Purpura: We have observed the same prolonged inhibition of visual cortical neurons following photic stimulation as has been observed following electrical stimulation of subcortical pathways. The reasons for the prolonged IPSP's have been suggested in my report. It should be recalled that all responses are composites of EPSP's and IPSP's, and if the EPSP's are absent or poorly represented in the overt response of a neuron recorded intracellularly then there will be less tendency for the IPSP to be "interrupted" by EPSP's.

It is necessary to emphasize that excitatory drives are by no means absent in immature cortex. Inhibition could not be expressed without excitation since IPSP's must be generated by inhibitory neurons which are themselves subjected to excitatory input. Consequently, there must be excitatory interneurons operating in immature cortex. There is probably no afferent pathway that enters cortex and generates monosynaptic inhibition in cortical neurons. Excitation, however weak or poorly developed, must occur at each subcortical cell station in a projection pathway. What is not known is the extent to which excitatory and inhibitory events at the thalamic level contribute to the properties of specific and nonspecific projection systems in the immature brain. For example, inhibition in the ventrobasal complex or in intrathalamic internuclear synaptic pathways may be much more prolonged than in the adult. In studies with Dr. Martin Feldman, it has been shown that, during evoked thalamocortical synchronization in the adult animal, conductance increases associated with IPSP's may persist for several seconds during the synchronization process. This indicates a continuing inhibitory transmitter liberation and action on thalamic neurons that may virtually short-circuit the soma-membrane during the period of induced spindle bursts. It may be that in younger animals thalamic inhibition may be even more powerful and prevent intermittent breakthrough of EPSP's required for the synchronized discharges of thalamic neurons.

We have emphasized the importance of the discovery of potent inhibitory pathways in the immature brain in order to call attention to the inadequacy of notions such as "fatigue" and "refractoriness" in consideration of the unique properties of evoked responses of immature brain. Inhibition is indeed an active process which must subserve some function, as yet unknown, in the immature brain.

Dr. Roberts: The development of the GABA system generally follows that of the acetylcholine system by some time. So that on the biochemical side, it would appear that the capacity to bring information into the organisms develops earlier than the capacity to modulate it (Roberts and Eidelberg, 1960; Roberts and Kuriyama, 1968).

Dr. Purpura: It is well established that the acetylcholine system (as defined by cholinesterase-staining of projection pathways or content of acetylcholine synthesizing or inactivating enzymes in cortex) is poorly developed in the neonatal period in altricial mammals. A more intriguing problem is why is the GABA content of immature cortex so high. Is GABA the inhibitory transmitter in cortex as has been suggested by several workers including Dr. Roberts? Although I have been involved with the GABA story for the past 13 years I cannot reach a definitive conclusion on this question. I would like you to be right, Dr. Roberts.

Dr. Sterman: I would like to ask a functional question. To the extent that sleep and wakefulness are cortical or neocortical processes, is the newborn cat capable of showing these functional states?

Dr. Scheibel: We have approached the problem from a slightly different point of view, asking the question "When can cortical activation and cortical synchrony first be demonstrated in the kitten?" We have found that the situation is unique during the first 7-10 days of postnatal life.

During this period, slow-frequency stimulation of the thalamic nonspecific system does not produce recruitment waves as it will in the adult. Depending on the strength of your stimuli, either nothing is seen in the cortical EEG, or else the trace flattens, almost like an activation response. Repetitive sensory stimuli, such as light flashes or clicks at 3-10/sec, similarly produce no time-locked wave phenomena. Again the cortical trace shows no response or else increasing degrees of flattening as the stimulus intensity increases. Between 10 and 14 days of postnatal life, larval responses in the cortical trace may begin to be seen and by the third to fifth week of life, well-developed cortical synchronous wave responses can be seen to develop in response to slow repetitive stimuli.

The phenomenon of cortical activation is also difficult to obtain in the newborn kitten. High-frequency stimulation (100/sec) in the brain stem reticular formation which will ordinarily flatten the adult cortical trace rich in slower wave components has, at best, a variable and inconstant effect during the first 7-14 days of life. In our experience, the first one or two stimulus bursts may flatten the EEG, but subsequent bursts of reticular stimulation have no discernible effect. Cortical EEG flattening may then continue to be unobtainable for 6-12 hr. Thereafter, one or two episodes of flattening may again be obtained. A reasonable explanation for this may lie in the rapid exhaustion of synaptic transmitter agents involved in cortical "activation," and the need for resynthesis in the very immature system. In any case, we assume from these data that the nature of sleep mechanisms at the cortical level must be quite different in the newborn cat.

Dr. Lindsley: Dr. Purpura, is it possible that more than one kind of inhibitory mechanism is operating here, contrasting the kitten with the adult cat, and pointing out that they both show prolonged inhibition? You also mentioned in relation to this that the neurons were densely packed, with very little glia, and I wonder if some possibility exists that acquisition of glia might be responsible for the change in basic inhibitory mechanisms of kittens vs the adult cat?

Dr. Purpura: The significance of the relatively late development of glia in the mammalian cerebral cortex is not known. At least one point is clear, however. Glia are not required for the evoked potentials observed in the neonatal period or for the intracellularly recorded EPSP's and IPSP's observed in young kittens. Glial maturation as indicated by myelination of corticofugal pathways is a relatively late event. A point of emphasis is that Golgi studies of cortex as well as electron microscopic studies indicate that maturation of neuronal elements and synaptic pathways is virtually completed before the peak maturational phase of glial proliferation. While glia do not seem to contribute to the events noted above, there has been evidence of a relationship between glial development and the cortical steady potential and the capacity of the immature brain to exhibit spreading depression.

The question raised, however, is whether the inhibition observed in the newborn and very young animal is the same as the inhibition observed in the adult animal. There is no doubt in my mind that the inhibition demonstrated in immature cortex neurons is postsynaptic inhibition initiated by transmitter-activated conductance increases. Presynaptic inhibition plays no role in this mechanism, since this type of inhibition has not been demonstrated in the cerebral cortex (nor have axoaxonic synapses of any variety been detected in the cerebral cortex). The conclusion is inescapable that the inhibition observed is postsynaptic in nature and the same as found in the adult animal.

Dr. Weitzman: Regarding Dr. Sterman's question, we found that by 34-36 weeks in the human premature infant one could clearly show a different auditory evoked response latency depending on whether the infant was having a continuous EEG pattern or an intermittent pattern. So, certainly in the relatively immature human nervous system there is evidence that one can show differences of sleep states, EEG patterns, and evoked responses. What is the maturational relationship of the newborn rat and cat to such an immature human nervous system?

Dr. Ellingson: The human brain is more mature at birth than that of the cat.

Dr. Weitzman: I am speaking of a 2-month premature infant.

Dr. Ellingson: In the cat and rat, you cannot see clearly identifiable EEG changes related to the wakefulness-sleep cycle at birth or for several days thereafter. There are behavioral changes which have been described and can be recorded by polygraphic methods (not EEG) in both species. At this epoch the stages of sleep are described as "quiet sleep" and "sleep with jerks," rather than "fast wave sleep" and "slow wave sleep." EEG differentiation does not become evident until several days after birth. In the human, EEG differentiation is present at least 1 month before term.

REFERENCES

Hubel, D. H. and Wiesel, T. N. (1963). Receptive fields of cells in striate cortex of very young, visually inexperienced kittens. *J. Neurophysiol.* **26**, 994-1002.

Hubel, D. H. and Wiesel, T. N. (1965). Binocular interaction in striate cortex of kittens reared with artificial squint. *J. Neurophysiol.* **27**, 1041-1059.

Huttenlocher, P. R., and Rawson, M. D. (1968). Neuronal activity and adenosine triphosphatase in immature cerebral cortex. *Exp. Neurol.* **22**, 118.

Roberts, E., and Eidelberg, E. (1960). Metabolic and neurophysiological roles of γ-aminobutyric acid. *Int. Rev. Neurobiol.* **2**, 279-332.

Roberts, E., and Kuriyama, K. (1968). Biochemical-physiological correlations in studies of the γ-aminobutyric acid system. *Brain Res.* **8**, 1-35.

3

Maturing Neuronal Subsystems: The Dendrites of Spinal Motoneurons*

Madge E. Scheibel and Arnold B. Scheibel

Ample documentation exists in the literature to support the concept that the histological structure of neural tissue undergoes changes with maturation. These changes may include one, or a combination, of the following: (1) enhancement in the complexity of patterning of individual elements such as the growth of the Purkinje cell dendrite system of the cerebellum (Ramón y Cajal, 1955); (2) linear extension of structures already, to some degree, present, such as the apical arches of cortical pyramidal cells (Ramón y Cajal, 1955; Scheibel and Scheibel, 1964); (3) replication or multiplication in numbers of structures present at birth, such as the terminal bouton systems in spinal cord (Kuypers, 1962; Tiegs, 1926); and (4) migration of neural entities, such as the descent of immature granule cells from Obersteiner's layer in cerebellum (Ramón y Cajal, 1955). Examples

*Supported by grants from NINDS (NS 01063) and NICHD (HD 00972).

49

may also be cited of changes in the relationship between already existing structures, although documentation here still lacks some degree of rigor. An example of this phenomenon appears to be the development of a "climbing type" of axodendritic relationship between corticipetal axons from brain stem and thalamic nonspecific systems with the apical dendrites of cortical pyramids (Scheibel and Scheibel, 1964).

In this chapter we want to report another example of developing interrelations between already existing neural structures, i.e., the dendrites of spinal motoneurons, together with a possible measurable physiological correlate.

TECHNIQUES

Structural observations are based on study of Golgi (chrome-silver)-impregnated preparations of spinal cords from approximately 200 animals of various ages. These include 2 adult and 3 newborn macaques, 50 kittens less than 1 week of age, 20 neurally mature cats of 3 months to 1 year, and more than 100 rats and mice of various ages. One adult human lumbosacral cord was also available for examination with Golgi modifications.

In previous communications we have considered the capabilities of the rapid Golgi variants (Scheibel and Scheibel, 1966a,b) as well as the problems inherent in the technique. It is probably sufficient to remind the reader that although the nature of the basic Golgi reaction remains unknown, the investigator can still exert some degree of control over the scope and quantity of elements visualized through manipulation of stain parameters. Relatively minor modifications of methodology also enable some degree of success in impregnating essentially adult tissue with the rapid Golgi method. The less sensitive but more widely staining Cox modification may also be used to provide further documentation in mature tissue.

We have also studied the electromyogram (EMG) at successive developmental epochs in an attempt to establish a possible functional correlate for the developing dendritic bundles. Kittens were suspended in a canvas sling arranged to support the body and head but allowing virtually unrestricted motion of the extremities (Fig. 1). Bipolar concentric recording electrodes were inserted subcutaneously over the gastrocnemius and anterior tibial muscles of one hind leg and led to the junction box of an Offner type T electroencephalograph. Each electrode consisted of a 34-gauge enameled stainless steel wire inserted into a ¾-in. long 27-gauge hypodermic needle, insulated except at the tip. A platform was usually placed under the hindquarters at such a height so as to allow some weight-bearing by the limb from which we were recording. In some of the later runs, the EMG was simultaneously taped on a 4-channel Ampex magnetic tape recorder and the outputs were integrated (Fig. 6).

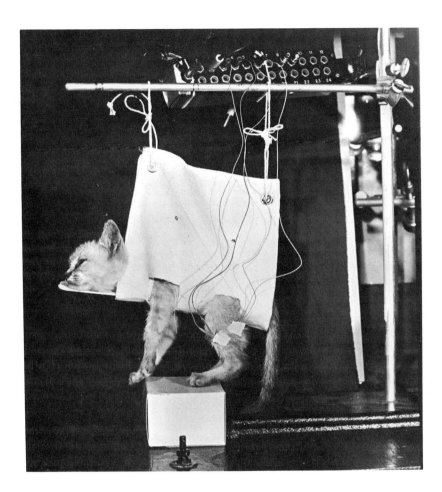

Fig. 1. Photograph of kitten in canvas harness with EMG leads in place.

RESULTS

Transverse sections through the spinal cord of the newborn cat reveal the radiating dendrite patterns of spinal neurons which have been familiar since the time of Ramón y Cajal (1955). These patterns are well developed by the third trimester of fetal life and further developmental changes which occur in the postnatal period consist largely in increase in the overall dimensions of grey and white matter and enhanced complexity of the neuropil field. While there is convincing evidence for segregation of motoneuron somata by functional groupings, and this organizational pattern becomes increasingly clear with maturation of the cord, it has not been possible to discover patterns of similar precision among the motoneuron dendrites. In fact, the mixing and interweaving of dendrites is such in the usual Golgi-stained section as to suggest either that the importance of function-specific somal groupings is largely subverted, or that the physiological properties of somata and dendrites are significantly different.

More recently, study of sagittal sections of cord has revealed aspects of dendrite patterning which could not have been predicted from analysis of cross sections alone. Dendrite systems of motoneurons appear organized largely in the rostrocaudal axis (Scheibel and Scheibel, 1969; Sterling and Kuypers, 1967), while most propriospinal neurons generate dendrite domains perpendicular to the long axis of the cord. Furthermore, when horizontal sagittal sections of mature spinal cord are examined with Golgi techniques, most of these longitudinally oriented dendrites appear to run in tightly organized bundles (Scheibel and Scheibel, 1970) which may maintain their identity for several hundred to several thousand microns. Each bundle consists of variable numbers (5 to 30) of dendrite shafts, and the same bundle often contains dendrites from several geographically discrete motoneuron pools. Comparison of the location of such pools with experimentally determined motoneuron groupings by Romanes (1951) leads to the conclusion that dendrite bundles usually represent combinations of shafts from nuclei of differing—often antagonistic—functions (Scheibel and Scheibel, 1970). Because of the obvious possibilities for physiological interaction in such structural complexes, it seemed useful to inquire whether they were completely formed at birth when levels of motor performance were still rudimentary, or developed coevally with increase in motor skills.

The nature of dendrite organization in the lumbosacral cord of the late fetal cat is illustrated in Fig. 2. It is clear that, although dendrites are already quite mature in appearance, the shaft patterns are primarily radiative and tend to show little of the sagittal orientation which will later characterize dendrite systems of the anterior horn.

In spinal cord specimens taken at the first postnatal day, the beginnings of sagittal organization of dendrite shafts is already apparent (Fig. 3). Measurements of 50 rostrocaudally oriented shafts compared with a similar number of transversely arranged dendrite branches shows that the former are now longer than the latter by an average 22%. The pair of EMG traces led from the region overlying gastrocnemius and anterior tibial muscles at this time (Fig. 6) shows a picture essentially without pattern. Both muscles produce records characterized

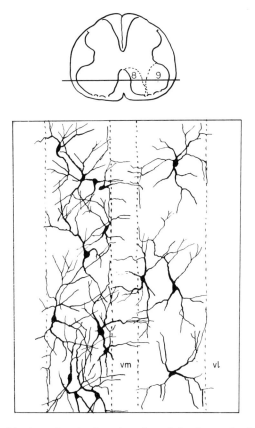

Fig. 2. Drawing of horizontal sagittal section through lumbosacral spinal cord of a late fetal cat (4-7 days before term). Neurons pictured on left and right sides probably represent a combination of motoneurons and propriospinal neurons. The dendrite pattern is essentially radiative in nature with no preferential orientation. Abbreviations: vm, ventromedial white matter; vl, ventrolateral white matter. Small cross section diagram of cord shows plane of section and identifies the position of Rexed's laminae 8 and 9. Most motoneurons are located in the latter. Rapid Golgi variant. × 200.

by low-to-medium voltage bursts of varying lengths, without discernible evidence of phasing of activity between the two muscles.

At 12 days of age, further lengthening of the dendrite system is apparent (Fig. 4) primarily along the long axis of the spinal cord. The length of dendrites extending in this direction surpasses that of transversely oriented shafts by a mean ratio of at least 2:1. Furthermore, as Fig. 4 shows, small groups of shafts, especially tips and the peripheral third of many dendrite branches, have begun to follow parallel courses in close apposition for intervals of 20-100 μ or more. In a few well-developed kittens, early evidence of this bundling phenomenon can be

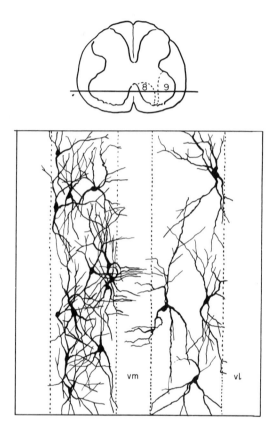

Fig. 3. Drawing of horizontal sagittal section through lumbosacral spinal cord of 1-day-old cat. The early development of a sagittal orientation of the dendrite shafts is especially noticeable in the case of the four isolated cells on the right side. Numerous commissural dendrite branches cross midline. Small cross section diagram of cord shows plane of section and identifies the position of Rexed's laminae 8 and 9. Abbreviations: vm, ventromedial white matter; vl, ventrolateral white matter. Rapid Golgi variant. × 200.

seen even earlier, between 7 and 14 days of age. The EMG taken at 12 days still shows a record essentially without organization. However, as indicated in Fig. 6, there is some hint of alternation in the bursts of EMG activity from gastrocnemius and anterior tibial muscles, especially in the latter half of this short strip. Since these appear temporally correlated with the initial appearance of bundling, and with the commencement of combined weight-bearing and walking movements of the extremities, it is tempting to speculate that a relationship exists among the three factors.

At 4 months of age the preponderance of sagittally directed dendrites seems fully stated while dendrite bundles are dense, numerous, and well-developed (Fig. 5). Individual dendrite shafts may continue as part of a bundle for 500-700

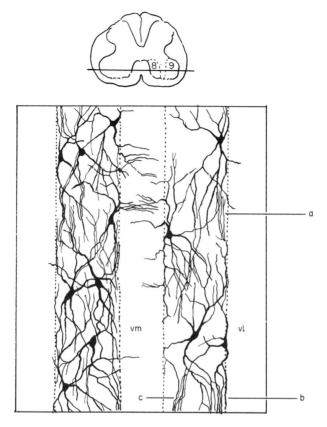

Fig. 4. Drawing of horizontal sagittal section through lumbosacral spinal cord of 12-day-old cat. Sagittal orientation of the dendrite systems is more marked and, in addition, the beginning of dendrite bundling can be seen at a, b, and c. Small cross section diagram of cord shows plane of section and identifies the position of Rexed's laminae 8 and 9. Abbreviations: vm, ventromedial white matter; vl, ventrolateral white matter. Rapid Golgi variant. × 200.

μ while the total bundle, with additions and subtractions, may maintain its identity for several millimeters. Individual dendritic components often run so closely apposed to each other that no space can be resolved between them with the light microscope (Scheibel and Scheibel, 1970). Dr. L. J. Stensaas (1970 personal communication) has informed us that motoneuron dendrites are unique among dendrite systems in the spinal cord, in cold-blooded vertebrate forms at least, for their almost complete lack of glial sheathing. If this should be applicable to the mammalian forms we are studying, the chances may be considerably improved for interaction between dendrites lying in virtual contact for hundreds of microns.

The EMG at 4 months (Fig. 6) shows alternating bursts of activity in the

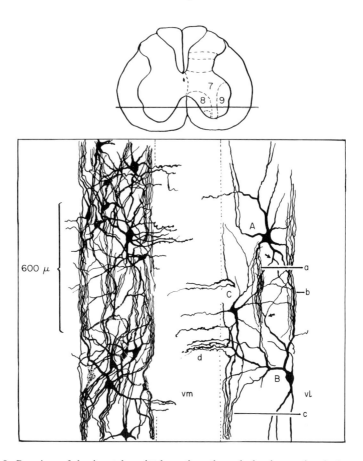

Fig. 5. Drawing of horizontal sagittal section through lumbosacral spinal cord of a 4-month-old cat. The bundling of motoneuron dendrites appears fully developed, as at a, b, and c. Arrows point to individual dendrite branches which bifurcate and send branches to join different bundles. Commissural dendrite branches are seen at d. Cells A and B represent large motoneurons of different motor pools while cell C is a large propriospinal neuron. Inset diagram shows cross section of spinal cord with plane of section, and Rexed's laminae 7, 8, and 9. Abbreviations: vm, ventromedial white matter; vl, ventrolateral white matter. Rapid Golgi variant. × 200. (Slightly modified from Scheibel and Scheibel, 1970.)

gastrocnemius, anterior tibial muscle pair during certain types of walking-weight-bearing movements. This does not represent the only pattern generated by the extensor-flexor pair and reciprocal sequencing of the two is often not apparent in the records. However, this particular type of record and its associated step-walk-weight-bearing continuum is of interest because of its possible relationship to dendrite bundling as a structural substrate. Clearly, if the relationship which we postulate actually exists, a good deal more must be learned about information-processing in dendrites.

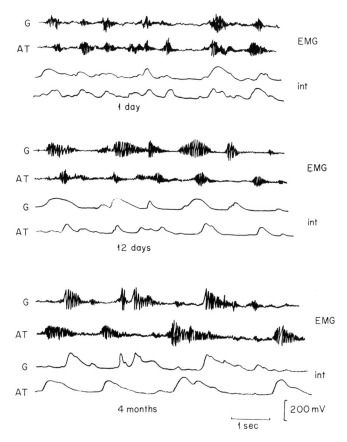

Fig. 6. Paired EMG traces from gastrocnemius (G) and anterior tibial (AT) muscles compared at 1 day, 12 days, and 4 months. Records taken while animal was attempting weight-bearing and walking or stepping movements against a platform slipped under his leg. Second pair of traces in each group represents integrate (int) of the first pair. There is a suggestion of sequencing or alternation of muscle bursts in the last few discharges in the 12-day record. Alternation is quite obvious in the 4-month record. Calibrations as shown.

DISCUSSION

The physiological significance of dendrite bundles has not yet been determined. In fact, the phenomenon of bundling in spinal motoneuron dendrites has apparently remained virtually unnoticed, or unmentioned, until very recently. Aside from our own description (Scheibel and Scheibel, 1970) we have been able to find only two other allusions to this phenomenon. The first occurs in a comment by Barron (1953) in which he refers to some rabbit spinal cord preparations of Laruelle where the dendrites were "absolutely interwoven." The second appears in a brief article by Marsh (1971) whose work is based on reconstructions from series of transverse Nissl sections showing groups of irregular oval profiles which he interprets as cross sections of bundles of dendrites.

However, if the physiological purpose of this structural figure remains enigmatic, there are several putative roles that it might fill. *Direct synaptic relations* between dendrites have been demonstrated in the olfactory bulb by Rall and his associates (1966). They have presented both anatomical and physiological data supporting the existence of presynaptic and postsynaptic relations between mitral and granule cell dendrites. Electron micrographs indicate adjacent synaptic areas organized for synaptic exchange in either direction on the basis of position of synaptic vesicles, subsynaptic thickening, etc. Inhibition is conceived as developing through nonpropagated depolarization of the dendritic tree. Although this represents an attractive model, some of whose features may be restated in retina (Kidd, 1962) and lateral geniculate body (Colonnier and Guillery, 1965), there are presently no data of this sort available in spinal cord. Electron microscopic analysis of spinal motoneuron dendrite systems is clearly indicated.

The possibility that *extrasynaptic modes of interaction* may play a significant role in anterior horn mechanisms has been considered by a number of workers. When Renshaw demonstrated that antidromic activation of certain groups of motoneurons condition reflex excitability in adjacent motoneuron groups (Renshaw, 1941), he suggested, as an alternative to the well-known recurrent collateral hypothesis, the possibility that perineuronal current flow might be the causative agent. More recently, Nelson and Frank (1964) have measured field potentials about active motoneurons for distances of at least 500 μ mediolaterally and 700 μ dorsoventrally. In some cases, the extracellular voltage gradients approached 100 mV/mm. Nelson (1966) has also reported short-latency facilitation representing as much as a 30% reduction in firing threshold of adjacent neurons. Brookhart and Kubota (1963) have also suggested a dendritic modulating effect on motoneuron firing capacity, while Garcia Ramos (1969) has suggested that dendritic potentials are largely responsible for the slow components of spinal cord potentials produced both by electrotonic and field effects.

He has also considered the dendrite system as capable of generating *discrete unitary potentials*, a position previously considered by Wall (1965) in the area of large spinal lamina IV cells and by a number of workers in other neural centers over the past decade.

Whatever the nature of spinal dendritic interactions is finally determined to be, we suggest that the information-processing capacity inherent in the motoneuron dendrite bundles in mature spinal cord will prove of considerable importance to motor mechanisms. Dendrites represent 80-90% of the available synaptic surface of motoneurons (Aitken and Bridger, 1961) and it now appears that much of this membrane area is packed into bundles in the mature cord. Furthermore, these bundles are of characteristically heterogeneous composition, clearly transcending the columnar grouping of motoneuron somata which also characterizes ventral horn organization.

The complex patterns of reciprocal activity between agonist and antagonist muscle pairs is an obvious feature of all motor activities of the extremities (Eccles, 1964; Lloyd, 1944; Sherrington, 1906; etc.). Despite a very large literature on the physiology and microphysiology of spinal motor behavior, there is still no clear idea as to the mechanisms involved in programming progressive components of motor acts such as stepping, walking, running, etc. We believe that the motoneuron dendrite bundle provides a structural substrate within which information processing necessary to these output programs can occur. Although many types of structural and biochemical changes are occurring in the first few postnatal months, we believe that the progressive bundling together of dendrite shafts from motoneurons with different and frequently opposed functional roles has particular significance. We suggest that the development of this structural complex, *pari passu* with the onset of increasingly integrated activity of the extremities, represents a more than fortuitous relationship.

CONCLUSION

In mature cats and in primates, it has been found that the dendrites of spinal motoneurons are gathered into bundles which run for long distances in the rostrocaudal axis of the cord. These bundles usually contain dendrite shafts from heterogeneous motoneuron groups including pairs of functional antagonists. The bundles are not present at birth but begin to appear between the first and second week of life (kitten). Bundling of motoneuron dendrites becomes progressively more obvious as stepping, walking, weight-bearing activities of the extremities become smoother and more effective, and apparently achieves the mature state between the third and fourth month of postnatal life (kitten). EMG's of functional antagonist pairs, such as the gastrocnemius and anterior tibial muscles, suggest that reciprocal sequencing of activity patterns appears at about the time that dendrite bundling can first be demonstrated. Despite the temporal congruence of these phenomena, the correlations we are suggesting are, at this point, only inferential. However, dendrite bundle complexes would appear to provide a promising substrate for extensive processing of information. The inclusion of shafts from motor groups of differing, often antagonistic, function suggest the possibility for programming activities centering about proper sequencing of functionally opposed muscle groups in the effective performance of motor acts.

It has been shown in a recently reported work (Matthews, *et al.,* 1971), using electron microscopy, that longitudinally oriented bundles or thickets of motoneuron dendrites can be interrelated in several ways. Whereas, in some cases, there were glial lamellae and/or fine fibers between the individual elements of the bundle; in others, the dendrite membranes were closely apposed either without detectable specializations, or with definite nonpolarized aggregates of electron dense material on each side of a gap of approximately 180 Å. No synaptic vesicles were seen. The authors concluded that this structural arrangement might serve as substrate for the weak electrical facilitation known to occur among motoneurons in cat spinal cord.

REFERENCES

Aitken, J., and Bridger, J. (1961). Neuron size and neuron population density in the lumbosacral region of the cat's spinal cord. *J. Anat.* **95**, 38-53.

Barron, D. H. (1953). Comment. *The Spinal Cord, Ciba Found. Symp., 1952,* p. 41.

Brookhart, J. M., and Kubota, K. (1963). Studies of the integrative function of the motor neuron. *Progr. Brain Res.* **1**, 38-64.

Colonnier, M., and Guillery, R. W. (1965). Synaptic organization in the lateral geniculate nucleus of the monkey. *Z. Zellforsch. Mikrosk. Anat.* **62**,, 333-355.

Eccles, J. C. (1964). "The Physiology of Synapses." Springer-Verlag, Berlin and New York.

Garcia Ramos, J. (1969). On the physiology of dendrites. *Curr. Mod. Biol.* **3**, 74-84.

Kidd, M. (1962). Electron microscopy of the inner plexiform layer of the retina in the cat and pigeon. *J. Anat.* **96**, 179-187.

Kuypers, H. G. J. M. (1962). Corticospinal connections; postnatal development in the rhesus monkey. *Science* **138**, 678-680.

Lloyd, D. P. C. (1944). Functional organization of the spinal cord. *Physiol. Rev.* **24**, 1-17.

Marsh, R. C. Matlovsky, L., and Stromberg, M. W. (1971). Dendritic bundles exist. *Brain Res.* **33**, 273-277.

Mathews, M. A., Willis, W. D., and Williams, V. (1971). Dendrite bundles in lamina IX of cat spinal cord: A possible source for electrical interaction between motorneurons? *Anatom. Rec.* **171**, 313-327.

Nelson, P. G. (1966). Interaction between spinal motoneurons of the cat. *J. Neurophysiol.* **29**, 275-287.

Nelson, P. G., and Frank, K. (1964). Extracellular potential fields of single spinal motoneurons. *J. Neurophysiol.* **27**, 913-927.

Rall, W., Shepherd, G. M., Reese, T. S., and Brightman, M. W. (1966). Dendrodendritic synaptic pathway for inhibition in the olfactory bulb. *Exp. Neurol.* **14**, 44-56.

Ramón y Cajal, S. (1955). "Histologie du Système Nerveux de l'Homme et des Vertébrés." Vols. I and II. Consejo Superior de Investigaciones Cientificas, Madrid.

Renshaw, B. (1941). Influence of discharge of motoneurons upon excitation of neighboring motoneurons. *J. Neurophysiol.* **4**, 167-183.

Romanes, G. J. (1951). The motor cell columns of the lumbosacral spinal cord of the cat. *J. Comp. Neurol.* **94**, 313-364.

Scheibel, M. E., and Scheibel, A. B. (1964). Some structural and functional substrates of development in young cats. *Progr. Brain Res.* **9**, 6-25.

Scheibel, M. E., and Scheibel, A. B. (1966a). The organization of the nucleus reticularis thalami: a Golgi study. *Brain Res.* **1**, 43-62.

Scheibel, M. E., and Scheibel, A. B. (1966b). Patterns of organization in specific and nonspecific thalamic fields. *In* "The Thalamus" (D. Purpura and M. Yahr, eds.), pp. 13-46, Columbia Univ. Press, New York.

Scheibel, M. E., and Scheibel, A. B. (1969). Terminal patterns in cat spinal cord. III. Primary afferent collaterals. *Brain Res.* **13**, 417-443.

Scheibel, M. E., and Scheibel, A. B. (1970). Organization of spinal motoneuron dendrites in bundles. *Exp. Neurol.* **28**, 106-112.

Sherrington, C. S. (1906). "Integrative action of the nervous system." Yale Univ. Press, New Haven, Connecticut.

Stensaas, L. J. (1970). Personal communication.

Sterling, P., and Kuypers, H. G. J. M. (1967). Anatomical organization of the brachial spinal cord of the cat. II. The motoneuron plexus. *Brain Res.* **4**, 16-32.

Tiegs, O. W. (1926). The structure of the neuron junctions of the spinal cord. *Aust. J. Exp. Biol. Med. Sci.* **3**, 69-79.

Wall, P. D. (1965). Impulses originating in the region of dendrites. *J. Physiol. (London)* **180**, 116-133.

INVITED DISCUSSION: PAUL D. COLEMAN

I would like to devote most of my discussion to pointing out environmental and genetic effects on the development of neuronal dendritic fields, as revealed by quantitative Golgi studies in the cortex.

The points that I wish to make are, first, that quantitative study of dendritic fields reveals environmental and genetic effects on dendritic development that may be relatively subtle and that certainly would escape us in a qualitative microscopic study; and second, I would like to suggest that these less obvious effects on dendritic development may be functionally significant as revealed by correlations between dendrite measures and behavior.

We previously reported a collaborative work with Austin Riesen (Coleman and Riesen, 1968) in which we showed effects of rearing cats in the dark (to age 6 months) on the development of dendrites in several regions of the brain. We examined layer IV stellate cells in area 17 and cingulate gyrus pyramids. Control measurements were taken from layer V pyramids in area 17. The measurements we took were pretty standard (e.g. Eayrs, 1955; Sholl, 1956). We traced out the dendrites with a camera lucida, measured length of dendrites as a function of order, counted numbers of dendrites as a function of order, put a bull's eye arrangement (Fig. 7) around the neuron and counted the location of branch points in the concentric bands. We also counted intersections of dendrites with the concentric circles. The results we got from rearing animals in the dark are shown in Figs. 8-15.

Figure 8 shows a count of intersections with the concentric circles in the control animals and the dark-reared animals, showing clear differences between the two groups. However, there seem to be no differences in the dendrites close to the cell body.

Figure 9 shows the number of dendrites as a function of order, again with clear effects of dark-rearing. Again, I would like to point out that there do not seem to be any group differences in the dendrites close to the cell bodies.

Counting branch points (Fig. 10), again there is no significant difference close to the cell body, but then when we get farther out, we do have some differences between groups.

Length, as a function of order, again shows no differences between groups close to the cell body, but farther from the cell body we get a big difference, which falls off at still greater distances from the cell body (Fig. 11).

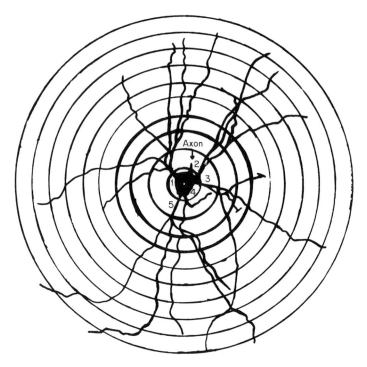

Fig. 7. Illustration of a stellate cell centered in a series of concentric circles. In this case, the radius of successive circles increases by 18 μ. (Data from S-1 and S-3 rats were taken using 20 μ increments.) Counts were taken of intersections of dendrites with successive circles and dendrite branchings in successive bands. Template used in counting had lines accurately drawn on plexiglas in a milling machine.

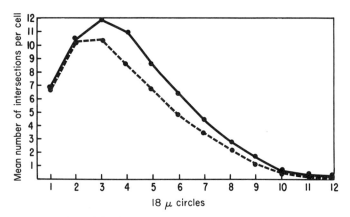

Fig. 8. Average number of dendrite intersections with concentric circles as a function of circle radius. (See Fig. 1.) Layer IV striate stellate cell dendrites in dark-reared and normally reared cats. (—) Control; (– –) experimental. (From Coleman and Riesen, 1968; courtesy of Cambridge University Press.)

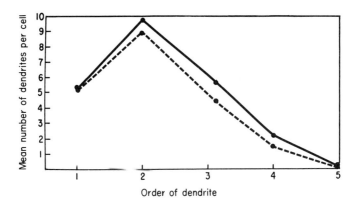

Fig. 9. Average number of dendrites per cell as a function of order of dendrite in dark-reared and normally-reared cats. Layer IV striate stellate cells. (—) Control; (– –) experimental. (From Coleman and Riesen, 1968; courtesy of Cambridge University Press.)

Figures 8-11 all show that dark-reared cats have had deficient dendritic development, and the nature of the deficiency appears to be largely a decreased probability of branching, particularly in the higher order dendrites.

We can see this in Fig. 12 which shows that in the dark-reared animals the individual dendrites of each order are longer than in the control animals. The circumferences of the dendritic fields are approximately the same for the two groups (Fig. 8), but within that area the dendrites of the dark-reared group are less likely to branch and are, therefore, longer. Consequently, within such a circumscribed area, these less branched, longer dendrites can only produce a less complex dendritic field.

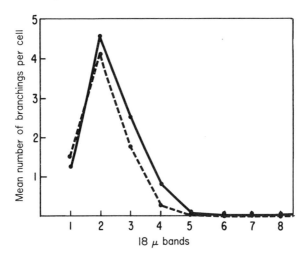

Fig. 10. Average number of branchings of dendrites in concentric circular bands as a function of distance of band from cell body. (See Fig. 1.) Layer IV striate stellate cells in dark-reared and normally reared cats. (—) Control; (– –) experimental. (From Coleman and Riesen, 1968; courtesy of Cambridge University Press.)

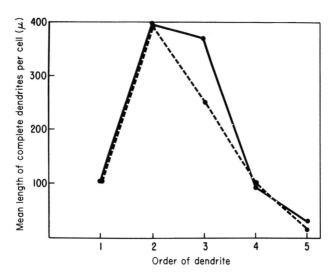

Fig. 11. Average length per cell of all uncut dendrites of each order in dark-reared and normally reared cats. Layer IV striate stellate cells. (——) Control; (– –) experimental. (From Coleman and Riesen, 1968; courtesy of Cambridge University Press.)

In our control measurements in layer V pyramids, the basal dendritic fields showed no differences between these groups of animals, suggesting that the differences we saw in layer IV are the direct result of the light deprivation, rather than being due to any generalized hormonal or nutritional effect.

The overall picture of the effects produced by our environmental manipulation is that there is relatively little effect on the dendrites close to the cell body, presumably dendrites that have developed earlier. Most of the effects appear to be on dendrites farther away from

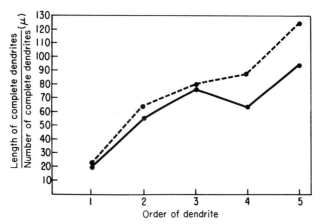

Fig. 12. Average length of individual dendrites (in microns) as a function of order in dark-reared and normally reared cats. Layer IV striate stellate cells. (——) Control; (– –) experimental. (From Coleman and Riesen, 1968; courtesy of Cambridge University Press.)

the cell body and the decreases in all the measures that we have shown here are attributable to decreased probability of branching.

Regarding controls outside of the area, we had thought that the cingulate gyrus might be a control but we in fact found an effect there. This makes sense in terms of the physiological studies, since visual evoked responses have been shown in that region (Harman and Berry, 1956). So, essentially, the area 17, layer V, pyramid basilar dendrites are serving as our control. We would like to do other regions in addition.

We had a very small sample. There were three animals in each group. We are confronted here with the problem of making extensive measurements of dendrites, a task so time-consuming that it severely limits the amount of data we can collect. We are presently developing a computer-controlled scanning microscope to speed up this task.

Genetic factors can also affect the development of dendritic trees. We have obtained from Dr. Mark Rosensweig at Berkeley some brains of the S-1 and S-3 strains of rats. These strains were derived from one set of parents whose offspring were mated on the basis of maze scores. This program was started in the mid-1920's. No selection pressure has been exerted for a number of years, but the strains are still quite different.

In a sample of these rats, we measured the dendritic fields of pyramids from CA-1 of the hippocampus in the same way we had previously measured the dendrites in the study of light-deprived animals. Results are shown in the next figures.

Figure 13 shows intersections of dendrites with concentric circles around the cell body. The data from the S-1 (presumably maze-bright) animals are represented by the squares and the data from the S-3 (presumably maze-dull) animals by the circles. The filled and unfilled symbols represent subgroups of each of these strains formed on the basis of scores in the Hebb-Williams maze as explained in the legend. For purposes of the present discussion of genetic factors, these subgroupings will not be considered. Figure 13 certainly shows that in terms of number of intersections with successive circles, the S-3 strain clearly has a more complex dendritic field. I do want to point out, in addition, that close to the cell body we have no differences and only when we get farther away from the cell body do the differences emerge.

In terms of branchings, again we have no particular differences close to the cell body (Fig. 14). As we get farther away, the differences emerge and we see again the S-3 strain has more branchings.

Figure 15 shows the numbers of dendrites and it is not quite so neat as some of the other figures, but again the S-3 animals seem to have dendrites in greater number, and again the difference, such as it may be, is largely farther away from the cell body.

Measures of dendrite length as a function of order do not show differences that are particularly striking upon visual inspection, but analysis by means of a Mahalanobis D-square shows significant strain differences in the fifth and sixth order dendrites; with the S-3 strain tending to have greater dendrite length.

We have done statistical analyses of all these data and, although these differences really do not appear to be as striking as those produced in the dark-rearing of cats, they are significant.

Once again, we have seen that the dendritic tree close to the cell body shows no differences between the groups as was the case with the dark-rearing experiment and the differences between the groups seem to lie in the characteristics of the dendritic tree at intermediate distances from the cell body, in this case between ~ 20 and $120 \, \mu$. Perhaps at a distance farther away from the cell body we might start to see more impressive differences in an EM study, but certainly it seems here that the primary dendrites do not show group differences in any of the situations we have looked at so far.

These differences in dendritic trees may be of functional significance, as suggested by regression analyses of the relations between dendrite measures, and maze scores of

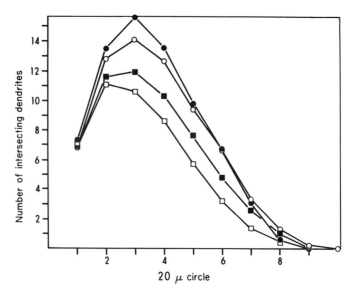

Fig. 13. Average number of intersections of dendrites of S-1 and S-3 rats with concentric circles. (See Fig. 1.) CA-1 hippocampus pyramid basal dendrites. The four groups are: (■) S-1S (45 cells, 3 rats) S-1 rats making few initial errors in the Hebb-Williams maze; (□) S-1D (45 cells, 3 rats) S-1 rats making many errors (○) S-3S (30 cells, 2 rats) S-3 rats making few errors; (●) S-3D (30 cells, 2 rats) S-3 rats making many errors.

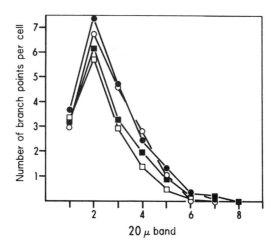

Fig. 14. Average number of branchings of dendrites in concentric circular bands as a function of distance of band from cell body. CA-1 hippocampus pyramid basal dendrites of S-1 and S-3 rats. Groups are the same as in Fig. 13.

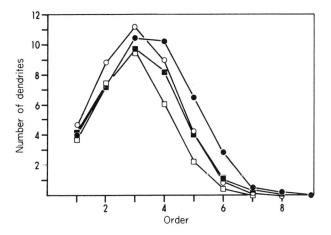

Fig. 15. Average number of dendrites per cell as a function of order of dendrite. CA-1 hippocampus pyramid basal dendrites of S-1 and S-3 rats. Groups are the same as in Fig. 13.

individual animals. The same animals were run in the Hebb-Williams maze at Berkeley before their brains were sent to us. The brains were coded and we measured them blind. We found some significant correlations between these dendritic measures and initial errors in the Hebb-Williams maze. The dendritic measures that we correlated with maze scores were: total numbers of dendrites, total dendritic length, total number of branch points, and total number of intersections, and, in addition, the number of branch points, number of dendrites, number of intersections, and dendrite lengths at that portion of the dendritic tree that showed the greatest differences between groups.

For example, when we were dealing with intersections as shown in the curve of Fig. 13, we would take the number of intersections at the region that showed the greatest difference between groups, which in the case of these hippocampal pyramids happened to be 60 μ away from the cell body. We had then eight dendrite measurements and the best possible measure in predicting (or the highest correlation between maze scores and dendrite measurements) was the number of dendrite branch points in the region between 20 and 40 μ from the cell body. The magnitude of this correlation was +0.57, not very large, but significant at the 0.05% level.

We derived a regression equation from this analysis and then on the basis of this regression equation, calculated maze scores for individual animals. We compared these calculated scores with the actual scores and found that the average difference between calculated and actual maze scores was 21%. In other words, we were off by an average of 21% in these calculated maze scores. If we throw more variables into the pot and do multiple regression analysis, we really do not improve things very much. The best combinations of three variables, when we do multiple regression analysis, was number of third-order dendrites, total number of branches, and total number of intersections with concentric circles. Using these best three variables the correlation went up to +0.70 with maze scores. Our error of so-called prediction (prediction is an imprecise term because in fact we are predicting on the same animals from which we got the measures) dropped from 21 to 19%, which is not a great improvement and if you add still more variables, the results would not be enhanced.

I think the studies outlined here suggest that both environmental and genetic variables may influence the development of dendrites in ways that can only be revealed by quantitative studies; and, in addition, that these effects may have significant relationships to the behavior of the organism.

REFERENCES

Coleman, P. D., and Riesen, A. H. (1968). Environmental effects on cortical dendritic fields. I. Rearing in the dark. *J. Anat.* **102**, 363-374.

Eayrs, J. T. (1955). The cerebral cortex of normal and hypothyroid rats. *Acta Anat.* **25**, 160-183.

Harman, P. J., and Berry, C. M. (1956). Neuroanatomical distribution of action potentials evoked by photic stimuli in cat pre- and mid-brain. *J. Comp. Neurol.* **105**, 395-416.

Sholl, D. A. (1956). "The Organization of the Cerebral Cortex." Methuen, London.

GENERAL DISCUSSION

Dr. Scheibel: Some few years ago, we were studying the effects of light deprivation on the cortex of newborn animals with our colleague, Dr. Globus. After making a great many dendrite counts, domain measurements, and the like, we came to the conclusion that following light deprivation instituted directly after birth and maintained for 1 month or more, the variations in dendrite length, bifurcations, and domain size might vary on either side of the previously established mean values. In the case of the stellate cells, at least, it was the variability in size and extent which appeared most impressive. We concluded that normal visual input, especially in the immediately postnatal period might be absolutely necessary to produce neurons of standard dimensions. Perhaps, in a sense, the input of visual stimuli serves to stabilize the genetic tape which originally lays out, only in rather crude fashion, the approximate dimensions of the cell population, the length and arrangement of components, etc. If this hypothesis has validity, it would serve as a most interesting example of the interaction of hereditary and environmental factors in the maturational process.

Dr. Coleman: Dr. Globus and I have discussed some of these differences at great length. When we compared individual animals (a small number) what we saw was not inconsistent with the notion of increased variability in the dark-reared animals, or decreased variability in normal controls.

I do think though that there are clearly some differences in the specific kinds of results that you got (Globus and Scheibel, 1967) and that we got, and in the discussions that I have had with Dr. Globus about this, we cannot arrive at any clear conclusion except perhaps to attribute it to differences in methodology.

As I understand from speaking to Dr. Globus, the way the lengths were measured in your laboratories was to superimpose concentric circles on the cells, and the way we measured the lengths was to actually follow them with a map mileage measurer.

When we superimpose this concentric circle kind of arrangement on the cell, we, too, find that dark-reared and normal animals are certainly no different in the extent to which the dendrites go away from the cell body. The length differences that we report only show up when we actually follow the tortuous or semitortuous trail of the dendrite away from the cell body.

Dr. Scheibel: That is interesting. In that regard we accepted four or five macaques that had been born and reared in darkness for 2 years. Counting went on in the laboratory 6 days a week for about a year and a half, and a tremendous amount of data was accumulated.

We could see no clear-cut changes in any of the parameters, either by visual inspection of the data, or with the help of a computer. We were very disappointed, because we had hoped to see something obvious come out of the data.

Dr. Clemente: What types of changes were you expecting—changes in the dendritic field, or number of synapses?

Dr. Scheibel: Not synapses. We looked at spine densities, length of stellate cell dendrites, the number of branch points, domain size, etc.

Dr. Coleman: I would like to throw in some information that I think is very interesting. In examinations of the retina that were done in Dr. Riesen's laboratory, he showed a species difference, using light-reared and dark-reared primates and cats (Riesen, 1966).

Dr. Lindsley: Weren't those monkeys given 1 hr. of diffuse illumination a day to prevent retinal ganglion cell degeneration?

Dr. Scheibel: One was so treated. The others were raised in complete darkness.

Dr. Coleman: That may be an important difference (in addition to the species difference) since our animals were always in total darkness. Results from the Berkeley group (Rosenzweig *et al.*, 1968) suggest that even short exposures to altered environment may be sufficient to influence brain changes.

Dr. Lindsley: I found the contribution by the Scheibels very interesting, especially the way in which the spinal dendrites develop their separate orientations followed by their bundling or cabling together at a later stage. Perhaps I am reading too much into this, but it reminded me of some older observations made in the 1920's, I believe, by Hooker, Minkowski, Coghill, and others on fetal behavioral development as well as on early postnatal development.

There was always an argument as to whether the earliest behavior patterns originated from a kind of mass responsiveness which later became differentiated into more specific patterns, or whether reactivity began with discrete, specific muscular actions and then became more massive and synergistic and eventually more differentially controlled as voluntary control emerged from a predominant reflex background.

It would seem to me that this latter idea, at least postnatally, would be more in line with what you have described with respect to the maturational organization of spinal dendrites, which are initially separate and somewhat isolated from one another but gradually come together, from diverse sources, in bundles. Thus, one might expect to find more discrete types of responses when they are separated and more massive responses when they are bundled together very closely, possibly in ephaptic relationships at the start. As further maturation takes place, with more medullation locally and with higher level (voluntary) nervous system control centrally one might expect there would be a separation into discrete action forms again. Is that too bizarre an interpretation?

Dr. Scheibel: That is an interesting idea, and one that we had not considered. But it seems, as we think about it, that the matrix of somata and dendrites which exists in the late prenatal phase should be sufficient substrate for the type of undifferentiated mass action effects which you describe. The bundling appears to be a very special structural stratagem which develops to fill a highly specific requirement of the maturing nervous system, the production of reciprocal motor outputs across paired muscle systems.

Dr. Lindsley: That was beautifully demonstrated by the EMG's.

Dr. Purpura: It has been well known in studies of dorsal and ventral root and cord potentials (Barron and Matthews, 1938; and more recently, Nelson, 1966; Decima and Goldberg, 1970) that electrotonic interaction between elements of the spinal cord can occur to varying degrees. It would be in error, however, to emphasize such factors of electrotonic or ephaptic interaction in the organization of spinal reflexes or their combination into coordinated movements during development. Perhaps a more important developmental point might be the way in which incoming afferents dip into the developing dendritic fields and are consequently organized in relation to these.

There are other factors, however, which seem to be more important and which occur well in advance of the morphological changes in dendritic organization in the kitten spinal cord. For one thing, it has been shown that EPSP's and IPSP's are relatively well developed in spinal motoneurons of newborn or young kittens, as indicated in the work of Naka (1964) and Wilson (1962). Studies of Eccles *et al.*, (1963) are also to the point here. The existence of well-established reflex activities in the young kitten would appear to be reflected in the capacity for newborn kittens to exhibit well-coordinated rhythmical movements of the extremities, particularly the forelegs. We have all observed newborn kittens engaged in such rhythmical and reciprocal activities while "pumping" for milk during suckling. Obviously, there is some mechanism built into the chassis of the spinal cord "half-centers" at birth which allows for these complex rhythmical activities to be expressed in the neonatal period. The entire behavior may be released in the food-seeking state. Whatever the elaboration of dendritic fields adds to these activities, it is clear that we shall not find this by examining EPSP's or IPSP's in spinal motoneurons, since these are already well developed in the young kitten.

In regard to Dr. Hoffer's work, I would like to ask whether he and his associates have been doing quantitative electron microscopic studies of developing synapses in the cerebellar cortex.

Dr. Hoffer: Dr. Bloom and Dr. Aghajanian have studied the cerebral cortex in hypothyroid animals, but the problem is that the diversity of synapses makes it difficult to delimit a specific synaptic deficit. We hope to repeat this study in the hypothyroid cerebellar cortex. Since the different classes of synapses can be readily identified in this brain area, specific developmental deficiencies may be more apparent.

Dr. Purpura: It would be possible to confine your observations to the upper 300 μ of cortex by skimming off the superficial regions in order to have a pure preparation of neuropil.

Dr. Clemente: Dr. Scheibel, were there segmental differences between cervical and lumbar motor cord zones?

Dr. Scheibel: We obviously have to compare the degree of development between cervical and lumbosacral cord. From the behavioral point of view at least, there is no question that the newborn kitten can produce effective pumping motions with his forelegs at a time when he can barely drag his hindlegs after him. So it would not be too surprising if the degree of maturity of lumbosacral neuronal structure was well behind that of the cervical region. The EMG seems a useful tool to us, since it gives some measure of the level of motor performance which may be quite a different matter than the apparent degree of maturity of structural and neurochemical substrate and the nature of the neuroelectrical phenomena.

Dr. Prescott: I would like to make a comment on Dr. Coleman's statistical analysis. Since you have utilized only one performance measure, it appears that you have unduly limited your ability to relate behavior changes to brain changes.

Dr. Coleman: Yes.

Dr. Prescott: If you had utilized multiple criterion measures, as well as multiple predictors, your possibilities of success would be enhanced, particularly if your criterion variables were related to the sensory system that has been deprived.

I am particularly intrigued by Dr. Hoffer's comment that the synaptic contacts begin to develop at day 5 and terminate at 10 weeks in the rat. In what part of the cerebellar cortex did you find this, since Altman (1969) has reported differential rates of maturation, and I wonder if a different story exists.

Dr. Hoffer: I think this is an important point. We work in lobules 6 and 7, which is the sagittal vermis just behind the primary fissure. By a happy quirk of fate, these are the parts that seem to mature the latest.

The anterior lobe and the pyramis mature considerably earlier; indeed, in the anterior lobe, you can get synapse formation by days 1 and 2.

Dr. Coleman: I would like to comment on this problem. I agree entirely with Dr. Prescott's comment on behavioral measures, and I think we have gotten ourselves into something of a mess; doing this kind of correlation study was not the primary purpose of our study. It is something that came out and looked interesting, but the kind of mess that we have gotten ourselves into is that the animals showing the more complex dendritic fields are the animals that are called the maze-dull animals—the dumb animals. And this, of course, is entirely against what one might hope. When you look at the behavior of these two strains in more detail (Searle, 1949), you find that the so-called maze-dull animals are very much superior behaviorally to the so-called maze-bright animals on many other kinds of tasks. And in part, because we do not have multiple behavioral measures, we really cannot be sure of what is correlating with what.

But I only wanted to make the point that doing this kind of correlational study of individual measures, be they anatomical or chemical or whatever, with individual behavior scores, is something that is very fruitful, and I would like to see it followed up, not only by people doing anatomical work, but all kinds of measures.

Dr. Prescott: Your observation that so-called maze-dull animals are superior on some behavioral tasks needs emphasis, since some maze-dull animal strains have been shown to be more emotionally reactive strains, and therefore stressful tasks could precipitate emotional reactions that would interfere with performance. A different type of test that did not elicit emotional reactivity could give different results.

Dr. Roberts: On that very same point, the original maze-bright animals were found to have higher cholinesterase activity than maze-dull ones. Then, when T. H. Roderick (1960) selected for cholinesterase activity he got the opposite association with maze performance.

Perhaps what Dr. Scheibel said is the most exciting thing, that the genetic potential is stabilized by the input that seems pertinent for the organism.

Is there any real reason for an assumption that a particular area of hippocampus should be related to something that is occurring in the learning of a task by an animal as opposed to other areas of the hippocampus?

Dr. Coleman: That, of course, opens another can of worms. There are many studies dealing with the relation between hippocampus and learning (Kaada *et al.*, 1961; Green, 1964; Douglas, 1967), as well as other behaviors, but precisely what they do show is problematical.

But certainly you have raised another very important point when you refer to the Roderick kind of study. I think it would behoove us to breed animals not on the basis of behavior but on the basis of dendritic measures, and then look at the behavior.

Dr. Chase: I would like to address a few remarks to Dr. Scheibel regarding the lack of reciprocal innervation of flexors and extensors in neonatal kittens.

In the young kitten, up to 2 weeks of age, stimulation of cutaneous exteroceptors from almost any area of the skin gives rise to bilateral flexor responses (Vlach, 1968; Ekholm, 1967). Only by 2 weeks of age are there inhibitory and excitatory cutaneous areas whose excitation is followed by responses which show local sign and reciprocal effects, such as crossed extension. After 2 weeks, there is a shift to a pattern of motoneuron discharge that is primarily driven by afferents of muscular rather than cutaneous origin.

The second point is that if a kitten is made decerebrate by the intercollicular method, flexor, rather than extensor rigidity results, and it has been shown that this is most likely due to the fact that γ motoneurons are not functional until kittens are approximately 2 weeks of age (Weed, 1917; Pollock and Davis, 1931; Skoglund, 1960).

Is it likely that your observations might reflect the development of the γ motoneurons and the subsequent bias of segmental systems toward more reciprocal effects, which are dependent upon the activity of muscle spindles and the γ motoneuron system?

Dr. Scheibel: Dr. Chase's suggestion is an interesting one. We have no definite answer. In presenting our data, we tried to make it clear that we were demonstrating a temporal relationship between development of a structural complex and a motor phenomenon. A cause-and-effect relationship certainly could not be proved at this point. Also, for lack of evidence, we omitted consideration of the possible effects of the developing γ system and of the entire range of suprasegmental controls which develop during the first few weeks of life. All of these systems are quite probably involved in the maturation of reciprocal motor activity between agonist-antagonist pairs.

Dr. Chase: Is it possible to examine differences between the dendritic bundling of large α motoneurons and γ motoneurons?

Dr. Scheibel: It is impossible to identify a small α from a large γ. They don't have little letters on them. And the Golgi is simply a visual tool. It has no physiological mark that we have been able to identify.

Some people claim that the γ's have no return collaterals, while the α do, and that you can differentiate on this basis. This is fine, except for the fact that 40-50% of the α's do not have recurrent collaterals either. So we still can't differentiate between them.

Dr. Metcalf: I want to comment on Dr. Coleman's presentation. I think what he did was very important and should be viewed as a model, not as an indication of relationship between maze-running and brain size, or what have you, but a model for future work that can be planned along a variety of directions.

McClearn (1970, personal communication), for instance, has bred rats and mice genetically true for a variety of these behaviors: maze-running, rope-climbing, free-field-running, changes in sleep-wake cycles, etc.

Because specific behaviors may therefore be partly genetically determined and also relate to functions in specific brain regions (as an expression of the genetic code), I wonder why you elected to study the hippocampus.

Dr. Coleman: As I mentioned before, I picked the hippocampus because there are studies showing relations between hippocampus lesions and maze-running. The studies are in a confused state, so we weren't really on firm ground. But if one is going to look, this is one place to look. We also looked at sensorimotor cortex, and we found the same sorts of differences there.

Dr. Gordon: My comment is directed toward what Dr. Coleman said. If I understand him, he said that the kittens that had been reared in the dark had longer dendrites but less branching. Is that right?

Dr. Coleman: Yes.

Dr. Gordon: And this is always talked about in terms of deprivation of light. Should we not consider that prematurely born babies are deprived of darkness? They should be floating around in dark, warm, relatively quiet waters for 4-8 more weeks and then emerge from the uterus, and because we are very much concerned about their respirations, we put them in incubators with bright lights and clicking monitors. Now, in order to lower serum bilirubin, we are exposing them to special phototherapy which may in itself carry dangers. We stopped swaddling them, which is the way we used to try to maintain body temperatures, when we got good incubators. So they are kicking around without the tactile support of clothing and blankets.

And the question is raised that these factors may not matter for babies born at 36 weeks gestation, but may matter for babies born after only 32 weeks gestation.

I am really asking whether the dendrites will get long enough before they start branching.

Dr. Coleman: I don't know. The kind of thing you are talking about sounds more like what Dr. Rose (see Chapter II) has been working on with stimulation, i.e., giving animals excess stimulation, light for 24 hr a day.

Dr. Himwich: I want to go back to what Dr. Scheibel said about stabilizing the genetic potential. This might explain the fact that we always find greater variability in our neurochemical data when we have interfered with the normal environment of the young animal, and we have been greatly at a loss to know why this was. We could not ascribe it to technical problems, but this might be the same thing that you were describing with the dendrites.

Dr. Weitzman: I would like to ask what role Dr. Purpura feels inhibition plays in the earliest responses obtained. I gather the earliest responses obtained are a large surface-negative response. Does he feel that this is swamping out the inhibitory response? Or does he feel that this is in some way a reflection of a combined inhibitory-excitatory response?

Dr. Purpura: Dr. Weitzman's question really relates to the issue of the nature of evoked potentials in general and the surface-negative primary response of the immature brain in particular. It is important to stress that all responses recorded from the cortical surface are composites of EPSP's and IPSP's and that when one notes a unit discharge limited to a particular phase of the evoked potential one rarely considers the possibility that prior to or after the discharge there may be a significant inhibitory synaptic action generated in the neuron under examination. This is what intracellular recording can reveal.

It must be recalled that the evoked potential is already an *averaged response* even before averaging many evoked potentials together. Hence, changes in amplitude of the evoked potentials reflect alterations in the algebraic summation of excitatory and inhibitory synaptic activities which contribute to the evoked potential. An increase in the amplitude of surface-negative waves could reflect an increase in EPSP's or a decrease in IPSP's locally generated, or the reverse of these in the cortical depths. In all instances, however, it is necessary to bear in mind the extent to which inhibition contributes to these gross surface-recorded activities. It is, in fact, remarkable how much inhibition contributes to the responses of other varieties of cells in the thalamus, caudate, or cortex. It is the most important of physiological processes, for without inhibition there can be nothing but chaotic operation in purely excitatory neuronal operations. It is to Ramón y Cajal's credit that he was able to sketch in broad outlines the basic wiring diagram of the neuraxis without regard to the process of inhibition.

Perhaps Dr. Roberts is anxious to have an answer to the meaning of evoked potential changes in terms of more or less inhibition or more or less excitation, but this cannot be done without knowledge of the synaptic transactions occurring during the evoked potential.

Dr. Roberts: I believe we have to think not only of inhibition per se, but also of inhibition of inhibition, or disinhibition.

I have been wondering for a long time why the projections of the reticular activating system, which are excitatory, release only inhibitory transmitters, or substances which are inhibitory when applied to neurons. The answer could be that these systems really are inhibiting inhibitory interneurons and, therefore, in effect are excitatory or "activating."

How would one interpret the electrical activity of inhibition carried out by the horizontal interneurons in the fourth cortical layer, and disinhibition of those by another set of inhibitory interneurons?

Dr. Purpura: Inhibition of inhibition is precisely the major synaptic mechanism operating in thalamic neuronal organizations during the transition from synchronized to desynchronized thalamocortical activity (Purpura, 1969). Thus, reticulocortical arousal essentially requires excitation of some pathways that activate inhibitory elements that in turn inhibit synchronizing IPSP's. That is the story of the reticular system. It acts differently upon different neuronal subsystems.

Dr. Lindsley: Dr. Purpura, I should like to reiterate the question I raised with you earlier that is, whether there are two kinds of inhibition. If I understand what you have said, there is initially in the kitten cortex only a manifestation of inhibition, and the excitatory drive does not come into play until later. This was shown in some work that Guenter Rose and I published (Rose and Lindsley, 1965, 1968) where initially a light flash caused only a long-latency negative wave, but by 10-15 days of age a short-latency positive-negative wave characteristic of the primary evoked response came in which was identified with excitatory influences over the specific or classical visual pathway via geniculostriate projections.

Do you feel that the development of the excitatory drive breaks up some kind of basic inhibition, which was already holding things in check, and creates IPSP's on top of what exists there? We know, of course, that there are negative DC shifts manifest over much of the cortex when an arousal stimulus leads to some expectancy.

I believe we must keep our thinking open to the possibility that in the newborn baby there may be mainly a pervasive inhibitory mechanism which has not been subjected to the excitatory drive that you say comes in later. This may account for the tendency of young animals to be under a kind of inhibitory mechanism which causes sleep so much of the time at that stage in the maturation of their brain and nervous system. We ought to use every opportunity to relate electrophysiological and other factors to sleep as a behavioral event.

Dr. Hoffer: I would like to second Dr. Lindsley's point. It has been emphasized that neonatal cells fire slowly. I think there is a danger of teleologically assuming that it is a baby cell so it sleeps a lot and is not very active. But in the cerebellum you can take the neonatal Purkinje cells, which fire slowly, and put on a depolarizing agent and increase the firing up to tenfold. Obviously, in the neonate, without any kind of synaptic input, Purkinje cells fire more slowly than they are capable of firing. One wonders about an inhibitory mechanism, intrinsic, perhaps biochemical, within the cell itself which is keeping the firing rate down. Such a mechanism may act apart from transsynaptic inhibition.

Dr. Purpura: In order to avoid any further misunderstanding of my position, I believe it is necessary to make a few concluding remarks. To begin with, it has been emphasized repeatedly that excitation and by inference excitatory synapses are *not* absent in the immature brain. But compared to inhibitory processes, excitatory synaptic drives are relatively weak. This brings us to one of the central issues on cortical maturation, i.e., the question of the status of interneurons in cortex. It is obvious that inhibitory neurons must be well-developed for them to exert the kind of prolonged IPSP's we have observed in intracellular recordings from neocortex and hippocampus in neonatal kittens. On the other hand, while excitatory interneurons are present in immature cortex their continuing development in the postnatal period must represent an important maturational event. Hence, interneuronal development is of crucial significance in the elaboration of cortical neuronal interconnectivity. We have probably overemphasized the development of pyramidal neurons at the expense of these interneurons which are more difficult to characterize. During the postnatal period, excitatory synaptic activities increase out of proportion to the inhibition, which is already prominent in the newborn animal. These are the observations that derive from intracellular studies, and these are the observations that must be incorporated into any notion of the maturation of behavior in general or sleep-wakefulness activity in particular.

REFERENCES

Altman, J. (1969). Autoradiographic and histological studies of postnatal neurogenesis. III. Dating the time of production and onset of differentiation of cerebellar microneurons in rats. *J. Comp. Neurol.* **136**, 269-294.

Barron, D. H., and Matthews, B. H. C. (1938). The interpretation of potential changes in the spinal cord. *J. Physiol.* **92**, 276-321.

Decima, E. E., and Goldberg, L. J. (1970). Centrifugal dorsal root discharges induced by motoneurone activation. *J. Physiol. (London)* **207**, 103-118.

Douglas, R. J. (1967). The hippocampus and behavior. *Psychol. Bull.* **67**, 416-442.

Eccles, R. M., Sheahy, C. N., and Willis, W. D. (1963). Patterns of innervation of kitten motoneurons. *J. Physiol. (London)* **165**, 392-402.

Ekholm, J. (1967). Postnatal development of excitatory and inhibitory skin areas for hindlimb muscles in kittens. *Acta Soc. Med. Upsal.* **72**, 20-24.

Globus, A., and Scheibel, A. B. (1967). The effect of visual deprivation on cortical neurons: a Golgi study. *Exp. Neurol.* **19**, 331-345.

Green, J. D. (1964). The hippocampus. *Physiol Rev.* **44**, 561-608.

Kaada, B. R., Rasmussen, E. W., and Kveim, O. (1961). Effects of hippocampal lesions on maze learning and retention in rats. *Exp. Neurol.* **3**, 333-355.

McClearn, G. (1970). Personal communication.

Naka, K. I. (1964). Electrophysiology of the fetal spinal cord. *J. Gen. Physiol.* **47**, 1003-1038.

Nelson, P. G. (1966). Interaction between spinal motoneurons of the cat. *J. Neurophysiol.* **29**, 275-287.

Pollock, L. J, and Davis, L. (1931). Studies in decerebration. VI. The effect of deafferentation upon decerebrate rigidity. *Amer. J. Physiol.* **98**, 47-49.

Purpura, D. P. (1969). Interneuronal mechanisms in thalamically induced synchronizing and desynchronizing activities. *In* "The Interneuron" (M. A. B. Brazier, ed.), pp. 467-496. U. C. L. A. Forum in Medical Sciences, Los Angeles, California.

Riesen, A. H. (1966). Sensory deprivation. *Progr. Physiol. Psychol.* **1**, 117-147.

Roderick, T. H. (1960). Selection for cholinesterase activity in the cerebral cortex of the rat. *Genetics* **45**, 1123-1140.

Rose, G. H., and Lindsley, D. B. (1965). Visually evoked electrocortical responses in kittens: Development of specific and nonspecific systems. *Science* **148**, 1244-1246.

Rose, G. H., and Lindsley, D. B. (1968). Development of visually evoked potentials in kittens: specific and nonspecific responses. *J. Neurophysiol.* **31**, 607-623.

Rosenzweig, M. R., Love, W., and Bennett, E. L. (1968). Effects of a few hours a day of enriched experience on brain chemistry and brain weights. *Physiol. Behav.* **3**, 819-825.

Searle, L. V. (1949). The organization of hereditary maze-brightness and maze-dullness. *Genet. Psychol. Monogr.* **39**, 279-325.

Skogland, S. (1960). On the postnatal development of postural mechanisms as revealed by electromyography and myography in decerebrate kittens. *Acta Physiol. Scand.* **49**, 299-317.

Vlach, V. (1968). Some exteroceptive skin reflexes in the limbs and trunk in newborns. *In* "Studies in Infancy, Clinic in Developmental Medicine" Number 27 (M. C. Bax and R. C. MacKeith, eds.), pp. 41-54. Heinemann, London.

Weed, L. H. (1917). The reactions of kittens after decerebration. *Amer. J. Physiol.* **43**, 131-157.

Wilson, V. J. (1962). Reflex transmission in the kitten. *J. Neurophysiol.* **25**, 263-276.

NEUROCHEMICAL FACTORS
IN THE MATURATION OF SLEEP BEHAVIOR

4

Coordination between Excitation and Inhibition: Development of the GABA System

Eugene Roberts

INTRODUCTION

All normal or adaptive activity is a result of coordination of excitation and inhibition in the nervous system within and between neuronal subsystems in a particular organism. The underlying principle of information-processing is a coordinated interplay of excitatory and inhibitory influences. Most communication that takes place between receptor and neuron, neuron and neuron, and neuron and effector probably occurs via the presynaptic liberation of substances that have either excitatory or inhibitory influences on postsynaptic membranes (see Roberts and Matthysse, 1970, for review and some pertinent general references). Several known naturally occurring substances have been implicated as potential excitatory or inhibitory transmitters. Acetylcholine and glutamic and aspartic acids may be excitatory transmitters. γ-Aminobutyric acid (GABA), glycine, the catecholamines, histamine, and serotonin may be inhibitory transmitters. Knowledge of the properties and distributions of the enzymes which form some of these substances and degrade them and of the neural circuits in which they exist is only now becoming available. Mechanisms of presynaptic release of transmitters and their modes of action on postsynaptic membranes are being studied. The transport mechanisms which have been identified in neuronal membranes and which, in most instances, may be the chief mechanisms for removal of the active substances from synapses also are only now becoming known.

Biochemical studies of development are difficult because there is superimposition of developmental variables onto experimental situations already interpretable with difficulty. Some of the developmental processes which take place during the early period are growth and arborization of dendritic neuronal processes; myelination of axons; growth and branching of the capillary bed; differentiation and proliferation of glial elements; and the differentiation, movement, and multiplication of the short-axoned granule cells or microneurons. In addition, the types and extent of sensory input during active postnatal cerebral growth might selectively enhance neural pathways that are used extensively; and therefore such pathways might have a greater probability of becoming important information-processing units than those which are used less or not at all. Thus, in a developing nervous system there is a mutual interplay of developmental and stimulatory variables. Minimally, all of the above factors must be kept in mind when one is studying a developing nervous system. Certainly, all of the cellular structures, as well as the extracellular compartment, must be considered when an assessment is being made of the existence of different metabolic "pools" and their changes during development and in different normal and abnormal functional states. To complicate matters even more, there are obvious differentiations even within a single given neuron. The morphology, chemistry, and function of the dendrites, soma, axon, and synaptosome differ from each other in the adult and change in different ways at varying rates during development.

In developmental studies, even more than in studies of fully developed structure, one must face the problem of obtaining chemical information that is *meaningful with regard to the information-processing in a particular structure,* and not just related to its maintenance metabolism. Most questions still remain to be answered about the transmitter biochemistry of the nervous system. The inescapable conclusion from the work done to date is that specific chemical, enzymic, or immunocytochemical probes will have to be developed for the localization of the transmitters and the enzymes of their metabolism at an ultrastructural level in functionally meaningful loci before completely conclusive data can be obtained with regard to their exact relationships. Until the latter is achieved, an experimenter who would study *only* the changes in some biochemical parameter of a whole brain or a dissected part of it as a function of development in a particular species often would be wasting his time, since the specificity of the information obtained would be of a low order and there would be little probability of eventual detailed correlation with morphological and physiological parameters. The question might be asked about what might be expected to be learned from studies during development of a variety of biochemical variables in brain homogenates, slices, or subcellular particulates from grossly dissected areas of brain. It appears to me that by and large such work will have to be redone when the neuronal systems studied become better known from physiological and morphological points of view.

It is extremely interesting that good coordination between excitation and inhibition generally is not present in early mammalian infancy. Certainly, in the human, capacity for coordinated movement and activity develops gradually until a maximal degree of coordination is attained somewhere between the ages of 18 and 23. It is at this age that one sees the best athletes, jet pilots, football players, etc., and people have the greatest capacity for mental productivity. As aging proceeds, the extent of coordination gradually decreases. I believe that the latter condition occurs largely because of the loss of small inhibitory interneurons that are found within the various neural systems and subsystems in the brain and spinal cord. It appears likely that a decreased effectiveness of circulation, such as one finds in arteriosclerosis, would be more damaging to the small interneurons than to the larger pyramidal neurons, which traverse a greater region in the brain. The shutting-off of a small capillary near a small neuron would be fatal to it, whereas the larger neurons would have a number of capillaries in their vicinity and the loss of one may have less far-reaching consequences.

There are data, ranging from suggestive to convincing, that implicate several known naturally occurring amino acids as potential excitatory or inhibitory transmitters. GABA and glycine may be inhibitory transmitters and glutamic and aspartic acids may be excitatory transmitters. The physiological and pharmacological properties of these substances have been studied in a variety of biological systems. Knowledge of the properties and distributions of the enzymes which form and degrade some of these and of the neural circuits in which they exist is becoming available. The transport mechanisms which have been identified in neuronal membranes and which, in most instances, may be the chief mechanisms for removal of the active substances from synapses also are becoming known.

The ultimate goals in the study of transmitters are to be able to identify the neurons that may employ the substances as transmitters, to localize at an ultrastructural level those synaptic junctions at which these substances are released and act, to elucidate the modes of action of the transmitters on neural membranes at a molecular level, and to define the roles of such neurons in the neural systems of functioning organisms.

We will consider here data about GABA as a potential transmitter which may be pertinent to the attainment of these goals. The reader may consult a number of recent reviews for more thorough coverage of various aspects of the literature

(Roberts and Eidelberg, 1960; Roberts and Kuriyama, 1968; Roberts and Matthysse, 1970; Iversen and Kravitz, 1968; Curtis and Johnston, 1970; Kravitz, 1967).

An outline of the chief known reactions of GABA is shown in Fig. 1, and those of major concern to the present discussion are emphasized. GABA is formed in the central nervous system (CNS) of vertebrate organisms to a large extent, if not entirely, from L-glutamic acid. The reaction is catalyzed by an L-glutamic acid decarboxylase (GAD), an enzyme found in mammalian organisms only in the CNS, largely in gray matter. This enzyme is inhibited by anions and carbonyl-trapping agents.* The reversible transamination of GABA with α-ketoglutarate is catalyzed by an aminotransferase, GABA-T, which in the CNS is found chiefly in the gray matter, but also is found in other tissues. Both GAD and GABA-T are B_6 enzymes requiring pyridoxal phosphate as coenzyme. The products of the transaminase reaction are succinic semialdehyde and glutamic acid. If a ready metabolic source of succinic semialdehyde were available, GABA could be formed by the reversal of the reaction. To date, however, no convincing evidence has been adduced for the formation of significant amounts of GABA by reactions other than the decarboxylation of L-glutamic acid. It has been shown that γ-hydroxybutyric acid can be formed enzymically by reduction of succinic semialdehyde. It also has been shown that rat brain *in vivo* is capable of converting intracisternally administered ^{3}H-GABA to γ-hydroxybutyrate to a small extent. Whether or not γ-hydroxybutyrate occurs in significant amounts in nervous tissue, however, is still a matter of controversy. Brain also contains a dehydrogenase which catalyzes the oxidation of succinic semialdehyde to succinic acid, which in turn can be oxidized via the reactions of the tricarboxylic acid cycle. Consistent with these relationships, glutamic acid, GABA, and succinic semialdehyde can be oxidized by various brain preparations and can support oxidative phosphorylation. Therefore, in both vertebrate and invertebrate nervous systems, as a whole, there can exist a metabolic "shunt" around the α-ketoglutarate oxidase system of the tricarboxylic acid cycle, the operation of which depends on the unique occurrence of GAD and GABA, a formulation consistent with all *in vitro* and *in vivo* studies performed to date. The occurrence and metabolism of homocarnosine, guanidinobutyric acid, and other possible metabolites of GABA is reviewed elsewhere (Baxter, 1970). The most recent assessment of the quantitative significance of the "GABA shunt" pathway in guinea pig cortical slices *in vitro* showed the GABA flux to be about 8% of the total tricarboxylic acid flux (Balázs *et al.*, 1970). It is not clear what this kind of calculation might mean in

---

*The α-decarboxylation of L-glutamic acid now has been shown to occur in kidney and several other nonneuronal tissues, including glial cells and cerebral blood vessels (Haber *et al.*, 1970a, b; Kuriyama *et al.*, 1970). The enzyme catalyzing the latter process requires high concentrations of anions for maximal activity and is activated by carbonyl-trapping agents.

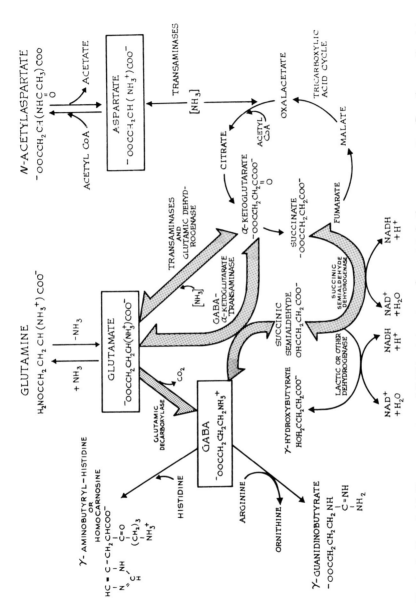

Fig. 1. Outline of chief known reactions of GABA, glutamate, and aspartate in the nervous system. Reactions pertinent to GABA metabolism are emphasized by large arrows.

terms of information-processing in the nervous system, since the components of the GABA system are not homogeneously distributed among all of the diverse cellular structures in the CNS or probably even among dendrites, somata, axons, and synaptosomes of individual neurons. It is doubtful that one can talk meaningfully about overall GABA metabolism.

Virtually all the data in the literature are consistent with the interpretation that the steady state concentrations of GABA in various brain areas normally are governed by the GAD activity and not by the GABA-T (Roberts and Eidelberg, 1960; Roberts and Kuriyama, 1968; Baxter, 1970). Pharmacological studies brought forth the first evidence that the above first two enzymes involved in the "GABA shunt" are not present in the same location in the vertebrate CNS (Roberts and Kuriyama, 1968). It was shown upon administration to animals of hydroxylamine or aminooxyacetic acid, substances which are potent inhibitors of both GAD and GABA-T *in vitro*, that only the GABA-T was inhibited, and that there were marked elevations of GABA content in the brains of the treated animals. One of the simplest possibilities was that the two enzymes are present in different cell types or in different intracellular sites in the same cells and that the inhibitors penetrate to the regions containing the transaminase but not to those in which the decarboxylase is located. This was consistent with the findings from all cell fractionation studies. Study of the distribution of the two chief enzymes of GABA metabolism indicated that both GAD and GABA-T are associated with particulate fractions. Work with subtle cell fractionation procedures and with electron microscopic monitoring has shown the GAD to be particularly rich in presynaptic nerve ending fractions, while the GABA-T is found largely in the free mitochondria. Since the free mitochondria, probably a mixture from neuronal perikarya and dendrites and from glial and endothelial cells, are relatively much richer in GABA-T than those prepared from isolated presynaptic nerve endings, it is reasonable to propose that the metabolism of GABA takes place chiefly at postsynaptic intracellular neuronal sites and at extraneuronal intracellular sites. In the case of GAD, only approximately 40% of the total enzyme activity in brain homogenates has been recovered in fractions containing the presynaptic endings. These findings strongly suggest the possibility that GAD also is present at other neuronal sites, as well as in presynaptic endings.

From data in the literature we may derive the tentative picture that, at least in some inhibitory nerves, both GAD and GABA are present and are distributed throughout the neuron, the GAD being somewhat more highly concentrated in the presynaptic endings than elsewhere. The GABA-T is contained in mitochondria of all neuronal regions, but it seems to be richer in the mitochondria of those neuronal sites onto which GABA might be liberated. Such regions would be expected to exist in perikarya and dendrites that receive inhibitory inputs and possibly in the glial and endothelial cells that are in the vicinity of inhibitory synapses.

It is believed that there is a presynaptic release of GABA on the stimulation of some inhibitory neurons. Stimulation of axons of several nerves inhibiting different lobster muscles was shown to result in the release of GABA in amounts related to the extent of stimulation, while stimulation of the excitatory nerve did not produce GABA release (Otsuka *et al.*, 1966). Data showing the liberation of GABA on stimulation of specific inhibitory neurons in the vertebrate nervous system are extremely difficult to obtain. More GABA and less glutamic acid were liberated from the perforated pial surface of the cortex of cats during sleep than in the aroused state (Jasper *et al.*, 1965). GABA also was shown to be specifically released from the surface of the posterior lateral gyri of cats during cortical inhibition produced either by stimulation of the ipsilateral geniculate or by direct stimulation of the cortex (Mitchell and Srinivasan, 1969). In cats pretreated with aminooxyacetic acid to block GABA metabolism, the rate of GABA release in a perfusate of the fourth ventricle was increased threefold over the control level during stimulation of the cerebellar cortex (Obata and Takeda, 1969). The GABA may be released in regions facing the fourth ventricle, where Purkinje cells synapse on neurons of cerebellar subcortical nuclei.

Considerable physiological evidence is available that suggests that GABA may be the inhibitory transmitter liberated on stimulation of the Purkinje cells. Depolarization of rat brain cortical slices preloaded with ^{3}H-GABA in the presence of aminooxyacetic acid (by high potassium concentrations or electrical stimulation) led to an enhanced release of GABA, which, in the case of the high potassium, was dependent on the calcium ions in the medium (Srinivasan *et al.*, 1969).

The ionic basis of the inhibitory effect of GABA on the postsynaptic regions of vertebrate and invertebrate neurons (Roberts and Eidelberg, 1960; Roberts and Kuriyama, 1968) appears to be an increase in the membrane conductance to Cl^- ions with the resultant "clamping" of the membrane potential near the resting level.

The first step in any action of a substance upon cellular structures must be through some physical or chemical association of the substance with those structures. The cessation of action of such a substance could be brought about by the removal of the substance from the sensitive sites by destruction, by transport, or by diffusion. In the case of GABA, it appears that uptake serves to terminate its physiological action by rapidly removing it from its sites of action in synaptic clefts. A reasonable picture of what happens to free extraneuronal GABA that is liberated into the extracellular region of the synapse is as follows (see Roberts and Kuriyama, 1968, for discussion and references): The membranes (presynaptic and postsynaptic and possibly glial) contain highly mobile binding sites for GABA which have an absolute Na^+ requirement for their activity and need a high Na^+ concentration (0.1 M) for maximal activation. Thus, GABA binds to membranes to a greater extent in a high Na^+ environment than in a low Na^+ concentration. The GABA bound on the outer surface of the membranes equilibrates rapidly with the GABA in solution in the extracellular medium. The GABA bound on the inside of the membranes equilibrates rapidly with GABA in solution intracellularly. The binding sites are partially restricted to one or the other side of the membrane by a barrier. The frequency with which the binding sites traverse the barrier may be dependent upon various asymmetries on the two sides of the membranes (redox; degree of phosphorylation; Na^+, K^+, and Cl^- ion concentrations; levels of sugars, amino acids, nucleotides, etc.). Under metabolic conditions, because of the lower concentrations of Na^+ ions present intraneuronally than extraneuronally, GABA tends to dissociate from the carrier on the intraneuronal side and to become available for mitochondrial metabolism. Thus, the asymmetric concentration of Na^+ ions sets up the conditions for a rapid removal of GABA from the extraneuronal synaptic environment into the intraneuronal environment and a rapid metabolism of the GABA therein. The energy for operation of carrier-mediated transport systems for amino acids (and possibly many other metabolites) is furnished by the Na^+ ion gradient that animal cells usually maintain. There would not be a requirement for the linkage of metabolically generated adenosine triphosphate (ATP) to each transport carrier, but a utilization of ATP for the operation of the Na^+ pump which maintains the gradient that could presumably enable the many Na^+-requiring membrane carriers to carry out active transport.

Specific pharmacological antagonists of putative neurotransmitters are extremely useful tools in helping establish neurotransmitter roles. Until recently, of all the many substances tested for possible antagonism to the inhibitory action of GABA, picrotoxin was found to be active in more of the test systems than any other substance. In crustacean muscle picrotoxin blocks, specifically, the action of the natural inhibitory transmitter and, similarly, that of GABA (Robbins and Van der Kloot, 1958; Takeuchi and Takeuchi, 1969). Picrotoxin-GABA antagonism also has been shown in cells of the cuneate nucleus (Galindo, 1969) and in oculomotor neurons (Obata and Highstein, 1970) in the vertebrate CNS. In general, however, the degree of specificity of action of picrotoxin is not high enough to establish it as the antagonist of choice to be used in analyses of particular inhibitory pathways for which GABA could be the transmitter. Only recently, bicuculline, a phthalide-isoquinoline alkaloid, has been shown to be a relatively specific inhibitor of GABA action in neurons in several regions of the mammalian CNS and in the crayfish stretch receptor system (Curtis *et al.*, 1970; McLennan, 1970). Both picrotoxin and bicuculline are currently being employed in many studies.

CEREBELLUM

Since one of the goals in the study of any transmitter is to understand its possible role in the function of particular neuronal systems, let us examine what is known of the function of GABA in the cerebellum, a structure believed by some even to play a role in sleep. Extensive correlative neuroanatomical and neurophysiological analyses have been made of the cerebellum (Eccles *et al.*, 1967; Fields and Willis, 1970; Fox and Snider, 1967; Llinás, 1969). A schematic presentation of neuronal relationships in the mammalian cerebellar cortex is shown in Fig. 2. The overall function of the cerebellum probably is entirely inhibitory, the only output cells of the cerebellum, the Purkinje cells, inhibiting in Deiters' and intracerebellar nuclei monosynaptically (Fig. 2). The basket, stellate, and Golgi cells are believed to play inhibitory roles within the cerebellum. The basket cells make numerous powerful inhibitory synapses on the lower region of the somata of the Purkinje cells and on their basal processes or "preaxons." The superficial stellate cells form inhibitory synapses on the dendrites of Purkinje cells. The Golgi cells make inhibitory synapses on the dendrites of the granule cells. Afferent excitatory inputs reach the cerebellum via the climbing and mossy fibers, which excite the dendrites of the Purkinje and granule cells, respectively. The latter are believed to be the only cells lying entirely within the cerebellum which have an excitatory function.

From the foregoing, and because of its conveniently layered structure, it appeared that in the vertebrate nervous system the cerebellum is a favorable site for chemical investigation of the possible substance (or substances) which may mediate the activity of neurons with inhibitory functions. After hand dissection of frozen dried sections, GABA content and GAD activity were determined in the molecular, Purkinje, and granular cell layers of the gray matter and in the subjacent white matter of the rabbit cerebellum (Kuriyama *et al.*, 1966). Also, the GABA-transaminase-succinic semialdehyde route (GABA-T-S), the metabolic pathway by which GABA is converted to succinic acid, was visualized histochemically. Measurements of GABA content and the histochemical procedure also were performed on cerebellar tissue from animals that had been injected previously with aminooxyacetic acid, which, *in vivo*, blocks GABA-T but not GAD activity, and causes elevation of GABA levels.

The GAD activity and GABA content of the layer containing the Purkinje cells are higher than those found in whole cerebellum or in the other cerebellar cortical regions (Fig. 2). The high values could be attributable to the Purkinje cell bodies themselves, to the numerous presynaptic endings from the basket cells on the somata of the Purkinje cells, or to both. The granular layer is significantly lower in both GABA and GAD; and the extensive dendritic arborizations of the Purkinje cells are largely found in the molecular layer, and the axons of the Purkinje cells lie in the granular layer and below. It is likely that the GAD might be somewhat concentrated in the presynaptic endings from the basket cell axons, since cell fractionation studies have shown it to be an enzyme contained in the synaptosomes in the cerebellum as well as other neural structures. However, it is likely that GAD also is found throughout neurons that

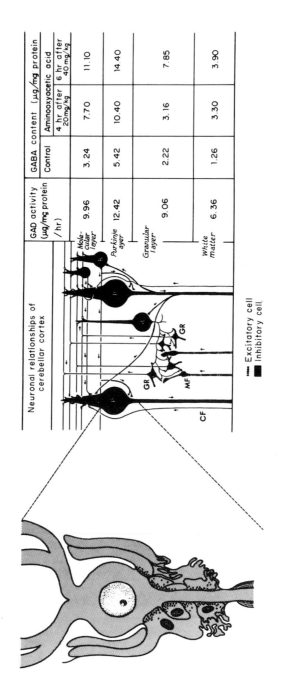

Neuronal relationships of cerebellar cortex	GAD activity (μg/mg protein /hr)	GABA content (μg/mg protein)			
		Control	Aminooxyacetic acid		
			4 hr after 20 mg/kg	6 hr after 40 mg/kg	
Molecular layer	9.96	3.24	7.70	11.10	
Purkinje layer	12.42	5.42	10.40	14.40	
Granular layer	9.06	2.22	3.16	7.85	
White matter	6.36	1.26	3.30	3.90	

Excitatory cell
Inhibitory cell

Fig. 2. Schematic presentation of neuronal relationships in the mammalian cerebellar cortex (from Eccles *et al.*, 1967) and some pertinent data on GAD activities and GABA content (from Kuriyama *et al.*, 1966). P, Purkinje cell; S, stellate cell; B, basket cell; GO, golgi cell; GR, granule cell; MF, mossy fiber; CF, climbing fiber.

contain this enzyme. A high level of the GABA-T-S, the GABA metabolizing system, was seen uniformly in the Purkinje cell cytoplasm. The nuclei of the cells and axons always were negative. A spatial separation of GAD and GABA-T activities is consistent with the findings that the latter enzyme is associated largely in free mitochondria in subcellular fractionation studies and that the mitochondria within nerve endings have lower GABA-T activity than those in a mixed mitochondrial population from neuronal perikarya and glial cells. The effects of the differential inhibition of the transaminase *in vivo* are shown in those instances in which aminooxyacetic acid was administered (Fig. 2). The inhibition was verified histochemically. The levels of GABA were raised in all areas studied, the extent of elevation being related to the control GAD level and being greatest in the Purkinje cell layer. Analyses of various types of individually dissected neurons from cat CNS showed the Purkinje cells to have the highest concentration of GABA (Obata *et al.*, 1970). However, since such dissected cells still have the large presynaptic basket cell terminals adhering to them, clear-cut assignment of the GABA and GAD on the basis of such determinations could not be made either to the Purkinje cells or to the basket cell terminals. However, recent experiments with intracellular recordings from Purkinje cells have shown that both the basket cell inhibition of these cells and their inhibition by iontophoretically applied GABA are blocked by bicuculline, a GABA antagonist (Curtis *et al.* 1970; Curtis and Felix, 1971). The evidence is strong, therefore, that basket cell inhibition of Purkinje cells is mediated by GABA. A reasonable interpretation of the above data, taken together with that from study of transport of GABA by subcellular particles, is that in the cerebellum GABA is formed and stored in the presynaptic endings of the basket cells and upon stimulation is released from them onto membranes of Purkinje cells. A part of the released GABA could be transported into the presynaptic endings, where most of it would be retained for subsequent release, or could be taken up by the Purkinje cell bodies, where it could be transported down the axons or metabolized by the GABA-T-S pathway. There also is the possibility of glial uptake and metabolism.

The granular layer had lower GAD and GABA levels than the other layers of the cerebellar gray matter and showed less elevation of GABA content in animals treated with aminooxyacetic acid (Fig. 2). The granule cells were completely negative for GABA-T-S, but the Golgi cells and the endings of the mossy fibers were strongly positive. There are numerous axosomatic synapses on the Golgi cell bodies, possibly inhibitory, at least some of which come from the Purkinje cells. The GAD-GABA system probably is located at the presynaptic endings of these sites, since the Purkinje cells probably are GABA neurons. The GABA-T-S activity in the Golgi cell bodies may serve the same function as postulated for the Purkinje cells. Likewise, the Golgi cells may liberate GABA at the mossy fiber-granule cell synapse, and the GABA-T-S system visualized at the postsynaptic sites would serve an intracellular degradative function. Golgi axon terminals probably have endings both on the dendrites of the granule cells and on the mossy fiber terminals.

GAD activity and GABA were found at the lowest levels in the cerebellar white matter (Fig. 2), while the GABA-T-S system was below the level of detection of the histochemical procedure. The principal constituents of this region are the efferent fibers of the Purkinje cells, the axons of the afferent climbing and mossy fibers, glial cells, and a small number of granule cells. Since the GABA system usually is not found in excitatory cells, it seems likely that in this region the GAD and GABA are present in the axons of the Purkinje cells, possibly in a state of transport from the cell body to the presynaptic endings of these cells on Deiters' neurons in the vestibular nucleus and the cells of the intracerebellar nuclei, where the Purkinje cells inhibit monosynaptically. GABA applied iontophoretically to neurons in Deiters' nucleus and in the surrounding reticular formation mimicked the effects of natural inhibition of these cells through the Purkinje cell input, producing a strong depressant effect involving an increase of membrane conductance and hyperpolarization of the cells. Both natural inhibition and GABA were found to act by producing an increase in the Cl^- conductance of the postsynaptic membranes in such cells (Obata *et al.*, 1967). The action of both natural inhibition and GABA on Deiters' neurons is blocked by bicuculline (Curtis *et al.* 1970a, 1970b). The above data make a very strong physiological case for GABA being the transmitter released by the Purkinje cells onto the postsynaptic membranes of recipient cells. In confirmation of this idea, GAD activity was found to be 2.5 times greater in the dorsal than in the ventral part of Deiters' nucleus; Purkinje cell axons terminate in the dorsal but not in the ventral part (Fonnum *et al.*, 1970). Destruction of the Purkinje cells in the anterior cerebellar vermis resulted in a loss of approximately two-thirds of the GAD activity in the dorsal region of Deiters' and no change in the ventral portion. Likewise, destruction of those Purkinje cells in the left cerebellar hemisphere that send their axons to the left nucleus interpositus resulted in an extent of loss of GAD similar to that above, while there was no decrease from the normal level in the right nucleus interpositus. Taken together, the anatomical and chemical observations suggest that there is a high concentration of GAD, and consequently GABA, within the Purkinje axon terminals. As would be expected from cells that receive a GABA input, cells in Deiters' and intracerebellar nuclei stain heavily for GABA-T-S activity (Kuriyama *et al.*, 1966).

GABA may be involved not only as an inhibitory transmitter within the cerebellum and as the substance mediating all signals that leave the cerebellum, but it also may take part in information-processing beyond the Purkinje cell synapses. Rabbit oculomotor neurons are inhibited by neurons found in the vestibular nuclear complex, and this inhibition is blocked by intravenously administered picrotoxin (Obata and Highstein, 1970). Picrotoxin administered electrophoretically onto oculomotor neurons blocks the inhibition from secondary vestibular neurons and also blocks the inhibition produced by the application of GABA (Obata and Highstein, 1970). Although glycine also inhibits the neurons tested, the inhibition by this amino acid is not affected by picrotoxin. On the other hand, strychnine blocks the action of glycine but not that of GABA on the oculomotor neurons. These latter observations suggest the possibility that inhibitory neurons utilizing GABA as a transmitter may play an important role in the changes in eye movements observed in different phases of sleep.

THE GABA SYSTEM IN THE CEREBELLUM
OF THE DEVELOPING CHICK

Because of its conveniently layered structure and the known progression of development of individual cell types within the cerebellum, it appeared that cerebellum of developing chick embryo might be a favorable site in which to begin to examine the development of the GABA system in correlative manner with the morphological development (Kuriyama *et al.*, 1968b). The time sequence of the development of components of the GABA system was correlated with development as observed at both light microscopic and electron microscopic levels. Study also was made of the changes of histochemically visualized GABA-T activity and of the subcellular distribution pattern of the GABA system with the age of the embryo.

Characteristic synaptic structures were noted in the chick cerebellum at 11 days of incubation, the degree of synaptogenesis at this early stage being small by comparison with that observed at subsequent stages of development. From the histological observations it was suggested that the synapses observed might be between Purkinje cell axons and the somata of cells of the intracerebellar nuclei and between Purkinje cell axon collaterals and the somata and dendrites of other Purkinje cells. Much further detailed work will be required to settle definitively the location of the electron microscopically observed synapses at this stage of development.

The chief enzymes of the GABA system, GAD and GABA-T, began to increase much later in development than did the weight and protein content of the cerebellum (Fig. 3). Likewise, the amount of material recovered in the synaptosome-rich fraction, P_2-B, also began to increase rapidly only at 17 days of incubation (Fig. 4). It appears that the development of the key components of the GABA system is temporally better correlated with the development of recognizable synaptic structures than with accretion of the total mass of the cerebellum. The fractionation data were consistent with the supposition that both GAD and GABA are present at least in some inhibitory nerves and are

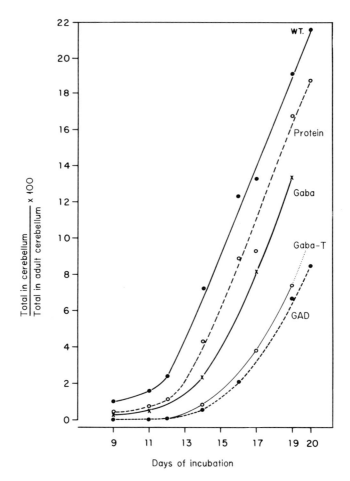

Fig. 3. Increases of weight, protein, and GABA contents, and GAD and GABA-T activities in cerebellum of chick embryo expressed as percentages of adult values (From Kuriyama *et al.*, 1968b.)

distributed throughout the neuron, the GAD being somewhat more highly concentrated in the presynaptic endings than elsewhere. The GABA-T was found to be particularly high in the free mitochondria, which probably come largely from those neuronal sites onto which GABA might be liberated, such as perikarya and dendrites that receive inhibitory inputs, and also from glial and endothelial cells in the vicinity of inhibitory synapses. GABA-T activity also was found to a small extent in the nerve endings, and this probably is attributable to the nerve ending mitochondria (see Roberts and Kuriyama, 1968, for discussion and pertinent references). A centrifugally derived preparation of presynaptic nerve endings is a mixture from inhibitory and excitatory nerves. In some brain

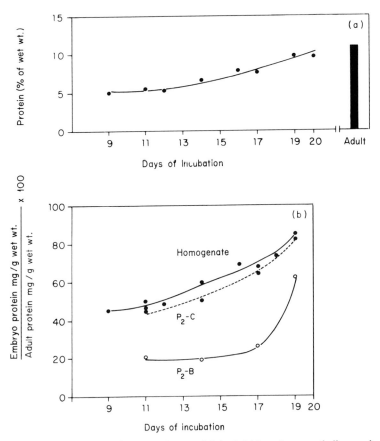

Fig. 4. (a) Protein content (percent of wet weight) of chick embryo cerebellum and adult chicken cerebellum. (b) Protein contents in whole homogenates of chick embryo cerebellum and of the P_2-B (synaptosome-rich) and P_2-C (mitochondrial) fraction as a function of age. (From Kuriyama *et al.*, 1968b).

areas, there are inhibitory presynaptic endings on nerve endings which, themselves, serve as excitatory presynaptic inputs on other postjunctional neuronal sites. It is, therefore, possible that the GABA-T found in the nerve ending fraction is located in those presynaptic endings that liberate excitatory transmitter, and which receive an input of GABA from inhibitory neurons; while the true inhibitory presynaptic endings may not contain any GABA-T at all. The results fit the *suggestion* that in the chick cerebellum GABA largely is formed at presynaptic sites and metabolized at postsynaptic sites onto which it is liberated. However, proof of this idea will only come when it is possible to visualize GAD, GABA-T, and GABA at an ultrastructural level in specific neuronal sites of ultrathin sections of the cerebellum.

Thus, in the above case, results obtained by methods at the limits of our current technical capabilities give us some meaningful information about the development of a much studied chemical transmitter system in the best known vertebrate neuronal system. Further advances will depend, in part, on the development of quantitative methods for measurement of synaptogenesis, and of methods for the identification of synapses that are inhibitory and excitatory, and the determination for each type of synapse of the major transmitter system with which it deals. The numerous connections of the cerebellum and its important role in orientation of mammalian organisms in space and time (Blomfield and Marr, 1970) unquestionably will implicate it in some of the phenomena associated with sleep and its regulation. Insofar as there is a great deal of cerebellar development that takes place postnatally, it will be interesting to learn whether any correlations exist between various aspects of its developmental features and the developmental sequence of changes in sleep behavior.

GABA IN OTHER VERTEBRATE NEURONAL SYSTEMS

Many studies have been made in the past of changes in GABA and GAD levels with development in whole brains or in specific brain regions of a variety of species (see Baxter, 1970). In all instances, progressive increases in the levels of components of the GABA system have been found during development which correlated well with other developmental features, such as increases in degree of dendritic arborization and synaptogenesis. Studies similar to those for the GABA system in the developing chick cerebellum could be performed for other biochemical systems and in other neuronal structures. Indeed, studies of some aspects of the biochemistry and physiology of the GABA system have been made in retina (Roberts and Kuriyama, 1968; Kuriyama *et al.*, 1968a; Kaita and Goldberg, 1969; Noell, 1959; Graham *et al.*, 1970), hippocampus (Curtis *et al.*, 1970b; Curtis, 1970; Fonnum and Storm-Mathisen, 1969), cortex (Curtis *et al.*, 1970b; Dreifuss *et al.*, 1969), and spinal cord (Albers and Brady, 1959; Salvador and Albers, 1959; Graham *et al.*, 1967; Graham and Aprison, 1969; Davidoff *et al.*, 1967), and it appears that the GABA system may be important in functional control in all of these structures. However, in none of the latter instances has the degree of knowledge with regard to structural and physiological organization begun to approach that available for the cerebellum, and years of combined effort might be required before a comparable degree of sophistication is attained.

COMMENT

Little could be learned about the actual participation of amino acid transmitters in ongoing information-processing in a nervous system, even if it were possible to measure the steady state concentrations of those portions of neuronally contained amino acids that are related to information transmission between neurons, to determine the maximal potential activities of all of the enzymes involved in their metabolism, and to assess the capacities of the transport processes associated with their removal from synapses. A more pertinent measurement would be the determination of that portion of the total turnover of these substances that can be attributable to the presynaptic release of postsynaptically effective amounts, preferably at individual synapses at which they act. From what has gone before, it is obvious that suitable experimental approaches are not yet available to measure such complex biophysical and biochemical phenomena.

A realization of the above may help prevent the reader from accepting too readily *causal interpretations of correlations* between increases or decreases in total concentrations in whole brains or in brain areas of one or another of the potential amino acid transmitters with alterations of physiological or behavioral states produced by environmental manipulation, by surgery or drugs, or those occurring during development. The biochemist cannot stand alone. To be meaningful, his results must be imbedded in a matrix of appropriate morphological, physiological, and behavioral information.

REFERENCES

Albers, R. W., and Brady, R. O. (1959). The distribution of glutamic decarboxylase in the nervous system of the rhesus monkey. *J. Biol. Chem.* **234**, 926-928.

Balázs, R., Machiyama, Y., Hammond, B. J., Julian, T., and Richter, D. (1970). The operation of the γ-aminobutyrate bypath of the tricarboxylic acid cycle in brain tissue *in vitro. Biochem. J.* **116**, 445-467.

Baxter, C. F. (1970). The nature of γ-aminobutyric acid. *In* "Handbook of Neurochemistry" (A. Lajtha, ed.), (Vol. 3), pp. 289-353. Plenum Press, New York.

Blomfield, S., and Marr, D. (1970). How the cerebellum may be used. *Nature (London)* **227**, 1224-1228.

Curtis, D. R. (1970). Personal communication.

Curtis, D. R., and Johnston, G. A. R. (1970). Amino acid transmitters. *In* "Handbook of Neurochemistry" (A. Lajtha, ed.), Vol. 4, pp. 115-134. Plenum Press, New York.

Curtis, D. R., Duggan, A. W., and Felix, D. (1970a). GABA and inhibition of Deiters' neurones. *Brain Res.* **23**, 117-120.

Curtis, D. R., Duggan, A. W., Felix, D., and Johnston, G. A. R. (1970b). GABA, bicuculline and central inhibition. *Nature* **226**, 1222-1224.

Curtis, D. R., and Felix, D. (1971). GABA and prolonged spinal inhibition. *Nature New Biology* **231**, 187-188.

Davidoff, R. A., Grahar, L. T., Jr., Shank, R. P., Werman, R., and Aprison, M. H. (1967). Changes in amino acid concentrations associated with loss of spinal interneurons. *J. Neurochem.* **14**, 1025-1031.

Dreifuss, J. J., Kelly, J. S., and Krnjevic, K. (1969). Cortical inhibition and γ-aminobutyric acid. *Exp. Brain Res.* **9**, 137-154.

Eccles, J. C., Ito, M., and Szentágothai, J. (1967). "The Cerebellum as a Neuronal Machine." Springer-Verlag, Berlin and New York.

Fields, W. S., and Willis, W. D., Jr., eds. (1970). "The Cerebellum in Health and Disease." Warren H. Green, Inc., St. Louis, Missouri.

Fonnum, F., Storm-Mathisen, J. (1969). GABA synthesis in rat hippocampus correlated to the distribution of inhibitory neurones. *Acta Physiol Scand.* **76**, 35A-37A (abstr.).

Fonnum, F., Storm-Mathisen, J., and Walberg, F. (1970). Glutamate decarboxylase in inhibitory neurons. A study of the enzyme in Purkinje cell axons and boutons in the cat. *Brain Res.* **20**, 259-275.

Fox, C. A., and Snider, R. S. (1967). *Progr. Brain Res.* **25**, 1-355.

Galindo, A. (1969). GABA-picrotoxin interaction in the mammalian central nervous system. *Brain Res.* **14**, 763-767.

Graham, L. T., Jr., and Aprison, M. H. (1969). Distribution of some enzymes associated with the metabolism of glutamate, aspartate, γ-aminobutyrate and glutamine in cat spinal cord. *J. Neurochem.* **16**, 559-566.

Graham, L. T., Jr., Shank, R. P., Werman, R., and Aprison, M. H. (1967). Distribution of some synaptic transmitter suspects in cat spinal cord: glutamic acid, aspartic acid, γ-aminobutyric acid, glycine, and glutamine. *J. Neurochem.* **14**, 475-472.

Graham, L. T., Jr., Baxter, C. F., and Lolley, R. N. (1970). *In vivo* influence of light or darkness of the GABA system of the frog (Rana pipiens). *Brain Res.* **20**, 379-388.

Haber, B., Kuriyama, K., and Roberts, E. (1970a). An anion stimulated L-glutamic acid decarboxylase in non-neural tissues: Occurrence and subcellular localization in mouse kidney and developing chick embryo brain. *Biochem. Pharmacol.* **19**, 1119-1136.

Haber, B., Kuriyama, K., and Roberts, E. (1970b). L-Glutamic acid decarboxylase: A new type in glial cells and human brain gliomas. *Science* **168**, 598-599.

Iversen, L. L., and Kravitz, E. A. (1968). The metabolism of GABA in the lobster nervous system—uptake of GABA in nerve-muscle preparations. *J. Neurochem.* **15**, 609-620.

Jasper, H. H., Khan, R. T., and Elliott, K. A. C. (1965). Amino acids released from the cerebral cortex in relation to its state of activation. *Science* **147**, 1448-1449.

Kaita, A. A., and Goldberg, A. M. (1969). Control of acetylcholine synthesis—the inhibition of choline acetyltransferase by acetylcholine. *J. Neurochem.* **16**, 1185-1191.

Kravitz, E. A. (1967). Acetylcholine, γ-aminobutyric acid, and glutamic acid: Physiological and chemical studies related to their roles as neurotransmitter agents. *In* "The Neurosciences: A Study Program" (G. C. Quarton, T. Melnechuk, and F. O. Schmitt, eds.), pp. 433-444. Rockefeller Univ. Press, New York.

Kuriyama, K., Haber, B., Sisken, B., and Roberts, E. (1966). The γ-aminobutyric acid system in rabbit cerebellum. *Proc. Nat. Acad. Sci. U.S.* **55**, 846-852.

Kuriyama, K., Sisken, B., Haber, B., and Roberts, E. (1968a). The gamma-aminobutyric acid system in rabbit retina. *Brain Res.* **9**, 165-168.

Kuriyama, K. Sisken, B., Ito, J., Simonsen, D. G., Haber, B., and Roberts, E. (1968b). The γ-aminobutyric acid system in the developing chick embryo cerebellum. *Brain Res.* **11**, 412-430.

Kuriyama, K., Haber, B., and Roberts, E. (1970). Occurrence of a new L-glutamic acid decarboxylase in several blood vessels of the rabbit. *Brain Res.* **23**, 121-123.

Llinás, R. (1969). "Neurobiology of Cerebellar Evolution and Development." A.M.A. Press, Chicago, Illinois.

McLennan, H. (1970). Bicuculline and inhibition of crayfish stretch receptor neurones. *Nature* **228**, 674-675.

Mitchell, J. F., and Srinivasan, V. (1969). Release of ³H-γ-aminobutyric acid from the brain during synaptic inhibition. *Nature (London)* **224**, 663-666.

Noell, W. K. (1959). The visual cell: Electric and metabolic manifestations of its life processes. *Amer. J. Ophthalmol.* **48**, 347-370.

Obata, K., and Highstein, S. M. (1970). Blocking by picrotoxin of both vestibular inhibition and GABA action on rabbit oculomotor neurons. *Brain Res.* **18**, 538-541.

Obata, K., and Takeda, K. (1969). Release of γ-aminobutyric acid into the fourth ventricle induced by stimulation of the cat's cerebellum. *J. Neurochem.* **16**, 1043-1047.

Obata, K., Ito, M., Ochi, R., and Sato, N. (1967). Pharmacological properties of the postsynaptic inhibition by Purkinje cell axons and the action of γ-aminobutyric acid on Deiters' neurones. *Exp. Brain Res.* **4**, 43-57.

Obata, K., Otsuka, M., and Tanaka, Y. (1970). Determination of gamma-aminobutyric acid in single nerve cells of cat central nervous system. *J. Neurochem.* **17**, 697-698.

Otsuka, M., Iversen, L. L., Hall, Z. W., and Kravitz, E. A. (1966). Release of gamma-aminobutyric acid from inhibitory nerves of lobster. *Proc. Nat. Acad. Sci. U.S.* **56**, 1110-1115.

Robbins, J. and Van der Kloot, W. G. (1958). The effect of picrotoxin on peripheral inhibition in the crayfish. *J. Physiol. (London)* **143**, 541-552.

Roberts E., and Eidelberg, E. (1960). Metabolic and neurophysiological roles of γ-aminobutyric acid. *Int. Rev. Neurobiol.* **2**, 279-332.

Roberts, E., and Kuriyama, K. (1968). Biochemical-physiological correlations in studies of the γ-aminobutyric acid system. *Brain Res.* **8**, 1-35.

Roberts, E., and Matthysse, S. (1970). Neurochemistry: At the crossroads of neurobiology. *Ann. Rev. Biochem.* **39**, 777-820.

Salvador, R. A., and Albers, R. W. (1959). The distribution of glutamic-γ-aminobutyric transaminase in the nervous system of the rhesus monkey. *J. Biol. Chem.* **234**, 922-925.

Srinivasan, V., Neal, M. J., and Mitchell, J. F. (1969). The effect of electrical stimulation and high potassium concentrations on the efflux of (^{3}H)-γ-aminobutyric acid from brain slices. *J. Neurochem.* **16**, 1235-1244.

Takeuchi, A., and Takeuchi, N. (1969). A study of the action of picrotoxin on the inhibitory neuromuscular junction of the crayfish. *J. Physiol. (London)* **205**, 377-391.

GENERAL DISCUSSION

Dr. Hoffer: I would like to direct a question to Dr. Roberts about the significance of the histochemical localization of GABA-T. We have studied it in developing rat cerebellum and we see essentially the same pattern you find in the chick.

When you study LDH and SDH histochemical localizations, you find that these are very similar to GABA-T. It is well known that there is a "GABA shunt" in the Krebs cycle. The problem, then, is that the presence of GABA-T may reflect a role in oxidative metabolism rather than transmitter function.

Dr. Roberts: The most recent estimate of the contribution of the "GABA shunt" to total brain oxidative metabolism is on the order of 8%. It is not possible to estimate how much of this is attributable to GABA undergoing a transsynaptic flux and how much to GABA remaining within particular neurons.

Dr. Hoffer: But if GABA-T activity is localized to an area, does this imply that GABA is a transmitter for this area?

Dr. Roberts: No, there is not necessarily any correlation. There may be, or there may not be. The Purkinje cells have high GABA-T activity and from this we inferred that maybe the Purkinje cell received an input of GABA. Recent experiments by Curtis indicate that, indeed, GABA may be the transmitter liberated by basket cells onto the Purkinje cells.

Dr. Hoffer: My point was, that in order to block basket-stellate inhibition of Purkinje cells, it was necessary to administer the blocking agent (bicuculline) parenterally. Since this route of administration distributes the drug throughout the brain, one may have excitation and inhibition through disinhibition and disfacilitation from a remote site. It is much more important to try to block the pathway with local (microiontophoretic) drug administration.

5

Contributions of Differential Housing to Brain Development: Some Implications for Sleep Behavior*

Walter B. Essman

A considerable amount of attention has been directed toward the early postnatal development of the brain and its functional implications, but there has been little concern given to those factors affecting the course of brain development, especially beyond postweaning maturation. One factor contributing to the postnatal development of brain cellular specificity and metabolism is differential housing, which may have direct relevance to the immediate question of sleep behavior, since it affects the same substrates of brain metabolism as those implicated in sleep, and at a behavioral level regulates responses that are similarly modified through sleep-wakefulness cycles. Some support for the behavioral and biochemical interaction apparently served by differential housing in mice (isolation vs aggregation) has been provided

*Supported in part by a grant from NICHD (HD-03493).

(Essman, 1971c) indicating that regional changes in biogenic amines, altered brain serotonin turnover, and cell number and ribonucleic acid (RNA) content thereof can be altered through isolation. With the presentation of environmental stimulation, isolated animals showed a marked decrease in cerebellar glial RNA, whereas the RNA content of cerebellar glia for aggregated mice given comparable stimulation did not change. In further studies (Essman, 1971a), it was found that isolated mice showed decreased activity of cholinesterases in somatosensory cortex, which was increased when such animals were provided with environmental stimulation; markedly elevated RNA levels in cerebellar glia, which became dramatically decreased by environmental stimulation; reduced cerebellar neuronal RNA content; elevated cerebellar glial RNA level as a decreased function of the age of onset of differential housing; and reduced cerebellar neuronal RNA levels as a decreased function of the age of onset of differential housing.

Those substrates altered by differential housing also have implications for sleep behavior: 1) serotonin (5-hydroxytryptamine; 5-HT) has emerged in its significance in that sleep can be induced by cells of the raphe nuclei that contain this amine (Jouvet, 1967), presumably leads to a state resembling slow wave sleep (SWS) with total paradoxical sleep (PS) suppression through increases in the amine brought about by 5-hydroxytryptophan (5-HTP) injection (Jouvet, 1967) and through its postulated correlation with SWS through an unknown deaminated 5-HT catabolite (Jouvet, 1969); 2) acetylcholine (ACh) in anesthetized rats was elevated from 14 to 42% above baseline levels (Crossland *et al.*, 1955), and when this amine was injected directly into the brain, SWS and PS were induced in the cat (Hernández-Peón, 1963); tryptophols, bearing structural similarity to ACh have been shown to induce sleep and may act at cholinergic receptor sites (Feldstein *et al.*, 1970); 3) RNA has been shown to be reduced during sleep (Palladin and Vladmirov, 1956; Smirnov, 1955), whereas sustained wakefulness induced by central nervous system stimulants also provides for increased regional RNA levels; the energy metabolism of neurons or glia specific to wakefulness or sleep states has been indicated (Hydén and Lange, 1965), and this could possibly also be reflected in altered lactate concentration with sleep (Shimizu *et al.*, 1966).

The hypotheses that isolation housing may represent a partial functional denervation in the somatosensory system and thereby provide for supersensitivity (lowered threshold) of components of this system (Prescott, 1967), seems particularly appropriate in the present context. Those components of the somatosensory system thus affected might be expected to provide for attenuation of effects which usually reduce stimulus input and potentiation of those effects tending toward activation of inputs. At a metabolic level, these differences could represent the cellular and synaptic requirements for excitation or quiescence, a continuum paralleled by the wakefulness-sleep dichotomy.

A variety of neurochemical measures, which previous study has suggested as being sensitive to differential housing, have been obtained, and these have been summarized in Table I. In all instances, mice weaned at 21 days of age were housed either singly or aggregated (five per cage) for 28 days, at which time the brain tissue was removed and prepared for the respective assays. Preparative and analytical procedures have been previously summarized (Essman, 1971b, c), and the data appear quite self-explanatory, in that the data presented represent, in all instances, statistically significant differences as a function of differential housing. In the case of neuronal-glial separations, morphological confirmation of enriched fractions was provided through phase-contrast light microscopy, and in the case of subcellular fractions both transmission and stereoscan electron microscopy provided for evidence of structural homogeneity. Standard spectro-photometric, spectrofluorometric, and bioassay methods were employed for all of the substrate and enzyme assays, and established subcellular fractionation procedures (Whittaker, 1969) were employed.

As a consequence of isolation housing, 5-hydroxyindoleacetic acid, the major metabolite of 5-HT in brain, was elevated, whereas 5-HT turnover time in at least two areas of the brain (with somatosensory inputs) was decreased. While neuronal RNA levels in cerebellar cortex were decreased in isolated animals, glial RNA in the same tissue was elevated; these findings add further support to the suggestion (Essman, 1969a) that isolation housing and functional denervation provided thereby to the somatosensory system can lead to cellular supersensiti-vity in that system. This threshold decrement to a cellular level may well be reflected in an acceleration of glial metabolism with reciprocal neuronal metabolic decrement. Cholinesterases, while apparently reduced in activity in the cerebral cortex tissue homogenates from isolated mice, were generally elevated in membrane fractions from the nerve ending, with the notable exception of the intraterminal mitochondrial fraction where acetylcholinesterase (AChE) was markedly lowered. The elevated ACh levels associated with cerebral cortex homogenate ("bound ACh") and with synaptosomes from isolated animals is perhaps a further suggestion of reduced neuronal activity. It is of further interest to note that synaptosomes fractionated from cerebral cortex, limbic system, and cerebellar cortex, as well as myelin fractions from the latter two areas, were not significantly different as a function of housing with respect to K^+/Na^+ ratios.

The RNA concentrations associated with various subcellular fractions of the cerebral cortex of differentially housed mice are summarized in Table II. It is of interest here to note that consistently significant differences in RNA level emerged, with the isolated mice having lowered RNA concentrations associated with myelin, synaptosomes, synaptic vesicles, external synaptic membrane, and intraterminal mitochondria fractions. Aside from its implications for attenuated neuronal and possibly synaptic activity as a consequence of isolation, there are

TABLE I *Summary of Representative Neurochemical Measures Showing Statistically Significant Differences between Isolated and Aggregated Mice*

	Housing condition			
	Isolation		Aggregation	
5-Hydroxyindoleacetic acid:				
diencephalon (μg/g)	0.307	(0.004)	0.264	(0.020)
5-Hydroxytryptamine turnover time (min)				
Olfactory bulbs	42		68	
Cerebral cortex	45		70	
"Free" 5-hydroxytryptamine (μg/g)	0.17	(0.02)	0.36	(0.04)
Diploid cell number ($\times$ 10^7)				
Mesencephalon	1.16		1.46	
Diencephalon	0.65		1.67	
Cerebellum	2.47		4.01	
Cellular RNA content: cerebellum (μg/cell)				
Neurons	19.5		34.1	
Glia	78.3		45.2	
Cholinesterases: cerebral cortex (moles/kg/hr)				
AChE	1.18	(0.32)	3.27	(0.43)
BuChE	0.33	(0.12)	0.77	(0.11)
Cholinesterases: cerebral cortex (moles/kg/hr)				
Frontal				
AChE	0.83	(0.21)	2.93	(0.47)
BuChE	0.34	(0.03)	0.76	(0.10)
Somatosensory				
AChE	1.40	(0.39)	3.23	(0.57)
BuChE	0.35	(0.04)	0.76	(0.11)
Auditory				
AChE	1.32	(0.23)	3.61	(0.63)
BuChE	0.31	(0.05)	0.82	(0.16)
Visual				
AChE	1.15	(0.14)	3.29	(0.63)
BuChE	0.35	(0.05)	0.76	(0.15)
Acetycholinesterase: cerebral cortex presynaptic nerve ending fractions (A.U./mg/min)				
External synaptic membrane	0.027	(0.01)	0.150	(0.04)
	0.032	(0.01)	0.004	(0.00)
	0.024	(0.01)	0.006	(0.00)
Incompletely disrupted synaptosomes	0.30	(0.09)	0.01	(0.00)
Intraterminal mitochondria	0.007	(0.00)	0.056	(0.01)
Acetylcholine: cerebral cortex (nmoles/g)				
Homogenate	16.00	(1.36)	6.66	(1.24)
Synaptosomes	4.00	(0.93)	2.40	(0.72)

TABLE II *Mean (±σ) RNA Concentration (μg/mg Protein) in Subcellular Fractions of Mouse Cerebral Cortex Following Differential Housing*

	Housing condition			
Subcellular fraction	Isolation		Aggregation	
Small myelin fragments	6.80	(0.14)	19.10	(0.10)
Synaptosomes	1.90	(0.18)	10.80	(0.17)
Mitochondria	6.80	(0.25)	4.50	(0.25)
Soluble cytoplasm	11.70	(0.20)	15.40	(0.53)
Synaptic vesicles	01.00	(0.02)	6.00	(0.11)
External synaptic	0.90	(0.01)	31.20	(0.31)
membrane	2.50	(0.14)	12.20	(0.44)
	2.10	(0.15)	16.80	(0.47)
Incompletely disrupted				
synaptosomes	0.31	(0.15)	19.70	(0.73)
Intraterminal				
mitochondria	0.17	(0.03)	09.80	(0.08)

further indications that these changes may modify the properties of storage pools for molecules of possible transmitter significance in the brain; this may be particularly appropriate for the vesicular- and membrane-associated RNA decrements. In previous communications (Bittman *et al.*, 1969; Bittman and Essman, 1970) we have suggested that certain putative transmitter molecules may be bound by RNA and that the subcellular sites at which this may be accomplished have direct relevance to synaptic transmission and protein synthesis.

The foregoing discussion and data have suggested that regional, cellular, and subcellular metabolic changes that can be brought about by differential housing, involve, in part, substrates and possible mechanisms relevant to sleep behavior, as well as the further possibility that the state of hypothesized functional denervation provided by isolation may also be expected to alter sleep behavior. Differences in barbiturate-induced sleep have been observed as a consequence of differential housing, periodicity of illumination (Davis, 1962), and other factors, such as strain, handling, and litter size (Vessell, 1968). Differences in uptake and metabolism of the drug have been suggested as accounting for the generally reduced effect of the drug among individually housed mice. At a behavioral level we have observed that isolated mice show increased locomotor activity (Essman, 1966a, 1968), are more susceptible to somatic changes induced by stress (Frisone and Essman, 1965; Essman, 1966a; Essman and Frisone, 1966; Caputo *et al.*, 1968), and demonstrate altered patterns of motivated competitive behavior (Essman and Smith, 1967; Essman, 1969a). Inasmuch as several classical pharmacological agents may be expected to exert predictable effects upon endogenous substrates of brain metabolism, and isolation, per se, may be expected to have effects on the same systems, this interaction was selected for study, utilizing a simple criterion for a sleep-wakefulness contingency. Earlier indications have been that those substrates considered in the present context can be altered by barbiturates and amphetamines; the former has been suggested as suppressing ACh synthesis (Mann *et al.*, 1938; Johnson and Quastel, 1953; McLennan and Elliott, 1951), elevating brain 5-HT levels (Bonnycastle *et al.*, 1962; Garattini *et al.*, 1960), and lowering brain RNA content (Pevzner, 1966), whereas the latter appears to exert effects in quite the opposite direction (Paasonen and Vogt, 1956; Lal and Chessick, 1964; Carlini and Carlini, 1965). Considering that isolation serves to modify the metabolism of some substrates in common with those acted upon by the drugs, one might generate some predictions on this basis concerning sleep induction and locomotor excitation. Barbiturates could be expected to have reduced efficacy, since those substrates affected by its action have already been modified through isolation. Amphetamines might exert a greater excitatory effect, since those substrates affected by its action have not been altered in the same direction through isolation; i.e., one could therefore predict less barbiturate-induced sleep and greater amphetamine-induced locomotor excitation. Mice, after either isolation or aggregation as previously described, were injected (i.p.) with either 50 mg/kg of amphetamine sulfate, or an equivalent volume of 0.9% saline. From the onset of injection, sleeping time (interval during which there was an absence of a righting response with the absence of both forefeet on the cage floor for 20 sec or more) was measured within a 120-min interval between 2 and 4 PM. Locomotor activity level was measured for amphetamine- and saline-treated mice in an apparatus designed to provide for necessary locomotion, the absence of which indicated complete immobility, or sleep (Essman, 1966b). Activity was measured from the onset of injection for 15 min, at approximately 2 PM.

Aggregated mice showed a mean barbiturate-induced sleeping time of 78 (±5.3) min during the 120 min following drug treatment, whereas isolated animals slept for 42 (±6.4) min during the same interval; it may also be noted that nondrug-induced sleeping time in the isolated mice (saline-treated) was 17% less than for aggregated animals.

Isolated mice showed 25% more spontaneous locomotor activity than did aggregates, and as a consequence of amphetamine treatment the aggregates showed a 16% locomotor activity increase to 94 (±7.9) counts in 15 min; the isolated mice showed a locomotor activity increase of 83% to 187 (±10.3) counts within the same interval, the difference between drug-treated animals being statistically significant ($p < 0.02$). The results concerned with drug-induced sleep and activation appear to be consistent with the predictions generated by the metabolic findings. One possible variable that could account for such differences is periodicity in the sleep-wakefulness cycle; if this were subject to modification through differential housing, either through changes in neurochemical metabolic periodicity, or behavioral change, or both, then differences, not only in drug effects but also in activation and/or quiescence peaks might be expected. Isolated and aggregated mice, from conditions identical with those previously described, were tested over a complete 24-hr period with cumulative locomotor activity recorded continuously through an electronic circuit providing for activity counts against a time base, the physical requirements of the apparatus allowed absent counts to be equated with sleep (Essman, 1966b). The cumulative records were summated for each of six 4-hr intervals, beginning at 8 AM. A reasonably high degree of interrelationship emerged between the sequences of activity and quiescence over the 24-hr sequence for isolated and aggregated mice ($\alpha = 0.60$). It is interesting to note that peak activity occurred for both conditions of housing with the same 4-hr interval, 4 AM to 8 AM, and there was no difference between conditions at this time (175.10 ± 77.45 vs 175.45 ± 63.51) peak quiescence (interval during which maximal sleep was apparent) for the aggregated mice occurred between 4 PM and 8 PM, at which time these animals averaged 54% less activity than isolated mice; however, the isolated animals showed peak quiescence in the 8 PM to 12 PM interval. This suggests that isolation can mediate a shift in the sleep cycle without modification of maximal wakefulness activity. To insure that the onset of the activation-quiescence measurement did not constitute a contributory variable, this was randomly initiated at each of the six 4-hr sequences, and was determined to be without effect.

The results discussed here are not intended as a definitive basis for relating changes in brain metabolism produced by isolation to sleep behavior; rather, they are intended as an example of how the biochemical plasticity of the young adult mouse brain provides avenues through which sleep behavior may be investigated, and for exploration of basic mechanisms through which sleep behavior can be modified environmentally and biochemically.

REFERENCES

Bittman, R., and Essman, W. B. (1970). 5-Hydroxytryptamine-nucleic acid interactions. Implications for physical and *in vivo* studies as a model for neural function. *Pap., 3rd Annu. Winter Conf. Brain Res., 1970.*

Bittman, R., Essman, W. B., and Golod, M. I. (1969). Studies of the interaction of 5-hydroxytryptamine with nucleic acids. *Abstr. Amer. Chem. Soc., 1969* p. 330.

Bonnycastle, D. C., Bonnycastle, H. F., and Anderson, E. G. (1962). The effect of a number of central depressant drugs on brain 5-hydroxytryptamine levels in the rat. *J. Pharmacol. Exp. Ther.* **135**, 17-20.

Caputo, D. V., Essman, W. B., Teitler, G., Lowe, G., and Frisone, J. D. (1968). Housing modification as a variable in fasting-induced ulcerogenesis. *J. Psychosom. Res.* **12**, 129-135.

Carlini, G. R. S., and Carlini, E. A. (1965). Effects of strychnine and cannabis sative (marihuana) on the nucleic acid content in brain of the rat. *Med. Pharmacol. Exp.* **12**, 21-26.

Crossland, J., Pappius, H. M., and Elliott, K. A. C. (1955). Acetylcholine content of frozen brains. *Amer. J. Physiol.* **183**, 27-31.

Davis, W. M. (1962). Day-night periodicity in pentobarbital response of mice and the influence of sociopsychological conditions. *Experientia* **18**, 235-237.

Essman, W. B. (1966a). Gastric ulceration in differentially housed mice. *Psychol. Rep.* **19**, 173-174.

Essman, W. B. (1966b). The development of activity differences in isolated and aggregated mice. *Anim. Behav.* **14**, 406-409.

Essman, W. B. (1968). Differences in locomotor activity and brain-serotonin metabolism in differentially housed mice. *J. Comp. Physiol. Psychol.* **66**, 244-246.

Essman, W. B. (1969a). Differential housing in mice—a source of behavioral neurochemical change. *Pap., Workshop Develop. Violence Pleasure Man, 1969.*

Essman, W. B. (1969b). Free and motivated behavior and amine metabolism in isolated mice. *In* "Aggressive Behavior" (S. Garattini and E. B. Sigg, eds.), pp. 203-208. Wiley (Interscience), New York.

Essman, W. B. (1971a). Neurochemical changes associated with isolation and environmental stimulation. *J. Biol. Psychiat.* **3**, 141-147.

Essman, W. B. (1971b). Some neurochemical correlates of altered memory consolidation. *Trans. N.Y. Acad. Sci.* **32**, 948-973.

Essman, W. B. (1971c). Isolation-induced behavioral modification—some neurochemical correlates. *In* "Brain Development and Behavior" (M. B. Sterman, D. J. McGinty, and A. M. Adinolfi, eds.), pp. 265-276. Academic Press, New York.

Essman, W. B., and Frisone, J. F. (1966). Isolation-induced facilitation of gastric ulcerogenesis. *J. Psychosom. Res.* **10**, 183-188.

Essman, W. B., and Smith, G. E. (1967). Behavior and neurochemical differences between differentially housed mice. *Amer. Zool.* **7**, 793 (abstr.).

Feldstein, A., Chang, F. H., and Kucharski, J. M. (1970). Tryptophol 5-hydroxytryptophol 5-methoxytryptophol-induced sleep in mice. *Life Sci.* **9**, 323-329.

Frisone, J. F., and Essman, W. B. (1965). Stress-induced gastric lesions in mice. *Psychol. Rep.* **16**, 941-946.

Garattini, S., Kato, R., and Valzelli, L. (1960). Biochemical and pharmacological effects induced by electroshock. *Psychiat. Neurol.* **140**, 190-206.

Hernández-Peón, R. (1963). Physiological basis of mental activity. *Electroencephalogr. Clin. Neurophysiol. Suppl.* **24**, 284.

Hydén, H., and Lange, P. W. (1965). Rhythmic enzyme changes in neurons and glia during sleep and wakefulness. *Progr. Brain Res.* **18**, 92-95.

Johnson, W. J., and Quastel, J. H. (1953). Narcotics and biological acetylation. *Nature (London)* **171**, 602-605.

Jouvet, M. (1967). States of sleep. *Sci. Amer.* **216**, 62-72.

Jouvet, M. (1969). Biogenic amines and the states of sleep. *Science* **163**, 32-41.

Lal, H., and Chessick, R. D. (1964). Biochemical mechanisms of amphetamine toxicity in isolated and aggregated mice. *Life Sci.* **3**, 381-384.

McLennan, H., and Elliott, K. A. C. (1951). Effects of convulsant and narcotic drugs on acetylcholine synthesis. *J. Pharmacol. Exp. Ther.* **103**, 35-43.

Mann, P. J. G., Tannenbaum, M., and Quastel, J. H. (1938). Mechanisms of acetylcholine formation *in vitro*. *Biochem. J.* **32**, 243-261.

Paasonen, M. K. and Vogt, M. J. (1956). Effect of drugs on the amount of substance P and 5-hydroxytryptamine in mammalian brain. *J. Physiol. (London)* **131**, 617-626.

Palladin, A. V., and Vladmirov, G. E. (1956). Use of radioactive isotopes in the study of functional biochemistry of the brain. *Proc. Int. Conf. Peaceful Uses At. Energy, 1955* vol. 12, p. 551.

Pevzner, L. Z. (1966). Nucleic acid changes during behavioral events. *In* "Macromolecules and Behavior," (J. Gaito, ed.), pp. 43-70. Appleton, New York.

Prescott, J. W. (1967). Central nervous system functioning in altered sensory environments. *In* "Psychological Stress" (M. H. Appley and R. Trumbull, eds.), pp. 113-117. Appleton, New York.

Shimizu, H., Tabushi, K., Hishikawa, Y., Kakimoto, Y., and Kaneko, Z. (1966). Concentration of lactic acid in rat brain during natural sleep. *Nature (London)* **212,** 936-937.

Smirnov, A. A. (1955). Content and exchange of phosphorus in various zones of cerebral cortex of dogs in rest and activity. *Dokl. Akad. Nauk SSSR* **105,** 185-187.

Vessell, E. S. (1968). Genetic and environmental factors affecting hexobarbital metabolism in mice. *Ann. N.Y. Acad. Sci.* **151,** 900-912.

Whittaker, V. P. (1969). The synaptosome. *In* "Handbook of Neurochemistry" (A. Lajtha, ed.), Vol. 2, pp. 327-361. Plenum Press, New York.

GENERAL DISCUSSION

Dr. Rose: I would like to ask Dr. Essman a question which I am certain he has been asked before. What kind of isolation or what variables do you think are producing these changes?

I can think of many possibilities. Is the effect due to social isolation? Is it a function of the reduced complexity of the environment? Is it associated with less heat than normally present when other animals are in the cage?

Would you get the same effect if you reared one animal isolated from his peers but in an environment that was very complex, with many kinds of sensory input? Have you attempted to fractionate any of these suggested variables?

Dr. Essman: We have done something of this nature. Animals, for example, have been raised in isolation, but then we provided them with a very complex environment consisting of a variety of novel stimuli, handling, exploration of mazes, manipulandae, etc. We felt that isolation per se was an extremely important variable that had been overlooked in previous experiments, and indeed it does contribute to those differences that we have observed. If these isolated animals (mice) are provided with more complex environmental stimulation, they seem to differ less markedly from group-housed animals that receive no such stimulation, and when the group-housed animals are environmentally stimulated, they show changes to a considerably lesser degree.

Dr. Rose: Isolation, then, may be too general a term.

Dr. Essman: It probably is. We are really not sure what they are isolated from, although I should say that the visual experience apparently does not, as far as what we have measured, seem to make very much difference.

Dr. Rose: Although there are many studies that have shown that differential rearing under various cues enhances learning ability at later stages.

Dr. Essman: I did not mean to say we provided the mice with some sort of enriched visual experience; we did not do this. These animals were housed under either isolated or grouped conditions with different gross levels of illumination, depending upon whether the cages were completely transparent, semitransparent, or completely opaque. We thought that perhaps differences in visual experience, with other animals as visual stimuli, could account for some of the stimulation. We found that this did not contribute in any way.

6

The Role of Biogenic Amines in Sleep

Oscar Resnick

Professor Jouvet (1969) has postulated that serotonin (5-hydroxytryptamine; 5-HT) may be involved in slow wave sleep (SWS), whereas, the catecholamines (CA) may be involved in paradoxical sleep (PS). This postulate was based on extensive neurophysiological and neuropharmacological studies, primarily in the cat, and is described in great detail. Of particular interest is the observation that Jouvet drew support for such a dualistic theory of sleep from ontogenetic studies derived from his laboratory and those of Shimizu and Himwich (1968), Roffwarg *et al.* (1966), and many others. The following is a summary of these investigations.

Newborn mammals (such as the cat, rat, and rabbit) whose central nervous system (CNS) is incompletely developed at birth manifest only the succession from waking to rapid eye movements sleep (REMS). SWS appears later on in development. In newborn mammals (such as the guinea pig and lamb) whose

CNS is well developed at birth, SWS and REMS alternate periodically. Thus, if 5-HT is involved in SWS and SWS is absent in the newborn cat, rat, and rabbit, what is the level of 5-HT in the CNS of such neonates? In addition, since SWS is present in the newborn guinea pig and lamb, what is the level of 5-HT in the CNS of such neonates? Bennett and Giarmin (1965) reported that animals such as the rat and rabbit, which are poorly developed at birth, possess low levels of brain 5-HT at birth, whereas the guinea pig and goat, species which are well developed and competent at birth, possess levels of brain 5-HT which approach or, in the case of the goat, exceed the adult levels. Thus, there is presumptive evidence that 5-HT may be involved, directly or indirectly, in the establishment and maintenance of SWS. However, it is also possible that the above correlations might be explained on the basis that those neonates which are poorly developed at birth possess a CNS whose maturation or development is at a primitive stage and whose enzymes, including those responsible for the formation of the biogenic amines, are not yet fully formed or operative. It is also possible that the biogenic amines once formed may regulate the maturation of the CNS. This would be in addition to the presumed role of the biogenic amines as neurotransmitters or neuromodulators. Evidence for this may be derived from studies of aminoacidurias, such as phenylketonuria (PKU).

One may now ask: What are the sleep patterns of the animal whose CNS has partially or completely lost its ability to synthesize 5-HT? Conversely, it would be of great interest to compare the sleep patterns of various strains of animals whose content of CNS 5-HT has been found to be normally different. For example, Sudak and Maas (1964a, b) found that there is a positive correlation between levels of brain 5-HT and emotionality in mice and rats.

Koe and Weissman (1966) reported the effects of p-chlorophenylalanine (PCPA) on brain amine levels. PCPA at optimum doses reduces brain 5-HT to about 10% of normal, while having only very slight effects on norepinephrine (NE) levels. PCPA was shown to be a potent inhibitor of phenylalanine hydroxylase (PAH) and tryptophan hydroxylase and thus interfered with the biosynthesis of 5-HT in brain and other tissues. Since PCPA inhibits both PAH and tryptophan hydroxylase, one might expect decreases in both 5-HT and NE. However, while tryptophan is the only precursor of 5-hydroxytryptophan (5-HTP) (which is then decarboxylated to 5-HT), there is sufficient tyrosine available from sources other than the hydroxylation of PA for a nearly normal CA biosynthesis. These investigators reported, in the rat, that after a single administration of PCPA the concentration of 5-HT in the brain remains at low levels for several days and then slowly returns to control levels in about 10 days. Since Jouvet and others have made extensive use of PCPA in their studies on the role of 5-HT in sleep, I would like to discuss the actions of PCPA in greater detail.

Lipton *et al.* (1967) reported that in animals treated with PCPA there is an elevated blood and tissue level of PA, with minimal effects on the levels of tyrosine. High levels of blood and tissue PA, essentially normal levels of blood and tissue tyrosine, and decreased levels of blood and tissue 5-HT are the distinguishing characteristics of experimental PKU produced in animals fed high doses of PA, and of clinical PKU. *In essence, PCPA treatment in animals results in a biochemical state of PKU.* It is of interest to note that PCPA is an inhibitor of PAH, the same enzyme which is absent or inoperative in experimental and clinical PKU. If Jouvet's hypothesis is correct, then those animals which have not yet developed SWS should not do so following treatment with PCPA or treatment with high levels of PA, which produces experimental PKU. Thus, the sleep patterns of animals made PKU by feeding PA and the sleep patterns of patients with PKU would be of great interest. When PCPA is administered to an animal, not only is the synthesis of 5-HT by the brain and other tissues of the body inhibited, but an amino acid imbalance characteristic of PKU is also produced. Therefore, are the effects reported following PCPA administration the result of the 5-HT depletion or the result of a state of PKU, or both? Certainly, in addition to measuring the 5-HT content of the brain, one should also assess the effects of PCPA administration as related to the characteristic amino acid imbalance produced in the blood and tissues. As already stated, PCPA produces an elevation of blood and tissue PA without an increase in tyrosine. Swaiman *et al.* (1968) induced an elevated plasma PA concentration in 7-day-old rabbits over a 6-hr period by an intraperitoneal (i.p.) injection of PA. ^{14}C-lysine was injected i.p. into these rabbits and into control animals. The rate of incorporation of ^{14}C-lysine into brain ribosomal protein was decreased during a 5-hr period in the presence of elevated plasma PA concentrations. Lysine transport from the peritoneum to the plasma was unaffected by the high plasma PA concentrations. Thus, Swaiman considers the possibility that aminoacidurias, such as PKU, produce abnormalities in protein metabolism in the CNS, thus accounting for cerebral dysfunction. Of course, one would expect the greatest cerebral dysfunction to be produced in the developing immature brain. What effect PKU has on the already developed and mature brain is not yet fully known or understood. In light of the similarities between experimental PKU and PCPA treatment, the following is of interest. Schlesinger *et al.* (1968) reported that PCPA "enhanced" the acquisition of a discriminated avoidance response in mature rats. In rats treated chronically with PCPA from birth and every third day thereafter until 41 days of age, there was a "retardation" in learning of a discriminated response. Thus, these authors observed a difference in PCPA effects between "mature" and "immature" rats.

A possible role of 5-HT depletion in the CNS deficits accompanying experimental PKU in the mouse has been suggested by Woolley and van der Hoeven (1965) and for clinical PKU in man by Pare *et al.* (1957, 1958). Woolley and van der Hoeven (1965) produced a 5-HT deficiency in mice in the following ways: (1) treatment with PA plus tyrosine to produce experimental PKU; (2) feeding reserpine; and (3) feeding chlorpromazine. The mice treated in the above manner from birth until maturity had a subnormal maze-learning ability. The mice treated in the above manner from weaning to maturity not only did not show a subnormal maze-learning ability, but actually displayed an increase in maze-learning ability. These results were interpreted to mean that the behavioral deficit seen in animals made PKU experimentally is attributable to the 5-HT deficiency imposed in early infancy. Experimental PKU induced in older mice did not produce any learning deficits. Recent work would seem to indicate that such an interpretation may be valid. Stevens *et al.* (1967) reported that "adult" male albino rats treated with PCPA learned two brightness discrimination tasks with fewer errors than did the control animals. Schlesinger *et al.* (1968) reported that chronic PCPA treatment begun 24 hr after birth and continued to 41 days of age retarded the performance of rats and mice in conditioned avoidance tasks. Thus, inhibiting the synthesis of brain 5-HT in animals by various methods (e.g., production of experimental PKU or treatment with PCPA) before the maturation of the CNS is completed produces CNS deficits. Similar treatments after the maturation of the CNS is complete not only do not produce CNS deficits but actually may enhance the learning ability of animals. This latter finding may possibly be explained by the role of 5-HT in emotionality. Sudak and Maas (1964a, b) found that there is a positive correlation in adult rats between levels of brain 5-HT and emotionality. Tenen (1967) and Stevens *et al.* (1969) have also reported less emotional reactivity in adult rats with depleted 5-HT, as a result of PCPA treatment.

The mature CNS is known to have a very vigorous protein metabolism, which has been implicated in learning, memory, and in response to stress. Way *et al.* (1968), working with mice, observed an association of tolerance and physical dependence to morphine with an increased protein synthesis in the CNS. This was suggested by the observation that tolerance and physical dependence to morphine could be prevented by cycloheximide, a protein synthesis inhibitor. This finding has been corroborated in rats (Cochin, 1970). These investigators also reported that 5-HT "turnover" is increased in the tolerant animals, and is unchanged in the untreated controls or in the withdrawn animals. They further reported that inhibition of 5-HT synthesis with PCPA markedly decreases tolerance and physical dependence development to morphine. Finally, these same authors reported that the rate of 5-HT turnover in the brains of morphinized mice treated with cycloheximide, a protein synthesis inhibitor, was similar to the control animals rather than to the morphinized animals. These authors concluded that the observation that the rate of synthesis of brain 5-HT increases with tolerance to morphine suggests that the protein involved may be associated with 5-HT synthesis.

Maynert and Klingman (1962) reported that the rate of brain NE turnover in animals also increases with tolerance to morphine. This has recently been corroborated by Clouet and Ratner (1970). Thus, there is evidence in animals that after chronic administration of morphine there is an increase in protein synthesis in the CNS, as well as an increased turnover of both 5-HT and NE. The observation that tolerance and physical dependence to morphine in mice can be prevented either by treatment with cycloheximide, a protein synthesis inhibitor, or by PCPA, a 5-HT depletor, becomes very important. Is the action of PCPA interpreted on the basis of a production of elevated plasma and tissue levels of PA which result in a decrease in protein synthesis by the morphinized brain, or is it the result of the 5-HT depletion? This question becomes even more important since Myers and Veale (1968) reported that the preference for ethyl alcohol was reduced or abolished in rats treated with PCPA. It would be of interest to ascertain if cycloheximide produced the same results. Thus, a study of the sleep patterns of patients with PKU and of patients tolerant to and addicted to various agents such as the hard narcotics, ethanol, tobacco, etc., is of great import. It would be especially important to try to correlate, where possible, the clinical state with blood and tissue levels of PA and 5-HT. The therapeutic potentialities are quite obvious.

It is also of interest to speculate that the circadian rhythms of sleep are correlated with circadian rhythms of protein synthesis in the CNS, which in turn may be reflected in the circadian synthesis of the biogenic amines. That a correlation between protein synthesis and the turnover of biogenic amines in the CNS may actually exist may be seen from the studies involving stress and the chronic administration of morphine or ethanol. For the past 20 years, the role of the biogenic amines in the CNS has been extensively investigated. Most of the work has been focused on the indoleamines, 5-HT and tryptamine, and on the CA's, dopamine, NE, and epinephrine (E). Dopamine is now attracting much attention because of its role in Parkinsonism. It is also well known that many additional biogenic amines are selectively synthesized by the CNS and one may assume that these compounds might also have biological roles in the CNS. Studies on the role of 5-HT and other endogenously occurring amines are made difficult by the fact that these substances do not enter the CNS in appreciable quantities when administered peripherally. Because of this, investigators have frequently made use of compounds which "do" enter the brain and there selectively affect the synthesis, transport, and degradation of the naturally occurring substances. Studies on 5-HT and on all of the other biogenic amines which made use of this technique were limited, however, by the fact that most compounds which affect 5-HT metabolism also either affect metabolism of other endogenous amines in the CNS or have pharmacological actions by themselves or are transformed into amines which are not naturally occurring but have biological potency.

The discovery of PCPA was hailed as a major breakthrough in neuropsychopharmacology. While not minimizing the importance of this compound as a research tool, I have tried to indicate that PCPA has other far-reaching effects in addition to inhibiting 5-HT synthesis.

5-HTP, the precursor of 5-HT, is administered to animals for the purpose of increasing the levels of tissue 5-HT. However, 5-HTP has been shown to decrease NE and dopamine in the brain as well as to increase 5-HT (Aprison and Hingtgen, 1965; Sourkes *et al.*, 1961).

Dopa, the precursor of dopamine, is administered to animals for the purpose of increasing the levels of tissue CA. However, dopa has been shown to deplete brain 5-HT as well as to increase brain dopamine. Everett and Borcherding (1970) reported that large doses of *l*-dopa given to mice produced marked increases in brain dopamine, no change in NE, and a remarkable decrease in brain 5-HT. Thus, dopa (a precursor of dopamine) and PCPA (an inhibitor of 5-HT synthesis) both result in a decrease in brain 5-HT. PCPA has been reported to produce hypersexuality in the rat (Tagliamonte *et al.*, 1969; Sheard, 1969) and in the cat (Ferguson *et al.*, 1970). Recently a small percentage of Parkinsonian patients treated with large doses of dopa have been reported to experience hypersexuality. It would be of great interest to determine if large doses of dopa also affect tolerance and addiction.

Disulfiram (Antabuse) is administered to animals for the purpose of inhibiting the synthesis of NE (by inhibiting dopamine-β-oxidase). However, Antabuse is an aldehyde dehydrogenase inhibitor and as such interferes with the metabolism of the endogenous biogenic amines (e.g., 5-HT, NE, E, and dopamine).

The decarboxylase inhibitors, such as α-methyl-*m*-tyrosine, are administered to animals for the purpose of inhibiting the formation of the biogenic amines. However, these inhibitors may themselves be decarboxylated to form false amines or neurotransmitters. The monoamine oxidase (MAO) inhibitors will have different effects on the metabolism of the biogenic amines in different species of animals and in different tissues of the same animal.

Despite all of the above-mentioned obstacles, it would seem from the work of Jouvet and others (Weitzman *et al.*, 1968) that the biogenic amines play a very important role in the genesis, as well as the maintenance, of the sleep patterns in mammals.

REFERENCES

Aprison, M. H., and Hingtgen, J. N. (1965). Neurochemical correlates of behavior. IV. Norepinephrine and dopamine in four brain parts of the pigeon during period of atypical behavior following the injection of 5-hydroxytryptophan. *J. Neurochem.* **12**, 959-968.

Bennett, D. S., and Giarmin, N. J. (1965). Schedule of appearance of 5-hydroxytryptamine (serotonin) and associated enzymes in the developing rat brain. *J. Neurochem.* **12**, 911-918.

Clouet, D. H., and Ratner, M. (1970). Catecholamine biosynthesis in brains of rats treated with morphine. *Science* **168**, 854-856.

Cochin, J. (1970). Possible mechanism in development of tolerance. *Fed. Proc., Fed. Amer. Soc. Exp. Biol.* **29**, 19-27.

Everett, G. M., and Borcherding, J. W. (1970). L-Dopa: Effect on concentrations of dopamine, norepinephrine and serotonin in brains of mice. *Science* **168**, 849-850.

Ferguson, J., Hendrikson, S., Cohen, H., Mitchell, G., Barchas, J., and Dement, W. (1970). "Hypersexuality" and behavioral changes in cats caused by administration of *p*-chlorophenylalanine. *Science* **168**, 499-501.

Jouvet, M. (1969). Biogenic amines and the states of sleep, *Science* **163**, 32-41.

Koe, B. K., and Weissman, A. (1966). *p*-Chlorophenylalanine: A specific depletor of brain serotonin. *J. Pharmacol. Exp. Ther.* **154**, 499-516.

Lipton, M. A., Gordon, R., Guroff, G., and Udenfriend, S. (1967). *p*-Chlorophenylalanine-induced chemical manifestations of phenylketonuria in rats. *Science* **156**, 248-250.

Maynert, E. W., and Klingman, G. (1962). Tolerance to morphine. I. Effects on catecholamines in the brain and adrenal glands. *J. Pharmacol. Exp. Ther.* **135**, 285-295.

Myers, R. D., and Veale, W. L. (1968). Alcohol preference in the rat: Reduction following depletion of brain serotonin. *Science* **160**, 1469-1471.

Pare, C. M. B., Sandler, M., and Stacey, R. S. (1957). 5-Hydroxytryptamine deficiency in phenylketonuria. *Lancet* **1**, 551-553.

Pare, C. M. B., Sandler, M., and Stacey, R. S. (1958). Decreased 5-hydroxytryptophan decarboxylase activity in phenylketonuria. *Lancet* **2**, 1099-1101.

Roffwarg, H. P., Muzio, J. N., and Dement, W. C. (1966). Ontogenetic development of the human sleep-dream cycle. *Science* **152**, 604-619.

Schlesinger, K., Schreiber, R. A., and Pryor, G. T. (1968). Effects of *p*-chlorophenylalanine on conditioned avoidance learning. *Psychom. Sci.* **11**, 225-226.

Sheard, M. H. (1969). The effect of *p*-chlorophenylalanine on behavior in rats: Relation to brain serotonin and 5-hydroxyindoleacetic acid. *Brain Res.* **15**, 524-528.

Shimizu, A., and Himwich, H. E. (1968). The ontogeny of sleep in kittens and young rabbits. *Electroencephalogr. Clin. Neurophysiol.* **24**, 307-318.

Sourkes, T. L., Murphy, G. F., Chavez, B., and Zielinska, M. (1961). The action of some α-methyl and other amino acids on cerebral catecholamines. *J. Neurochem.* **8**, 109-115.

Stevens, D. A., Resnick, O., and Krus, D. M. (1967). The effects of *p*-chlorophenylalanine, a depletor of brain serotonin, on behavior. I. Facilitation of discrimination learning. *Life Sci.* **6**, 2215-2220.

Stevens, D. A., Fechter, L. D., and Resnick, O. (1969). The effects of *p*-chlorophenylalanine, a depletor of brain serotonin on behavior: II. Retardation of passive avoidance learning. *Life Sci.* **8**, 379-385.

Sudak, H. S., and Maas, J. W. (1964a). Behavioral-neurochemical correlation in reactive and nonreactive strains of rats. *Science* **146**, 418-420.

Sudak, H. S., and Maas, J. W. (1964b). Central nervous system serotonin and norepinephrine localization in emotional and non-emotional strains in mice. *Nature (London)* **203**, 1254-1256.

Swaiman, K. F., Hosfield, W. B., and Lemieux, B. (1968). Elevated plasma phenylalanine concentration and lysine incorporation into ribosomal protein of developing brain. *J. Neurochem.* **15**, 687-690.

Tagliamonte, A., Tagliamonte, P., Gessa, G. L., and Brodie, B. B. (1969). Compulsive sexual activity induced by *p*-chlorophenylalanine in normal and pinealectomized male rats. *Science* **166**, 1433-1435.

Tenen, S. S. (1967). The effects of *p*-chlorophenylalanine, a serotonin depletor, on avoidance acquisition, pain sensitivity and related behavior in the rat. *Psychopharmacologia* **10**, 204-219.

Way, E. L., Loh, H. H., and Shen, F. (1968). Morphine tolerance, physical dependence and synthesis of brain 5-hydroxytryptamine. *Science* **162**, 1290-1292.

Weitzman, E. D., Rapport, M. M., McGregor, P., and Jacoby, J. (1968). Sleep patterns of the monkey and brain serotonin concentration: Effect of *p*-chlorophenylalanine. *Science* **160**, 1361-1363.

Woolley, D. W., and van der Hoeven, T. (1965). Serotonin deficiency in infancy as a cause of a mental defect in experimental phenylketonuria. *Int. J. Neuropsychiat.* **1**, 529-544.

GENERAL DISCUSSION

Dr. Schulte: Table I and Fig. 1 show results which might challenge current theories about 5-HT, its role in the maintenance of sleep, and the distribution of active vs quiet sleep. We studied infants with PKU, since these infants are known to have a very low 5-HT level: 22 untreated infants and young children with PKU, from 4 weeks to 4 years of age, were compared with 22 normal infants and children of exactly the same age. Furthermore, 13 untreated PKU infants were compared with 13 infants equal in age but with PKU under dietary control. In all untreated infants, PA levels were markedly elevated, the $FeCl_3$ urine test was positive, and plasma 5-HT was low. In all infants under dietary treatment, the corresponding values were normalized. Then 2-3-hr polygraphic recordings were made under identical conditions and the records were analyzed in a single blind fashion, i.e., the interpreter did not know the infants' condition. No difference could be detected in the distribution of active vs quiet sleep between normal and PKU infants as well as between treated and untreated infants (Table I).

I would like to have your comments on these as yet unpublished results. For me, it is difficult to make a case for the role of 5-HT in the distribution of sleep states, since PKU is really a good natural experiment with a remarkably disturbed 5-HT metabolism normalizing under dietary treatment.

Dr. Metcalf: Twenty-two infants were not treated?

Dr. Schulte: Twenty-two untreated PKU infants were matched for age with 22 normal control infants, and 13 untreated PKU infants were matched for age with 13 PKU infants under biochemically successful dietary control.

Dr. Metcalf: Were those significant differences?

Dr. Schulte: No, no significant differences could be detected in the distribution of active vs quiet sleep in the corresponding groups of infants.

Dr. Purpura: Do you have the 5-HT levels?

Dr. Schulte: Yes, 5-HT always significantly increased during therapy. This is also well known from other studies.

Dr. Metcalf: I would like to comment on our longitudinal studies of children with PKU. We have not studied sleep cycles developmentally but find there is an earlier age of onset of K-complex sleep spindle development in these children. We see certain configurations (distorted K-complex spindle combinations) a year or two earlier with PKU than is the case with control infants. I think this must be a very complex cortical control relationship and I wonder what you are going to find in these children.

Dr. Schulte: As you know, some years ago, we published results on spindle development in infants and young children with PKU (Gross and Schulte, 1969). They have significantly more and longer sleep spindles than normal infants of the same age (Fig. 1).

Dr. Resnick: It appears from your slide that there is a marked difference in the second cycle between the untreated and treated infants.

TABLE I *Sleep Cycles in Phenylketonuria (PKU)*

Infants	Quiet sleep (%)		
	Cycle I	Cycle II	Cycles I and II
PKU-untreated	57.0 ± 20.5	66.2 ± 17.2	59.6 ± 19.8
N = 22	n = 21	n = 8	n = 29
Control	58.2 ± 19.7	55.6 ± 16.2	57.4 ± 18.5
N = 22	n = 21	n = 8	n = 29
PKU-untreated	60.4 ± 18.2	71.1 ± 9.9	63.5 ± 16.7
N = 13	n = 12	n = 5	n =17
PKU-treated	64.9 ± 17.2	55.0 ± 18.3	62.0 ± 17.7
N = 13	n = 12	n = 5	n = 17

Dr. Schulte: There are certainly differences between one or the other individual sleep cycles. In some infants, we had a little less quiet sleep in the first cycle, but after that, a little more in the second one. If one combines all cycles recorded there is no significant difference between normal vs abnormal and treated vs untreated infants. As a matter of fact, the percentages are almost exactly the same. I am tempted to say they are almost too identical to be true.

Dr. Dement: With regard to the effect of PCPA, we have studied the problem in cats extensively, utilizing chronic administration as opposed to acute administration from both a biochemical and physiological point of view. Chronic administration produces a very complicated but very consistent syndrome, not simply an effect on SWS.

Very briefly, the phasic activity of REMS is enhanced early in the treatment period. For 2 days, there is minimal effect on SWS. Then a profound insomnia develops which lasts 3-4 days. At the same time, phasic activities—PGO spikes of REMS—cease to be regulated at all. They are discharged continually in wakefulness, REMS and NREMS. Around the sixth or seventh PCPA day, there is a return of NREMS and REMS. Thus, in the virtual absence of brain 5-HT, there can be almost normal levels of SWS.

The transient insomnia is very consistent and there are some interesting findings in connection with it. For example, during this period barbiturates will not induce NREMS, whereas thorazine will induce a dramatic return of essentially normal-looking SWS. Pargyline will also produce profound sleep in the PCPA animal but not in the normal. The question that really intrigues us, however, is, why does sleep return? The first point to make is that it is not totally normal sleep. There are spindles and slow waves, but the configuration of sleep stages is quite different.

The usual sequence of wake to NREM to REM is reversed in the chronic PCPA cat. It tends to be wake to REMS to NREMS. This may be a very important point when we compare results in the cat to results obtained by other investigators in humans with chronic PCPA treatment, and in the rat. In addition, the more or less unregulated discharge of phasic activity in REMS and in SWS in the chronic PCPA-treated cat continues. We feel that the best bet for explaining the return of sleep in the cat is really a readjustment of some 5-HT antagonist.

Jack Barchas and his colleagues at Stanford have obtained evidence that there is a change in turnover of noradrenaline (NA), which is not surprising. However, this change in turnover of NA is below controls in resting PCPA-treated rats and higher than controls in PCPA rats who are fighting. So there is probably some marked alteration in the way these two systems interact, which is clearly seen in the evidence of *l*-dopa having a depleting effect of 5-HT in mice that was mentioned before.

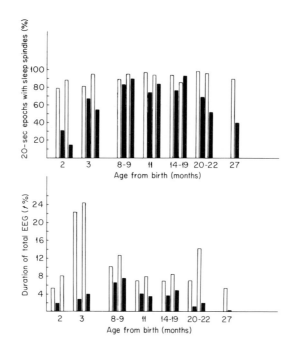

Fig. 1. Occurrence and duration of sleep spindles during quiet (NREM) sleep in normal vs. PKU infants and young children. (■) Control infants; (□) infants with PKU.

We are not interested in PCPA effects, of course. We are really interested in what is happening in normal animals. If we assume that 5-HT mediates SWS, the turnover must be more active in SWS and less active in wakefulness or REMS. If this were true, we might expect small changes in 5-HT levels as a function of these states. Arabinda Sindha and Steve Henriksen have been doing studies in cats with cannulae implanted in the heart, so they can be killed instantly with potassium injections.

They kill the animal after 5 min of REMS—pure REMS—or 20 min of SWS or 20 min of wakefulness. You can't do this in the rat because the sleep stages are too brief. Pilot results suggest that brain stem 5-HT is higher in the cat killed during the REM phase or wakefulness as opposed to SWS.

This could be some evidence supporting Jouvet's hypothesis.

Dr. Clemente: Are you saying that 5-HT levels are lower following SWS?

Dr. Dement: Utilization is higher, we presume; that is why the level goes down. In REMS, the level goes up.

Dr. Clemente: I just wonder how far the defenders of the serotonergic concept of the onset of SWS wish to carry their idea. It is very difficult for me to conceive of levels of almost any humor changing so rapidly in the nervous system, to account for an almost instantaneous onset of sleep, especially in a conditioning situation. For example, the lights are on in this room and all of us are awake; suddenly the lights go out and a slide goes on the board and our jaws become relaxed, our eyes droop, and off we go to sleep. Are you saying that within a matter of seconds or a minute 5-HT levels can change to be the trigger for the onset of sleep? Is this what Jouvet is saying?

Dr. Dement: No, I am merely suggesting that if serotonergic neurons are more active during NREMS and more 5-HT is utilized at the synapse, then there might be a relatively small drop in the level because synthesis never quite catches up. Similarly, there might be a relative rise in the level during REMS if serotonergic neurons are not so active as synthesis gets ahead of synaptic utilization. We assume that this kind of change may need a little time, which is why we have begun the experiments in the cat whose sleep phases persist for longer periods of time.

Dr. Purpura: I don't know why you are surprised that enzyme levels can change rapidly. Anybody who has tried to remove brains for biochemical studies is aware of this.

Dr. Clemente: I can appreciate that serotonergic pathways might be involved in sleep behavior, but it is hard for me to understand that levels of 5-HT in the brain become radically changed so quickly as to alter our behavior, and that this substance is the responsible trigger mechanism for the onset of SWS.

Dr. Dement: First, we are not talking about radical differences in level. Secondly, we are not talking about trigger mechanisms. We are assuming, perhaps wrongly, that serotonergic activity is what produces the unique properties of NREMS and that when this state is present, we can assume that serotonergic neurons are more active. Conclusive results, let alone the pilot data I have mentioned, would not prove the 5-HT hypothesis, but it would be a step in that direction.

Dr. Weitzman: One must differentiate the problem of the initiation of sleep, either because of environmental determinants or circadian rhythmic events from the continuation or maintenance of sleep, once having been initiated. I don't think anyone has postulated that 5-HT is concerned with the initiation of sleep or is the specific determinant of the circadian rhythm or initiates SWS or NREMS.

The evidence is supportive of the notion, but certainly not proved, that once an animal goes to sleep, if one alters 5-HT the amount of SWS decreases. In our studies, we recorded monkeys for 24 hr/day and continuously defined their sleep-wake state (Weitzman *et al.,* 1968). There were 12 hr with lights on and 12 hr with lights off. The monkeys went to sleep when the lights went out. In the monkey, one can differentiate stages 1 through 4 NREMS, as in man. When we compared the amount of stage 3-4 with stage 1-2, there was significantly less 3-4 than 1-2 sleep, whereas REMS was not changed in absolute amount. Therefore, the percentage of REM to total sleep actually increased.

Dr. Kleitman pointed to this problem years ago, that we have to talk about initiation as well as maintenance of sleep. Little attention has been paid in the field to what is the determinant of the dominant 24-hr sleep-wakefulness cycle. Most people are concerned with the mechanisms that allow the phenomenon to persist once initiated. These may well be different mechanisms.

Dr. Sterman: Whether we like it or not, we are stuck with the neurochemical model Jouvet has given us. To my knowledge, there is no solid evidence that electrical stimulation of the raphe nuclei produces any change that could be interpreted physiologically as the onset of sleep.

Moreover, with regard to PCPA-induced changes in the amount of sleep, I have always been struck by the fact that the human subjects studied by Cremata and Koe (1968), showed no striking sleep disturbances, but reported dizziness, nausea, and a number of other unpleasant symptoms in response to PCPA. I know, from our work with cats, that emesis, respiratory difficulties, or other such disturbances cause a profound decrease in both patterns of sleep. So I wonder if the administration of drugs which disturb physiology in these numerous ways might not be expected to produce such changes in sleep.

Dr. Roberts: I want to try on for size a hypothesis about what 5-HT and NE might be doing at membranes. If these latter substances activate membrane adenyl cyclases, one of the results may be that this will give a faster rate of delivery of ATP to the sodium pump. In this manner, these substances would be inhibitory, because they would allow a membrane segment to repolarize or resist depolarization more effectively than before the substances were delivered onto the membrane. Is that okay?

If that is the case, we should be able to affect sleep mechanisms by things that affect the sodium pump. Substances which, for example, inhibit the sodium pump might inhibit sleep, an effect opposite to that of 5-HT.

Dr. Himwich: Someone has tried with an adult brain.

Dr. Purpura: It produces seizures.

Dr. Resnick: Can't they be excitatory?

Dr. Roberts: Only if they inhibit.

Dr. Resnick: For example, in the isolated aorta, NE will cause sodium ions to enter and potassium ions to leave the muscle cells, thus producing depolarization.

Dr. Roberts: But has it been shown in neurons?

Dr. Purpura: Which neurons? In helix cells it can both excite and inhibit.

Dr. Roberts: In a vertebrate organism?

Dr. Purpura: No, in the snail. It has not been so identified in the vertebrate.

Dr. Hoffer: In the cerebellum, we have been able to record intracellularly from Purkinje cells during extracellular application of NE. NE produces hyperpolarization of the membrane associated with a decreased conductance, opposite to classical IPSP's. If NE action is mediated by cAMP, these effects might be considered to be a "metabolic hyperpolarization." We are still investigating the mechanism for the potential change.

Dr. Roberts: If the sodium pump is set at submaximal level, normally, you could push it up to a higher level of activity by 5-HT or NE.

Dr. Hoffer: It is interesting that Gessa and Brodie (Gessa *et al.,* 1970) have been able to induce sleeping behavior by injection of cAMP into the cerebellum of cats and rats. I don't think they have done the EEG analysis to determine whether it is SWS or REMS.

Dr. Purpura: What was the membrane potential of the cells studied?

Dr. Hoffer: We have studied over 40 cells. Our membrane potentials have varied from ~25 to 80 mV.

Dr. Purpura: NE increased this above that level?

Dr. Hoffer: We have done i.v. curves and haven't been able to get the hyperpolarization to reverse during an i.v. curve.

Dr. Purpura: Did you measure the membrane conductance?

Dr. Hoffer: Yes, there is an increased membrane resistance.

Dr. Purpura: If you are correct in this, I believe it would be the first demonstration in the vertebrate CNS of a putative transmitter activation of an electrogenic sodium pump. Of course, one must be very careful about this, as recent experience in invertebrate neuronal systems has indicated, since the conductance change may be at remotely located synapses and reversal potentials may be difficult to establish to prove or disprove an electrogenic pump mechanism.

Dr. Hoffer: This is a difficult problem to attack in mammals, since one has to be able to manipulate extracellular and intracellular ions to prove that an electrogenic sodium pump is involved. While activation of an electrogenic pump is one possibility, these changes might also be produced by reduction of a resting sodium conductance, as has been found in the turtle retina.

Dr. Resnick: Dilantin markedly inhibits the sodium pump. What effect has Dilantin on sleep?

Dr. Dement: There are similar data from both humans and cats. Dilantin does not affect NREMS at a dose of 9 mg/kg. After 10 days on this dose, the cat starts to show toxicity.

Dr. Essman: It also elevates GABA, which goes up with sleep deprivation.

Dr. Roberts: It is hard to say what that means. The GABA neurons may not be firing continually, and increased levels could be attributable to a block in release or decrease in destruction after release. It can be very deceptive to talk about GABA levels. When one builds up the levels in brain by treating with aminooxyacetic acid and thus blocking GABA degradation by the transaminase pathway, there is only a slight and brief decrease in susceptibility to electroconvulsive seizures in the presence of a sixfold increase in brain GABA levels. This probably can be attributed to the accumulation of GABA largely in postsynaptic and glial sites, while the synaptically effective GABA in presynaptic sites may not be increased greatly. We need to develop a procedure by which the turnover of synaptic GABA can be measured.

Dr. Resnick: What are the effects of steroids on sleep? As you know, aldosterone is the most active regulator of ion transport in and out of the cell.

Dr. Weitzman: We have not studied the effects of steroids on sleep, but we have studied the effect of sleep on steroids.

Dr. Dement: We gave rats enormous doses of dexamethasone. There was no effect at all and we were surprised. Some of the rats died of massive infection, which I am sure was the effect of the drug.

Dr. Resnick: Steroids are also quite effective as MAO inhibitors.

Dr. Weitzman: After inversion of the sleep-waking cycle in one normal human adult, essentially no cortisol was found in the plasma for a 7- or 8-hr sleep period during the day. We obtained samples every half hour via a catheter, and the subject slept quite well.

Dr. Gordon: I am glad somebody mentioned that, because in the interpretation of some of the slides shown, such as those of Dr. Roberts, there were marked increases in enzyme activity right after birth. With some enzymes, there are big changes after birth and they are really not ontogenetic; they are a reflection of being born, sometimes a reflection of how one is born (Gordon, 1967). I wonder whether the animals that were being studied were delivered by caesarean section or were born vaginally.

We have information on this in a field that has nothing to do with sleep. In babies who were born to diabetic mothers, Cornblath and I (Cornblath *et al.*, 1961) were trying to raise blood sugar with glucagon. We found we could not raise it in the babies of diabetic mothers, but we could in normal babies.

We looked further, and it turned out that babies of diabetic mothers had been born by caesarean section, for the most part, and the normals had been born vaginally. We went back and obtained adequate controls and found glucagon ineffective in babies born by caesarean section to mothers who did not have diabetes and had not labored.

So it was not a question of diabetes; it was the question of the mode of delivery and whether the mother had labored. Dr. Migeon at the time was showing that a woman in labor had high corticoids in her blood, and that was easy to understand. So Dr. Cornblath took the babies born to mothers by caesarean section—nondiabetic and without labor—and when we gave them cortisone, their response to glucagon was the same as in infants born vaginally.

In the interpretation of some of the curves, with rises of enzyme activity after birth, one has to consider the effect of this and maybe other hormones.

Dr. Anders: We have done a study on plasma cortisol and growth hormone levels during the first month of life in human infants during different states of sleep and wakefulness. We obtained peripheral blood by heel stick during four behavioral states—NREMS, REMS, quiet wakefulness, and crying—after the infant had sustained the state for 20 min.

Figure 2 demonstrates a dramatic and highly significant elevated plasma cortisol response during the state of crying in all infants. This response is presumably a stress or activation response and is clearly present as early as the first week of life. The plasma cortisol levels were not significantly different during the other behavioral states, though there was a trend toward higher levels during more active states.

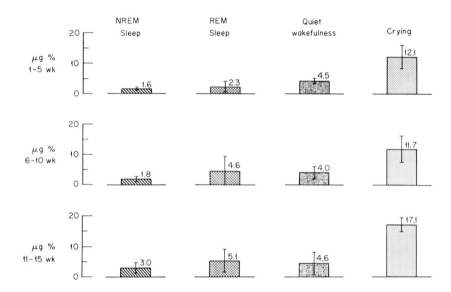

Fig. 2. Plasma cortisol, age, and behavioral state in human infants (mean and S.D.).

Figure 3 demonstrates that crying did not produce a significant increase of plasma growth hormone during the early weeks, though this has been described for adults (Reichlin, 1968). Further, despite previous reports that growth hormone is markedly elevated in the first weeks of life (Cornblath *et al.*, 1965), even our youngest subjects had adult basal levels during the state of quiet wakefulness.

We conclude from this that different hormone responses mature at different rates, and more importantly, that behavioral state is an important variable that needs to be controlled when studying these responses in the newborn.

Dr. Gordon: You have to get back into the delivery room; that is where the mother's cortisol affects the responses.

Dr. Roberts: Doesn't secretion of growth hormone increase during SWS and get shut off during REM?

Dr. Weitzman: The evidence is that during the first 2 hr of sleep in an adult, there is a significant secretion of growth hormone. During the latter part of the night, when most of the REMS is occurring, there is a decrease or absence of growth hormone, although there are occasionally little bursts of growth hormone. It is still premature to say that this is related to a specific sleep stage. It is clearly related to a time period of 1-2 hr following sleep onset.

We have some data also on growth hormone in the newborn period (Shaywitz *et al.*, 1970). We tried to correlate growth hormone to sleep state in the newborn and were unable to do so. We did not find that there was a clear relationship between a sleep state and the growth hormone elevation. However, we did find, as Dr. Anders just mentioned, that during the first 2 or 3 days after birth, the infants have high growth hormone values (80-100 ng/ml). By the fourth through the eighth day, the oldest we studied, the hormones were down to the fairly normal range (10-20 ng/ml).

Dr. Essman: Just a casual observation on growth hormone and sleep: we observed a number of years ago that from 19 to 20 days of daily growth hormone administration to male mice, individually housed, produced a very high incidence of nest-building by these

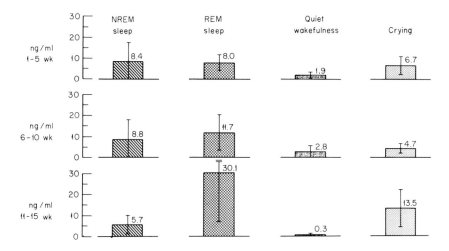

Fig. 3. Plasma growth hormone, age, and behavioral state in human infants (mean and S.D.).

animals; these were a shallow type of sleeping nest in which the mice spent a considerable amount of time during the 8 AM to 6 PM period of the day during full illumination.

Dr. Purpura: This subject relates to the whole problem of biogenic amines and sleep and wakefulness behavior. May I remind you that we know very little about the morphology of these systems.

REFERENCES

Cornblath, M., Ganzon, A. F., Nicolopoulos, D., Baens, G. S., Hollander, R. J., Gordon, M. H., and Gordon, H. H. (1961). Studies of carbohydrate metabolism in the newborn infant. III. Some factors influencing the capillary blood sugar and the response to glucagon during the first hours of life. *Pediatrics* 27, 378-389.

Cornblath, M., Parker, M., Reisner, S., Forbes, A., and Daughaday, W. (1965). Secretion and metabolism of growth hormone in premature and full-term infants. *J. Clin. Endocrinol. Metab.* 25, 209-218.

Cremata, V. Y., and Koe, B. K. (1968). Clinical and biochemical effects of fenclonine: A serotonin depletor. *Dis. Nerv. Syst.* 29, 147-152.

Gessa, G. Krishna, G., Fron, J., and Brodie, D. (1970). Behavioral and vegetative effects produced by dibutyryl cyclic AMP injected in different areas of the brain. *In* "The Role of Cyclic AMP in Cell Function" (P. Greengard and E. Costa, eds.), pp. 371-381. Raven Press, New York.

Gordon, H. H. (1967). Some biological aspects of premature birth, *In* "A Symposium on the Child" (J. A. Askin, R. E. Cooke, and J. A. Haller, Jr., eds.), pp. 233-253. John Hopkins Press, Baltimore, Maryland.

Gross, H. P., and Schulte, F. H. (1969). Über vermehrte Spindelaktivität im Schlaf-EEG bei Kindern mit Phenylketonurie. *Z. Kinderheilk.* 105, 324-333.

Reichlin, S. (1968). Hypothalamic control of growth hormone secretion and the response to stress. *In* "Endocrinology and Human Behavior" (R. P. Michael, ed.), p. 256. Oxford Univ. Press, London and New York.

Shaywitz, B., Finklestein, J., Hellman, L., and Weitzman, E. D. (1970). Human growth hormone in newborn infants during sleep-wake periods. *Psychophysiol.* **7**, 322.

Weitzman, E. D., Rapport, M. M., McGregor, P., and Jacoby, J. (1968). Sleep patterns of the monkey and brain serotonin concentration: Effect of *p*-chlorophenylalanine. *Science* **160**, 1361-1363.

7

Developmental Changes in Neurochemistry during the Maturation of Sleep Behavior

Williamina A. Himwich

Ontogenetic variation in the amount of time occupied by paradoxical sleep (PS), slow wave sleep (SWS), and the waking state is a gradually changing but nevertheless clear-cut phenomenon affording the opportunity to correlate biochemical changes in the developing brain with concomitant neurophysiological events. Jouvet (1969) demonstrated through the use of drugs and brain lesions in a series of elegant experiments a relationship of biogenic amines to the states of sleep in the adult animal. However, we do not yet have enough data on the biochemical changes in pertinent discrete areas of the brain in immature animals to determine whether the same or similar mechanisms are involved in concomitant decreases in PS occurring during development. In the young animal the lack of homeostasis militates against the use of lesion-producing techniques. Furthermore the relative inactivity of enzymes for the pathways which metabolize drugs modifies the effects of drugs in the neonate (Fouts and

Adamson, 1959; Nyhan, 1961). Nor has it been determined to what extent the earlier maturation of the caudad portions of the brain may be responsible for the predominance of PS in the newborn of species born immature, a predominance which diminishes perceptibly as the adult level of integration is achieved in the forebrain.

The records of Shimizu and Himwich (1968b) show the EEG, EMG, and respiration during periods of wakefulness, SWS, and activated sleep, called, respectively, calm or tranquil sleep and sleep with jerks in the neonate, for at this age it is the absence or presence of jerking movements rather than the EEG activity which distinguishes the two states. The traces show episodes typical of the two kinds of sleep (Fig. 1) and of wakefulness. In the studies in the kitten by Shimizu and Himwich (1968a, b, 1969) the patterns of sleep and of wakefulness (Fig. 2), and the changing relationships between the two types of sleep and wakefulness followed a developmental course essentially the same as that later described by Madame Jouvet and colleagues (Jouvet-Mounier *et al.*, 1970). However, Shimizu and Himwich presented most of their data as percentage of total recording time, whereas Jouvet-Mounier *et al.* (1970) used the ratio % $[(SP/ST)NN] / [(SP/ST)A]$ (SP = paradoxical sleep; ST = total sleep; NN = neonate; and A = adult). The change in the sleep cycle in the kitten consists primarily of a decrease in activated sleep and an increase in SWS. It is interesting to note that Shimizu and Himwich (1969) found a decrease in wakefulness in the older kitten which they attributed to the recording situation in that younger kittens need to be fed more often than older ones and so became hungry and were, therefore, awake a greater percentage of the time. However, Jouvet-Mounier *et al.* (1970), recording continuously for 24 hr from kittens left with the mother, also found decreased wakefulness in kittens from the 1st to the 15th postnatal day.

In the rabbit the same changes in the relationship between SWS and PS occur, but the mature relation is attained at an earlier age (Shimizu and Himwich, 1968b) (Fig. 3). As maturation is achieved, the proportions of SWS and activated sleep comprising total sleep alter, i.e., the percentage of time spent in SWS increases while that of activated sleep decreases. The number of episodes of both kinds of sleep occurring during 1 hr decreases (Fig. 4), but it should be noted that that of SWS decreases moderately during only the first postnatal week and then remains fairly constant, while that of PS falls sharply between 1 and 10 days, then decreases moderately up to about 23 days. The duration of the single episodes of SWS shows a steady increase, while that of episodes of activated sleep increases slightly during the first week, then decreases (Fig. 5).

We have been interested in studying the development of biogenic amines (Table I) in the brains of young animals (Agrawal *et al.*, 1966b). In general, the levels of noradrenaline (NA), dopamine, and serotonin (5-HT) increase from birth to adulthood in all of the species we have studied. Of these three biogenic amines,

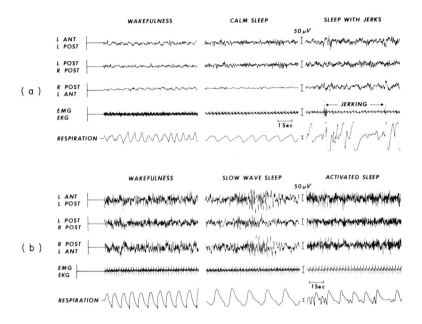

Fig. 1 Wakefulness and sleep in rabbit with implanted electrodes. Bipolar recordings of anterior and posterior cortical activity, EMG, EKG, and respiration (a) 3-day-old rabbit; (b) 10-day-old rabbit. (Shimizu and Himwich, 1968c.)

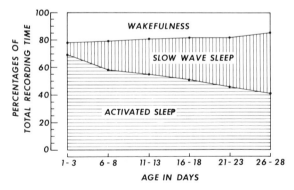

Fig. 2. Ontogeny of sleep and wakefulness as percentages of total recording time in kitten during the first 28 days of life. (Shimizu and Himwich, 1968c.)

dopamine is the last to attain the adult level, at least in the rat and the mouse (Agrawal *et al.*, 1968). Unfortunately, in only a few instances have we been able to correlate changes in the levels of these biogenic amines with concomitant determination of sleep in the same species.

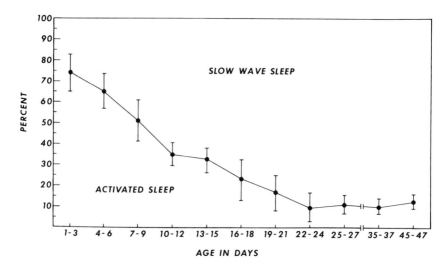

Fig. 3. Relation of activated sleep and slow wave sleep as percentage of total sleeping time in the developing rabbit. (Shimizu and Himwich, 1968c.)

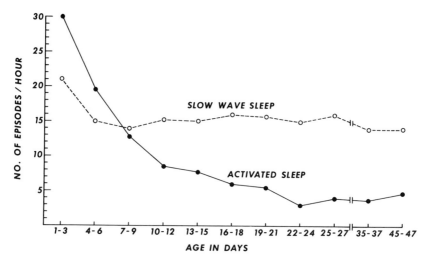

Fig. 4. Number of episodes per hour of activated and slow wave sleep during development in the rabbit. (Shimizu and Himwich, 1968c.)

To facilitate the observation of concomitant biochemical and neurophysiological events, we have attempted to depict graphically the levels of the biogenic amines and other biochemical constituents as well as a comparison of the ratios of PS to total sleep in the developing and the adult animal. The data for the rat, rabbit, and cat are presented in separate graphs in which the ordinate represents

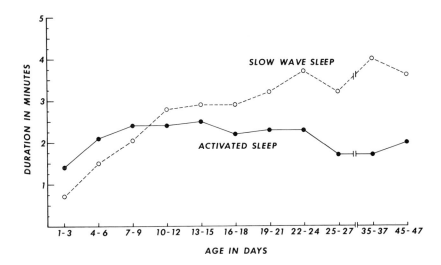

Fig. 5. Duration in minutes of single episodes of activated and slow wave sleep in the developing rabbit. (Shimizu and Himwich, 1968c.)

TABLE I *Changes of Monoamines of Rat and Mouse Brain during Development[a]*

Age (days)	Serotonin[b]		Dopamine[b]		Norepinephrine[b]	
	Rat[c]	Mouse[d]	Rat[c]	Mouse[d]	Rat[c]	Mouse[d]
0	0.16 ± 0.03	0.21 ± 0.02	0.28 ± 0.15	0.30 ± 0.10	0.06 ± 0.03	0.07 ± 0.01
5	0.17 ± 0.03	0.22 ± 0.05	0.29 ± 0.16	0.32 ± 0.10	0.13 ± 0.05	0.15 ± 0.03
10	0.19 ± 0.05	0.24 ± 0.04	0.31 ± 0.07	0.26 ± 0.10	0.16 ± 0.00	0.14 ± 0.03
15	0.19 ± 0.03	0.39 ± 0.04	0.31 ± 0.08	0.33 ± 0.05	0.18 ± 0.00	0.14 ± 0.03
20		0.31 ± 0.04		0.50 ± 0.05		0.19 ± 0.04
25	0.29 ± 0.03	0.38 ± 0.05	0.39 ± 0.15	0.60 ± 0.09	0.23 ± 0.09	0.25 ± 0.04
30		0.32 ± 0.05		0.85 ± 0.10		0.26 ± 0.05
35	0.33 ± 0.05		0.44 ± 0.11		0.31 ± 0.00	
40	0.29 ± 0.06		0.67 ± 0.19		0.41 ± 0.00	
Adult	0.33 ± 0.05	0.41 ± 0.04	0.90 ± 0.15	1.33 ± 0.24	0.41 ± 0.00	0.31 ± 0.09

[a]From Agrawal and Himwich, 1970.
[b]Values are expressed as $\mu g/gm$ wet weight tissue ± SD.
[c]Each value is the average of 8 determinations.
[d]Each value is the average of 6 determinations.

the period from birth to adulthood (Figs. 6-8). This correlated graph necessitated an adjustment of the values to fit the scale, in some cases expanding the curves and in others contracting them. I am uneasy about the graphs for this reason, and also because the actual values of the brain constituents cannot be calculated from the curves.

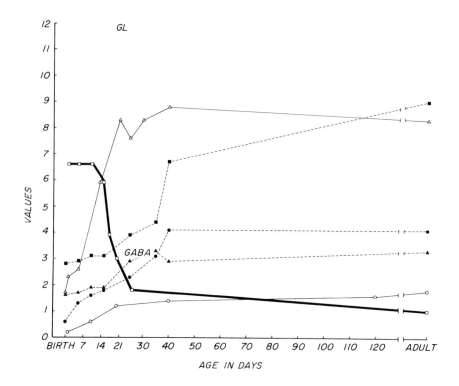

Fig. 6. Biochemical development of the rat correlated with changes in sleep patterns between birth and adult life. In this and in the two figures which follow the GL and GABA squares mark the attainment of the peak values of glutamic acid and GABA, respectively. (□)Ratio % [(SP/ST)NN] /[(SP/ST)A] ; (▲) serotonin, μg/g × 10 wet wt. tissue; (●) norepinephrine, μg/g × 10 wet wt. tissue; (■) dopamine, μg/g × 10 wet wt. tissue; (△) acetylcholinesterase, [mmoles/(hr − g)] /100 wet wt. tissue; (○) protein, mg/100 × absolute wt. (Serotonin, norepinephrine, and dopamine data from Agrawal *et al.* (1966b). GABA and glutamic acid data from Agrawal *et al.* (1966a); sleep ratio from Jouvet-Mounier *et al.* (1970); protein data from Donaldson (1924); acetylcholinesterase, Himwich (1969).

If we look at such a compiled graph for the rat (Fig. 6), it is apparent that the proportions of SWS and activated sleep characteristic of the adult sleep pattern appear before the adult levels of the biogenic amines, acetylcholinesterase (AChE), and protein are achieved. We have included cholinesterase because of the implication of acetylcholine in sleep by Jouvet (1969). These data were determined on whole brain and are, therefore, less applicable to our problem than data obtained from the pontine area would be. It is of course obvious that at the time of the height of PS the concentrations of both 5-HT and NA are low in whole brain. These values do not reach the adult levels until the rat is approximately 40 days of age. In the case of this animal, it is interesting that while dopamine continues to increase to adulthood, the other two compounds, NA and 5-HT, do not increase after approximately 40 days. Essentially, the same picture is seen in the mouse. If the relative maturity of the caudad portions of the brain is considered, it may well be that the serotonergic and the adrenergic cells of this area possess their mature complement of these neurotransmitters, but the concentrations determined in whole brain may be so diluted by the presence of other less mature tissue in which the levels are still low that no valid conclusions can be drawn. The best way to approach this problem may not be through direct chemical analyses, but rather through histochemical techniques, which would give reasonable qualitative analyses of the contents of the biogenic amines in various nuclei. Just for comparison, I have included in the graphs two small squares, one for glutamic acid and one for GABA, which mark the attainment of the peak concentrations of these substances (Agrawal *et al.,* (1966a) and show the relation of these peaks to the development of the sleep cycle. A curve for GABA would be similar to those for the other constituents in that GABA reaches the mature level after PS has approached the mature proportion of total sleep.

The graphic representation of similar data in the rabbit leads us to approximately the same conclusions (Fig. 7). The later maturation of the chemical substances as compared to that of the pattern of sleep is perhaps not so obvious in these data for the rabbit as in those for the rat. I should point out that in this species, in contrast to the rat, the levels of 5-HT are higher than those of norepinephrine (NE) throughout development (H. E. Himwich *et al.,* 1967).

In the cat, the experimental animal par excellence for the study of PS as attested by the many excellent works that have appeared using this animal, we see the development of a mature sleep pattern some time after 70 days of age (Fig. 8). Previous to this time, change in the pattern is slow as compared to the very marked change which occurs fairly early in both the rat and the rabbit. The neonatal cat also differs in that it spends less time in PS than do the newborn rat and rabbit (Jouvet-Mounier *et al.,* 1970). In comparison with this, the biogenic amines in the pons-medulla reach mature levels at about 30 days, although there are further slight changes after that time (H. E. Himwich *et al.,* 1967). In contrast, in the hypothalamus there is a second spurt in the concentration of 5-HT occurring at about 180 days. NE reaches its peak in that area at about 30 days and then falls to the adult value. Although in this case we do have data on pons-medulla, we are still unable to make a good correlation between the maturation of the sleep patterns and the concentrations of the biogenic amines. Unfortunately the excellent study of tyrosine hydroxylase by McGeer *et al.,* (1967) casts little effective light on the role of catecholamines (CA) in the sleep pattern of immature animals.

The administration of chlorpromazine, 10 mg/kg orally in a single dose

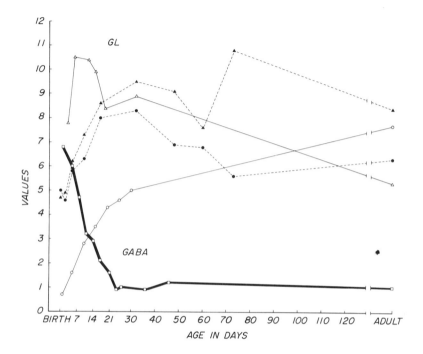

Fig. 7. Biochemical development of the rabbit correlated with changes in sleep patterns between birth and adult life. ($\triangle$) Cholinesterase, mmoles acetylthiocholine hydrolyzed/g wet tissue (hr $\times$ 10); ($\bigcirc$) protein, (mg/whole brain)/100; ($\square$) ratio % [(SP/ST)NN]/[SP/ST)A]; ($\blacktriangle$) serotonin, μg/g $\times$ 10 wet wt. tissue; ($\bullet$) norepinephrine, μg/g $\times$ 10 wet wt. tissue. (Sleep ratio adapted from Shimizu and Himwich (1968b); norepinephrine and serotonin data from H. E. Himwich *et al.* (1967); glutamic acid and GABA data from Agrawal *et al.* (1966/1967); cholinesterase data from McCaman and Aprison (1964); protein values from Chanda and Himwich, 1969.)

repeated no oftener than every 5 days, had little effect on wakefulness in the kitten until the age of 21-23 days when wakefulness was significantly decreased (Shimizu and Himwich, 1969). This decrease was accompanied by an increase in SWS (Fig. 9). You can see that the increase in SWS occurred as early as 1-3 days and that this change was reflected in a decrease in activated sleep even at this early age. In the 16- to 18-day-old animal when the effect on wakefulness was just beginning to appear, there was a marked increase in SWS and a decrease in activated sleep. Propericiazine, a phenothiazine which does not have the sedating effect of chlorpromazine, had no effect on wakefulness (Fig. 9), but increased SWS and decreased activated sleep. Haloperidol acted somewhat similarly to chlorpromazine in that it reduced wakefulness and increased SWS (Shimizu and Himwich, 1969) (Fig. 10). In the case of imipramine (Fig. 11) wakefulness was

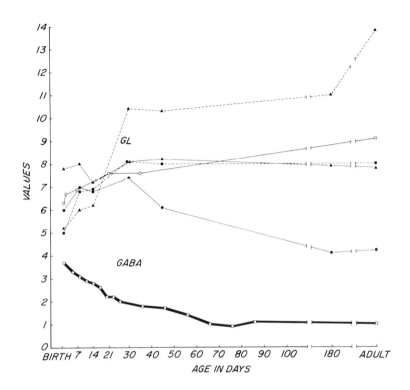

Fig. 8. Biochemical development of the cat correlated with changes in sleep patterns between birth and adult life. (– –) Hypothalamus; (—) pons-medulla; (▲) serotonin, $\mu g/g \times 10$; (●) norepinephrine, $\mu g/g \times 10$; (□) ratio % $[(SP/ST)NN]/[(SP/ST)A]$; (○) protein, % protein in mesodiencephalon. (Serotonin and norepinephrine data from H. E. Himwich *et al.* (1967); GABA and glutamic acid data from Berl and Purpura (1966); sleep ratio adapted from Shimizu and Himwich (1968b); protein data from Berl (1966).)

slightly increased in young animals and decreased in older ones. SWS increased at the expense of activated sleep. For the sake of comparison, it is helpful to look at the effects of these drugs in Fig. 12. As you can see, the effects on wakefulness are greatest in the chlorpromazine- and imipramine-treated groups with some effects also being present in the haloperidol-treated animals (Shimizu and Himwich, 1969). In regard to activated sleep, imipramine caused the greatest reduction and haloperidol the least. The changes in activated sleep are mirrored by those in SWS with imipramine causing the biggest increase in SWS and haloperidol the least. Amphetamine (Shimizu and Himwich, 1968a) was given at two dose levels, both of which increased wakefulness and SWS while markedly depressing activated sleep (Fig. 13).

The results of Shimizu and Himwich (1969) suggest that the effects of

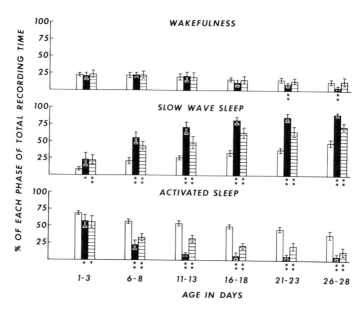

Fig. 9. Effects of two phenothiazines, administered orally, on phases of the sleep-wakefulness cycle in growing kittens. (☐) Control; (■) chlorpromazine, 10 mg/kg; (⊟) propericiazine, 3 mg/kg. (Taken from Shimizu and Himwich, 1969.)

psychotropic drugs are less apparent in neonates and become more marked during the growth period. The same was observed for amphetamine. At 21-28 days of age the effects of the drugs are similar to those in the adult cat. The action of imipramine in diminishing the percentage of time spent in wakefulness was not evident until the kittens were 16-18 days of age and became more prominent by 26-28 days. The effect of chlorpromazine in decreasing wakefulness was not apparent at 11-13 days, became noticeable at 16-18 days, but not significant until 21-23 days. It seems possible that the effects of these drugs on activated sleep are established at an earlier age than those on SWS and on wakefulness. These data may be explained by the relative immaturity of those neural structures and systems which are responsible for the development of the adult sleep-wakefulness cycle (Valatx *et al.,* 1964). Although we might expect that the drugs would be more potent in the younger animals, due to the lack of metabolizing enzymes, they seem actually, in this case, to be less effective.

These data suggest that these drugs, amphetamine as well as the tranquilizers, disturb the 5-HT-NE relationship so that, in general, calm sleep is increased at the expense of activated sleep even as early as 1-3 days. This may mean, as hypothesized by Jouvet (1969), that in the presence of drugs the "serotonergic mechanisms involved during slow sleep" do not "act as primary mechanisms" to trigger the PS to as great an extent as in the nonmedicated animal. On the other

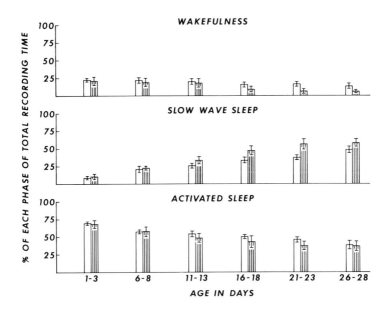

Fig. 10. Effects of haloperidol on phases of the sleep-wakefulness cycle in growing kittens. (☐) Control; (▥) haloperidol, 3 mg/kg orally. (Taken from Shimizu and Himwich, 1969.)

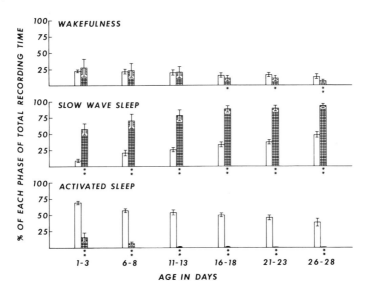

Fig. 11. Effects of imipramine on phases of the sleep-wakefulness cycle in growing kittens. (☐) Control; (▦) imipramine, 5 mg/kg orally. (Taken from Shimizu and Himwich, 1969.)

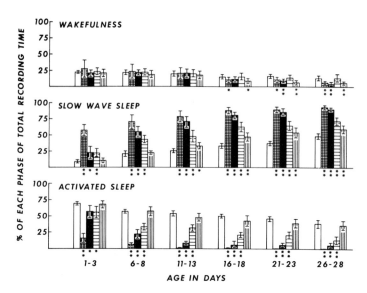

Fig. 12. Effects of four psychotropic drugs, administered orally, on phases of the sleep-wakefulness cycle in growing kittens. (☐)Control; (▦) imipramine, 5 mg/kg; (■) chlorpromazine, 10 mg/kg; (☰) propericiazine, 3 mg/kg; (▥) haloperidol, 3 mg/kg. (Shimizu and Himwich, 1969.)

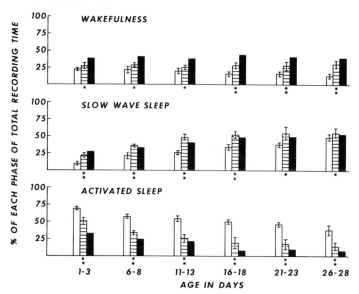

Fig. 13. Effects of amphetamine, administered orally, on phases of the sleep-wakefulness cycle in growing kittens. (☐) Control; (☰) 0.3 mg/kg; (■) 0.5 mg/kg. (Shimizu and Himwich, 1968a.)

hand, the action of the drugs may be upon the noradrenergic mechanisms in the locus coeruleus and the partial loss of these mechanisms may be responsible for the depression of PS. It has been reported (Gey and Pletscher, 1961; Pletscher and Gey, 1962) that two of the drugs used, imipramine and chlorpromazine, block membrane permeability and that haloperidol blocks NA (van Rossum, 1965) and lowers dopamine in the caudate (W. A. Himwich and Glisson, 1967). The administration of 12 mg/kg of chlorpromazine has no demonstrable effect on the biogenic amines in whole brain. Propericiazine, however, at a dose of 10 mg/kg in the adult rat, reduces NA from 0.42 ± 0.07 to 0.32 ± 0.05 $\mu g/g$ (Leiner, K. Y., and Himwich, W. A., 1969, unpublished data). This difference is statistically significant ($P < 0.01$). Amphetamine also depletes NA but only in large doses (8-20 mg/kg) (Glowinski and Axelrod, 1965). Smaller doses do not appear to affect NA (Javoy *et al.*, 1968).

However, the effects of these drugs on wakefulness in young animals are not seen until 16-18 days of age. Is there a degree of maturation necessary before wakefulness can be influenced by drugs? To examine the present biochemical status of some aspects of the developing brain, we shall return to Fig. 8. The time period, 16-18 days, precedes the nadir of the sleep ratio and also the peak of the concentrations of NE, 5-HT, or other constituents. It must also be kept in mind in interpreting these data that the environmental conditions of the experiment tend to promote sleep.

As Valatx *et al.*, (1964) have pointed out: "Paradoxical sleep is qualitatively different from, and ontogenetically older than slow sleep. Furthermore, it is probable that the neural structures which are responsible for the fast cortical activity during paradoxical sleep come into play sooner after birth than the neural structures responsible for cortical arousal during waking. Finally the onset of the high voltage slow waves of slow sleep appears to be contemporaneous with the achievement of cortical maturation."

REFERENCES

Agrawal, H. C., and Himwich, W. A. (1970). Amino acids, proteins and monoamines of developing brain. *In* "Developmental Neurobiology" (W. A. Himwich, ed.), pp. 287-310. Thomas, Springfield, Illinois.

Agrawal, H. C., Davis, J. M., and Himwich, W. A. (1966a). Postnatal changes in free amino acid pool of rat brain. *J. Neurochem.* 13, 607-615.

Agrawal, H. C., Glisson, S. N., and Himwich, W. A. (1966b). Changes in monoamines of rat brain during postnatal ontogeny. *Biochim. Biophys. Acta* 130, 511-513.

Agrawal, H. C., Davis, J. M., and Himwich, W. A. (1966/1967). Postnatal changes in free amino acid pool of rabbit brain. *Brain Res.* 3, 374-380.

Agrawal, H. C., Glisson, S. N., and Himwich, W. A. (1968). Developmental changes in monoamines of mouse brain. *Int. J. Neuropharmacol.* 7, 97-101.

Berl, S. (1966). Glutamine synthetase. Determination of its distribution in brain during development. *Biochemistry* 5, 916-922.

Berl, S., and Purpura, D. P. (1966). Regional development of glutamic acid compartmentation in immature brain. *J. Neurochem.* 13, 293-304.

Chanda, S. K., and Himwich, W. A. (1969). Unpublished data.

Donaldson, H. H., ed. (1924). "The Rat." Wistar Inst. Press, Philadelphia, Pennsylvania.

Fouts, J. R., and Adamson, R. H. (1959). Drug metabolism in the newborn rabbit. *Science* 129, 897-898.

Gey, K. F., and Pletscher, A. (1961). Influence of chlorpromazine and chlorprothixene on the cerebral metabolism of 5-hydroxytryptamine, norepinephrine and dopamine. *J. Pharmacol. Exp. Ther.* 133, 18-24.

Glowinski, J., and Axelrod, J. (1965). Effect of drugs on the uptake, release, and metabolism of H^3-norepinephrine in the rat brain. *J. Pharmacol. Exp. Ther.* 149, 43-49.

Himwich, H. E., Pscheidt, G. R., and Schweigerdt, A. K. (1967). Comparative studies on development of biogenic amines in brains of growing rabbits and cats. *In* "Regional Development of the Brain in Early Life" (A. Minkowski, ed.), pp. 273-296, Blackwell, Oxford.

Himwich, W. A. (1969). Unpublished data.

Himwich, W. A., and Glisson, S. N. (1967). Effect of haloperidol on caudate nucleus. *Int. J. Neuropharmacol.* 6, 329-332.

Javoy, F., Thierry, A. M., Kety, S. S., and Glowinski, J. (1968). The effect of amphetamine on the turnover of brain norepinephrine in normal and stressed rats. *Commun. Behav. Biol., Part A* 1, 43-48.

Jouvet, M. (1969). Biogenic amines and the states of sleep. *Science* 163, 32-41.

Jouvet-Mounier, D., Astic, L., and Lacote, D. (1970). Ontogenesis of the states of sleep in rat, cat, and guinea pig during the first postnatal month. *Develop. Psychobiol.* 2, 216-239.

McCaman, R. E., and Aprison, M. H. (1964). The synthetic and catabolic enzyme systems for acetylcholine and serotonin in several discrete areas of the developing rabbit brain. *In* "The Developing Brain" (W. A. Himwich and H. E. Himwich, eds.), *Progr. Brain Res.* vol. 9, pp. 220-223.

McGeer, E. G., Gibson, S., Wada, J. A., and McGeer, P. L. (1967). Distribution of tyrosine hydroxylase activity in adult and developing brain. *Can. J. Biochem.* 45, 1943-1952.

Nyhan, W. L. (1961). Toxicity of drugs in the neonatal period. *J. Pediat.* 59, 1-20.

Pletscher, A., and Gey, K. F. (1962). Action of imipramine and amitriptyline on cerebral monoamines as compared with chlorpromazine. *Med. Exp.* 6, 165-168.

Shimizu, A., and Himwich, H. E. (1968a). The effects of amphetamine on the sleep-wakefulness cycle of developing kittens. *Psychopharmacologia* 13, 161-169.

Shimizu, A., and Himwich, H. E. (1968b). The ontogeny of sleep in kittens and young rabbits. *Electroencephalogr. Clin. Neurophysiol.* 24, 307-318.

Shimizu, A., and Himwich, H. E. (1968c). Unpublished data.

Shimizu, A., and Himwich, H. E. (1969). Effects of psychotropic drugs on the sleep-wakefulness cycle of the developing kitten. *Develop. Psychobiol.* 2, 161-167.

Valatx, J. L., Jouvet, D., and Jouvet, M. (1964). Evolution électroencéphalographique des différents états de sommeil chez le chaton. *Electroencephalogr. Clin. Neurophysiol.* 17, 218-233.

van Rossum, J. M. (1965). Different types of sympathomimetic α-receptors. *J. Pharm. Pharmacol.* 17, 202-216.

GENERAL DISCUSSION

Dr. Ellingson: Is the cat brain a lot less susceptible to amphetamine than the human brain? You said 5 mg/kg. Even 0.5 mg/kg would make a total dose of 35 mg in a 70 kg man, which is a large dose for man.

Dr. Himwich: I had not thought about that. I was thinking in terms of using 3 mg/kg in the mouse.

Dr. Ellingson: They must be less susceptible than man.

Dr. Akiyama: I would like to ask a question about the sleep criteria which were used in drug-treated animals. Did the animals always fit your criteria for quiet sleep or activated sleep, or did you see another kind of sleep that did not seem to fit the criteria?

Dr Himwich: As far as I know, after they are 3 or 4 days old, there seems to be a little problem. Up to this age, Dr. Shimizu based his decision not only on the EEG record but also on respiration and on the EMG.

Dr. Resnick: Did you observe a correlation between the effects of the phenothiazines in reducing REMS with their ability to produce extrapyramidal side effects?

Dr. Himwich: We had seen this, not in the young animal, but in the adult dog. Never as consistently as I wished, however. I do believe that Dr. Kleitman and Dr. Dement are the people to answer that. I might throw this in to muddy things further. We have determined NA and 5-HT on cat, dog, rabbit, rat, and mouse, routinely. But we have never managed to get decent dopamine values for discrete areas of the brain, apart from the caudate nucleus. The values are completely inconsistent for some reason we cannot determine. Caudate values are consistent, however, at any age level.

Dr. Resnick: If the phenothiazines produce their effects by competing with the biogenic amines, then age differences in response to the psychotropic drugs may be determined by the stage of ontogeny and the concomitant levels of the cerebral biogenic amines.

Dr. Roberts: As I recall the experiments, the effective concentration is on the order of 10^{-7}. I would guess that phenothiazines may prolong effectiveness of NA by prolonging the lifespan of NA molecules within the synaptic gap.

Dr. Himwich: It might.

Dr. Roberts: I do not know of any data that show that imipramine or phenothiazines compete for the receptor with the NA or with the other CA's.

Dr. Resnick: I am referring to drug-induced Parkinsonism.

Dr. Roberts: I do not know any evidence that it competes at a receptor. You are talking about a symptom. I am talking about electrophysiological observations.

Dr. Resnick: I believe there are such data.

Dr. Roberts: I do not know what the reaction on the receptor is. In other words, when NE is liberated onto a nerve cell, an inhibitory effect is produced, presumably because of the activation of membrane adenyl cyclase. If the latter is the case, we would really expect that the effect would be accentuated if the lifespan of the NE molecule were prolonged. Thus, a given amount of liberated NE would be more effective per unit time on the receptor if imipramine were present to block its inactivation via reuptake.

Dr. Himwich: You would have to assume the normal complement of active enzymes or the lack of them in order to say that. Maybe Dr. Resnick or Dr. McGinty know if there are data showing that chlorpromazine inhibits at the cellular membrane, whereas imipramine inhibits uptake at the vesicular membrane.

Dr. Resnick: When the phenothiazines competitively inhibit the uptake of the biogenic amines, iatrogenic or drug-induced Parkinsonism occurs.

Dr. Himwich: Of course, with Parkinsonism, one problem seems to be the failure of uptake of tyrosine into the caudate nucleus.

Dr. Sterman: You must remember that the dependent variable here is something that we call sleep. We may be using this term in a far too restrictive manner. I like to think of the term sleep the way psychiatrists think of schizophrenia. We see many different patterns which probably reflect the fluctuating involvement of numerous neural mechanisms. Drugs may affect these mechanisms selectively, thereby changing some aspect of the manifestation, but not the process.

Dr. Himwich: After 10 days in the rabbit, you get nicely defined spindles.

Dr. Hoffer: I would like to say a few words in support of Dr. Roberts' suggestion on imipramine. I think there are good data from the peripheral nervous system that the imipramines act to block the membrane pump for NA and 5-HT. We have data from the cerebellum showing that after destruction of the adrenergic presynaptic terminals, desmethylimipramine is no longer effective. Since there are considerable data that reuptake is the major mechanism of termination of transmitter action at adrenergic synapses, one would predict that reuptake blockade would have very potent electrophysiological sequelae.

Dr. Himwich: Except Dr. Resnick was pointing out that the enzyme systems actually would destroy the NA very rapidly.

Dr. Roberts: Which enzymes are you talking about?

Dr. Himwich: COMT.

Dr. Hoffer: At peripheral adrenergic synapses, blocking reuptake greatly potentiates transmitter action, while blocking MAO and COMT has little physiological effect.

Dr. Anders: Was there any recovery of the REMS that seemed to be suppressed?

Dr. Himwich: Not during the recording period. These were uniform recording periods of 90 min, and during that time there was none.

Dr. Anders: An important developmental question is the age at which a recovery of response first appears. Our work with human infants and the work of Berger and Meier (1966) suggests that this response does not occur during the immediate newborn period.

Dr. Weitzman: May I add a clinical note. Dr. Bedrich Roth from Prague (Roth *et al.*, 1969) has reported that imipramine reduces symptoms of the type of narcolepsy associated with sleep onset, REM periods, as well as recurring REM periods, during the day. It had little effect on the NREM type of narcolepsy.

Dr. Purpura: I think Dr. Himwich has opened up here—and I must say it has been a major concern to us—this whole problem of developmental psychopharmacology.

REFERENCES

Berger, R., and Meier, G. (1966). The effects of selective deprivation of states of sleep in the developing monkey. *Psychophysiology* **2**, 354-371.

Roth, B., Bruhová, S., and Lehovský, P. (1969). REM sleep and NREM sleep in narcolepsy and hypersomnia. *Electroencephalogr. Clin. Neurophysiol.* **26**, 176-182.

8

Maturation of Neurobiochemical Systems Related to the Ontogeny of Sleep Behavior*

Peter J. Morgane

If I had to pick one neural system complex which seems to hold clues to a host of physiological and behavioral mechanisms, and might be a key element in establishing a neurology of motivation, I would certainly start with the medial forebrain bundle. This system welds the midbrain to the limbic system, basal forebrain area, and septum across a hypothalamic bridge in reciprocating circuits. As is well known, these channels have already been closely tied to feeding and sexual behavior, sleep, and a variety of instinctual drives, in addition to forming the substrate of the positive reinforcing (self-stimulation) systems in the brain. With respect to sleep mechanisms, the limbic structures linked to the brain stem via the medial forebrain bundle might well be considered important in the expression of basic biological drives forming the crucial link between the primitive mechanisms of dreaming sleep and the emotionally charged experi-

*Supported by grants from NIMH (MH-02211), NSF (GB-8066), NINDS (NS-03097), and USAF (AFOSR-62-364).

ences of dreaming (Snyder, 1963). There is little doubt that this bundle, heterogeneously organized into cholinergic, serotonergic, adrenergic, and dopaminergic systems, can only be fractionated by histochemical studies and chemitrode mapping of neurobehavioral systems, and these are already indicating a close link between this system complex and the states of sleep.

There are several remarks I wish to make relating especially to Dr. Himwich's chapter (Chapter 7), and I will do so while discussing certain topics and presenting our own related data at the same time. I shall begin with some general observations pertaining to ontogenetic studies in neurobiochemical systems and their interpretation.

One of the obvious values of the developmental approach lies in the possibility of relating the appearance of biochemical processes during maturation of the nervous system to the emergence of some well-defined functional phenomena, each identified by specific criteria of its own. However, with respect to the biochemical development of the neonate brain, it is obvious that a temporal sequence does not necessarily imply any causal connection or, in other words, correlation is most certainly not causation. In sleep states this becomes a most complex problem, as we really do not know how many possible states we are dealing with since definitions and criteria have been relatively inexact. Furthermore, it is not known whether each state, even as defined by electrographic and behavioral criteria, has its own privately wired circuit and biochemical substrate.

It has often been pointed out that the two central problems in relating biochemistry to behavior are those of quantification and correspondence. Biochemical data are practically always parametric, consisting of real numbers, and the variable can usually be expressed in explicit, operationally defined units. On the other hand, many important behavioral variables are nonparametric without these properties. Some are essentially generic names for an entire class of loosely related behavioral complexes and, as most commonly used, are both unitless and dimensionless. This makes things rather difficult when one gets into problems of thinking in terms of unified vs complex multiples of neural operations that are involved in such things as behavioral motivation, the sleep states, and disease states such as that constellation of neural events often termed the schizophrenias.

With respect to sleep, it is essential to observe that it is practically impossible to dissect the entire sleep continuum or group of states into quantifiable units appropriate for biochemical studies. It is obviously an oversimplification to speak of the three general states, i.e., wakefulness, slow wave sleep (SWS), and fast wave (rapid eye movement) sleep (REMS), assuming that each of these has a dominant biochemical correlate.

It was Hobson (1969) who observed that in the history of behavioral physiology other examples of anatomofunctional dualisms such as we see in sleep have come and gone. He observed that it is reminiscent of the sympathetic-parasympathetic dualism of Cannon and of the ergotropic-trophotropic subdivisions of hypothalamic function put forward by Hess. Thus, at the start, I think it is especially well to observe that the biogenic amine hypothesis of sleep is probably another heuristically useful but short-lived oversimplification. Certainly, the trend toward the dichotomization of NREMS and REMS has been developed to a further extent by Snyder (1963, 1965) in which he pointed out that state REM is sufficiently different from NREMS that it should not be considered "sleep" at all but rather as a qualitatively unique "biological mode of existence." Of course, the REM state itself is not a homogeneous event as shown by the studies of Moruzzi (1963) in which the distinction between tonic and phasic characteristics of stage REM was made. As emphasized by Molinari and Foulkes (1969), the tonic-phasic distinction thus undermines the previous NREM/REM model by seeming to require qualitatively different kinds of mechanisms for the explanation of the tonic events and for that of the phasic events occurring within stage REM. Additionally, Pompeiano (1967) has shown that the tonic and phasic characteristics of stage REM in the cat are probably mediated by distinct anatomical structures in the brain stem. Further, with respect to biochemical correlations, it seems more appropriate to assume that a specific chemical event may be related to a small segment of behavior, such as phasic or tonic intra-REM activities, rather than to some larger behavioral heterogeneous constellation comprised of many aspects. Or, this specific chemical event may trigger processes in a concatenation of neurons thus generating "complexes" of behavior with some clock mechanism controlling the periodicities and oscillations. I hope to relate many of these points to Dr. Himwich's chapter (Chapter 7) at the end of some data I want to present bearing on our approaches to studying sleep from the standpoint of interacting neural circuits and their biochemical underpinnings.

Certain pertinent questions that need to be asked are: (1) When do biochemical systems, with their many substrates and metabolic products, begin to appear in the brain and in what regional pattern do they appear? (2) What is their qualitative and quantitative relationship to each other? (3) What is the effect of a newly appearing substance during ontogeny upon an already existing biochemical system?

It is unfortunate that most of the biochemical analyses of the brain have been carried out on whole brain. It is important, in the light of knowledge concerning the organization of brain systems and subunits in behavior, that particular parts of the brain subserving different functions be looked at with respect to their changing biochemical profiles. Obviously, the comparative approach will be a most productive method of getting at some mechanisms where, for example, the sleep states evolve differently in animals showing either different brain development at birth or different regional biochemical profiles.

Since numerous species of animals have been studied with respect to neural and behavioral ontogenesis, one immediate question that might be asked in comparing, for example, the rat and cat with the guinea pig and goat is whether the postnatal neurochemical profile is similar in these different species who show different degrees of maturity at the time of birth. Linear relations in these biochemical systems are often looked for, but any straightforward growth curves toward adult concentrations of chemical agents and the relation of these to specific behavior is hard to come by. With respect to the so-called "maturity hypothesis" of the brain in relation to brain chemistry, I would point out that the idea of a linear growth curve toward adult concentrations is often implied, whereas such is not usually the case. Again, relating to some of the morphological criteria for "brain maturity," it should be mentioned that charting the parameters of postnatal ontogeny chronologically, such as the EEG in sleep with respect to dendritic maturity, becomes even more of a correlative problem. It is, of course, likely that the presence of chemical modulators and transmitters at terminals in the brain would relate most closely to development of synaptic contacts and branching. Overall, it is probable that the best and most precise analysis that can be made at present concerns the temporal relations of the EEG and other neuronal manifestations of the sleep states with regional development and rhythmic changes in serotonin (5–HT) and norepinephrine (NE) content. It is important to consider this as the different systems (catechol systems, indole systems, and even cholinergic systems) probably mature at different rates in different brain areas. This differential maturity could, then, account for the progressive changes that are seen in the sleep states as "balances" are developed between the neural systems resulting in the establishment of homeostasis seen in maturity.

The above general remarks will be touched on again. However, I would like to first present some material comparing the effects on sleep of p-chlorophenylalanine (PCPA) administration with that following lesions in the anterior raphe nuclei in cats. Fig. 1 shows the particular raphe nuclei I want to call your attention to, i.e., the nucleus raphe dorsalis and the nucleus raphe medialis. It is of special interest to note that these anterior raphe nuclei are anatomically a part of the limbic midbrain area and that limbic projections to this region are very powerful. Similarly, this region projects strongly to the hypothalamus, preoptic area, and entire limbic forebrain regions including the basal forebrain area. This fact is usually overlooked in discussions relating the raphe system to sleep in large part because the relations of the raphe complex, based on histofluorescence studies (Dahlstrom and Fuxe, 1964, 1965), use a terminology of numbering histofluorescing areas not easily or directly translatable into anatomical regions. Nevertheless, two nuclei of the anterior raphe group, particularly the nucleus raphe dorsalis and the nucleus raphe medialis, are part and parcel of the limbic midbrain field, a fact which deserves special reemphasis in the light of some of the discussions to follow. When lesions are confined to the nucleus raphe dorsalis, with a slight extension into the nucleus raphe medialis (Fig. 1) the sleep profiles are markedly altered as shown in Table I. It can obviously be seen from this latter figure that the effects of raphe lesions and of PCPA treatment seem to significantly increase the amount of waking time primarily at the expense of SWS.

On the basis of the work of Jouvet (1967, 1969) and others (Torda, 1967; Weitzman *et al.*, 1968) it might be thought that these two procedures act on sleep mechanisms by depleting certain brain areas of 5-HT. It is interesting that both the PCPA treatment and the limited anterior raphe lesions produce almost the same findings with respect to quantitative changes in the sleep profiles (Table I).

Figure 1 interprets, in parasagittal profile, three of five raphe lesions in this series and shows the lesions to involve, in one case, the anterior part of the nucleus raphe dorsalis, in a second case the posterior part of the same nucleus and the area just below it, while the third lesion involves the center of the nucleus raphe dorsalis and also extends into most of the nucleus raphe dorsalis. Table I represents a summary of the means of 6 days (23-hr recordings each day) for all five cats in the series. I am presenting this figure to show how remarkably similar effects on sleep profiles can be produced by a pharmacological agent and a well-defined and limited central nervous system (CNS) lesion, both of which presumably act by depleting the brain of 5-HT.

I am sure, in the light of the organization of the raphe circuits and the multiple links between the limbic midbrain area and the basal forebrain areas via the medial forebrain bundle systems, that one might well expect that preoptic lesions could affect the sleep states in a manner similar to that I just showed. For example, Nauta (1946) found that lesions in the preoptic area of rats produced chronic wakefulness to the point of death in the animals with absolutely no recovery of function. Later on McGinty and Sterman (1968) reported similar findings in cats. Since the preoptic region is bound via the medial forebrain bundle with the raphe nuclear complex, it would appear that it is all part of the same neural system and that similar effects from lesioning this system rostrally and caudally might be predicted. On the other hand, it is somewhat puzzling why we do not see chronic wakefulness with lesions in the lateral hypothalamic area, although I suspect the peculiar types of syndromes following lateral hypothalamic lesions, especially those associated with death ascribed to lack of feeding and drinking, may relate to some of the present findings. Thus, I could have indeed added at least a preoptic column to my table but not any others that I know of. I do not think the impression ought to be given that there are many areas in the nervous system in which chronic wakefulness can be produced following ablation. However, I have intended not to review the literature with respect to brain lesions which result in chronic wakefulness, but rather to

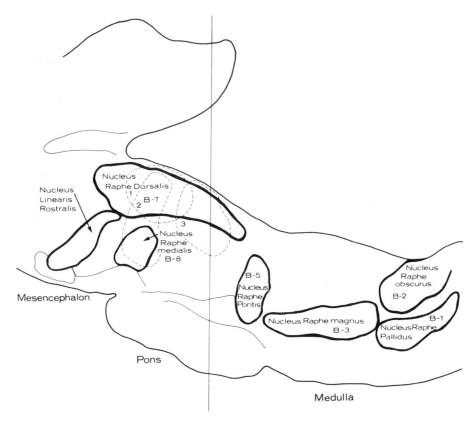

Fig. 1. Parasagittal schematic representation of the lower brainstem of the cat illustrating the raphe nuclei. Lesions in this study are shown as: 1, confined to the nucleus raphe dorsalis; 2, involving the nucleus raphe dorsalis and most of the nucleus raphe medialis; and 3, involving the posterior part of the nucleus raphe dorsalis. The other two lesions in this series (not shown) correspond closely to lesions 1 and 3. The nucleus raphe dorsalis and nucleus raphe medialis are in the limbic midbrain field and are represented as B-7 and B-8, respectively, in the histofluorescence studies of Dahlstrom and Fuxe (1964, 1965).

compare a drug effect (which, purportedly, specifically depletes the brain of 5-HT by blocking tryptophan hydroxylase, the rate-limiting step in 5-HT synthesis) and a brain lesion destroying nuclear formations which produce and store great concentrations of 5-HT and which link the basal forebrain areas primarily via serotonergic circuits within the medial forebrain bundle.

Much work indicates that the medial forebrain bundle system regulates both NE and 5-HT in the entire basal forebrain area (Moore and Heller, 1967; Heller and Moore, 1968). It has, therefore, become of interest to know if these changes in forebrain chemoarchitecture relate to changes in the sleep states following raphe, hypothalamic, or preoptic lesions. We have been able to show that there

TABLE I *Effects of Anterior Raphe Lesions and pchlorophenylalanine (PCPA) on Sleep Profiles[a]*

	Means and standard deviation		
	Average values from Delorme, Sterman, and Morgane	Effects of raphe lesions	Effects of PCPA (150 mg/kg i.p.)
Waking/total recording time	28.8 ± 5.5	82.6 ± 9.6[b]	87.3 ± 8.3[c]
Total sleep/total recording time	71.2 ± 4.8	17.4 ± 4.5	12.7 ± 3.6
Slow wave sleep/total recording time	54.8 ± 5.9	2.8 ± 1.3	2.1 ± 1.2
Fast wave sleep/total recording time	16.3 ± 2.3	14.6 ± 2.7	10.6 ± 2.2
Slow wave sleep/total sleep	74.6 ± 5.4	16.1 ± 2.5	16.5 ± 3.2
Fast wave sleep/total sleep	25.3 ± 4.3	83.9 ± 5.1	83.5 ± 6.5
Mean duration of fast wave sleep episodes (min)	5.7 ± 1.4	7.9 ± 3.2	8.4 ± 4.8

[a]From Sterman *et al.* (1965), Delorme *et al.* (1964) and Morgane (1971).

[b]6 day means of 5 cats beginning 36 hr after operation.

[c]6 day means of 5 cats beginning 36 hr after PCPA administration.

are amine-specific fiber components within the medial forebrain bundle complex wherein particular lesions selectively affect either 5-HT or NE in the basal forebrain area. Figure 2 represents a schematic interpretation of two amine-specific pathways in the lateral and medial components of the medial forebrain bundle. Although much more needs to be done in this series, the preliminary results indicate that lesions predominantly lowering 5-HT in the basal forebrain result in selective depression of SWS while those lesions lowering forebrain NE increased the percentage of SWS. Large lesions in the medial forebrain bundle, involving both systems simultaneously, had no significant effects on sleep profiles. It then appears that raphe lesions and lesions in the more medial components of the medial forebrain bundle lower 5-HT, while lateral mesencephalic lesions and lesions in the lateral components of the medial forebrain bundle selectively lower NE in the basal forebrain. If I might speculate for a moment, it is almost as if we have two systems in the medial forebrain bundle maintaining some NE-5-HT "balance" in the basal forebrain regions. It might be that 5-HT levels in this region are most important with respect to SWS. Thus, if this agent is lowered by medial forebrain bundle or raphe lesions then SWS is depressed. It also seems that lesions lowering NE selectively are not directly important in themselves other than that they change the relative amounts of these chemicals in the forebrain, with 5-HT now predominating, resulting in an increase in SWS. Large lesions that depress both 5-HT and NE might maintain the relative "balance" between the two and result in no changes in sleep. This is, of course, highly speculative but emphasizes one line of approach we are taking.

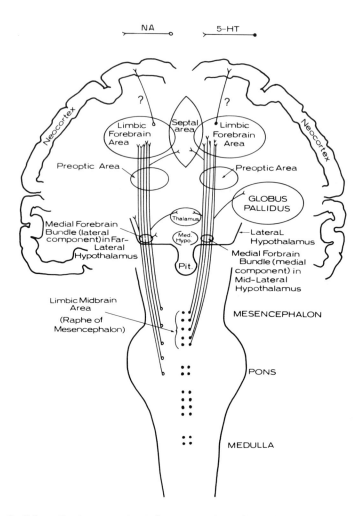

Fig. 2. Schematic interpretation of serotonergic and noradrenergic systems in the medial forebrain bundle. On the left is shown the noradrenergic (NA) system originating in the lateral mesencephalic tegmentum and projecting, via the lateral component of the medial forebrain bundle, into preoptic and limbic forebrain areas. On the right is shown the serotonergic (5-HT) system originating in the raphe nuclei and projecting, via the medial component of the medial forebrain bundle, to these same forebrain fields. Lateral mesencephalic tegmental or far-lateral hypothalamic lesions lower norepinephrine in the basal forebrain areas while limbic midbrain area (anterior raphe) or midlateral hypothalamic lesions lower serotonin in the basal forebrain areas. Thus, it appears that amine-specific pathways exist in the medial forebrain bundle.

As mentioned later, however, this type of "balance" theory does not hold up when considering relative recovery between chronic PCPA-treated animals and lesioned animals. Our results also are somewhat different from those of McGinty and Sterman (1968) in which they reported that preoptic lesions depressed both SWS and REMS. I have no preoptic lesions in this series, but it would seem that lateral hypothalamic lesions might have been comparable. Of course, more work will be necessary to resolve this matter.

The animals were maintained usually for about 30 days. In both the raphe and PCPA columns (Table I) the figures represent recordings for six 23-hr periods within the 30-day time before sacrifice. These measurements began 3 days after the lesion or first PCPA treatment and represent recordings for the next 6 days, sequentially. Following this, in the period up to 30 days, there was a clear tendency to "recover" with values approaching by day 30 the normal sleep profile data of column 1 in both the raphe-lesioned group as well as the PCPA-treated group. This recovery occurred even though the PCPA group still continued to receive the 5-HT-depleting drug. This is interesting because raphe-lesioned animals keep a lowered forebrain 5-HT and NE level, whereas the chronic PCPA administration presumably only lowers forebrain 5-HT. So, "recovery" occurs with 5-HT depressed with respect to NE in the PCPA group, while the lesion lowers both 5-HT and NE. This then, tends to confound any "balance" theory of these two chemical agents in the forebrain.

Although the animals were kept for a full 30 days, the values in the table represent essentially the mean profiles for days 3 through 9 following the procedure. In the period from day 9 to day 30 there was gradual recovery of function as noted above. Actually, it might have been good to keep these animals a bit longer in the light of the work of McGinty and Sterman (1968) in which they noted that recovery was complete in the period 6-8 weeks.

There was a recovery of sleep processes in both the raphe-lesioned cats and in the animals receiving PCPA, but somewhat different time courses were observed. There was a definite tendency for the lesioned animals to take a longer time to return to control sleep profile levels, but "recovery" of sorts did occur in both groups. In two of the raphe-lesioned animals that were kept 30 days, there were still rather marked alterations in the sleep profiles with slow sleep still significantly below control levels with wakefulness proportionally increased. We did not see this in the case of PCPA-treated animals which tended to be back to control levels within about a 2½-3-week period. Recovery of sleep in lesioned animals having low forebrain 5-HT and in chronic PCPA-treated animals having almost no whole brain 5-HT certainly does make one wonder about the direct relation of 5-HT to sleep. In the lesioned group there is regional depression (raphe area and basal forebrain) of 5-HT but the PCPA-treated group the entire brain would be depleted of 5-HT. Thus, "compensatory" theories of recovery of function do not seem to hold up either.

The animals were kept in plexiglass chambers where they were observed regularly and were recorded for periods of 23 hr a day. Both lesioned and PCPA-treated animals seemed agitated a good part of the time. They paced around the cage, and were quite difficult to handle. They were definitely more intractable as compared to their preoperative or predrug state. I noticed a clear-cut sham-rage syndrome in most of the animals, but after 2 weeks or so, when the sleep profiles were beginning to return to control values, this tended to diminish rather markedly and the animals could again be handled without danger of attack. In the raphe-lesioned group, the rage and hyperirritability appeared to persist for a longer period of time coincident with the longer persisting abnormal sleep profiles in this group. But these also returned to rather normal behavior as the profiles began to reach control values. It is of interest that Nauta (1946) also mentioned a syndrome which resembled sham-rage in his rats showing chronic wakefulness following preoptic lesions. I would definitely emphasize that this rage phenomenon seen in our cats was much more clear-cut in the raphe-lesioned animals than it was in the chronic PCPA-treated group even though both groups, as shown in Fig. 2, tended to show essentially the same effects with respect to alterations of the sleep profiles.

One thing is rather interesting. Some of the animals tended to remain transfixed, walking to the side of the chamber and standing there in catatonic-like stances. These animals oscillated between a state of relaxed wakefulness and SWS with definite periods of slow waves and spindle bursts in the EEG. Other than that, there were no special motor disturbances of note.

If I might move into a slightly different area, I would like to briefly touch on the matter of the morphological indices of maturation. I think we can agree that the developing brain can tell us much about sleep or any other behavior, since structural, physiological, and biochemical changes occur in a developing organ in established sequences and chronology, and can be studied under normal and altered conditions. There are several comments I wish to make extending somewhat Dr. Scheibel's remarks into the realm of another correlation or concomitant of development of function in parallel with morphological changes in specific neural pathways. These remarks also relate to Dr. Himwich's paper in that she has several times referred to "maturation of the brain," and I think the more morphologically minded in this group might consider certain additional structural indices that may relate to maturing patterns of function in the CNS. Flechsig (1962) long ago noted that myelination of the brain stem and cerebral hemispheres takes place according to systems of fibers rather than as a regional phenomenon, and also that when fiber systems mature at different times, insofar as their myelination is concerned, each system has a different functional significance. There seems to be a sequence in which separate bundles of fibers become myelinated and the myelination of the cortex to which these bundles project appears to take place in the same sequence. In general, the more recently acquired areas phylogenetically mature latest in ontogenetic sequence. Of course, this could relate to the delayed development of forebrain inhibitory pathways acting on lower brain stem centers. It certainly would be of great interest to compare the maturation also of afferent cortical systems in different species. We have to have regional morphological indices like these defined more rigorously and quantitatively and match these with the maturation of sleep patterns or other behaviors. In Chapter 3 the Scheibels have presented a discussion of their Golgi preparations and some rather elaborate development of dendritic geometry, such as the bundling of heterogeneous dendritic systems into single packets in the spinal cord and the relationship of this to evolving motor function. There is a parallel myelogenetic finding that links closely with this bundling of heterogeneous fibers in the spinal cord. This is illustrated by a study of the medial lemniscus (Yakovlev and Lecours, 1967) which shows that while the intensity of staining is increasing rapidly, the size of this bundle and density of the fibers increases much more slowly, suggesting the bundle contains fibers of a heterogeneous origin which myelinate at different rates and have different cycles. Thus, I think this other indicator of neural maturity, i.e., the cycle of myelogenesis is an important parameter of regional brain maturation and it may be assumed that the cycle reflects and, in a sense, defines the position of a fiber system or region in the hierarchy of functional organization of the developing nervous system. Figure 3, modified from Yakovlev and Lecours (1967), indicates many examples of different myelogenetic cycles in specific neural systems. Myelination is thought to be an orderly process in which the functionally allied systems of fibers are synchronized in an orderly sequence and tempo of their myelination. By using the Loyez modification of the Weigert technique and studying the tinctorial character of fetal material, newborns, and older animals, definite cycles of myelogenesis in specific neural pathways can be mapped and related to development of specific functions these paths are known to mediate. This type of maturational index, if taken system by system in longitudinally organized columns in the developing and differentiating brain, would follow the "logic" of the evolving nervous system as opposed to "maturing" segmentally and consecutively in some artificial, hierarchical manner.

Analysis of Fig. 3 shows that these myelogenetic cycles begin in motor roots first and then in sensory roots. It also shows that myelination of fiber systems mediating sensory input to the thalamus and cerebral cortex generally anticipate myelination of the fiber systems of correlation and integration of sensory data into movement. The cycles of myelination of the specific and nonspecific thalamic projection fibers to the respective cortical areas appear to be synchronized with the cycles of myelination of the corticofugal fibers from these areas in which the respective afferents and efferents conjugate as limbs of an arc (Yakovlev and Lecours, 1967).

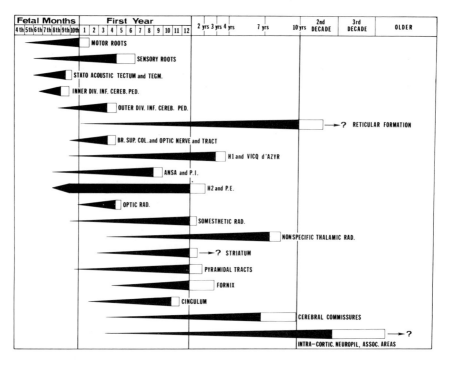

Fig. 3. Systems analysis of myelogenetic cycles in the brain. The width of the graphs indicate progression in the intensity of staining and density of myelinated fibers. The white areas at the end of each graph indicate the approximate age range of termination of myelination estimated from comparison of the fetal and postnatal material with material from adults in the third and later decades of life.

In addition to the interpretation of cycles of myelogenesis in specific neural circuits, an important facet of these studies might be termed zonal myelination. This is illustrated in Fig. 4 which shows the three zones of the cerebral wall, the median zone, the paramedian zone, and dorsolateral zone. This same figure shows that each of these zones has its own cycle of myelination. Each zone myelinates as a tectogenetic and myeloarchitectonic unit and exhibits a different cycle of myelination. The median zone (representing the diffusely reticulate, allocortical pediment of the cerebral hemisphere) has an extraordinarily protracted cycle. The paramedian zone, including the striatum, pallidum, and paramedian thalamus (lemniscal and limbic nuclei and center median) presents a sharp contrast to the median zone and exhibits a short cycle of myelination of its fiber systems. The myelination of the paramedian zone appears to be harmonized in sequence and tempo with the myelination of the pyramidal tract fibers in the internal capsule and of the striatum, pallidum, subthalamic region, and the specific thalamocortical projections. In the supralimbic zone, the

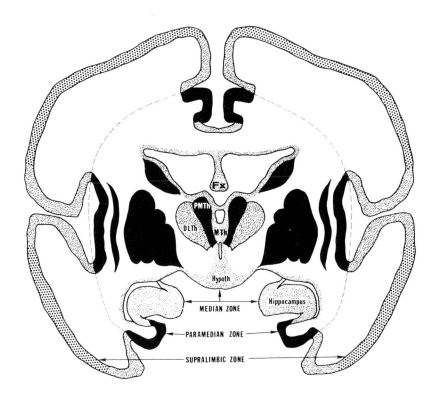

Fig. 4. The three primary zones of the cerebral wall. The median zone: light grey stipple; the paramedian zone: black; the dorsolateral zone: heavy dots are the supralimbic association areas, while medium grey stippling represents the opercular and paralimbic areas. The comparative cycles of myelination of these respective myeloarchitectonic zones are shown in the graph.

myelination of these cortical areas appears to be synchronized with the myelination of the diffuse cortical projections from the dorsolateral and posterior nuclei of the thalamus and of the corticopontine tracts, and the cycle of myelogenesis in this system is quite protracted. Certain of these areas even exhibit an exponential cycle of myelination, the end of which is not specifically definable. In terms of function, the protracted cycle of myelination of the median zone of the forebrain appears to correlate with the protracted ontogenetic development of the reflex and behavioral patterns in the sphere of visceral motility and metabolic, enzymic, and hormonal processes, which change slowly through the years of reproductive life (Yakovlev and Lecours, 1967). In contrast, the somatic motility of the outward expression of the internal states and movements of the body on the body itself, such as mimicry, gestures, postural habitus, and vocalizations, become definitive of the individual makeup already by the end of the second decade and change very little thereafter. The shorter cycle of myelination of the paramedian zone appears to correlate with the more rapid maturation of the reflex and behavioral patterns in the sphere of innate or instinctive movements conventionally assigned to basal ganglia and extrapyramidal systems. There is also some evidence that the exponential myelination of the supralimbic division of the hemisphere and cerebral cortex correlates with the exponential maturation of the behavioral patterns in the sphere of motility of the effective, societal transactions, i.e., symbolized thought, language, and of learning from individual experience.

These remarks about myelogenetic cycles in relation to maturing systems in the brain obviously cannot account for the many neural circuits and centers that are not myelinated. Other indices, such as histofluorescence techniques applied to the developing brain, could conceivably fill in as maturational indices in these areas. One of these, of special importance to the present discussions, is the medial forebrain bundle system which is very poorly myelinated and therefore myelogenetic techniques cannot be used to study its development. On the other hand, this bundle does contain noradrenergic, cholinergic, and serotonergic fiber systems which can be detected and "mapped" by application of suitable histochemical techniques (Dahlstrom and Fuxe, 1964, 1965; Shute and Lewis, 1966; Lewis and Shute, 1967). Mapping of systems by histochemical techniques has had some of the same disadvantages as the study of the myelogenetic cycles, i.e., the difficulty in quantitating the degree of fluorescence in the one case or amount of myelin in the other. However, in the case of histofluorescent techniques, Lichtensteiger (1969) has clearly shown that such quantitation is now possible. Such quantitative chemomorphogenetic methods applied to the developing brain might conceivably be important in relating respective development of serotonergic, noradrenergic, and cholinergic systems to the developing phases of the sleep states. Probably no neural system can be considered to be fully functional until it gets its neural linkages established, and it is likely that the chemoarchitecture of each region is closely tied to such indices of maturity as myelogenesis and amount of neurochemical agents in neural centers and circuits.

Other beginnings in this direction have also been carried out by Loizou (1969) who pointed out that monoamine-containing cell groups such as described by Dahlstrom and Fuxe (1964, 1965) in the adult brain could be visualized at birth in the rat. He showed that the intensity of fluorescence was lower than in adult animals, but that it increased gradually up to the fourth week to attain the adult pattern by the fifth week. Virtually, no noradrenaline (NA) or 5-HT-containing terminals were present at birth, but low density, weakly fluorescent dopamine-containing terminals were present in the neostriatum, tuberculum olfactorium, and other forebrain areas. He also emphasized that dopamine-containing terminals were found to proliferate gradually during development, and that NA terminals developed slowly over the first 2 weeks and thereafter their content of NA increased rapidly until an adult pattern of distribution, density, and intensity was obtained by the fourth to fifth week of life. The 5-HT-containing terminals developed at a somewhat faster rate and attained an adult pattern by the third week. Inhibition of catecholamine (CA) synthesis at the tyrosine hydroxylase step by the administration of α-methyl-*p*-tyrosine induced a time-dependent depletion of CA's from cell bodies and terminals in the newborn, as well as in older animals, suggesting that conduction and transmission of impulses in the dopaminergic pathways and axoplasmic flow of storage granules actually occurs from the time of birth. He also found that young animals were more sensitive to the blocking of the storage granules by reserpine and recovery of fluorescence was much slower. Up to about 2 weeks of age the monoamines could cross the blood-brain barrier and be taken up by mono-aminergic-containing neurons. These types of developmental histofluorescence studies certainly are needed and will, I think, shed a great deal of light on the development of the neurobiochemical systems with respect to indices of maturation in the sleep state. More particularly, they illustrate the dynamics of the chemical substrates during morphogenesis, especially synaptogenesis in neural pathways. This fits well with the postulations of Karki *et al.*, (1962) who observed that the development of behavioral maturity is related to the elaboration of neuronal pathways perhaps modulated by monoamines.

The collection of sleep data on which to assess the very minute changes in sleep states are, of course, based on the development of quantitative sleep profiles. (This is not emphasized by Dr. Himwich in Chapter 7 but is, of course, taken for granted.) Table II illustrates that sleep is indeed a biological constant having rigorous baselines for quantitative analysis of any drug changes or other manipulations that might affect the sleep states. It is also pertinent to point out here that these profiles are stabilized rather early in life and are maintained remarkably constant, showing that powerful, regulatory mechanisms are operative in maintaining these states. Indeed, here, as in other physiological mechanisms, we are dealing with many problems of regulatory physiology.

There are several additional remarks I would like to make with respect to "matching" brain chemistry with any behavior, be it sleep or otherwise. First of

TABLE II *Quantitative Aspects of Sleep-Wakefulness in Cats (Method of Continuous Polygraphic Recordings) Showing the Stability of Sleep Patterns in Three Different Laboratories*[a]

	Means and standard deviation (%)		
	Lyon, France[b]	Los Angeles, Calif.[c]	Shrewsbury, Mass.[d]
Waking/total recording time	31.5 ± 7	28 ± 4	27 ± 5
Total sleep/total recording time	68.5 ± 6.5	72 ± 4	73 ± 4
Slow wave sleep/total recording time	52.5 ± 7	56.5 ± 5.3	55.5 ± 6
Fast wave sleep/total recording time	16 ± 2	15.5 ± 2.2	17.5 ± 2.4
Slow wave sleep/total sleep	77 ± 4	72.4 ± 4.2	74.5 ± 4.5
Fast wave sleep/total sleep	23 ± 4	27.5 ± 4.2	25.5 ± 4.6
Mean duration of fast wave sleep episodes (min)	5.8 ± 1.3	5.8 ± 1.3	5.6 ± 1.7

[a] These quantitative data serve as baselines on which to assess changes in the states of sleep following brain lesions or pharmacological manipulation.
[b] Means of 9 cats.
[c] Means of 8 cats.
[d] Means of 6 cats.

all, it is almost impossible to get a clear and direct relation between any behavior (and concomitant electrographic indices) and multiple chemical profiles of the whole brain and, even more so, with respect to the chemoarchitectonic profiles of regional areas of the brain which is, perhaps, even more important. Although it is not made clear, I assume, in Dr. Himwich's studies (see Chapter 7) that the amine analyses were done on animals killed either during a sleep stage or immediately thereafter. Most studies do not emphasize when animals were sacrificed or whether the sacrifices were done by killing the animal within or immediately after a particular sleep phase. This might be important in light of the fact that in correlating brain biochemistry with behavior it is not often stressed that a particular sleep state may actually be running on some biochemical "fuel," thus lowering that agent in the brain as that state progresses. It might then be expected that a chemical agent would be high in a certain region during a defined state, whereas, in reality, as that state develops, this particular chemical may be almost completely expended.

Figure 5 represents a gathering of data from the literature showing developmental changes in some chemicals and enzymes in whole brain of the rat (cf. the data of Dr. Himwich in Chapter 7, Figs. 6-8, showing the curves of development of several enzymes and substrates in the brain). If one tries to correlate curves of this sort with what is going on behaviorally and electrographically with respect to the evolving sleep states during this period, it becomes a really confounding experience. Similarly, in looking at Dr. Himwich's graphs, no clear trends are obvious with respect to a biogenic amine theory of

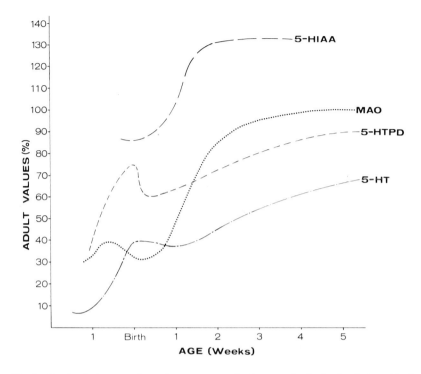

Fig. 5. Graph of changes of certain enzymes and substrates in the brain of the rat in the period immediately preceding birth up to approximately 5 weeks postnatal. From a study of this figure it is not possible to correlate these changes with development of the sleep profiles during this period. 5-HT, serotonin; 5-HTPD, 5-hydroxytryptophan decarboxylase; MAO, monoamine oxidase; 5-HIAA, 5-hydroxyindoleacetic acid.

sleep, and it is consequently difficult to come up with an adequate biochemical definition of immaturity or maturity with respect to sleep behaviors.

The generality that needs to be made here is that if one looks at the overall curve for behavioral development (in this case with respect to ontogeny of the sleep states), it must be stressed that beneath this lie all the biochemical and physiological vicissitudes of appearance, disappearance, and regulation. The vector line for "sleep" thus has beneath it multiple interacting, out-of-phase, regional biochemical phenomena, the overt behavior being the vector of these many fluxes. I do not see in these data of Dr. Himwich biochemical correlates of the gradual but linear decrease in the proportion of total sleep time spent in fast wave sleep from the time of birth on. Also, work from Dr. Himwich's laboratory has indicated that the sleep pattern of the cat reaches mature levels at about 70 days, but that biogenic amines do not attain their complete maturation until approximately 1 year. Thus, again, correlations become somewhat difficult to make. I think it is of special interest, in light of the possible caudal-rostral maturation gradients, to note that Dr. Himwich shows "mature" pons-medulla levels of biogenic amine at 30 days of age in the cat. Related to these same problems is the work of Himwich *et al.* (1967) who reported that during growth of the brain the accumulation of amines is proportional to brain weight. They showed a linear relationship between growth of the brain and accumulation of amine content both in different parts of the brain and in whole brain. It is noteworthy, then, that Bennett and Giarman (1965) showed that levels of 5-HT, monoamine oxidase, and 5-hydroxytryptophan decarboxylase increased in the rat brain at a rate which is "irregular" and markedly different from the increase in brain weight. This would be more in line with the special, regional accumulations of neurochemical agents and not merely related to an increase in brain weight.

One of the other problems to be considered also with reference to Fig. 5, and with particular reference to Dr. Himwich's data, is that practically all measures she refers to have been carried out on whole brains or in some cases pons-medulla combinations, and I think this is another confounding problem. More information might be derived if analyses were done regionally in the brain, because we know these chemical agents have special patterns of cycling in regions already related to sleep, such as the raphe, locus coeruleus, medial forebrain bundle, hypothalamus, basal forebrain area, etc. Looking at whole brains simply will not give us the best correlations we can get, especially if we consider interacting regions that might be reciprocally balanced, such as the basal forebrain areas and midbrain, etc. In whole brain determinations special biochemical regional differentiations often go unnoticed or are "buried." Since the individual brain areas have their own unique patterns of indole and catechol development, when one looks at whole brain the real issues which are being decided in local areas related to sleep are masked. Looking at the whole brain can be, as Kety (1967) once pointed out, somewhat like correlating the whole animal concentration of 5-HT with behavior, all the time realizing that as much as 98% of the 5-HT in the body is in the gut and not likely to be relevant.

If interactions between adrenergic, cholinergic, and serotonergic neural circuits, for example, produce behavioral resultants, then it is critical to examine the interactions between the rhythms of chemistry in regions interlocked and woven together by these neural systems. The resultants of these constant interactions between circuits obviously represent fluctuations in the excitability of the central response pathways. Regardless of how we may eventually solve the problem of analyzing the development of the chemoarchitecture of the brain and the interaction of chemospecific systems, I do think whole brain analyses will not give us much useful data with respect to the ontogeny of any behavior. Therefore, if one thinks in terms of interacting neural pathways, one obviously cannot "dissect" these out for chemical analyses, but one can manipulate these systems, especially by chemical stimulation and then study the regional effects on brain chemistry and behavior.

Relative to the topic of "maturity across species," I would like to recall the study of Fox (1966) in Dr. Himwich's laboratory. I bring this up because this paper by Fox refers to so-called "levels" of maturation in different regions of the brain, from the spinal cord up to the cortex, as the indicator of the maturity "level" of a particular species at birth. It assumes a presumably caudal to rostral maturation gradient in the rat to rabbit to guinea pig, but it also implies that each species at birth has a brain developed "up to a particular segmental level," as though brains are put together by adding one block on another, irrespective of the fact that the level below is not "immature" across species but is developing itself and especially is changing due to its developing interactions with higher centers. I think this kind of segmenting of brain areas, based on anatomical "levels" ("building-block theory") in the brain stem, as though each brain in phylogeny is only a direct ascent along the stem, does not represent the correct case with respect to a maturity index across species. If, for example, to use the myelin index again, myelination of the brain stem and cerebral hemispheres takes place according to systems of fibers, rather than as a regional segmental phenomenon, then it is important to remember that when fiber systems mature at different times, insofar as their myelination is concerned, each system has a different functional significance. As noted by Friede (1959), the observation of a caudal-rostral process of biochemical maturation in various parts of the nervous system does not allow proper recognition of the changes in particular nuclei within a part. Confirmation of this concept can be found in the elegant quantitative and qualitative histochemical studies on homologous cell populations in various areas of the nervous system (Kuhlman and Lowry, 1956; Robins and Lowe, 1961; Robins *et al.*, 1961; McCaman and Aprison, 1964).

Dr. Himwich also observed (Chapter 7) that Jouvet mentions a cholinergic link in his proposed sleep system, but it might be emphasized that he was referring to a neural link from the posterior group of raphe nuclei to the locus coeruleus, which is an entirely different circuit complex in the lower brain stem. However, just so the descending cholinergic hypnogenic systems (Hernández-Peón *et al.*, 1963; Hernández-Peón, 1965) in the medial forebrain bundle do not get lost in these discussions of monoaminergic systems, I would stress that it also needs to be looked at in more detail in future studies. Of course, adding a cholinergic sleep system further complicates matters and brings us again into the problems of how "checks and balances" between multiple chemospecific neural systems can be analyzed. It is particularly pertinent to point out that these cholinergic descending hypnogenic circuits in the medial forebrain bundle are the cardinal links between the basal forebrain areas and the limbic midbrain area. These chemical systems may be out of phase in development in a particular link in the system complex thus perturbing regulatory "balance" of the entire circuit. The ontogenetic histofluorescence studies of Loizou (1969) indicate, as noted above, different sequences of maturation in these biochemical systems. It is, as Kety (1967) notes, not so much that one amine determines a "behavior" as that several acting in concert in specific areas of the brain establish a primitive substrate for that behavior that must be activated by, as yet, unknown factors. Of course, the particular site of a chemical reaction in the brain may well be a parameter of equal importance to substrate and enzyme activity in determining the outcome in the nervous system.

Finally, and specifically with reference to Dr. Himwich's chapter, I would say that she has presented a vast amount of data in developing animal species, but, just as she has noted, when it is fractionated and distilled, we still do not come up with anything remotely proving a biogenic amine hypothesis of sleep based on manipulation of these amines by pharmacological agents in developing animals. Some of the data shows a temporal relationship between drug-induced biochemical changes in monoamines and altered sleep states, but this by no means proves that one was causative of the other. Obviously, pharmacological experiments such as these give only the most indirect evidence. As a generality, Kety (1967) and others have emphasized that when we get into biochemical effects there appears to be no crucial, direct evidence that an action on behavior is produced by a "transmitter" or "modulator" acting locally at specific sites in the brain. Most of the evidence depends upon many pharmacological studies which have utilized drugs as tools in studying behavioral effects of amines in the CNS. Major drawbacks of this approach must be stressed, the most important of these being that no pharmacological agent produces only one effect. Thus, there might be a desired effect and a whole host of side effects, and it is practically impossible to separate these. Pharmacological studies to get at something like the sleep states are, therefore, simply not going to provide unambiguous answers to the main questions. Throwing multiple brain systems entirely out of balance by drugs that obviously affect many chemical systems in the brain is just not producing many clear-cut answers. It seems obvious that until we know more about the kind of structural and chemical changes that normally occur regularly and rhythmically in the nervous system in such a complicated series of processes as are involved in the sleep states, then little more than "shotgun" progress is being made toward relating biochemistry to behavior. Therefore, we are nowhere near a "biochemistry of behavior" as yet, and attempting to get at this by systemic administration of drugs that affect many brain areas and systems simultaneously and indiscriminately will not give us conclusive answers.

REFERENCES

Bennett, D. S., and Giarman, N. J. (1965). Schedule of appearance of 5-hydroxytryptamine (serotonin) and associated enzymes in the developing rat brain. *J. Neurochem.* **12**, 911-918.

Dahlstrom, A., and Fuxe, K. (1964). Evidence for the existence of monoamine-containing neurons in the central nervous system. I. Demonstration of monoamines in the cell bodies of brain stem neurons. *Acta Physiol. Scand.* **62**, Suppl. 232, 1-55.

Dahlstrom, A., and Fuxe, K. (1965). Evidence for the existence of monoamine neurons in the central nervous system. II. Experimentally induced changes in the intraneuronal amine levels of bulbospinal neuron systems. *Acta Physiol. Scand.* **64**, Suppl. 247, 1-86.

Delorme, F., Vimont, P., and Jouvet, D. (1964). Etude statistique du cycle veille-sommeils chez le chat. *C. R. Soc. Biol.* **158**, 2128-2131.

Flechsig, P. (1962). *In* "The Growing Brain. An Essay in Developmental Neurology" (M. C. H. Dodgson, ed.), p. 163. John Wright & Sons, Ltd., Bristol.

Fox, M. W., (1966). Neuro-behavioral ontogeny. A synthesis of ethological and neurophysiological concepts. *Brain Res.* **2**, 3-20.

Friede, R. L. (1959). Histochemical investigations on succinic dehydrogenase in the central nervous system. I. The postnatal development of rat brain. *J. Neurochem.* **4**, 101-110.

Heller, A., and Moore, R. Y. (1968). Control of brain serotonin and norepinephrine by specific neural systems. *Advan. Pharmacol.* **6A**, 191-209.

Hernández-Peón, R. (1965). Central neuro-humoral transmission in sleep and wakefulness. *Prog. Brain Res.* **18**, 96-117

Hernández-Peón, R., Chávez-Ibarra, G., Morgane, P. J., and Timo-Iaria, C. (1963). Limbic cholinergic pathways involved in sleep and emotional behavior. *Exp. Neurol.* **8**, 93-111.

Himwich, H. E., Pscheidt, G. R., and Schweigerdt, A. K. (1967). Comparative studies on development of biogenic amines in brains of growing rabbits and cats. *In* "Regional Development of the Brain in Early Life" (A. Minkowski, ed.), pp. 273-296. Blackwell, Oxford.

Hobson, J. A. (1969). Sleep: Physiologic aspects and Sleep: Biochemical aspects. *N. Engl. J. Med.* **281**, 1343-1345 and 1468-1470.

Jouvet, M. (1967). Mechanisms of the states of sleep: A neuropharmacological approach. *In* "Sleep and Altered States of Consciousness" (S. S. Kety, E. V. Evarts, and H. L. Williams, eds.), pp. 86-126. Williams & Wilkins, Baltimore, Maryland.

Jouvet, M. (1969). Biogenic amines and the states of sleep. *Science* **163**, 32-41.

Karki, N., Kuntzman, R., and Brodie, B. B. (1962). Storage, synthesis, and metabolism of monoamines in the developing brain. *J. Neurochem.* **9**, 53-58.

Kety, S. (1967). The central physiological and pharmacological effects of the biogenic amines and their correlations with behavior. *In* "The Neurosciences" (G. C. Quarton, T. Melnechuk, and F. O. Schmitt, eds.), pp. 444-451. Rockefeller Univ. Press, New York.

Kuhlman, R. E., and Lowry, O. H. (1956). Quantitative histochemical changes during the development of the rat cerebral cortex. *J. Neurochem.* **1**, 173-180.

Lewis, P. R., and Shute, C. C. D. (1967). The cholinergic limbic system: Projections to hippocampal formation, medial cortex, nuclei of the ascending cholinergic reticular system, and the subfornical organ and supra-optic crest. *Brain* **90**, 521-540.

Lichtensteiger, W. (1969). Cyclic variations of catecholamine content in hypothalamic nerve cells during the estrous cycle of the rat, with a concomitant study of the substantia nigra. *J. Pharmacol. Exp. Ther.* **165**, 204-215.

Loizou, L. A. (1969). The development of monoamine-containing neurones in the brain of the albino rat. *J. Anat.* **104**, 588.

McCaman, R. E., and Aprison, M. H. (1964). The synthetic and catabolic enzyme systems for acetylcholine and serotonin in several discrete areas of the developing rabbit brain. *Prog. Brain Res.* **9**, 220-233.

McGinty, D. J., and Sterman, M. B. (1968). Sleep suppression after basal forebrain lesions in the cat. *Science* **160**, 1253-1255.

Molinari, S., and Foulkes, D. (1969). Tonic and phasic events during sleep. Psychological correlates and implications. *Percept. Motor Skills* **29**, Monogr. Suppl. 1, 343-368.

Moore, R. Y., and Heller, A. (1967). Monoamine levels and neuronal degeneration in rat brain following lateral hypothalamic lesions. *J. Pharmacol. Exp. Ther.* **156**, 12-22.

Morgane, P. J. (1971). Integration from biochemical to behavioral processes: Relationship of sleep to neuroanatomical circuits, biochemistry, and behavior. *Ann. N.Y. Acad. of Sci.* (in press).

Moruzzi, G. (1963). Active processes in the brainstem during sleep. *Harvey Lect.* **58**, 233-297.

Nauta, W. J. H. (1946). Hypothalamic regulation of sleep in rats. An experimental study. *J. Neurophysiol.* **9**, 285-316.

Pompeiano, O. (1967). The neurophysiological mechanisms of the postural and motor events during desynchronized sleep. *In* "Sleep and Altered States of Consciousness" (S. Kety, E. V. Evarts, and H. L. Williams, eds.), pp. 351-423. Williams & Wilkins, Baltimore, Maryland.

Robins, E., and Lowe, I. P. (1961). Quantitative histochemical studies of the morphogenesis of the cerebellum. I. Total lipids and four enzymes. *J. Neurochem.* **8**, 81-95.

Robins, E., Fisher, H. K., and Lowe, I. P. (1961). Quantitative histochemical studies of the morphogenesis of the cerebellum. II. Two beta-glycosidases. *J. Neurochem.* **8**, 96-104.

Shute, C. C. D., and Lewis, P. R. (1966). Cholinergic and monoaminergic systems of the brain. *Nature (London)* **212**, 710-711.

Snyder, F. (1963). The new biology of dreaming. *Arch. Gen Pyschiat.* **8**, 381-391.

Snyder, F. (1965). Progress in the new biology of dreaming. *Amer. J. Psychiat.* **122**, 377-391.

Sterman, M. B., Knauss, T., Lehman, D., and Clemente, C. D. (1965). Circadian sleep and waking patterns in the laboratory cat. *Electroencephalogr. Clin. Neurophysiol.* **19**, 509-517.

Torda, C. (1967). Effect of brain serotonin depletion on sleep in rats. *Brain Res.* **6**, 371-375.

Weitzman, E. D., Rapport, M. M., McGregor, P., and Jacoby, J. (1968). Sleep patterns of the monkey and brain serotonin concentration: Effect of *p*-chlorophenylalanine. *Science* **160**, 1361-1363.

Yakovlev, P. I., and Lecours, A. R. (1967). The myelogenetic cycles of regional maturation of the brain. *In* "Regional Development of the Brain in Early Life" (A. Minkowski, ed.), pp. 3-70. Blackwell, Oxford.

DEVELOPMENT OF EEG AND ACTIVITY PATTERNS IN RELATION TO SLEEP

9

Development of Wakefulness-Sleep Cycles and Associated EEG Patterns in Mammals*

Robert J. Ellingson

The early development of electroencephalographic (EEG) patterns related to the wakefulness-sleep cycle has been described in some detail for a number of species in recent reviews of the ontogenesis of the electrical activity of the nervous system (Ellingson, 1967; Ellingson and Rose, 1970; Scherrer *et al.,* 1970). These species include the chicken, rabbit, rat, mouse, guinea pig, cat, dog, sheep, pig, monkey (macaque), chimpanzee, and man. Detailed descriptions of EEG pattern development will therefore not be undertaken here. Rather, in order to provide a background for succeeding articles in this volume, a number of generalizations will be presented, with brief discussion in several instances, followed by some statements about interspecies differences.

*Supported by a grant from NICHD (HD-00370).

INTERSPECIES SIMILARITIES

There are a number of common features in the course of wakefulness-sleep pattern development among the various mammalian species which have been studied:

Generalization 1.

No wakefulness-sleep cycle can be detected at the time at which EEG activity makes its first appearance.

Generalization 2.

The wakefulness-sleep cycle can usually be differentiated by means of non-EEG observations before EEG pattern differences related to the two states can be detected (Jouvet-Mounier *et al.,* 1970; Shimizu and Himwich, 1968). The non-EEG variables which are usually involved are respiration, heart rate, eyelid position, eye movements, and somatic muscle activity (gross body jerks and other movements, nuchal muscle twitches, and masticatory muscle twitches, often rhythmic in nature).

Generalization 3.

Two stages of sleep are distinguished from the time at which sleep can first be clearly distinguished from wakefulness. The regular alternation of these stages is characteristic of all mammalian species thus far studied. On the basis of their behavioral characteristics, these stages have been referred to as "sleep with jerks" or "active sleep" on the one hand and "quiet sleep" on the other (Fig. 1). When related EEG patterns differentiate, it is found that "active sleep" tends to be primarily associated with low-voltage fast activity in the EEG, but in the early developmental period in some species higher voltage fast activity and other variations may be displayed. "Quiet sleep" tends to be associated with slower activity of higher voltage (Fig. 2). Thus, active sleep is often referred to as "low-voltage fast wave sleep" or more cryptically as "fast sleep," and quiet sleep is referred to as "slow wave sleep" or "slow sleep." Active or fast wave sleep is also widely referred to as "paradoxical sleep," after Jouvet. The terms "quiet sleep" (QS) and "paradoxical sleep" (PS) will be used to identify the two stages of sleep in the nonhuman mammal. Rapid eye movement (REM) episodes tend to occur during PS.

The situation is somewhat different in human newborns than in subprimates. In humans, QS is associated with an intermittent burst EEG pattern, most often

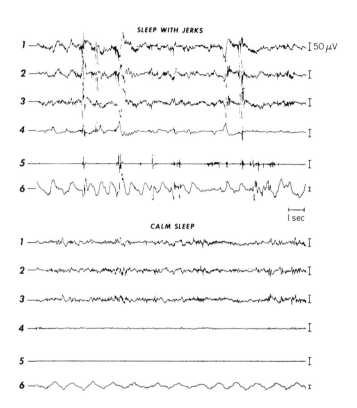

Fig. 1. Sleep with jerks and calm (quiet) sleep in the young kitten (under 10 days of age). Muscle potential bursts associated with jerks are recorded in all channels (above). Most REMs occur simultaneously with jerks. Note lack of clear differences between EEG tracings in the two states. (1) anterior cortex-reference; (2) posterior cortex-reference; (3) anterior cortex-posterior cortex; (4) electrooculogram; (5) EMG of posterior neck muscles; (6) respiraogram. (From Shimizu and Himwich, 1968.)

called *tracé alternant* but also called episodic sleep activity. Active sleep in the human newborn tends to be associated with continuous relatively low voltage, mixed fast and slow activity, but with the slow features predominating. REMs occur episodically during this period. There is a transitional period of higher voltage slower waves, which gradually break up into bursts as the *tracé alternant* pattern is achieved. REMs never occur during the *tracé alternant* pattern. These developments are described more fully and are illustrated in the chapter by Parmelee.

It should be noted that very early in the development of the EEG, before wakefulness-sleep pattern differences emerge, an alternating burst pattern similar to, but not identical with the *tracé alternant* pattern of human QS (Ellingson,

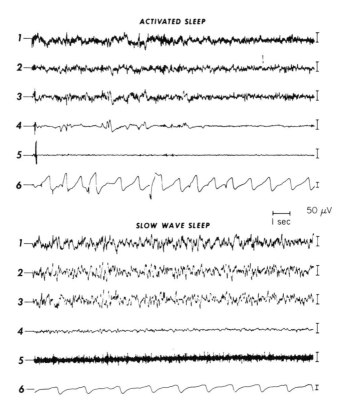

Fig. 2. Activated (fast wave) sleep and slow wave sleep in an older kitten. The patterns are similar to those of the adult. Labeling same as in Fig. 1. (From Shimizu and Himwich, 1968.)

1967), is present continuously. The topographical distribution of the bursts is different, the waveform configurations are different, and associated spindle bursts are usually of different frequencies from postnatal sleep spindles (σ activity) and are probably unrelated to the latter. Dreyfus-Brisac (1968) has expressed the opinion that the premature human infant, who displays this pattern at 24-27 weeks of conceptional age, more or less, is in a continuous state of immature or atypical sleep. A similar early intermittent burst pattern stage has been seen in all mammalian species in which the entire ontogenetic evolution of the EEG has been studied (Ellingson and Rose, 1970).

Generalization 4.

Sleep spindle bursts (σ activity) tend to appear relatively late, after most of the other elements of the EEG sleep pattern are established. Some weak and evanescent σ-like activity can sometimes be seen in the EEG of the full-term human newborn, and is very likely the anlage of σ activity, which is seen clearly from about 1 month postterm.

Verley (1965) has described a rich variety of spindle burst activity in the early EEG's of several species, which differs from mature sleep spindle activity in several respects and is possibly analogous to that seen in the early human premature discussed above.

Generalization 5.

The amplitude of all frequency components of the EEG, both during wakefulness and sleep, increases with age through the period of infancy, then decreases somewhat again as puberty is approached and continues to decrease gradually into old age.

Generalization 6.

Total sleep time (TST) is high in the newborn, often increases for a few days after birth, but then decreases gradually with age.

Generalization 7.

The number of wakefulness-sleep cycles per day decreases with increasing age. This occurs first as a result of consolidation of sleep periods, with lengthening of single periods of wakefulness occurring later (Kleitman, 1963).

Generalization 8.

PS as a percentage of TST is high in the newborn and decreases with age, for example, from 90% in the newborn kitten to 25% in the cat (Jouvet-Mounier *et al.,* 1970).

Generalization 9.

Conversely, QS as a percentage of TST is relatively low in the newborn and increases with age.

Generalization 10.

The number of sleep phases (that is, shifts from one stage of sleep to another) is high in the newborn as compared with the adult of a species, and the average durations of sleep phases are low.

Generalization 11.

A basic rest-activity cycle exists within the wakefulness-sleep cycle, or perhaps rather the wakefulness-sleep cycle is superimposed upon a basic rest-activity cycle (Kleitman, 1963, 1967). The duration of this cycle appears to increase both as the phylogenetic scale is ascended and within species from birth to maturity. Dr. Sterman elaborates on some aspects of this cycle in Chapter 10.

INTERSPECIES DIFFERENCES

There are considerable similarities in the ontogenesis of the wakefulness-sleep cycle and its EEG correlates in the various species thus far studied. In this section we will discuss interspecies differences, which can also be looked upon as phylogenetic variables.

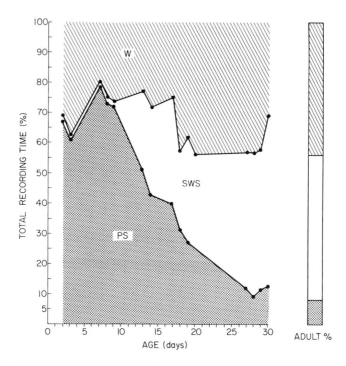

Fig. 3. Changes in mean percentages of wakefulness (W), slow wave sleep (SWS) ("quiet sleep" during the first 12 days), and paradoxical sleep (PS) during 8-hr recordings as a function of age in the rat. $N = 48$; number of animals = 18. The column at the right shows the 24-hr percentages of W, SWS, and PS in the adult. (From Jouvet-Mounier *et al.*, 1970. Courtesy of John Wiley & Sons, Inc.)

First, PS either does not occur (Hermann *et al.*, 1964) or is rare and evanescent (Ellingson, 1967; M. Jouvet, 1965a, b) in submammalian species.

Second, it would be idle to attempt to describe interspecies similarities and differences in EEG frequencies during sleep stages, since virtually no quantitative work has been done, and data given in the literature represent no more than rough estimates by the investigators in most cases. In fact, wakefulness and sleep were not even differentiated in many early studies of the ontogenesis of the animal EEG (Ellingson and Rose, 1970).

Marked interspecies differences in behavioral maturity at birth are largely reflected in differences in central nervous system maturity, both anatomical and physiological, including the maturity of EEG patterns. For example, as would be expected, the guinea pig displays relatively mature patterns at birth, and the rabbit, rat, and others relatively immature patterns (Ellingson and Rose, 1970).

Again, man requires a special note. The unusual association of the *tracé alternant* pattern with QS in the human infant has already been mentioned. It tends to disappear by 1-2 months after birth as the more familiar patterns seen throughout the remainder of life evolve.

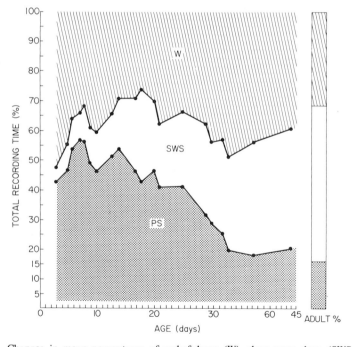

Fig. 4. Changes in mean percentages of wakefulness (W), slow wave sleep (SWS), and paradoxical sleep (PS) as a function of age in the kitten. The column at the right shows the 24-hr percentages of W, SWS, and PS in the adult. (From Jouvet-Mounier *et al.*, 1970. Courtesy of John Wiley & Sons, Inc.)

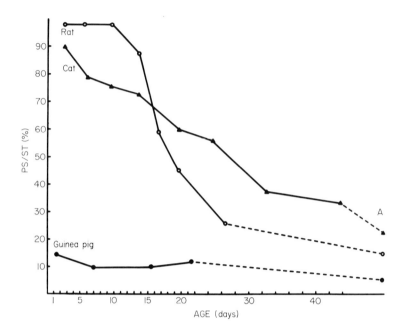

Fig. 5. Percentage of total sleep time (ST) of time spent in paradoxical sleep (PS) expressed as a function of age in the rat, cat, and guinea pig. (o) Rats; (●) cats; (▲) guinea pigs. The dotted lines connect with the percent value in the adult (A). (From Jouvet-Mounier *et al.,* 1970. Courtesy of John Wiley & Sons, Inc.)

Another distinctive feature of the EEG of the young human (at roughly 6 months to 8 years of age) is hypersynchronous intermediate slow (3-5/sec) activity during drowsiness (stage 1 sleep in the Kleitman-Dement classification). This is sometimes called "hypnagogic" or "oscitant" activity (Ellingson, 1967). Very similar activity has been observed during stage 1 in the macaque from age 1 week to age 15 months (Caveness, 1962). This has been described for no other species, except for a suggestively similar phenomenon in the dog, reported only by Fox (1967).

While TST as a proportion of total time decreases from birth to adulthood, there are marked interspecies differences. For example, the decrease in the cat is slight, while in man the decrease is from approximately 70% to approximately 30%. Another striking contrast in sleep pattern development concerns the proportions of QS time to PS time, and the changes in these ratios with age in different species. A recent paper by Jouvet-Mounier *et al.,* (1970) provides excellent examples. In the rat, for example, almost all sleep time is PS at birth (Fig. 3), but at maturity about 85% of sleep time is QS. In the cat (Fig. 4) there is a bit more QS at birth, and less QS at maturity (about 75%). Fig. 5 shows the developmental changes in PS time as a proportion of TST in three species. Figure

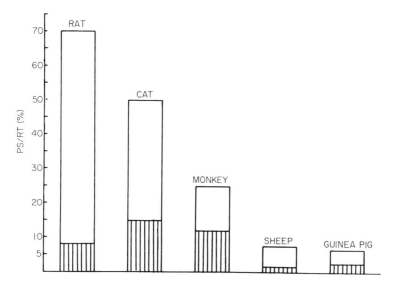

Fig. 6. Percentages of paradoxical sleep (PS) calculated for total recording time (RT) a'
7-8 days of age and in the adult of different mammals. The white columns show the PS
values in the young animals and the hatched columns show them in the adults. Data for PS
in rhesus monkey from Meier and Berger (1965). (From Jouvet-Mounier *et al.*, 1970.
Courtesy of John Wiley & Sons, Inc.)

6 shows PS time as a proportion of total recording time in infant and adult
animals in five species. This aspect of the development of sleep patterns seems to
be influenced by weaning (Astic and Jouvet-Mounier, 1968) and other
alimentary factors (D. Jouvet and Valatx, 1962; Jouvet-Mounier and Astic,
1966; Pellet and Béraud, 1967; Ruckebusch, 1962, 1963).

Several investigators have noted that these changes in PS in proportion to QS
do not follow a consistent phylogenetic pattern (Jouvet-Mounier *et al.*, 1970; M.
Jouvet, 1965a, b; D. Jouvet and Valatx, 1962; Pellet and Béraud, 1967). Rather,
species seem to fall into three groups with high, medium, and low percentages of
PS at maturity. Carnivores appear to retain the greatest percentage of PS time,
herbivores the least, and omnivores fall between (Jouvet-Mounier *et al.*, 1970;
Pellet and Béraud, 1967). Pellet and Béraud (1967) have presented two
hypotheses to explain these observations, of which they favor the hypothesis
that the differences are primarily related to diet and food-seeking habits.

REFERENCES

Astic, L., and Jouvet-Mounier, D. (1968). Effets du sevrage en fonction de l'âge sur le cycle
    veille-sommeil chez le cobaye. *J. Physiol. (Paris)* **60**, 389.
Caveness, W. F. (1962). "Atlas of Electroencephalography in the Developing Monkey:
    Macaca mulatta" Addison-Wesley, Reading, Massachusetts.

Dreyfus-Brisac, C. (1968). Sleep ontogenesis in early human prematurity from 24 to 27 weeks of conceptional age. *Develop. Psychobiol.* 1, 162-169.

Ellingson, R. J. (1967). The study of brain electrical activity of infants. *Advan. Child Develop. Behav.* 3, 54-98.

Ellingson, R. J., and Rose, G. H. (1970). Ontogenesis of the electroencephalogram. *In* "Developmental Neurobiology" (W. A. Himwich, ed.), pp. 441-474. Thomas, Springfield, Illinois.

Fox, M. W. (1967). Postnatal development of the EEG in the dog. II. Development of electrocortical activity. *J. Small Animl Pract.* 8, 77-107.

Hermann, H., Jouvet, M., and Klein, M. (1964). Analyse polygraphique du sommeil de la tortue. *C. R. Acad. Sci.* 258, 2175-2178.

Jouvet, D., and Valatx, J. L. (1962). Etude polygraphique du sommeil chez l'agneau. *C. R. Soc. Biol.* 156, 1411-1414.

Jouvet, M. (1965a). Etude de la dualité des états de sommeil et des mécanismes de la phase paradoxale. *In* "Aspects Anatomo-fonctionnels de la Physiologie du Sommeil," pp. 397-499. CNRS, Paris.

Jouvet, M. (1965b). Les bases neurophysiologiques et l'ontogénèse du sommeil chez l'animal. *Ann. Médico-Psychol.* 123, 481-482.

Jouvet-Mounier, D., and Astic, L. (1966). Etude du sommeil chez le cobaye adulte et nouveau-né. *C. R. Soc. Biol.* 160, 1453-1457.

Jouvet-Mounier, D., Astic, L., and Lacote, D. (1970). Ontogenesis of the states of sleep in rat, cat, and guinea pig during the first postnatal month. *Develop. Psychobiol.* 2, 216-239.

Kleitman, N. (1963). "Sleep and Wakefulness," rev. ed. Univ. of Chicago Press, Chicago.

Kleitman, N. (1967). Phylogenetic, ontogenetic and environmental determinants in the evolution of sleep-wakefulness cycles. *Res. Publ. Ass. Res. Nerv. Ment. Dis.* 45, 30-38.

Meier, G. W., and Berger, R. J. (1965). Development of sleep and wakefulness patterns in the infant Rhesus monkey. *Exp. Neurol.* 12, 257-277.

Pellet, J., and Béraud, G. (1967). Organisation nycthérmérale de la veille et du sommeil chez le cobaye (*Cavia porcellus*). Comparaisons interspécifiques avec le rat et le chat. *Physiol. Behav.* 2, 131-137.

Ruckebusch, Y. (1962). Evolution post-natale du sommeil chez les ruminants. *C. R. Soc. Biol.* 156, 1869-1873.

Ruckebusch, Y. (1963). Etude poligraphique et comportementale de l'évolution postnatale du sommeil physiologique chez l'agneau. *Arch. Ital. Biol.* 101, 111-132.

Scherrer, J., Verley, R., and Garma, L. (1970). A review of French studies in the ontogenetical field. *In* "Developmental Neurobiology" (W. A. Himwich, ed.), pp. 528-549. Thomas, Springfield, Ill.

Shimizu, A., and Himwich, H. E. (1968). The ontogeny of sleep in kittens and young rabbits. *Electroencephalogr. Clin. Neurophysiol.* 24, 307-318.

Verley, R. (1965). Recherches sur le développement des activités électro-corticales avec des électrodes corticales radiaires. *J. Physiol. (Paris)* 57, 407-436.

10

The Basic Rest-Activity Cycle and Sleep: Developmental Considerations in Man and Cats *

M. B. Sterman

For the past two decades, sleep research has proceeded under the notion that the state of sleep consists of two qualitatively and quantitatively distinct patterns. These patterns are defined by *composite* polygraphic and behavioral criteria, a fact reflected in the curious multiplicity of labels applied to them. These include, for example, *slow wave* vs *activated sleep*, with reference to the EEG; *REMS* (rapid eye movement sleep) vs *NREMS* (non-REM sleep), with reference to eye movements; and *quiet* vs *active sleep*, with reference to behavior. This fact has produced a chronic condition of semantic confusion in the sleep literature, a condition which is compounded when we consider sleep in immature organisms. To avoid this problem here, I will attempt to be consistent

*Supported by the United States Veterans Administration and by a grant from NIMH (MH-10083). Bibliographic assistance was received from the UCLA Brain Information Service which is part of the Neurological Information Network of NINDS and is supported under Contract DHEW PH-43-66-59.

by utilizing my own favorite labels for the two patterns, quiet sleep and REMS; although, as will become clear below, the latter term is suspect. The list of criteria which defines these patterns is by now familiar to the interested reader. Today, this list of behavioral and physiological measures is used with confidence to distinguish these two patterns of sleep from each other and from different behaviorally quiescent states, such as resting wakefulness, hypnotic trance, anesthesia, or coma.

These established criteria, with all of their reliability for defining sleep in the adult, are of little use, however, when we consider functional states in the infant. In the human newborn, many of the distinguishing characteristics of the pattern of quiet sleep are absent or sufficiently altered so as to require an entirely new set of standards. To be sure, the infant shows a state of quiescence resembling adult quiet sleep. However, this state is not comparably sustained, shows no systematic temporal distribution, is characterized by unusual behavioral manifestations, such as sucking and startle, and has few stable physiological correlates. These facts suggest that the similarity is misleading. Physiological criteria are particularly altered in comparison to adult definitions. EEG patterns are unique and poorly correlated with quiescent behavior. Spindle burst activity, an important EEG aspect of quiet sleep in the adult, does not appear in infant tracings until 1-3 months of age. Parmelee and Stern (see Chapter 11) indicate that some correlation does exist between EEG patterns and other criteria of state in the newborn, primarily due to more stable configurations in the REM state, but still find this measure to be one of the least reliable as a determinant. Additionally, excitability in sensory and motor pathways during quiescent periods is often indistinguishable from other states, or does not show the same consistent relationships characteristic of quiet sleep in the adult, even though some similarities are observed (Hrbek *et al.*, 1969; Vlach *et al.*, 1969; Rose, 1971; see also Chapters 12 and 14, this volume). The modulation of motor response threshold to sensory stimuli clearly does not distinguish between quiescent periods and so-called wakefulness periods in the neonate (Ellingson and Ellis, 1970); Finkelstein *et al.* (1971) have failed also to find in the infant the recently described changes in pituitary hormone secretions which accompany quiet sleep in the adult. Therefore, behavioral quiescence, and its reversibility, provide the only sound basis upon which one can ascribe quiet sleep to the human newborn. Yet we know that behavior alone cannot serve as a meaningful definition of state, at this or any other age.

It would seem, therefore, that the quiescent state in the newborn represents, in comparison to the adult, an altered state of consciousness. This altered or, perhaps more appropriately, unique state may be preliminary to a more dynamic adult quiet sleep. Such a position is supported by the extensive neurophysiological evidence for a multifaceted sleep mechanism in the adult (Hernández-Peón, 1967; Sterman and Clemente, 1968) and by the immature if not altered status of its probable neural substrates in the newborn (see Purpura, Chapter 1, this volume). Until a suitable criterion for quiet sleep can be established, which provides for a valid comparison between adult and newborn, it seems advisable to avoid a functional label at this point in development. Such an approach provides for the possible determination of a gradually emerging and developmentally plastic quiet sleep state, and for the study of the neural maturation associated with it.

Unlike quiet sleep, the REMS state is clearly present in the newborn. This state recurs regularly and without interruption throughout the first weeks of life, regardless of whether the infant is quiet or engaged in such activities as sucking, crying, or fussing (Emde and Metcalf, 1970). In fact, the continuous and intensified manifestations of the REM state in the infant led Kleitman (1963, 1969) to propose that this state represents a more fundamental recurrent process than sleep itself, a process which continues also during wakefulness. He attributed this cycle in central nervous system (CNS) activity to the coalescence during development of several primary physiological periodicities, and termed it the *basic rest-activity cycle*. This concept implies that the REM state, or the physiological process which it reflects, bears no specific relation to sleep. *How, indeed, can one study sleep in the infant?*

I would have viewed such a conclusion as unlikely several years ago. However, an increasing amount of evidence, much of it from our own studies, has led us to a serious reconsideration of the concept of a basic rest-activity cycle, and its implications for the study of functional states in the infant. The implied dissociation of the REM state from the process of sleep is an important departure from current interpretations and will require much substantiation in order to redirect the thinking of the sleep research establishment. I would like to describe some of our findings which are pertinent to this point, and which have convinced us that the REM state does reflect a functionally independent phenomenon.

Numerous studies, many of which are reviewed by Parmelee and Stern (Chapter 11) have shown that the unusual patterns of motor activity which accompany the REM state in the infant are its earliest and most reliable manifestation in ontogeny. The close correlation of one aspect of this activity, gross body movement, with other polygraphic criteria is shown in Fig. 1 (Roffwarg *et al.*, 1966). We have utilized this fact in an attempt to trace the REM state into the prenatal period by recording intrauterine fetal motility continuously from the abdomen of the resting or sleeping mother. The method employed is described in detail elsewhere (Sterman, 1967; Sterman and Hoppenbrouwers, 1971) and is reviewed in Fig. 2. Eight pregnant women were adapted to the laboratory recording situation and then studied monthly in the second and third trimesters during all-night recording sessions. The measurements included 5-9 hr of fetal activity, recorded through pressure electrodes

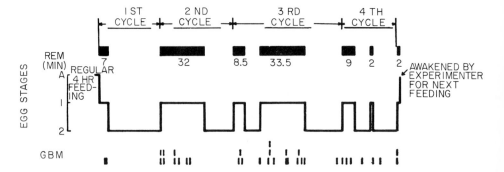

Fig. 1. Physiological and behavioral correlates of the REM cycle in a 4-day-old infant as reported by Roffwarg *et al.* (1966). Periods of REM are accompanied by stage 1, or low-voltage fast EEG patterns, and by gross body movements (GBM). The close correlation established between periods of gross body motility and other state criteria in the infant was pertinent to the study of this cycle in the human fetus.

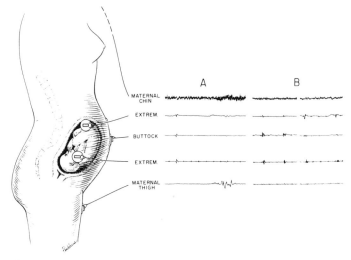

Fig. 2. Procedure for recording fetal activity is shown here utilizing a lateral representation of a pregnant subject and her fetus. Pressure-sensitive electrodes were placed systematically on the abdominal surface in relation to the position of the fetus within the uterus. A similar electrode was placed on the dorsal surface of the maternal thigh, together with chin EMG and other sleep-monitoring leads. Typical polygraphic recordings obtained from the fetal electrodes and those monitoring maternal movements are shown in A and B. Generalized fetal movement can be distinguished from maternal activity in A, and different patterns of fetal activity can be detected from the tracings in B. (From Sterman and Hoppenbrouwers, 1971).

placed over the estimated fetal head, extremities and buttock, and maternal EEG, eye movements, chin EMG, and gross body movements. The earliest recordings obtained were at 21 weeks gestation age, the latest at 40 weeks. All but one of the mothers slept more or less normally during these recording periods.

Fetal movements were counted and compiled for both cross-sectional and longitudinal analysis. These data were inspected visually and then subjected to power spectral analysis utilizing BMDX92 program from Dixon (1969), with bin widths of 1, 2, and 5 min and, in the case of data combined across subjects, with several different subject orders. This analysis provided for the determination of periodicities in these time series data and controlled for some of the errors which could occur with the linking of time series samples. Every test performed disclosed the existence of two consistent cycles of fetal activity. The cross-sectional analysis indicated that these periodicities were consistent throughout gestation. The analysis of data collected at 27-31 weeks gestation age is shown in Fig. 3 for two subject orders, and indicates two periodicities peaking at 38 and 83 min, respectively. Longitudinal analysis was made feasible by the absence of any gestational trend and had the advantage of reducing variability resulting from differences between infants. Such an analysis is shown in Fig. 4. Summary data for the eight subjects studied and mean cycle values obtained from each are shown in Table I. From these data an overall mean of 39.6 ± 11.8 min was obtained for the faster of the two cycles and a value of 96.4 ± 13.2 for the other.

Several of these infants participated as newborns in a study of sleep cycles by Stern *et al.* (1969), and their sleep patterns were followed for several years by Parmelee's group. At term, these infants displayed REM state cycles, determined by polygraphic and direct visual observation, which were virtually identical to the faster cycle derived from the analysis of fetal motility. We conclude, therefore, that these recurrent periods of motor activity observed in the fetus are a prenatal manifestation of the REM state or basic rest-activity cycle. Since this cycle was observed as early as 21 weeks gestation age and the existence of functional sleep and waking states at this and even later points in fetal development is most unlikely, a differentiation of the rest-activity and sleep-waking cycles is indicated in ontogeny.

The slower of the two cycles detected in fetal activity is not manifest in the newborn. This suggested that its origin may reside within the intrauterine environment, and implicated the mother as a possible physiological source. A comparison of fetal activity data with simultaneously recorded maternal sleep physiology has provided some evidence that the slower motility cycle is related to the REM cycle of the mother (Fig. 5). A similar conclusion was stated

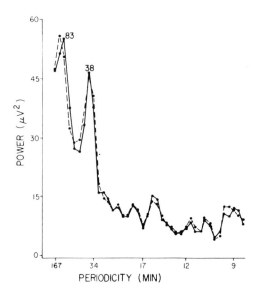

Fig. 3. Data from four subjects recorded between 27 and 31 weeks gestation were combined into separate, randomly determined time series and subjected to power spectral analysis. Combination was based upon visually detected modulation of activity and was required to achieve an adequately extended time sample for the determination of slow periodicities. This control procedure indicated that the order in which subject data were linked did not affect the periodicities detected by this analysis. In all orders and at all gestational periods sampled, two distinct peaks of cyclic activity were observed. (–) Order A; (– –) order B. (From Sterman and Hoppenbrouwers, 1971.)

TABLE I   *Summary of Fetal Recordings and Mean Periodicities in Fetal Motility Obtained by Power-Spectral Analysis[a]*

Subject	No. recording nights	Gestation period (weeks)	Cycles (min)	
			1	2
EL	2	21-23	20.0	96.0
PS	5	21-37	38.7	89.5
SW	5	21-39	57.0	105.0
JS	5	23-39	34.3	87.8
KK	3	25-35	50.3	121.3
HL	4	29-40	39.3	85.3
EM	3	31-37	47.0	81.2
SP	3	32-36	30.0	104.2
$N = 8$	$N = 30$	Range = 21-40	$\bar{x} = 39.6$	$\bar{x} = 96.4$
			SD = 11.8	SD = 13.2

[a]From Sterman and Hoppenbrouwers, 1971.

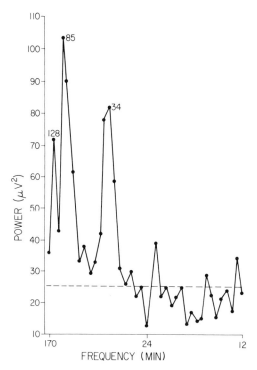

Fig. 4. Power spectral analysis utilizing five longitudinal samples of fetal activity data obtained from one subject between 23 and 39 weeks gestation age. Visual analysis of these data disclosed clear periodicities which were utilized in linking noncontinuous samples (i.e., last period of quiescence in one record was overlapped with first period of quiescence in the next). This procedure provided for a valid quantitative analysis, which for every subject disclosed two general clusters of periodicity, as indicated by peaks of spectral density in the analysis shown above. Dotted horizontal line indicates mean baseline density.

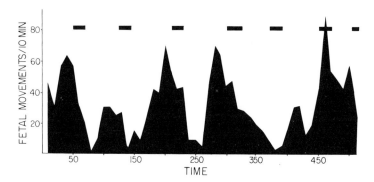

Fig. 5. Comparison of slower fetal activity cycle, enhanced for visual representation by the use of longer time intervals, with the maternal REM cycle as indicated by solid bars. Male subject, 35 weeks gestational age. The correspondence between peaks of fetal activity and periods of maternal REM sleep seen here was observed in approximately 65% of the comparisons and indicated a degree of relationship between these events. (From Sterman and Hoppenbrouwers, 1971.)

recently by Jeannerod (1969) from fetal studies carried out in France, but initiated in collaboration with our laboratory. It is interesting to note also that the slower fetal cycle of 96.4 ± 13.2 min compares favorably with the normative value of 101.5 min reported recently by Globus (1970) for the adult REM cycle.

We can conclude, tentatively, that this component of periodicity in fetal activity is related in some way to changes in physiology attendant upon the maternal rest-activity cycle. That this cycle continues during wakefulness was suggested by its clear manifestation in fetal activity data obtained from the one subject who could not sleep in the laboratory recording situation, but was willing to spend the greater part of four nights awake in the interest of science (Fig. 6).

Other indications of a differential development of the sleep-waking and rest-activity cycles can be found by relatively simple descriptive and normative comparisons. Figures 7 and 8 show developmental changes observed in sample EEG tracings taken from birth to 2 years of age in the same infant during the REM and quiescent states, respectively. Inspection of Fig. 7 suggests that very little change occurs in the polygraphic pattern of the REM state during development. Conversely, Fig. 8 demonstrates a dramatic developmental change in the quiescent state which is marked, particularly, by the appearance of sustained high amplitude slow waves and periodic spindle-bursts at 3 months of age. The maturation of thalamocortical systems between 1 and 3 months of age may parallel the emergence of an essentially adult quiet sleep mechanism, which contrasts with the presence of the REM state even prior to birth.

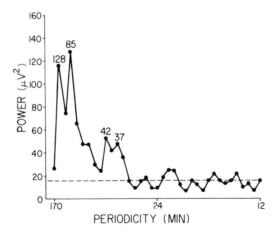

Fig. 6. Power spectral analysis of four longitudinal activity samples obtained from a subject (25-38 weeks gestation) who showed only minimal sleep during each of the 8-hr recording periods. Note that distribution of spectral densities, indicating fetal activity cycles, is very similar to that obtained from sleeping subjects. (From Sterman and Hoppenbrouwers, 1971.)

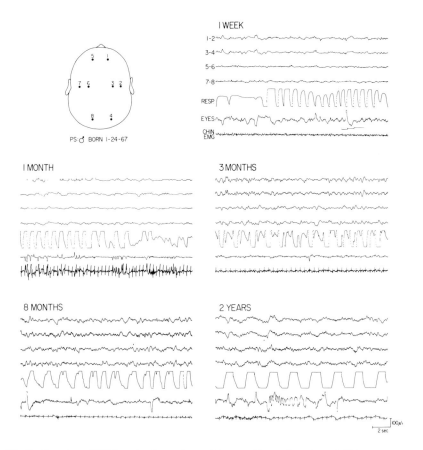

Fig. 7. Samples of EEG and other polygraphic recordings taken from REM state periods in the same male infant from 1 week to 2 years of age. Comparison of these samples indicates that the low voltage, fast EEG activity, irregular respiration, REM, and low submental muscle tone constitute a rather stable composite polygraphic pattern for this state throughout this period of dynamic CNS development. The slight but consistent increase in EEG modulation evident from 3 months on may be attributed to the maturation of neural systems not directly related to the brain stem mechanism underlying the occurrence of this state. (Data obtained through the courtesy of A. Parmelee and co-workers.)

The temporal distribution of states represents another dimension in which developmental comparison can be made between the sleep-waking and rest-activity cycles. A circadian rhythm of diurnal waking and nocturnal sleep is first manifest in the human infant during the second or third week of life (Rutenfranz, 1961) and becomes stabilized by 6 months of age (Kleitman and Engelmann, 1953). While the duration of the sleep and waking components of

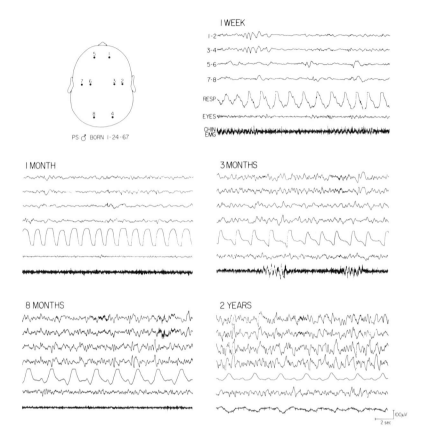

Fig. 8. Polygraphic samples taken at the same intervals from infant described in Fig. 7, but showing instead characteristic patterns during periods of quiescence. A dramatic change in EEG configuration can be noted between 1 month and 3 months of age. At 3 months well-developed slow waves and rudimentary spindle burst activity are present, a pattern which progresses to an essentially adult configuration by age 2 years. The relatively abrupt appearance during ontogeny of EEG and other manifestations (see text) of adult quiet sleep suggests the maturation of a dynamic sleep mechanism during this period, in contrast to the more or less constant manifestation of the REM state.

this rhythm will continue to change with age, the approximate 24 hr periodicity of each does not. In contrast with this, a survey of the available literature, combined with our findings derived from fetal studies, indicated that the temporal maturation of the rest-activity cycle follows a different course (Fig. 9). Stability in this cycle appears to wait upon developments occurring at 5-10 years of age, and perhaps later. This observation raises the possibility that the maturation of the rest-activity cycle is related to important changes in hypothalamic and pituitary functions which occur generally during this same developmental period.

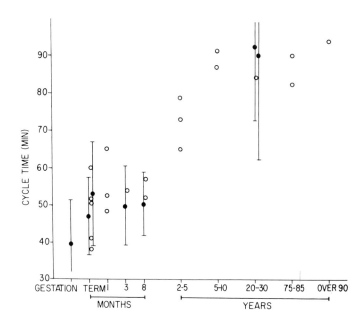

Fig. 9. Survey of the development of the human rest-activity or REM state cycle during ontogeny. Solid dots indicate reliable sample means for which adequate sample size and statistical description were available in the articles reviewed. Bars indicate standard deviation of these means. Open circles represent mean values derived from other data presented or merely stated without further statistical information. Collectively, these data indicate a slight trend toward lengthening of the cycle from the prenatal sample to 8 months of age; however, it is impossible to determine the statistical validity of this trend from these data, and the overlapping variabilities suggest no reliable developmental change during this period. A clearly significant increase in cycle duration is evident by 20-30 years of age, which appears to be sustained into senility. The precise period during which this shift occurs cannot be determined here, but the data suggest a transition between 2 and 10 years of age. Sources: gestation, this paper; term (●), Stern *et al.*, 1969, Roffwarg *et al.*, 1966 (statistics derived), (◯), Prechtl, 1968, Monod and Pajot, 1965, and other data from Roffwarg *et al.*, 1966; 1 month, Roffwarg *et al.*, 1966, Monod and Pajot, 1965, Kleitman, 1963; 3 months and 8 months, Roffwarg *et al.*, 1966; 2-5 years, Kohler *et al.*, 1968, Roffwarg *et al.*, 1964, Garvey, 1939; 5-10 years, Feinberg *et al.*, 1967, Roffwarg *et al.*, 1964; 20-30 years (●), Globus, 1971, this paper, (◯), Kahn and Fisher, 1969; 75-85 years, Feinberg *et al.*, 1967, Kahn and Fisher, 1969; over 90, Kahn and Fisher, 1969.

Animal studies in our laboratory have provided additional evidence for a separation of sleep-waking states from the rest-activity cycle. In a series of brain-transected preparations we have observed, as have others, that the isolated forebrain can continue to manifest EEG and other indications of quiet sleep, including slow waves and spindles, pupillary myosis, relaxation of the nictitating membranes and increased sensory thresholds (Batsel, 1960; Villablanca, 1966;

Slosarska and Zernicki, 1969). Also observed in these preparations is the simultaneous manifestation from the remaining hindbrain of an almost unaltered REM cycle, as indicated by recurrent periods of rapid eye movements, pontine spindle bursts, and neck muscle atonia. The occurrence of the REM state is clearly independent of the physiological pattern present in the forebrain at any given moment (Fig. 10). Thus, again, we find evidence that the brain mechanisms responsible for sleep on the one hand, and the REM state on the other, may indeed be separate and capable of independent function. We would agree with Jouvet (1967) in ascribing to structures in the pons an essential role in the manifestation of the REM cycle, but would place responsibility for sleep in the forebrain.

In other experiments with intact, behaving cats we have sought evidence for a continuous modulation of CNS excitability similar to the REM cycle, but occurring in the waking state. In order to approach this question, it was necessary to study a behavior the nature of which might reflect periodicity in sensory, motor, or cognitive functions. Previous studies carried out in our laboratory have developed the technique of EEG autoregulation in the cat (Sterman and Wyrwicka, 1967; Wyrwicka and Sterman, 1968). Animals are trained to receive food by producing specific localized EEG patterns. In the present context, this procedure was utilized to provide for the detection and automatic reinforcement with food of a discrete EEG pattern localized to sensorimotor cortex in the cat. This pattern has been termed the sensorimotor rhythm (SMR) (Fig. 11). Cats learn this instrumental EEG response rather quickly and show reliable levels of performance after several weeks of training (Fig. 12). The SMR seemed desirable since it is a centrally generated EEG pattern which at the same time is closely associated in behavior with the suppression of movement. Thus, in order to produce the SMR response, animals learn to adopt characteristic immobile postures. The resulting suppression of phasic motor behavior is a constant correlate of the SMR, but is not itself sufficient to produce this EEG pattern. We felt that such a central manifestation of performance might provide a meaningful assessment of the proposed CNS modulation during wakefulness.

An analysis of the intervals between sequential SMR responses disclosed a periodicity in the production of this EEG response. When plotted in relation to subsequent sleep, and compared with the REM cycle therein, periods of peak performance were found to describe a cycle, the duration of which was comparable to the REM cycle in sleep and the timing of which appeared to be continuous with that cycle (Figs. 13 and 14). When sleep followed more or less immediately upon the termination of performance, the initial REM period occurred at approximately the same time as the next predicted performance peak, based upon the preceding performance cycle (Fig. 13). On occasion, sleep was terminated at this point and the REM epoch replaced by a period of

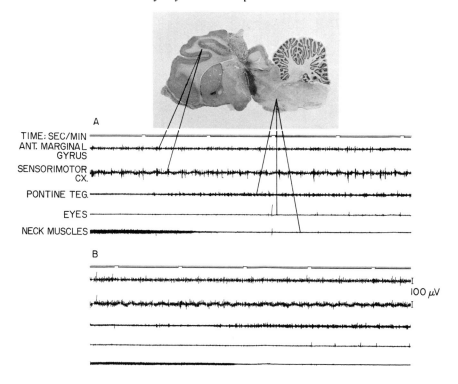

Fig. 10. Polygraphic tracings from a brain-transected adult cat. Saggital section of transected neuraxis at top indicates level at which forebrain and midbrain were separated by blunt transection and tissue aspiration. In this preparation, the tectum and tegmentum of the midbrain, as well as the remaining caudal portions of the CNS, are intact. Rostrally, the posterior diencephalon is damaged, but most middle and anterior thalamic and hypo-thalamic, as well as limbic, neostriatal, and telencephalic structures are intact. In A, large slow waves and spindle activity characterize the EEG pattern displayed by the isolated forebrain, particularly from recordings taken over sensorimotor cortex as is the case during sleep in normal animals. Pupillary myosis and relaxation of the nictitating membranes were observed also at this time. Recordings obtained simultaneously from the isolated hindbrain show a clear onset of the REM state, as indicated by pontine tegmental spindles, bursts of eye movements, and neck muscle atonia. In B, a similar initiation of the REM state is shown, but in this case occurring simultaneously with a desynchronized EEG pattern, pupillary mydriasis and contraction of the nictitating membranes in the separated forebrain. A functional and anatomical dissociation of forebrain sleep cycle and hindbrain REM cycle mechanisms is indicated.

performance *at peak levels*, with subsequent REM periods indicating an ongoing periodicity (Fig. 14). A comparison of performance and REM cycles from six animals is shown in Table IIA. No reliable differences were found between the mean values presented. A second paradigm was utilized to explore this question further. Animals trained to obtain food through instrumental SMR response

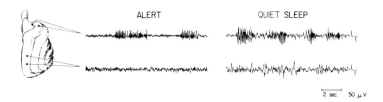

Fig. 11. Sample tracings of the 12-14 Hz rhythm recorded from sensorimotor cortex in the cat during wakefulness and sleep. The former has been termed the *sensorimotor rhythm* and the latter will be recognized as the familiar sleep spindle-burst. The functional relationship between these slow wave patterns has been established. The manifestation during wakefulness of the mechanism involved was utilized here as an instrumental response for the study of periodic modulation in CNS function. (Sterman *et al.*, 1970. Copyright 1970, American Association for the Advancement of Science.)

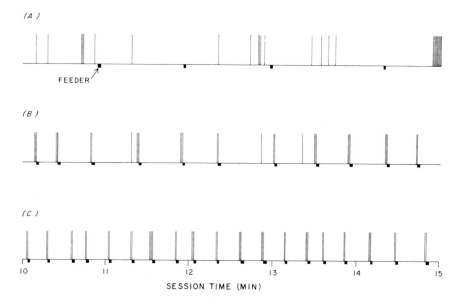

Fig. 12. Development of conditioned sensorimotor rhythm response in the cat. Vertical bars indicate distribution of quarter-second epochs of this rhythm (A) during random milk reinforcement, (B) during first session in which rhythm was reinforced by milk, and (C) 20 daily sessions later. Data samples were taken, in each instance, during a continuous 5-min period, 10 min after the initiation of a given test session. (From Wyrwicka and Sterman, 1968.)

were recorded from continuously for periods of 24 hr. These animals were not deprived of food prior to observation and, therefore, seldom demonstrated long periods of sustained performance. Instead, performance was episodic; however, these episodes occurred systematically, and described a cycle which was similar

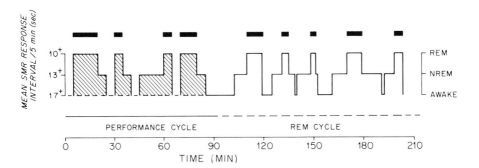

Fig. 13. Graphic representation of the sequential modulation of conditioned sensorimotor rhythm performance rate together with subsequent stages of wakefulness and sleep in the cat. Performance rate is indicated here as the mean interval between EEG responses in continuous 5-min epochs. Black bars during work indicate periods of peak performance and during sleep indicate REM periods. Note the similarity between intervals indicated by bars under waking and sleeping conditions and the apparent continuity of the cycles so described.

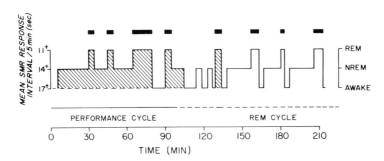

Fig. 14. Representation of performance cycle and REM cycle in the cat similar to that described in Fig. 13. In this animal, a sustained sleep did not develop following the initial termination of performance for food. The period of performance was brief and response output was at peak level. This performance epoch occurred at the expected time of the first REM period and was followed by a rather systematic series of evenly spaced REM periods. Both quantitative and visual analysis indicated a continuity in CNS modulation across wakefulness and sleep.

to and continuous with the REM cycle during sleep (Figs. 15 and 16). Mean REM cycle, performance cycle, and transition periods for four animals studied in this manner are presented in Table IIB. No reliable differences were obtained from *t*-test comparisons of these means.

We conclude from these findings that performance as measured here was modulated by a somewhat variable central timing mechanism whose period was similar to and continuous with the REM cycle during sleep. We assume a

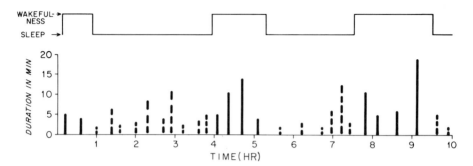

Fig. 15. Analysis of performance and sleep modulation during prolonged observation under *ad lib* food condition. The sleep-wakefulness cycle of this cat is indicated in the upper portion of figure and was determined by standard scoring of polygraphic data. Periods of instrumental performance (conditioned sensorimotor rhythm for food) are shown as solid vertical bars, the height of which indicates their duration. REM state periods during sleep and their duration are similarly indicated by broken vertical bars. Note the similarity in the distribution of work periods during waking to the distribution of REM periods during sleep. Viewed in this manner, the continuity of these cyclic manifestations is particularly apparent.

TABLE II   *Comparison of Performance Cycle, REM Cycle and Transition Period Means and Standard Deviations Obtained in Two Experiments Outlined in Text*

	Cycle duration		
	REM	Performance	Transition
A. Continuous Performance and Sleep (2-4 hr observation)			
(Group Data, $N = 6$)			
	23.6 ± 8.9	23.4 ± 8.9	30.5 ± 9.4
B. Alternating Performance and Sleep (24 hr observation)			
(Individual Data, $N = 4$)			
1	21.6 ± 6.4	19.5 ± 6.6	16.7 ± 4.7
2	19.9 ± 5.8	20.2 ± 9.2	23.3 ± 15.5
3	21.1 ± 7.7	27.8 ± 15.0	26.1 ± 8.6
4	29.0 ± 10.9	36.0 ± 15.3	21.0 ± 11.2

common central mechanism for these periodicities under the concept of a basic rest-activity cycle. As such, performance provides a measure of this cycle during wakefulness. A similar conclusion has been drawn from studies of the REM cycle and performance modulation in humans (Globus *et al.*, 1971).

The sleep-waking rhythm and REM cycle are being compared also before and after EEG conditioning (Lucas and Sterman, 1971). We have found, thus far, that the sleep-waking rhythm is shortened significantly by the introduction of a task during the 24-hr period of observation. This shift reflects an increase in the amount of time spent awake and a decrease in sleep. Overall food intake is not increased with performance, since the baseline condition also provides free access to food. Therefore, it would seem that the cat can definitely get by with less sleep when some meaningful task is available during wakefulness. One is tempted to explore the implications of this finding with regard to human sleep patterns.

While the sleep-waking rhythm of trained animals was significantly altered in comparison to pretraining measures, the rest-activity cycle, as indicated by the recurrence of REM periods, was not. This is another indication that the two periodicities can vary independently. Some of these trained animals were administered low doses of amphetamines, orally, in half portions mixed with solid food and presented at 12-hr intervals. Sleep-waking behavior was monitored continuously during the intervening periods. With doses as low as 0.35 mg/kg of amphetamine, sleep was severely curtailed. In spite of the obvious disruption of the sleep-waking rhythm produced by this drug, many animals continued to show normal performance of the trained EEG response for food (Fig. 16). While few REM epochs were observed, their period, as well as the cycle of performance demonstrated during prolonged wakefulness, did not differ from baseline values previously obtained. Therefore, amphetamine altered the sleep-waking rhythm without apparently affecting the rest-activity cycle. This dissociation of these two phenomena again suggests their independent modula-

TABLE III *Comparison of 24-hr Sleep-Waking Rhythm and Rest-Activity Cycle Data Obtained Before (Control) and After (Performance) the Acquisition of an Instrumental EEG Response for Food[a]*

Cat no.	Sleep-wakefulness rhythm		Rest-activity (REM) cycle	
	Baseline	Performance	Baseline	Performance
1	147.33	104.67	25.81	18.78
2	128.33	111.67	22.74	22.18
3	130.67	113.33	28.65	24.90
4	110.33	92.67	18.68	16.64
$\bar{x}$	129.17	105.58	23.97	20.62
S.D.	15.14	9.38	4.27	3.65
	$t = 2.294, df = 6$		$t = 1.03, df = 6$	
	$p < 0.05$		NS	

[a]Values presented are mean cycle times measured from four different cats during 24-hr observations. The rest-activity cycle was determined during sleep by reference to REM state periodicity.

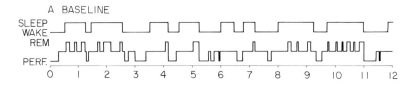

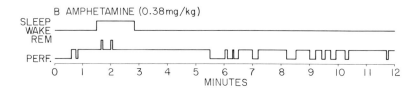

Fig. 16. Comparison of sleep-waking and rest-activity cycles (the latter indicated by performance and REM state periodicity as in Fig. 15) in a cat before and after the oral administration of time-released amphetamine. In both (A) and (B) the sleep-waking cycle is shown above a similar representation of the rest-activity cycle, indicated by REM periods as upward bars and work periods as downward bars. A normal modulation, similar to that shown in Fig. 15, is apparent in the predrug recording at (A). As seen in (B), amphetamine abolished sleep within 3 hr after administration. However, the REM cycle during the one sleep period was essentially normal, as was the performance cycle, after some delay in onset.

tion by the CNS. If the REM state is specifically rooted in the physiology of sleep and a fundamental aspect of the expression of that process, it would be expected that any influences which alter sleep would affect also the temporal manifestation of the REM state. Yet in the two instances described above, and in experiments relating the occurrence of REM to sleep onset (Globus *et al.*, 1969) or to previous REM deprivation (Kales *et al.*, 1964), this was not the case.

The rest-activity cycle is most easily studied during sleep, where the contrasting patterns of physiology provide for a facile discrimination of alternating states. The findings reported above lend renewed importance to this physiological periodicity and have led us to examine it more closely. Figure 17 presents data from Lucas and Sterman (1971) showing the distribution of intervals between REM epochs recorded during sustained sleep periods in 15 cats. It is essential that the determination of normative values for the distribution of intervals between REM epochs, and thus the rest-activity cycle, be made during continuous sleep. Measurement of this temporal dimension is made impossible by any prolonged break, as it were, in the ruler. Wakefulness represents a change in baseline state. According to the position taken here, it is possible to measure this cycle across states only when a suitable means of detection is continuously available. In the present analysis, we wished only to measure manifestations of the rest-activity cycle during sleep. It can be seen from Fig. 17 that this cycle is subject to normal variation. The distribution is gaussian, with a slight positive skew. The mean value obtained for the cat was 22.3 ± 4.3 min and the modal interval 20-30 min. Subsequent studies with more animals have produced a somewhat shorter mean cycle of 19.20 ± 2.20 min (Sterman *et al.*, 1972).

We have made an attempt to follow the ontogenetic development of this cycle in the cat by compiling *reliable* data points at various ages. Unfortunately, the sleep literature is sparse on this measure, and we have found it necessary to collect much of the required information ourselves. The limited data obtained thus far, together with less complete information from the kitten literature and several solid values from adult studies, are presented in Fig. 18. These combined data suggest that the kitten has a significantly shorter cycle than the adult for at least the first 3 weeks of life. It appears as though adult values are achieved by 1 month of age, but the estimates shown do not provide measures of variability and may represent limited samples. A definitive determination of this developmental sequence awaits further data.

DISCUSSION

It has become increasingly clear in recent years that the sleep process represents the interplay of many variable neural influences. Contrary to previous conceptions, which portrayed sleep as a homogeneous, all-or-none kind of phenomenon, more recent findings indicate a heterogeneous process responsive to essentially every aspect of biological function, and taking, accordingly, a number of distinguishable configurations (Sterman and Wyrwicka, 1967, 1970; Jacobs *et al.*, 1971); see also Dement, Chapter 15 this volume). Perhaps this

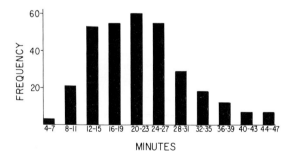

Fig. 17. Distribution of the durations of 320 REM period cycles obtained in equitable amounts from 15 adult cats during sleep. Cycle times were taken exclusively from periods of sustained sleep, as explained in text. They were measured as the time elapsing from the start of one REM period to the start of the next. *N* = 320.

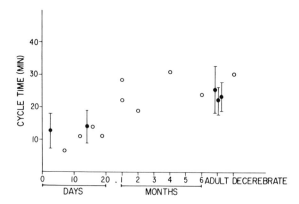

Fig. 18. Survey of the development of the feline rest-activity cycle in ontogeny, as indicated by measures of REM state periodicity. Solid dots and bars indicate means and standard deviations from studies carried out in our laboratory. The last of the three statistically described samples from the adult cat is, however, from Ursin (1968). Open circles indicate values reported without statistical reference. These data points show a clear lengthening of cycle duration between kitten and adult cat, and suggest a transition at the end of the first month. Values determined in our laboratory from one adult decerebrate preparation suggest that the cycle was not markedly altered by the removal of forebrain structures. (Sources for open circles: Jouvet-Mounier *et al.*, 1970; Chase and Sterman, 1967.)

fact is responsible for the frustration encountered in attempts to define this process and to specify its function.

In the present discussion, I have taken the rather unorthodox position that sleep does not exist in the newborn infant. From an objective standpoint, in which one applies the criteria for the distinction of sleep from other altered states of consciousness in the adult, this position would seem to be quite valid. However, I would rather interpret the unequivocal differences between adult and infant sleep as strengthening and extending the position elaborated above, namely, that sleep is a multifunctional process which accomplishes different objectives according to varying biological requirements. In the infant, where the complex adaptive functions of the forebrain are rudimentary and superseded by predetermined reflex patterns organized at lower levels of the neuraxis, the luxuries of choice and social obligation are still lacking, and the primary function of sleep is, most likely, restoration and growth. With the emergence of higher nervous capacities, additional neural components are added to the integration which determines both the control and the expression of this process. It is the development of these forebrain influences which conveys to sleep its adult complexities and thus its altered configuration and expanded utility. From this point of view, the primitive "sleep" of the newborn, the fetus, and the decerebrate cat is relegated to a more circumscribed, albeit fundamental, role.

A common feature of brain physiology in the presence of such a depressed or nonfunctional forebrain is the clear emergence of a more or less continuous rest-activity cycle, as manifest by alternating REM and NREM states. This is certainly the case in the decerebrate cat where the forebrain is removed, and in the fetus and newborn where the immature status of descending forebrain influences is documented. In the adult, this condition develops to some extent during sleep, a state serving complex functional needs, but also characterized neurophysiologically by the withdrawal of both facilitatory and inhibitory forebrain influences. These facts establish the rest-activity cycle as a fundamental aspect of physiology, both functionally and in terms of the structural evolution of the CNS. The controlling mechanism has been localized to the brain stem, and in the absence of forebrain integration expresses its influence overtly as a periodic modulation of neuronal excitability. The source of stimulation which modulates this brain stem "gain control" mechanism may be as basic as metabolism, residing in the accumulation or depletion of various biochemical precursors, enzymes, or by-products. Its function in the immature state may be simply homeostatic, but with the development of higher nervous activities it may, fortuitously, provide a unit of biological time. Kleitman (1967) has expressed this latter interpretation, pointing out that man has organized his waking day into roughly 2-hr units of work, feeding, and rest. He has suggested further that the onset and termination of sleep itself is influenced by this same unit, since sleep is always most successfully initiated during a trough in this cycle and terminated during a peak (i.e., a REM period). Our data from the study of sleep in cats support this position.

The recognition of a basic periodicity manifest in mammalian physiology and reflected also in behavior poses several important research challenges. What aspects of biological function provide the pendulum for this clock? How does disease modify this pendulum and how does the pendulum influence disease patterns? If the "hands" of this clock, to use Richter's (1965) term, are expressed in physiology and behavior, how can we use this knowledge to human advantage? Finally, can cognizance of this primary neural manifestation aid us in monitoring human development?

REFERENCES

Anders, T., Sachar, E., Kream, J., Roffwarg, H., and Hellman, L. (1971). Behavioral state and plasma cortisol response in the human newborn. *Psychophysiol.* 7, 323.

Batsel, H.L., (1960). Electroencephalographic synchronization and desynchronization in the chronic "cerveau isolé" of the dog. *Electroencephalogr. Clin. Neurophysiol.* 12, 421-430.

Chase, M. H., and Sterman, M. B. (1967). Maturation of patterns of sleep and wakefulness in the kitten. *Brain Res.* 5, 319-329.

Dixon, W. J. (1969). "BMD Biomedical Computer Programs," X-Ser. Suppl. Univ. of California Press, Los Angeles.

Ellingson, R. J., and Ellis, R. R. (1970). Motor response thresholds to electrical stimulation at the wrist in human newborns. *Develop. Psychobiol.* 2, 202-206.

Emde, R. N., and Metcalf, D. R. (1970). An electroencephalographic study of behavioral rapid eye movement states in the human newborn. *J. Nerv. Ment. Dis.* 150, 376-386.

Feinberg, I., Koresko, R. L., and Heller, N. (1967). EEG sleep patterns as a function of normal and pathological aging in man. *J. Psychiat. Res.* 5, 107-144.

Finklestein, J., Anders, T., Sachar, E., Roffwarg, H., and Hellman, L. (1971). Behavioral state, age, and plasma growth hormone levels in human neonates. *Psychophysiol.* 7, 322.

Garvey, C. R. (1939). "The Activity of Young Children During Sleep." Univ. of Minnesota Press, Minneapolis.

Globus, G. G. (1970). Quantification of the REM sleep cycle as a rhythm. *Psychophysiol.* 7, 248-253.

Globus, G. G., Gardner, R., and Williams, T. A. (1969). Relation of sleep onset to rapid eye movement sleep. *Arch. Gen. Psychiat.* 21, 151-154.

Globus, G. G., Phoebus, E., and Moore, C. (1971). REM "sleep" manifestations during waking. *Psychophysiol.* 7, 308.

Hernández-Peón, R. (1967). Neurophysiology, phylogeny and functional significance of dreaming. *Exp. Neurol., Suppl.* 4, 106-125.

Hrbek, A., Hrbkova, M., and Lenard, H. (1969). Somato-sensory, auditory and visual evoked responses in newborn infants during sleep and wakefulness. *Electroencephalogr. Clin. Neurophysiol.* 26, 597-603.

Jacobs, B. L., Harper, R. M., and McGinty, D. J. (1971). Neuronal coding of motivational level during sleep. *Physiol. Behav.* 5, 1139-1143.

Jeannerod, M. (1969). Les mouvements du foetus pendant le sommeil de la mère. *C. R. Soc. Biol.* 163, 1843-1847.

Jouvet, M. (1967). Neurophysiology of the states of sleep. *Physiol. Rev.* 47, 117-177.

Jouvet-Mounier, D., Astic, L., and Lacote, D. (1970). Ontogenesis of the states of sleep in rat, cat, and guinea pig during the first postnatal month. *Develop. Psychobiol.* 2, 216-239.

Kahn, E., and Fisher, C. (1969). The sleep characteristics of the normal aged male. *J. Nerv. Ment. Dis.* 148, 477-494.

Kales, A., Hoedemaker, F. S., Jacobson, A., and Lichtenstein, E. L. (1964). Dream deprivation: An experimental reappraisal. *Nature (London)* 204, 1337-1338.

Kleitman, N. (1963). "Sleep and Wakefulness," Univ. of Chicago Press, Chicago.

Kleitman, N. (1967). Phylogenetic, ontogenetic and environmental determinants in the evolution of sleep-wakefulness cycles. *Res. Publ., Ass. Res. Nerv. Ment. Dis.* 45, 30-38.

Kleitman, N. (1969). *In* "Sleep Physiology and Pathology" (A. Kales, ed.), pp. 33-38. Lippincott, Philadelphia, Pennsylvania.

Kleitman, N., and Engelmann, T. (1953). Sleep characteristics of infants. *J. Appl. Physiol.* 6, 269-282.

Kohler, W. C., Coddington, R. D., and Agnew, H. W. (1968). Sleep patterns in 2-year-old children. *J. Pediat.* 72, 228-233.

Lucas, E. A., and Sterman, M. B. (1971). To be published.

Metcalf, D. R. (1970). EEG sleep spindle ontogenesis. *Neuropaediatrie.* 1, 428-433.

Monod, N., and Pajot, N. (1965). Le sommeil du nouveau-né et du prématuré. *Biol. Neonatorum* 8, 281-307.

Prechtl, H. F. R. (1968). Polygraphic studies of the full-term newborn: II. Computer analysis of recorded data. *In* "Studies in Infancy" (M. C. Bax, and R. C. MacKeith, eds.), pp. 22-40. Heinemann, London.

Richter, C. P. (1965). "Biological Clocks in Medicine and Psychiatry," p. 80. Thomas, Springfield, Illinois.

Roffwarg, H. P., Dement, W. C., and Fisher, C. (1964). Preliminary observations of the sleep-dream pattern in neonates, infants, children and adults. *Monogr. Child Psychol.* **2**, 60-72.

Roffwarg, H. P., Muzio, J. N., and Dement, W. C. (1966). Ontogenetic development of the human sleep-dream cycle. *Science* **152**, 604-619.

Rose, G. H. (1971). The relationship of electrophysiological and behavioral indices of visual development in mammals. *In* "Brain Development and Behavior" (M. B. Sterman, D. J. McGinty, and A. M. Adinolfi, eds.), pp. 145-181. Academic Press, New York.

Rutenfranz, J. (1961). The development of circadian system functions during infancy and childhood. *In* "Circadian Systems," pp. 38-41. Ross Laboratories, Columbus, Ohio.

Slosarska, M., and Zernicki, B. (1969). Synchronized sleep in the chronic pretrigeminal cat. *Acta Biol. Exp. (Warsaw)* **29**, 175-184.

Sterman, M. B. (1967). Relationship of intrauterine fetal activity to maternal sleep stage. *Exp. Neurol.* **19**, 98-106.

Sterman, M. B., and Clemente, C. D. (1968). Basal forebrain structures and sleep. *Acta Neurol. Latino Amer.* **14**, 228-249.

Sterman, M. B., and Hoppenbrouwers, T. (1971). The development of sleep-waking and rest-activity patterns from fetus to adult in man. *In* "Brain Development and Behavior" (M. B. Sterman, D. J. McGinty, and A. M. Adinolfi, eds.), pp. 203-225. Academic Press, New York.

Sterman, M. B., and Wyrwicka, W. (1967). EEG correlates of sleep: Evidence for separate forebrain substrates. *Brain Res.* **6**, 143-163.

Sterman, M. B., Howe, R. C., and Macdonald, L. R. (1970). Facilitation of spindle-burst sleep by conditioning of electroencephalographic activity while awake. *Science* **167**, 1146-1148.

Sterman, M. B., Lucas, E. A., Macdonald, L. R. (1972). Periodicity within sleep and operant performance in the cat. *Brain Res.* (in press).

Stern, E., Parmelee, A. H., Akiyama, Y., Schultz, M. A., and Wenner, W. H. (1969). Sleep cycle characteristics in infants. *Pediatrics* **43**, 65-70.

Ursin, R. (1968). The two stages of slow wave sleep in the cat and their relation to REM sleep. *Brain Res.* **11**, 347-356.

Villablanca, J. (1966). Behavioral and polygraphic study of "sleep" and "wakefulness" in chronic decerebrate cats. *Electroencephalogr. Clin. Neurophysiol.* **21**, 562-577.

Vlach, V., von Bernuth, H., and Prechtl, H. F. R. (1969). State dependency of exteroceptive skin reflexes in newborn infants. *Develop. Med. Child Neurol.* **11**, 353-362.

Wyrwicka, W., and Sterman, M. B. (1968). Instrumental conditioning of sensorimotor cortex EEG spindles in the waking cat. *Physiol. Behav.* **3**, 703-707.

11

Development of States in Infants*

Arthur H. Parmelee, Jr. and Evelyn Stern

Study of fetal activity *in utero* and state organization in prematures, term newborns, and young infants gives us some insight into behavioral organization from its beginning. The dramatic changes in the complexity of behavior during the first weeks of life would appear to present us with the problem of redefining the organization of behavior each week and each month. The behavior of newborns and young infants seems chaotic and unpatterned in comparison to that of older infants and children, especially if only a single point in time is taken for study. But, if several points are compared, the chaotic quality can be seen to diminish, and patterning emerges. The rapidity of development in infants allows us to follow the evolution of behavioral organization over a relatively

*Supported in part by grants from NICHD (HD-00351 and HD-04008). Computing assistance was obtained from the Health Sciences Computing Facility, UCLA, sponsored by a grant from NIH (FR-3).

199

short time span. When we can correlate these observations with increases in the complexity of neural elements and brain neurochemistry, we will have a better understanding of how the nervous system influences behavior.

I will address myself to the problem of defining states and describing their maturational characteristics in the prematurely born, the full-term newborn, and the very young infant. According to Ashby (1956), "by states of a system is meant any well-defined condition or property that can be recognized if it occurs again." Prechtl (Prechtl, *et al.*, 1968) has rephrased this for behavioral studies of infants: "by the term state, one tries to describe constellations of certain functional patterns and physiological variables which may be relatively stable and which seem to repeat themselves." Thus, states represent sustained levels of organization of brain function that occur spontaneously or are induced and may recur cyclically. Understanding the organization of states is important for studies of induced behavioral responses, because the organism's state is a constraint on its response capabilities and state changes are likely to interact with stimulus properties, especially in the case of repetitive stimulation.

COMPONENTS OF STATE

In our behavioral studies of prematures and newborns we decided to use eyes open and eyes closed and amount of body activity as one measure of state. This was a practical decision based on the fact that these criteria can be readily observed and used over a wide age range, including the fetus and premature. These two variables were combined into one scale used for coding directly observed, not electronically monitored, behavior (see tabulation below).

	0.	No body movement
	1.	Facial movements only
Eyes closed	2.	Hand, foot, arm, or leg movements
	3.	Total body movements
	4.	Eyes opening and closing, with or without body movement
	5.	No body movement
	6.	Facial movement
Eyes open	7.	Hand, foot, arm, or leg movements
	8.	Total body movement
	9.	Crying (eyes open or closed)

For conventional description, we have designated the eyes closed periods as sleep and eyes open as wakefulness. For the 2- or 3-month-old infant there is little difficulty defending these designations. In the term newborn, the determination of sleep and wakefulness on the basis of eyes open or closed is less clear, but the stimulation studies of Wagner (1937) and Wolff (1959, 1966) would support this. In the premature infant, decisions about sleep and wakefulness on the basis of eyes open or closed become increasingly difficult with increasing prematurity (Gesell and Amatruda, 1945).

As our second measure of state, we chose respiratory pattern, which is probably only useful in defining states during sleep. When the eyes are open, respirations are almost always irregular, whereas during sleep a cycling of regular and irregular respiratory pattern as well as cycling of rate (Denisova and Figurin, 1926; Prechtl and Beintema, 1964) can be seen. Wagner (1937), Wolff (1959), and Prechtl *et al.* (1968) have used respiratory patterns in conjunction with eyes closed and body activity in their state definitions.

Finally, presence or absence of eye movements, observed under the closed eyelids or electronically recorded, is an important state criterion for us and most current investigators in this field. Kleitman (1963) credits Denisova and Figurin (1926) with first describing the cycling of eye movement activity in conjunction with changes in body activity and respiratory rate during sleep in babies (Fig. 1). Kleitman and Aserinsky's extension of these observations has been the basis for most of our current interest in the eye movement state in infants (Aserinsky and Kleitman, 1955).

Respiratory pattern and eye movements are also easily observed state parameters but are not as useful with the fetus and premature of low gestational age as body movements.

DEVELOPMENT OF STATE VARIABLES

We have been impressed by two major maturational changes in the organization of states, which appear to be manifestations of growth of brain inhibitory and feedback controlling mechanisms. They parallel the rapidly increasing complexity of dendritic interactions at all levels of the maturing central nervous system (CNS). One is the increasing proportion of quiescent periods in each parameter, that is, respiratory regularity, and absence of body activity and eye movements. The second is the increasing association of the various state criteria with each other, from almost complete dissociation in the 24-week fetus to close coherence and rhythmic cycling by 3 months past term.

The first fetal movement that can be elicited occurs at 7-8 weeks of postmenstrual age (Windle and Fitzgerald, 1937) and the first spontaneous movement at 9-10 weeks (Hooker, 1953). Therefore, potential for activity exists very early in fetal life. Sterman (Chapter 10) has demonstrated rhythmic activity cycling in the fetus *in utero* by 5 months gestation, the earliest age at which he recorded. Dreyfus-Brisac (1968) observed and recorded activity in the previable premature of 24-26 weeks gestation and reports almost continuous movement,

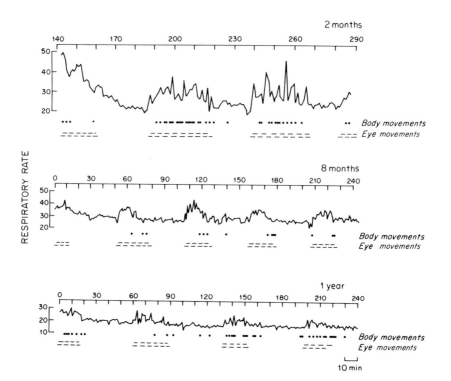

Fig. 1. Cycling of eye movements, body activity and respiratory rate in a 2-month-, 8-month-, and 1-year-old infant. Respiration ranges are 20-50 breaths/min (top and middle) and 10 to 30 (bottom). (From Denisova and Figurin, 1926.)

generally localized to the extremities. There is some rhythmic fluctuation in this activity, evident in her illustrations, but it is not pronounced (Fig. 2). At 28-30 weeks, very brief quiet periods begin to appear (Dreyfus-Brisac, 1967). These have some periodicity as illustrated by Eckstein and Paffrath (1928), (Fig. 3), who also emphasized that this periodicity is very unstable. By 32 weeks conceptional age, body movements are absent in 53% of the 20-sec epochs of our 2-3-hr sleep recordings. The modal observation score is taken for each 20 sec; thus a period scored as no movement may include a brief body jerk or other short lasting movement. The number of no movement epochs increases to 60% at term and 81% at 8 months. The frequency of periods with movement decreases accordingly. These changes indicate a rapid growth in inhibition of body activity in sleep during this period (Fig. 4).

We do not know when eye movements first appear in the fetus. Dreyfus-Brisac (1967) reports that they are very infrequent at 24-26 weeks and never appear in bursts. At 28-30 weeks they are sparse, occurring at a rate of 1-4/min, but

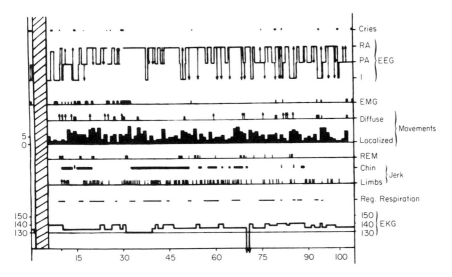

Fig. 2. Polygraphic sleep record of a 26-hr-old, 815-g infant born at 25 weeks gestation. Note the continuous localized body movements. (From Dreyfus-Brisac, 1968.)

almost continuously present. Continuous periods without eye movements are generally short; the longest was 12 min. By 32 weeks, the infant displays periods of much denser eye movement activity. In our study, 9 or more eye movements were seen in 13% of 20-sec epochs and 1-6 eye movements in 37%. Periods of no eye movements constituted 50% of the record at 32 weeks, 56% at term, and about 70% by 8 months past term (Fig. 5). Eye movement activity progresses from being almost totally absent at the earliest age, to infrequent and widely scattered, to clustered by 32 weeks; after 40 weeks conceptional age, a marked decrease in amount occurs. This progression also supports the concept of increasing cerebral inhibition.

Respiratory efforts of the fetus delivered at 9 weeks gestation are confined to occasional gasps; rhythmic respiratory movements can be observed by 17 weeks (Bergström and Bergström, 1963). Dreyfus-Brisac (1968) describes the respiration of the 24- to 26-week premature as predominantly irregular or semiregular and without change during movement. By 28-30 weeks, the respirations are almost exclusively irregular (1967). We scored 6% of 20-sec epochs as having regular respiration at 32 weeks, 24% at term, and 54% at 8 months. Again, there is evidence for the increasing development of a CNS controlling mechanism.

We have not done detailed analyses of chin EMG activity, primarily because there are so few periods of tonic activity in the premature before 36 weeks conceptional age. From term on, clearly contrasting and sustained periods of EMG activity and inactivity are frequent enough to make it a useful parameter of state.

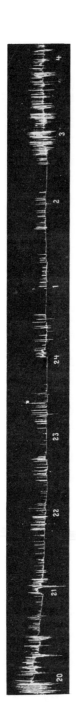
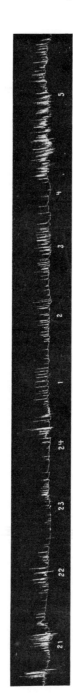

Fig. 3. Cycling of body activity in prematures. Top: infant of 1790 g birth weight. Bottom: infant of 1908 g birth weight. Hours indicated below each actogram record. (From Eckstein and Paffrath, 1928.)

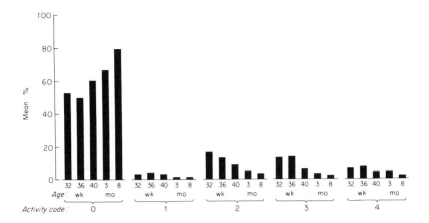

Fig. 4. Distributions of activity codes during sleep recordings at each age. See text for explanation of code numbers.

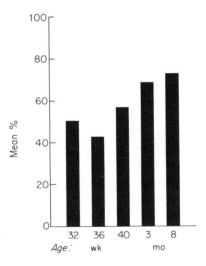

Fig. 5. Age distribution of 20-sec periods without eye movements during sleep recordings.

EEG activity in the 24- to 26-week premature infant consists solely of discontinuous bursts of activity. With maturation, an increasing number of readily discernible patterns evolve, so that by 8 months there are six sleep EEG patterns (Parmelee *et al.*, 1968a, b).

In summary, we can say that the parameters are not all equally useful in attempting to arrive at definitions of state in the young premature, because some show little or no variability before term. The ages and the degree to which each is applicable are shown schematically in Table I.

TABLE I *A Schematic Organization of the Usefulness of Measures in Defining State in the Premature and Young Infant*

	Weeks conceptional age					Months past term	
	24	28	32	36	40	3	8
Body movements	±	+	++	+++	++++	++++	++++
Eye movements		+	++	+++	++++	++++	++++
Respiration pattern			±	++	+++	++++	++++
EEG			±	++	+++	++++	++++
Chin EMG				+	+++	++++	++++

Thus, as the infant matures, he has a greater number of quiescent periods which, in addition, become consolidated into progressively longer, continuous periods. While in the older infant or adult, quiescence or activity on one parameter is very likely to occur simultaneously with quiescence or activity on other parameters, this does not hold true for the newborn or premature infant. The development of this concordance among parameters constitutes the second major maturational change which we feel is a function of the increasing complexity of the brain during this period.

DEVELOPMENT OF SLEEP STATES

On the basis of our own and other data, we defined two major sleep states in infancy: (1) quiet sleep, characterized by eyes closed and no eye movements, no body movements and regular respiration; (2) active sleep, characterized by eyes closed with eye movements, frequent body, limb, or face movements and irregular respiration pattern. Additional variables which we and others commonly record, besides observed behavior, eye movements, and respirations, are EKG, chin EMG, and EEG.

In the previable premature of 24 to 26 weeks gestation, the criteria are not met for either quiet or active sleep, causing Dreyfus-Brisac (1968) to conclude that these infants are always in an atypical sleep state. The continuous body motility and chin hypotonia are otherwise consistent with active sleep, but there are almost no eye movements. On the other hand, the absence of eye movements and the unvarying, discontinuous EEG are consistent with quiet sleep, but the rare regular respiration and the constant movements are not.

In slightly older premature infants of 28 to 30 weeks, the criteria for active sleep are met occasionally, because eye movements appear more often and in association with body movements and irregular respiration, which predominate. Quiet sleep is practically nonexistent, due to the paucity of periods during which regular respiration is present (Dreyfus-Brisac, 1967).

TABLE II *Concordance between Two out of Three Quiet Sleep Parameters*

	Percent of sleep record meeting criteria of:		
	Observed activity = 0	Observed activity = 0	Eye movements = 0
Age of Subject	Eye movements = 0	Respiration pattern = regular	Respiration pattern = regular
32 weeks	33	5	4
36 weeks	26	8	6
40 weeks			
Prematures	48	27	24
Full terms	44	25	22
3 months			
Prematures	59	40	38
Full terms	59	37	33
8 months			
Prematures	60	59	49
Full terms	76	51	47

From our own data we have calculated the percentage of the sleep record that meets the criteria for quiet sleep. In Table II, it can be seen that the frequency of any two criteria occurring simultaneously in a 20-sec epoch increases markedly from 32 weeks to 8 months past term. The requirement of regular respiration is a severe constraint at 32 and 36 weeks. Despite the fact that body activity is absent during half the record at 32 weeks and eye movements are also absent 50% of the time, these phenomena occur simultaneously only 33% of the time. By 40 weeks, they coincide more often, 48% of the time out of a possible 60%.

We have plotted the percentage of the record meeting all three criteria of active or quiet sleep, as well as the proportion of the record which did not meet the criteria for either state and was called transitional sleep (Fig. 6). The progressive decline in the amount of transitional sleep indicates the change in the amount of the record that can be classified as active or quiet sleep, that is, the greater concordance of parameters with maturation (Parmelee *et al.*, 1967; Petre-Quadens, 1967). Adding EEG criteria as a fourth parameter does not change these figures for us, since EEG patterns appropriate to each state were determined on the basis of the other three criteria. The relation between EEG patterns and states, however, shows the same maturational progression as that among the other physiological and behavioral variables (Parmelee *et al.*, 1968a, b).

Quiet sleep, as defined by our criteria, emerges after 36 weeks gestational age and continues to increase until it dominates at 3 months past term and thereafter. This is true not only for total sleep time but also for percentage of each sleep cycle (Table III; Stern *et al.*, 1969; Dittrichova, 1969).

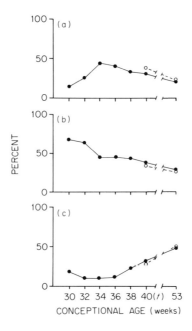

Fig. 6. Concordance among sleep state parameters. All three criteria of quiet and active sleep had to be met simultaneously. 53 weeks conceptional age is approximately 3 months past term birth. (a) Active sleep; (b) transitional sleep; (c) quiet sleep. (●) premature; (○) term. (From Parmelee *et al.*, 1967.)

TABLE III   *Relation of Sleep Cycle Components in Short (2-3 hr) Records*

Age	Number of infants	Sleep cycle (%)		P
		Active sleep	Quiet sleep	
Term	11	44	37	n.s.
3 months	15	25	49	< 0.01
8 months	14	28	56	< 0.01

SLEEP AND WAKING STATES

Thus far, I have discussed only the evolution of states within sleep, the growth of sustained, integrated patterns of events reflecting the maturational changes taking place in the brain, particularly the increasingly apparent role of inhibitory processes. Parallel evidence for these changes can be found in the maturational characteristics of the relation between sleep and wakefulness, taken as grossly defined contrasting states that occur in the course of a 24-hr period.

The data to be discussed next come from records kept by the infants' mothers. All 46 infants were on self-demand feeding schedules. Important changes in sleep-wake patterns appear during the first 3 months of life. At birth, total sleep time per 24 hr is only 16-17 hr, and this decreases very slowly during the first 16 weeks of life to 14-15 hr with another small decrease to 13-14 hr at 6-8 months (Kleitman and Engelmann, 1953; Parmelee *et al.*, 1964; Parmelee, 1961). The major changes are in the duration of single sleep periods and their placement in a 24-hr day. By 6 weeks, infants begin to sustain long 5- to 6-hr sleep periods, though not necessarily at night. Gradually this lengthens to 8-9 hr and shifts to nighttime, so that a diurnal pattern is well established by 12-16 weeks. However, a gradual shift to a diurnal pattern actually starts soon after birth. After 3 months of age there is a continuing development of the diurnal cycle and consolidation of daytime sleep into well-defined naps (Figs. 7 and 8; Parmelee *et al.*, 1964; Parmelee, 1961).

Although the decisions about the babies' states were made by the mothers using their own criteria, the results are similar to those obtained by means of actograms and observers' reports (Kleitman and Engelmann, 1953; Hellbrügge, 1960).

Waking patterns change only slightly in comparison to sleep patterns. At first, infants awaken about every 4 hr and stay awake for 1-2 hr. The longest sustained wakeful period increases slowly from 2-3 hr at 1 week to 3-4 hr at 16 weeks (Parmelee *et al.*, 1964; Parmelee, 1961).

Within the broad state "wakefulness," defined as those periods when infants' eyes are open, subclassifications have been made. Wolff (1965) studied the maturation of states he called quiet-awake, active-awake and crying. Infants seem to be most attentive, in the sense of selective looking or visual following, during the quiet-awake periods, which double in length during the first 4 weeks. Conversely, the amount of crying decreases, especially after 4-6 weeks (Fig. 9; Brazelton, 1962). As crying decreases, other waking behaviors, such as babbling and manual toy manipulation, increase in frequency (Fig. 10; Dittrichová and Lapáčková (1964). During the first 3 months primitive reflexes also become suppressed and social interaction emerges (Gesell and Ilg, 1943).

The development of attentive behaviors proceeds simultaneously with the development of quiet sleep and sustained sleep periods. These concurrent events again suggest the development of inhibitory and controlling feedback mechanisms made possible by the increasing complexity of the neural network and neurochemical development.

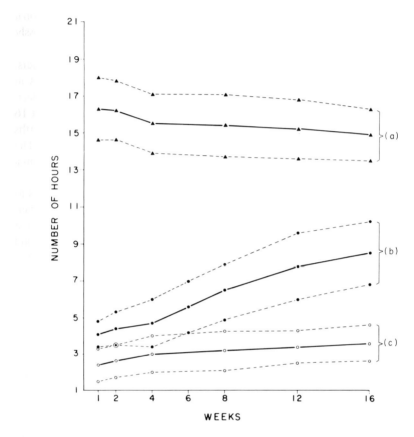

Fig. 7. Age-related changes in total amount of sleep per day and continuous periods of sleep or wakefulness. (A) total sleep per day; (B) daily longest sleep; (C) daily longest wakeful (− −) 1 S.D.; (—) mean. (From Parmelee *et al.*, 1964.)

ANIMAL STUDIES

Studies of sleep and waking states in human infants necessarily remain descriptive, although study of their evolution helps us make inferences about CNS controlling mechanisms. More detailed understanding of the neurophysiological control of states will have to come from experimental studies with newborn and infant animals. Several studies of infant animals indicate that the evolution of states within sleep, as well as sleep and wakefulness and their parameters, follows the same course as in the human infant (Garma and Verley, 1969; Jouvet-Mounier, 1968; Valatx *et al.*, 1964; Meier and Berger, 1965).

The newborn rat and rabbit are very immature and like the premature infant

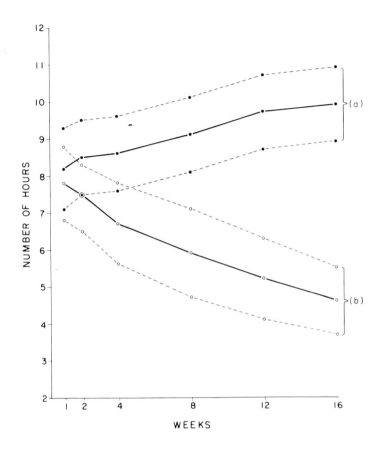

Fig. 8. The beginnings of a diurnal sleep-wake cycle can be seen in the night and day sleep during the first 4 months of life, although a strictly diurnal cycle is not established for several more years when day sleep is abolished. (A) night sleep; (B) day sleep. (− −) 1 S.D.; (−) mean. (From Parmelee *et al.*, 1964.)

of low gestational age. Garma and Verley (1969) have suggested that the newborn rabbit is like the 24-26 weeks previable premature infant. Both the rabbit and rat at birth, and for the first several days, have almost constant twitching body movements, no eye movements, no tonic neck muscle activity, and an unvarying discontinuous EEG pattern. With maturation, eye movements appear, first sporadically and then in bursts, EEG activity becomes continuous with varying voltage and frequency patterns, and periods of tonic neck muscle activity occur. The kitten is slightly more mature at birth, since eye movements are present, but the other parameters follow the same maturational changes as in the rat and rabbit. All three have predominately an atypical active sleep for the first few days and no identifiable quiet sleep. As in the human infant, quiet sleep

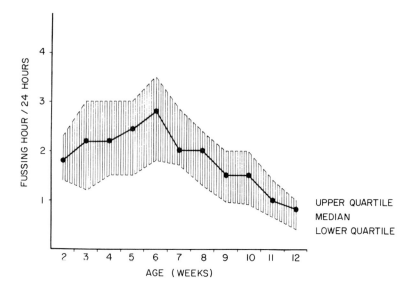

Fig. 9. Summary of the total crying time of 80 infants studied. (From Brazelton, 1962.)

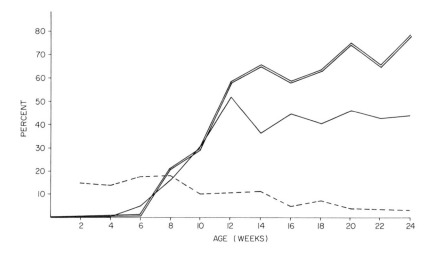

Fig. 10. Incidence of babbling (—), crying (– –), and hand manipulation of toys (=) in infants from 2 to 24 weeks of age. (From Dittrichová and Lapáčková, 1964.)

rapidly increases in amount as the infant animal matures. That this increase is largely a function of maturation of the nervous system and not environmental experience is demonstrated by the guinea pig which is very mature at birth. The newborn guinea pig displays easily identifiable active and quiet sleep comparable

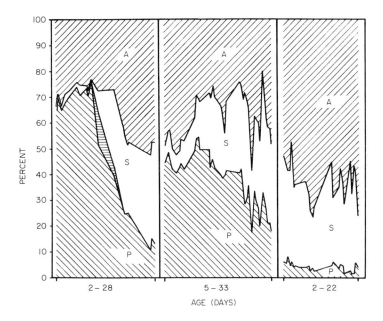

Fig. 11. Evolution of states in the rat, kitten, and guinea pig. A, awake; S, slow wave sleep; P, paradoxical sleep. Percentages based on 12-hr recordings. (From Jouvet-Mounier, 1968.)

to the adult's in form and amount (Fig. 11; Jouvet-Mounier, 1968). In these animals, as in the human infant, the development of wakefulness is concomitant with the development of quiet sleep.

CONCLUSIONS

We regard active sleep as a primitive anarchic state and quiet sleep as a more mature highly controlled state. Quiet sleep is considered the more important state for the study of the evolution of central nervous system control of behavior, because each parameter shows evidence of the development of inhibitory and feedback controlling mechanisms. Furthermore, the concordance of these parameters for sustained quiet sleep periods requires complex interaction of the brain stem and higher centers for some unity of control.

It is tempting to speculate that the progressive development of this highly controlled state is a manifestation of the development of cortical control. This idea is supported by the evidence for cortical control of slow wave sleep in animals, particularly the forebrain inhibiting area (Sterman and Clemente, 1962). However, it must be kept in mind that facilitory and inhibitory mechanisms are maturing at all levels of the CNS during infancy so that not all the changes in sleep states can be attributed to the cortex. Further lesion and stimulation experiments on appropriately selected newborn and infant animals are necessary to help clarify this problem.

REFERENCES

Aserinsky, E., and Kleitman, N. (1955). A motility cycle in sleeping infants as manifested by ocular and gross bodily activity. *J. Appl. Physiol.* 8, 11-18.
Ashby, W. R. (1956). "An Introduction to Cybernetics." Chapman & Hall, London.
Bergström, R. M., and Bergström, L. (1963). Prenatal development of stretch reflex functions and brain stem activity in the human. *Ann. Chir. Gynaecol. Fenn.* 52 Suppl. 117, 1-21.
Brazelton, T. B. (1962). Crying in infancy. *Pediatrics* 29, 579-588.
Denisova, M. P., and Figurin, N. L. (1926). Periodic phenomena in the sleep of children. *Nov. Refl. Fiziol. Nerv. Sistemy* 2, 338-345.
Dittrichová, J. (1969). Development of sleep in infancy. *In* Development in the Fetus and Infant. "Brain and Early Behavior": (R. J. Robinson, ed.), pp. 193-204. Academic Press, New York.
Dittrichová, J., and Lapáčková, V. (1964). Development of the waking state in young infants. *Child Develop.* 35, 365-370.
Dreyfus-Brisac, C. (1967). Ontogénèse du sommeil chez le prématuré humain: étude polygraphique. *In* "Regional Development of the Brain in Early Life" (A. Minkowski, ed.), pp. 437-457. Blackwell, Oxford.
Dreyfus-Brisac, C. (1968). Sleep ontogenesis in early human prematurity from 24 to 27 weeks of conceptional age. *Develop. Psychobiol.* 1, 162-169.
Eckstein, A., and Paffrath, H. (1928). Bewegungsstudien bei frühgeborenen und jungen Säuglingen. *Z. Kinderheilk.* 46, 595-610.
Garma, L., and Verley, R. (1969). Ontogénèse des états de veille et de sommeil chez les mammifères. *Rev. Neuropsychiat. Infant.* 17, 487-504.
Gesell, A., and Amatruda, C. S. (1945), "The Embryology of Behavior." Harper, New York.
Gesell, A., and Ilg, F. L. (1943). "Infant and Child in the Culture of Today." Harper, New York.
Hellbrügge, T. (1960). The development of circadian rhythms in infants. *Cold Spring Harbor Symp. Quant. Biol.* 25, 311-323.
Hooker, D. (1953). "The Prenatal Origin of Behavior." Univ. of Kansas Press, Lawrence.
Jouvet-Mounier, D. (1968). Ontogénèse des états de vigilance chez quelques mamifères. Thesis, J. Tixier & Fils, Lyon.
Kleitman, N. (1963). "Sleep and Wakefulness," rev. ed., Univ. of Chicago Press, Chicago.
Kleitman, N., and Engelmann, T. G. (1953). Sleep characteristics of infants. *J. Appl. Physiol.* 6, 269-282.
Meier, G. W., and Berger, R. J. (1965). Development of sleep and wakefulness patterns in the infant rhesus monkey. *Exp. Neurol.* 12, 257-277.
Parmelee, A. H., Jr. (1961). Sleep patterns in infancy. A study of one infant from birth to eight months of age. *Acta Paediat.* 50, 160-170.
Parmelee, A. H., Jr., Wenner, W. H., and Schulz, H. R. (1964). Infant sleep patterns from birth to 16 weeks of age. *J. Pediat.* 65, 576-582.
Parmelee, A. H., Jr., Wenner, W. H., Akiyama, Y., Schultz, M., and Stern, E. (1967). Sleep states in premature infants. *Develop. Med. Child Neurol.* 9, 70-77.

Parmelee, A. H., Jr., Akiyama, Y., Schultz, M. A., Wenner, W. H., Schulte, F. J., and Stern, E. (1968a). The electroencephalogram in active and quiet sleep in infants. *In* "Clinical Electroencephalography of Children" (P. Kellaway and I. Petersen, eds.), pp. 77-88. Almqvist & Wiksell, Stockholm.

Parmelee, A. H., Jr., Schulte, F. J., Akiyama, Y., Wenner, W. H., Schultz, M. A., and Stern, E. (1968b). Maturation of EEG activity during sleep in premature infants. *Electroencephalogr. Clin. Neurophysiol.* 24, 319-329.

Petre-Quadens, O. (1967). Ontogenesis of paradoxical sleep in the human newborn. *J. Neurol. Sci.* 4, 153-157.

Prechtl, H. F. R., and Beintema, D. (1964). "The Neurological Examination of the Full-Term Newborn Infant." Heinemann, London.

Prechtl, H. F. R., Akiyama, Y., Zinkin, P., and Grant, D. K. (1968). Polygraphic studies of the full-term newborn. 1. Technical aspects and qualitative analysis. *In* "Studies in Infancy" (M. C. Bax and R. C. MacKeith, eds.), pp. 1-21. Heinemann, London.

Sterman, M. B., and Clemente, C. D. (1962). Forebrain inhibitory mechanisms: sleep patterns induced by basal forebrain stimulation in the behaving cat. *Exp. Neurol.* 6, 103-117.

Stern, E., Parmelee, A. H., Akiyama, Y., Schultz, M. A., and Wenner, W. H. (1969). Sleep cycle characteristics in infants. *Pediatrics* 43, 65-70.

Valatx, J. I., Jouvet, D., and Jouvet, M. (1964). Evolution électroencéphalographiques des différents états de sommeil chez le chaton. *Electroencephalogr. Clin. Neurophysiol.* 17, 218-233.

Wagner, I. F. (1937). The establishment of a criterion of depth of sleep in the newborn infant. *J. Genet. Psychol.* 51, 17-59.

Windle, W. F., and Fitzgerald, J. E. (1937). Development of the spinal reflex mechanism in human embryos. *J. Comp. Neurol.* 67, 493-509.

Wolff, P. H. (1959). Observations on newborn infants. *Psychosom. Med.* 21, 110-118.

Wolff, P. H. (1965). The development of attention in young infants. *Ann. N.Y. Acad. Sci.* 118, 815-830.

Wolff, P. H. (1966). The causes, controls, and organization of behavior in the neonate. *Psychol. Issues* 5, Monogr. 17, 1-105.

INVITED DISCUSSION: NATHANIEL KLEITMAN

I will discuss the basic rest-activity cycle first, and then the duration of sleep and wakefulness.

As I see it, the basic rest-activity cycle (BRAC) is entirely independent of sleep and wakefulness. As we learn more and more about the BRAC, we find that it occurs also during nonsleeping hours. So it is something which stirs us up from time to time to activity.

The duration of the BRAC is related to the size of the animal. Thus, we find that small animals, both young and adult, have short cycles, and larger animals have longer cycles. It was shown that the elephant has a longer cycle, 2 hr, as compared to the 90-min BRAC seen in man.

There is no mystery about the increase in the duration of the cycle itself from birth to maturity, from small animals to large animals. The element to remember is that it is an activity cycle. After a certain amount of rest, one becomes active. There are two basic reasons for being active: one is to fill one's stomach, which is, of course, a feeding phase of the cycle; the other is a sexual phase. There is a penile erection phase in the BRAC, which has been detected during sleep. From time to time the animal is urged into activity.

From the self-demand arrangement of feeding of the newborn, it was found that the infant asked for food at intervals representing a number of cycles—three, five, or more. There is no mystery about the infants' waking up, crying, and asking for food. It has actually been demonstrated to be a gastric cycle which tends to stir them into activity, and if this does not occur at the end of the second BRAC, it will at the end of the third or fourth. Wada (1922) published early data on human infants in which she demonstrated the operation of the gastric cycle, both in infants and adults. Thus, there is nothing mysterious about the cycle and it has no relationship to sleep and wakefulness, except that, when we are stirred into activity during sleep, we are likely to dream, if we are capable of dreaming. I do not believe the newborn infant dreams. But infants at the age of 12 or 18 months do dream at night during the activity phase of the BRAC, and seem to do bizarre things, just as we do when our brain does not function properly. Actually, the performance of the dreaming brain can be likened to the performance of the waking brain when under the influence of alcohol or when one is quite senile.

So, if we are talking about the maturation of sleep, we really should stop at the age of 1 year, when every sleep type of behavior seems completely established. To go beyond that, and I trust that the brain is not quite mature at the age of 1 year, we do have to consider the wakefulness fraction, and this is the thing that is really intriguing. It takes an infant about 4-6 weeks to learn to sleep through the night—8, 9, 10 hours, that is about as much as any adult would sleep. There is very little training required for that purpose. It takes a child 5 or 6 years to develop long continuous waking periods, such as when the child gives up the afternoon nap and stays awake from morning to bedtime in the evening. That is what I call wakefulness capability and is something that develops with brain maturation. Apparently, wakefulness capability is not easily attained. Not all animals develop it equally. Some animals sleep most of the time.

Dr. Sterman indicated that the cat needs to have something to be awake for. Well, this is also true of man. If you have nothing to do, you are likely to sleep much more. The ability, of course, to stay awake is something with which we are concerned. The figures given by Dr. Parmelee brought that out. An infant which he studied at the age of 16 weeks was capable of increasing his longest sleep period from 4.1 to 8.5 hr, on the average, or over 100%. The increase in his waking period from 2.4 hr, on the average, to 3.6 hr was only a 50% increase in wakefulness. And we know, of course, that children raised in orphanages, not given the care mothers would give them, will sleep much more than children stimulated into activity. So, to make a long story short, it is our ability to stay awake that really depends upon the maturation of the brain, rather than our ability to go to sleep and sleep through the night.

It was found that the adult gorilla in its natural habitat, in the African rain forest, with plenty of leafy material for food, would sleep as much as 17 of every 24 hr—about 13 or 14 hr during the night when it is dark, and maybe about 3 or 4 hr of siestas, after breakfast, lunch, and dinner. This is because there is really nothing for the animal to do. I imagine that if the gorilla had to forage for food as some other animals do, it would stay awake more. You need something to stay awake for, and you have to have the capability of staying awake.

REFERENCE

Wada, T. (1922). Experimental study of hunger in its relation to activity. *Arch. Psychol.*, 8, 1-65.

INVITED DISCUSSION: DAVID R. METCALF

These comments are primarily in the direction of reemphasizing Sterman's contention that it is undesirable to speak of sleep and wakefulness in the fetus or newborn without consideration of the obvious differences from their adult manifestations.

Our own data (Emde and Metcalf, 1970; Metcalf and Emde, 1969) and those of many others indicate that there is a relatively loose coupling, during the first 3 months, among the various physiological and behavioral parameters generally considered in evaluating sleep and wakefulness. In my work with Emde (Emde and Metcalf, 1970; Metcalf and Emde, 1969), we have found REM state physiology (as measured by EEG, EMG, and respiration) not only during behavioral sleep, but also often associated with the behavioral states of drowsiness, nutritional sucking, fussing, and crying in the human neonate. Closer coupling among these many variables as well as between patterned physiology and behavior is not well established in the infant until around the age of 3 months. Thus, it would be preferable to avoid or to qualify categorical statements about wakefulness and sleep in young infant. By the same token, careful specificity and attention to both behavioral and physiological parameters are called for when identifying sleep stages during early development. I would not deny the existence of globally defined awake and sleep states and only two sleep stages during early infancy, but find this way of viewing wakefulness and sleep incomplete and therefore potentially misleading. We do not as yet know how best to name these states, but certainly a Procrustean choice between awake or asleep prejudges the situation when applied to the relatively primitive maturational status of the infant.

We have in the past used the term "behaviorally undifferentiated REM states" to refer to some of these indeterminate behavioral states between wakefulness and sleep. The concept "sleep" does have consensual and research value, but this value tends to be diluted if we ignore details of behavior and physiology. Thus, a problem arises, when during a state judged to be wakefulness by behavioral criteria, the physiological variables satisfy the criteria for sleep. Complexity of another sort is introduced when expected patterning within a parameter category (i.e., among physiological variables) is absent, as might be the case during behavioral sleep with eye movements and high voltage slow EEG. Therefore, it appears important not to risk the distortion that could result from the application of global categorization. In a different vein, the strengths of the global view may become a weakness if it leads to ignoring conflicting data, distortions of observations, or limitation of conceptualization.

The work of Danielle Jouvet-Mounier (Jouvet-Mounier *et al.*, 1970), drawn upon by Dr. Ellingson, contains data indicating her observations of an intimate relationship between nutritional sucking, grooming, and REM states in the kitten and the rat. Jouvet-Mounier also reports on the relationship in cats between weaning and paradoxical sleep (PS). Early abrupt weaning resulted in a prompt decrease in PS, whereas gradual, "natural" weaning, as well as abrupt weaning after 10 days, did not interfere with the regularly decreasing proportion of REMS. These findings suggest an important developmental interconnection between grooming (a "nonsleep" behavior), feeding, and REM physiology. We are interested in these data because they are not dissimilar from our observations of "behaviorally undifferentiated REM states" and because we find a group of major changes at about 3 months. After this time, REM physiology shows a predictable physiological patterning and is no longer found in association with nonsleep behavioral states, such as drowsiness, sucking, and crying (i.e., undifferentiated REM states are no longer seen). At about this age, sleep onset is characterized by a NREM rather than a REM state as was the case earlier. A critical investigation of early weaning in the human infant in relation to REM state development has not yet been reported; such a study would represent an important contribution to the understanding of interactions of innate and experiential factors in development. The situation is quite complex when one considers our observation that breast-fed babies during feeding tend to show REM activity with sucking for 1 or 2 months longer than do bottle-fed babies.

It has been noted in this conference, and it is well established in the literature, that the relative proportion of REMS decreases with increasing age from infancy to maturity. However, it should be stated unequivocally that the age-related details of this development are incompletely known for *any* species. In man, the decline is *not gradual*, but is probably more rapid in the first 3 months and continues at a less rapid rate until about 1 year. The major decrease in REM sleep takes place during the first year (reaching about 30%). This and other relative discontinuities in sleep stage and REM state development in man, partially related to feeding, and possibly related to other behavioral and physiological developments, indicate a need for further investigations of behavioral-physiological relationships for human infants in the first year of life.

We are interested in considering REM and NREM aspects of sleep as providing possible inbuilt prototypes for future behaviors. The role of REM states in this sense is not yet clear, although Roffwarg's ontogenic hypothesis appears to be the best heuristic model to date. In terms of NREMS, which may represent in some sense a more basal state, we have recently reported on sleep-cycle changes in the neonate following stress (Emde *et al.*, 1970). Infants, after circumcision, were found to have a significant increase in amount of NREM sleep, as well as a trend toward NREMS onset rather than the normal REMS onset. These findings are tentatively seen as fitting Engel's conservation-withdrawal hypothesis of preadapted CNS structuring and may, therefore, furnish another lead in understanding primitive rest-activity cycles in relation to observed behavior.

Lastly, and at a different level, with regard to our work on sleep spindle ontogenesis (Metcalf, 1970), we have recently completed computer analysis of infant sleep EEGs for the specific purpose of detecting and evaluating rudimentary spindles and their relations to more mature spindle bursts. Before spindle bursts are detectable and become mature during the 4-11-week age period, some type of rudimentary spindle activity is probably present as a virtually constant 16-17 Hz vertex rhythm. We are not the first to have commented on the existence of this activity (Ellingson, 1958), but we now believe it to be a true ontogenic precursor of 12-14 Hz sleep spindles. When grade I spindles (Metcalf, 1970) first develop at about age 4 to 6 weeks, autocorrelation and power spectral density analysis reveal that they coexist in locus and time with rudimentary spindle activity. Thus, the earliest sleep spindles can now be seen to consist of an almost continuous 16-18 Hz, 5-10 μV vertex rhythm. Grade I spindles occur as brief, low amplitude 12-14 Hz, vertex dominant bursts which, however, include a 16-18 Hz spectral line. The 16-18 Hz activity is not evident visually, or to computer analysis after grade II spindles develop at about 5-8 weeks. I would suggest that a shift in balance between inhibitory and excitatory pontine-thalamic-cortical integrative mechanisms at about 4-5 weeks in term infants is responsible, in part, for the rapid ontogenesis of obvious sleep spindle bursts at this age. This would mark not necessarily an upsurge, as it were, in leverage exerted by excitatory mechanisms, but rather the development and coming into play of an oscillating balance between inhibitory and excitatory mechanisms. This speculation, if demonstrated in terms of these or comparable data, would add relevance at the human level to Purpura's elegant description of the early primacy of inhibitory cortical functions in terms of neuroanatomical and neurophysiological ontogenesis.

We do not believe that the 4-6-week age for spindle maturation is an ontogenetic accident unrelated to behavioral development. It is likely that a number of behavioral developments in sleep and other areas can be meaningfully linked to maturational changes in the EEG. It is implied that these EEG changes indicate CNS maturations (whose precise natures are not known) which necessarily underlie behavioral development. This is the age when sleep-awake cycles begin to be predictably established in terms of sleeping-through-the-night, as well as being the average age of an upsurge in fussiness as already noted here by Kleitman and by Parmelee. The complex relation of this fussy period to EEG ontogenetic and other behavioral and neurological variables is under active investigation by our group (Tennes *et al.*, 1972). Neurophysiological plasticity at this age has already been demonstrated (Metcalf, 1969) in the finding that spindle ontogenesis can be influenced by experience; prematurely born infants (with longer extrauterine experience) have an earlier postconceptual age of onset of sleep spindles than do term infants.

In summary, although wakefulness and sleep are differentiable and remain useful concepts in reality and in theory, the traditional sleep-awake dichotomy does not apply unequivocally to infants under age 3 months. We have described a number of behaviorally undifferentiated REM states during this period. The poor patterning among behavioral and physiological variables at this time suggests the operation of a number of loosely related, poorly controlled, multilevel, relatively plastic systems whose "final common pathway" or "surface" manifestation may be viewed as "wakefulness" or "sleep;" closer coupling of these systems with predictably integrated physiological-behavioral patterning is seen after age 3 months. This is a fruitful area for future investigation of human development.

REFERENCES

Ellingson, R. J. (1958). Electroencephalograms of normal, full-term newborns immediately after birth with observations on arousal and visual evoked responses. *Electroencephalogr. Clin. Neurophysiol.* **10**, 31-50.

Emde, R. N., and Metcalf, D. R. (1970). An electroencephalographic study of behavioral rapid eye movement states in the human newborn. *J. Nerv. Ment. Dis.* **150**, 370–376.

Emde, R. N., Harmon, R. J., Metcalf, D. R., Koenig, K. L., and Wagonfeld, S. (1972). Effects of stress on neonatal sleep. *Psychosom. Med.* (in press).

Jouvet-Mounier, D., Astic, L., and Lacote, D. (1970). Ontogenesis of the states of sleep in rat, cat, and guinea pig during the first postnatal month. *Develop. Psychobiol.* **2**, 216-239.

Metcalf, D. R. (1969). The effect of extrauterine experience on the ontogenesis of EEG sleep spindles. *Psychosom. Med.* **31**, 393-399.

Metcalf, D. R. (1970). Sleep spindle ontogenesis. *Neuropaediatrie* **1**, 428-433.

Metcalf, D. R., and Emde, R. N. (1969). Ontogenesis of sleep in early human infancy. *Psychophysiol.* **6**, 264.

Tennes, K., Emde, R., Kisley, A., and Metcalf, D. (1972). The stimulus barrier in early infancy: an exploration of some formulations of John Benjamin. *In* "Psychoanalysis and Contemporary Science," Vol. 1. Free Press, New York. (In press.)

GENERAL DISCUSSION

Dr. Morgane: I would like to second the remarks of Dr. Metcalf regarding sleep and feeding behavior in young animals. Kittens will suckle for many hours in one of the sleep states, including REM, so that the "need to feed" hypothesis of kittens staying awake for reasons of having to feed so often does not apparently hold. The suckling mechanisms are apparently so innate that they do not in any way compete with other systems in the brain necessary for the sleep states to prevail. Indeed, the term "sucking REM" describes this situation quite well.

Dr. Prescott: Although this is a discussion of the subject of basic sleep mechanisms, it would seem appropriate to suggest the importance and relevance of certain clinical pediatric problems. As you are all aware, the phenomenon of infant crib deaths remains a mystery. A finding that should be of particular concern to members of this conference is the observation that most of these infants die during their sleep and the peak incidence is at 2 months of age. Is there anything we know about sleep mechanisms at 2 months of age that might account for crib deaths?

In this same context, the observation of Dr. Metcalf that neonatal life experiences can influence the development of several EEG sleep characteristics is worthy of emphasis. His finding that sleep spindle ontogenesis in prematures has an earlier postconceptual age of onset than term infants may have important implications for the study of hospitalized prematures, as does his observation that breast-fed babies tend to show REM activity during sucking for 1 or 2 months longer than bottle-fed babies. Whether these indicators have predictive value for later behavioral function and capacity is unknown; however, in this respect, it is known that certain sensory stimulation experienced by the premature is beneficial to its health status and developing behavior.

Neal (1968) provided vestibular stimulation in the form of rocking motion to 31 prematures (28-32 weeks gestational age) in their incubators. Stimulation began on the fifth day after birth and continued through the 251st day of total age (gestational age plus living age) or 36 weeks total age. Infants received the motion stimulation for a maximum of 56 days. Utilizing Rosenblith's modification of the Graham "Behavioral Test for Neonates," all experimental and control infants were tested at the attainment of 36 weeks or 252 days total age (gestational plus living age). The rocked prematures were found to be significantly superior to nonrocked controls on measures of general maturation (ability of infant to raise head in prone position; crawl in the same position; and weight that can be pulled by grasping; on responses to auditory and visual stimulation, e.g., orientation, fixation, and vertical and horizontal pursuit; and on muscle tension, as measured by a pull-to-sitting test, displacement of limbs, body activity, and body position). Additionally, the rocked group had significant weight gains as compared to the control group.

One question pertinent to this discussion is whether this rocking stimulation and corresponding significant improvement in health status and behavioral functions could be reflected in EEG sleep characteristics. In particular, questions can be raised as to the relevance of this study of the effects of breast-feeding vs bottle-feeding, as reported by Dr. Metcalf. Did the breast-fed babies receive more physical handling and rocking than bottle-fed babies? If breast-feeding is of longer duration and more frequent than bottle-feeding, as might be expected, then the prolonged REM activity during sucking could be attributable to differences in somatosensory stimulation rather than breast-bottle differences. These issues might be related to the findings reported by McGinty (in this volume) on the effects of isolation rearing upon EEG sleep characteristics. Elsewhere, I have provided arguments for interpreting the behavioral abnormalities resulting from isolation rearing as attributable to somatosensory deprivation (Prescott, 1970). Further, it might be appropriate to consider the premature infant in an incubator as being subjected to conditions of isolation rearing, particularly deprivation of somatosensory stimulation. This becomes particularly cogent when the sensory environment of the fetus is considered. Movement stimulation of the fetus is predominant, due to the movements of the mother.

At birth, this relatively continuous movement during waking hours is abruptly terminated. Thus, the dramatic reduction of *levels* of movement stimulation, as well as the drastic alteration of the *cyclic* or rhythmic characteristic of movement stimulation at birth, cannot but have some influence on the continuing ontogeny of CNS development and behavior. It is perhaps sufficient to emphasize the importance of relating EEG sleep characteristics to functional behavioral capacities as influenced by early life experiences, and to suggest that many applied problems in clinical pediatrics and behavioral development offer natural laboratories that can be fruitfully exploited to advance basic knowledge in the fundamental sciences.

Dr. Morgane: In answer to Dr. Prescott, I think it could be said that studies of sleep states represent, in a broader sense, examples of development of biological regulations involving maturing processes at all levels of the brain. In other words, sleep states are regulated because physiological mechanisms tend to keep them constant. If we can understand how these processes evolve and begin to interact with each other, we will answer fundamental problems applicable to disturbed homeostasis in a variety of spheres. Thus, collection of so-called "vast amounts" of data on something called "sleep" is not the only thing going on here—it has relevance to understanding how brains begin to work in the first place and how imbalances in their clocking mechanisms may tend to become cumulative errors resulting in mental disease.

Dr. Parmelee: My interests are clinical and in the early detection of deviation in development, and I think that these studies may provide us the potential for identifying early changes, particularly in longitudinal study. If a child does not proceed as expected in the development of sleep and waking states, we are justified in being concerned. When we study already identified grossly abnormal babies, we find they are deviant in their sleep cycles and in the parameters of their sleep cycles. So I think that there is no question we can approach this problem of brain and behavioral development in this way.

In hypothyroid infants, we have already found that in quiet sleep, as identified by our three non-EEG parameters, there are no sleep spindles until after a period of treatment. This had not been described before in the literature simply because it was easy to think the subjects studied had not arrived at this state of sleep. Lack of spindle development during quiet sleep in hypothyroid patients may be a model for study of other factors interfering with brain growth, such as malnutrition. In fact, two other babies who did not develop spindles in quiet sleep were hypoxic at birth. What this means in terms of what is going on in the brain has to be elucidated by the animal studies. Nevertheless, I think the potential for early detection and identification of etiological factors in delayed brain development in newborns and young infants is enormous, but the lag time is going to be great before this is practical enouh for daily use. We are still groping for definitive criteria.

Dr. Gordon: I am against high infant mortality, too. We all are. But we also have many concerns with the babies who do not die, whose personalities may not develop properly, and who may grow up and want to shoot people. I just hope that studies in this area might give us some better understanding of personality development which might be of importance to us with respect to survival of our species.

Dr. Sterman: Responding to Dr. Prescott's call for relevance, I think we have seen some new concepts emerging here. For instance, it has been suggested that the processes of sleep and wakefulness are products of maturation and experience and, therefore, are vulnerable to developmental modification. Early experience could be an extremely important determinant of later patterns, both of waking and sleeping behavior. I see here a means of studying the plasticity of the nervous system which could be utilized extensively.

Dr. Clemente: I wish to change the direction of the discussion, if I may. This morning, Dr. Sterman presented a new approach to our consideration of REM. In fact, he suggests that the use of the term REMS today might be questioned and that those brain mechanisms related to REM might not be the same as those related to the sleep process.

Dr. Roberts: I would like to ask Dr. Sterman to elaborate on the forebrain inhibition of brain stem activity, the areas he might think are involved, the possible role of the hypothalamus which he mentioned and some of the metabolic implications he indicated might be there.

Dr. Weitzman: I have a question for Dr. Sterman. I am much interested in this 80- or 90-min cycle measured in the fetus and mother. During maturation of the fetus, there was little change. If I understood you correctly, you implied that the mother superimposed this 80-90-min cycle on a 21- or 22-week-old fetus as well as on a 39-week-old fetus. It would be difficult to consider that the infant has a 90-min cycle which generates the mother's pattern. Are there uterine muscle contractions which can occur, particularly during the latter half of pregnancy? I wonder whether during REMS in the mother, the uterus might contract in response to the mother's 90-min sleep cycle? In addition to the uterine muscles, perhaps gut muscle contractions might occur. In other words, are there other muscle phenomena which occur during REMS in the mother which might explain the remarkable constancy of 90-min cycles in your measurement?

Dr. Sterman: We have studied uterine contractions and we are convinced that these are not contributing to our measure of movement in the fetus. Whether or not they are influencing the fetus is a question of interest. However, they do not become a serious consideration until the later part of gestation. We are seeing the slower cycle in the second and third trimester. We know that no movements, or records indicative of movement, are observed in the nonpregnant female.

Dr. Weitzman: Dr. Sterman has, in a sense, posed the issue of the tautology. That is, we either are or are not. We are either awake or asleep. He has challenged that concept and said we are in a different state. The infant who is in REMS is in a different state. He is not awake and he is not asleep. One could argue that the fertilized egg is clearly not awake or asleep, but somewhere along the line this developing organism does enter these states. The question is, where in time does this occur? The full-term newborn can be stimulated and put into an aroused state. An adult man during all stages of sleep can be aroused to wakefulness. I would propose that this indicates to me that the infant does wake up, and, therefore, he is asleep when he is not awake.

Dr. Sterman: With regard to Dr. Kleitman's concept of a basic rest-activity cycle, I feel that we are beginning to put our finger on a biological phenomenon which will allow us to understand the more basic organization of nervous function and perhaps to utilize this understanding to facilitate human performance. Dr. Kleitman pointed out that we do operate according to this cycle, to a certain extent, but we do not do it intentionally and we do not utilize the potential efficiency that it implies. If we accept this new approach, in many ways we have a new ball game with a whole new set of rules. Perhaps Dr. Dement will expand on some of these points later.

Dr. Roberts inquired about the forebrain mechanism implicated here in the development of sleep. Later on in this meeting Dr. McGinty will describe some studies from our laboratory on the development of descending forebrain influences upon brain stem mechanisms. I believe this also related rather pertinently to what Dr. Kleitman said. It was his feeling that the basic rest-activity cycle was a more recent phylogenetic development than sleep and wakefulness. I think, actually, the data suggest this is not true. It is rather clear now that the mechanism for this process is localized to the brain stem, specifically to the pons. If we consider the concept of encephalization, anatomically, this must be a more primitive mechanism. In addition, I would like to mention studies in such animals as the salamander, which does not really show what can be interpreted as sleep by mammalian standards, but which does show a very clear rest-activity cycle of approximately 2 hr. We have mapped the cycle and it is impressive. There are some indications from phylogenetic comparisons and manipulation of body temperature in decerebrate cats that the cycle may be related to metabolism. We have confirmed Jouvet's earlier finding that at higher temperatures the cycle is faster and at lower temperatures, slower than normal. I would suggest therefore that the rest-activity cycle is a phylogenetic antecedent to the sleep-waking cycle and a cycle which still exerts a basic temporal influence upon the more highly developed mammalian brain, helping to organize encephalized processes.

What does forebrain inhibition do in this organization? From my point of view, both wakefulness and sleep are manifestations of higher neural processes, of mechanisms in the diencephalon and neocortex. As they emerge, they exert then a modulating influence on these more primitive mechanisms. During sleep, at least in certain stages of sleep, a baseline state is established which is roughly comparable to the state we see in the infant and in the decerebrate cat, namely, the brain stem is released from this forebrain modulation. Under these circumstances, the rest-activity cycle is expressed in its more primitive manifestation. If some of the pathways responsible for this modulation are severed, some very dramatic changes in the physiology of these states can be seen. For example, monosynaptic motor reflex depression, which is very characteristic of the REM state in the adult, turns into reflex facilitation in a mesencephalic cat preparation. And, interestingly, this is exactly what is observed in the kitten, as Dr. Chase will tell us. By removing these forebrain influences in the adult, it appears that one can produce ontogenetically more primitive manifestations of organization. Obviously, we put a lot of stock in the pathways extending from the preoptic, basal forebrain area to the brain stem in this regard.

Dr. Morgane: Dr. Sterman, you might wish to elaborate on these circuits. I am sure you are thinking of the medial forebrain bundle with respect to the pathways extending to the preoptic area, so it might be well to tentatively name it as such. Also, I think it is not adequate to view brain stem segments as phylogenetically constant formations but, rather, to observe that these have changed due to developing telencephalic relations in phylogeny and, of course, also in ontogeny. Thus, mere severing of these connections in the adult animal, after the processes of regulation and adult cyclicities of phenomena have developed, does not return the brain stem back to some so-called "primitive" preparation equivalent to what it was phylogenetically before the telencephalic relations were built in the first place or ontogenetically before these telencephalic relations were wired-in during development of the individual. Thus, the lower brain stem itself evolves ontogenetically and phylogenetically, and just because the animal is low in the phylogenetic scale and has almost no neocortex or simply primitive allocortex or paleocortex predominating (and is, thus, in a sense, a "stem" preparation) does not mean that removing the inhibitory mantle in some way reduces the more evolved animal back to some earlier model. An adult animal cannot be reduced to the same "stem" levels of mechanism it had in its early ontogeny before the cortical controls developed, or to a phylogenetic equivalent whose cortical controls were minimal or of an entirely different order. I mention this because these brain stem-transected preparations, which are little more than brain stem tissue cultures, have often been looked at as "immature" in both the ontogenetic and phylogenetic sense. The new relations that have developed between the telencephalon and other brain centers with the stem have fundamentally changed the stem in ontogeny, and it cannot be changed back to what it was before. In other words, the lower brain stem itself becomes "adult" and one does not "revert" them to an immature stage by sectioning the stem and removing contact with forebrain structures that developed later in ontogeny. A stem which has been ontogenetically changed by the development of relations with higher structures is not the same stem that it was and never can be. I think it is a rather common phylogenetic error to look at the brain as though the numerators are expanding while the denominators are remaining constant.

Dr. Dement: I don't want to add to Dr. Sterman's burdens, but I would like to get settled for the record what the relationship is between the sensory motor rhythm and the sleep spindle. I remember an abstract in the EEG journal where the authors were studying various derivations and found that sleep spindles were recorded better when electrodes were moved farther and farther apart on the cortex. We have done extensive work in the cat, comparing scalp recordings vs cortical recordings, and it seems clear to us that the sleep spindle, that unique wave form which really differentiates sleep behavior vs waking behavior, is far better recorded from the scalp. Now, I have thought for a long time that probably the sensorimotor rhythm was simply accentuated when the animal behaviorally slept. But now, in terms of the data you presented this morning, it seems that this probably is not true.

Production of sensorimotor rhythm can be a very high level type function in the waking state. Yet, we *never* see spindles, as we record them to measure sleep stages, in the waking state when the cat is motionless or still for long periods. So, can you answer the question at this time?

Dr. Sterman: As you know, we think the sensorimotor rhythm reflects a mechanism in the central nervous system which is related to phasic motor inhibition. When an animal voluntarily suppresses movement, it creates a condition which we think involves cerebellar and proprioceptive afferent feedback and which releases a cortical circuit related to the sensorimotor rhythm. A state of motor inhibition, in fact, is one of the criteria for quiet sleep. Therefore, it is not surprising that among the manifestations of quiet sleep, we see both this spindle and a degree of motor inhibition. The sensorimotor rhythm also appears during the REM State. When it does so, it is accompanied by a complete cessation of phasic motor manifestations, including eye movements. Apparently the process of motor inhibition related to forebrain influences and indicated by this rhythm extends through all states of consciousness.

Dr. Dement: I tend to agree with the comments about motor inhibition; what I am asking is strictly an EEG question. Do you think it is a matter of recruitment, participation of more cortical area in that rhythm?

Dr. Sterman: Why is the spindle different? In experiments with Dr. Howe, in our laboratory we have found evidence for a shift in thalamocortical networks active in relation to the sensorimotor rhythm as compared with the sleep spindle. The sensorimotor rhythm involves primarily interactions between the nucleus ventralis posterior of the thalamus and postcruciate or somatosensory cortex of the cat. The sleep spindle, on the other hand, is related to simultaneously increased excitability in nucleus ventralis lateralis and precruciate or motor cortex. We feel that the changes in excitability which we have observed reflect the release of these various structures from other inhibitory influences. During wakefulness, the release is associated with proprioceptive stability, and during sleep with stability in corticocerebellar interactions. The similarity probably results from the fact that phasic motor inhibition in the waking state involves both proprioceptive and corticocerebellar stability. During sleep, however, proprioceptive input is depressed at the thalamic level, apparently shifting dominance to cerebellar systems.

Dr. Dement: Why do you see a spindle at the scalp level during sleep which has all of the characteristics of sensorimotor rhythm, and you *never* see it during wakefulness, if in fact the two are identical, or at least related? The only answer I can think of is that more elements must be recruited in sleep or that wider areas participate in the generation of the rhythm.

Dr. Roffwarg: On this subject I would like to remind you of certain facts in regard to the proportions of REM and NREM throughout life. If one forces all sleep in the infant into the "procrustean bed" (as Dave Metcalf calls it) of REM and NREM because "transitional sleep" is really not a separate "state" but generally a short intermediary sequence, a time of transition from REM to NREM, then one observes as we did that there are about 8 hr of REM and NREM in the newborn.

It might come as a surprise to some of you to hear that the amount of NREM sleep per day does not change at all until age 10; it stays at about 8 hr. As long as the child sleeps about 10 or 11 hr a night, he gathers about 8 hr of NREMS. Later, when he sleeps about 7 or 8 hr a night, the amount of NREM falls from 8 hr to about 6. But that is about a 25% reduction, whereas quite early in life REMS falls from 8 hr to about 2 hr, a 75% reduction. I agree with Dr. Metcalf, that this sharp drop is completed, if not within the first year, then sometime before a year and a half, rather than by age 2 or 3, as we used to believe.

I am trying to bring this back to one of Dr. Sterman's points about cycle length. He talked about cycle length being 38-40 min and not changing *in utero*. I think that is a fascinating finding. I had assumed that cycle length would increase with maturation *in utero,* and as it continued to increase would finally approach cycle length in the neonate. The fact of the matter is, as mentioned, cycle length has not been studied systematically. It is my impression that, after birth, cycle length does not change very quickly for a while, but I doubt that it takes until puberty to reach the adult cycle lengths of 90 min, because the changes in sleep-waking behavior, REM and NREM proportions, around the time of puberty are dramatically undramatic. But somewhere it begins to change, probably in the first year of life when stage 3-4 comes in. What I am getting at is that the finding of nonaltering cycle duration in the fetus is perhaps less important than the proportions of the cycle taken up by activity vs quiet. Did the proportions stay constant or did they change with maturation? I would doubt that they stayed constant. My speculation is that when we have an opportunity to study prematures, we will see that the ratio of REM to NREM will diminish and that this will be true of all mammalian species. So, it is the proportions of this somewhat fixed (for a while) cycle that may reflect REM and NREM quantities. Of course, it is also possible that all this activity may not be REM. Perhaps some fetal activity *in utero* is carried out in a rudimentary waking state which is possible in late pregnancy. Since the fetus has a fine oxygen support system plugged in at the placenta, it may be possible during portions of the activity period for him, as it is for an undersea diver with an air pipe, to sustain wakefulness while immersed in water.

Dr. Kleitman: I wish to comment about the very last item concerning cycle length in children. In preschool children, it is definitely about 70-80 min. We do need longitudinal studies in that respect, and I think some are going on.

The other question, Dr. Weitzman, regarding the mother and child—the very fact that the long cycle disappears immediately upon birth shows that it was the mother's. You asked what was the mother's part in that longer cycle, the 85-min cycle. It was definitely imposed upon the infant by the mother, because as soon as the child is born it disappears. What better proof do you want?

Dr. Weitzman: My question is, was he measuring the infant or was he measuring something as yet undefined in the mother?

Dr. Kleitman: Undoubtedly both. You cannot take away the mother's cycle.

Dr. Weitzman: I am asking, really, a very simple question, which may not be so simple to answer: Is he measuring with his devices the mother's uterine contraction or the mother's gut contraction or abdominal contraction sometimes, and not measuring the infant's movement?

Dr. Sterman: We are not measuring uterine contractions. After seeing Dr. Bodian's film, I think some of the strange patterns of activity we recorded could have been generated by the kind of movements we were able to visualize. It was interesting, also, that some of the infants were active in the amnion and when taken out became quiescent, while others were quiet in the amnion but became active when removed. One explanation for this paradox is found in the concept of a rest-activity cycle which was not influenced by the manipulations. The 90-min cycle represents some extension of the mother's physiology to the fetus, whatever its nature.

Dr. Petre-Quadens: I want to refer to Dr. Sterman's data which show the superimposing of fetal activity cycles with the mothers' REM. Three out of five cycles show a decrease in fetal activity in the middle of the mothers' REM. I wonder if these data show an interaction between mother and fetus in the sense of an *inhibition* coming from the mother and acting upon fetal movements, something similar to the presynaptic inhibition found in the trigeminal nerve during PS. I agree with your idea that it is not the peak of fetal activity which is important, but the slowing down of this activity.

Dr. Himwich: After hearing Dr. Kleitman, I realized that in our laboratory we may be heavily weighing our studies toward sleep. Perhaps we are boring our young animals to the point where they must sleep because there is nothing else to do.

Dr. Roberts: Is it fair to say there is a rest-activity cycle and also a consciousness-unconsciousness cycle and that the two can be disassociated by drugs like amphetamines? Is it possible that this consciousness-unconsciousness cycle is attributable to diurnal environmental variations such as light, and that it is only fortuitously associated with the rest-activity cycle?

Dr. Kleitman: When you bring in consciousness in relation to sleep and wakefulness, you get into trouble.

Dr. Lindsley: Dr. Kleitman and I worked four or five years on problems of consciousness in connection with Macy Conferences in the early 1950's.

Dr. Purpura: There are several points that require additional emphasis in considering the reports presented today. My concern is with the basic neurobiology of the problem of defining sleep-wakefulness mechanisms in the immature animal and how we go about this. I have indicated in my report that if one were to examine the neuronal organizations implicated in REM states in the newborn, these would probably be found to be as mature as they would ever be. But the problem is, where are these organizations and will they show basically mature appearing electrophysiological activities. Many of us have recorded from brain stem reticular neurons in very young kittens. I have personally not found such precociously developed functional activities in the kitten brain stem, but then again the experiments carried out did not have as their main objective the comparative development of neuronal organizations in different brain stem nuclei.

One point raised by Dr. Sterman concerned the shifting of spindle waves. This requires rather complex operations in reticulodiencephalic projection pathways, especially in the nonspecific systems which regulate spindle facilitation and suppression. The question of what happens in cortical efferent neurons, such as pyramidal tract neurons, during spindle waves should also be considered. Whenever inhibitory processes predominate, there appears an increase, not a decrease, in metabolic activity, since inhibition is a process requiring widespread interneuronal involvement. This brings into sharp focus again the role of inhibition in cortex and at the diencephalic level. Do you have data on the effects observed in unit discharges during the motor cortex rhythms shown in your presentation?

Dr. Sterman: We have some data on these points. We have been recording extracellular single-unit activity in chronic behaving animals, and we have stimulated the pyramidal tracts and recorded antidromic potentials at the motor cortex. There is no evidence from these studies of any change in the excitability of motor cortical units during the sensorimotor rhythm. What we do find, however, are rather significant changes in other extrapyramidal structures. For example, certain cells in VPL show an increased rate of discharge specifically during this rhythm, and other cells show a decrease. One of our most dramatic findings relates to the red nucleus where we find a marked depression of unit discharge in association with the sensorimotor rhythm. So I agree that the origins of phasic motor inhibition reside in the activity of extrapyramidal structures. They are responsible for the active process of voluntary somatic inhibition.

Dr. Scheibel: We are very much in agreement with Dr. Purpura's request for a higher degree of resolution in our studies of these phenomena of sleep and wakefulness, of rest and activity. Some time ago, Mila and I began to do long-term recording from individual reticular units in the medulla and pons in acute preparations (Scheibel and Scheibel, 1965). We found that a number of these units, when continuously recorded for 10-12 hr each, followed regular cycles of activity. Periods of reactivity to stimuli to the surface of the body were followed by periods in which the units were totally nonresponsive to the same type of stimulation. During these latter epochs, the units often appeared to follow rhythms of internal origin, such as the respiratory cycle. The length of time spent in the sensory reactive and nonreactive phases of each complete cycle were always remarkably similar ($\pm$1-3 min) and each of the approximately 12 units in this early group followed its own unique time sequence.

Interestingly enough, during the interoceptive or nonreactive phase of unit activity, it was often possible to reset the cycle by a brief stimulus train administered to the mesencephalic tegmentum. In these cases, we usually found that the unit cycle was reset to the sensory reactive phase and then followed out the same time sequence from the new starting point. We wondered whether this indicated the presence of a pacemaking system in the tegmentum, and we are now looking for such a system. In any case, it would seem as though, in cats at least, the rest-activity cycle is operating, in a sense, at the single-unit level.

Dr. Rosen: The question of uterine contractions has been raised many times. In almost every hollow smooth muscle organ, there are contractions of some rhythmicity. In the nonpregnant human female, uterine contractions occur in relation to her menstrual cycle. They occur in the pregnant woman in both the first trimester and second trimesters. Although they become apparent to her only after the sixth month of gestation, they are always taking place. I am sure Dr. Sterman has looked at this closely. If you spread out the wave by increasing the recording chart speed during the interval of fetal movements, you could probably see that this waveform has a frequency and a rise time which would distinguish it from the slower uterine contractions. These contractions would have a different duration, amplitude and shape.

There is another interesting way to look at this. If there is an influence from the external system on the developing internal (*in utero* fetal) system, perhaps the rhythmicity of the contractile pattern contributes in some way to the environment of the developing fetus, and you have a fixed cycling time in one state. I would think, as an outgrowth of these studies, you should also be measuring the uterine contractile pattern.

In our laboratory we have taken a small sound receiver and placed it next to the fetal sheep ear; we hear many maternal sounds such as heartbeat and bowel contractions. These are apparent and may be considered forms of stimuli.

Along a different line of thought, Dr. Sterman, have you looked at the interval between fetal heartbeats during your activity cycle and your nonactivity cycle; is there a statistical difference in the interval between heartbeats during one cycle and the other?

Dr. Sterman: Heartbeat is one of the worst measures of this cycle, in our experience. Dr. Roffwarg, would you agree, that heart rate in the newborn does not seem to differentiate the quiet and active states?

Dr. Roffwarg: I do not agree that it does not differentiate REM and NREM in the newborn.

Dr. Sterman: I have seen records of yours that show no change in heart rate.

Dr. Roffwarg: Most of the records I have show a hump in frequency with every REM period; even though the rate throughout sleep is downward, you get a hump with every REM period. You can distinguish the REM period from the NREM that precedes it and follows it.

Dr. Gordon: I want to make a comment with respect to Dr. Ellingson's and Dr. Parmelee's work having to do with attempts at prolonged recording of sleep cycles in prematurely born babies. They run up against what might be called a cultural heritage, or, more mundanely, nursery practices. One of these derives from our worry that some babies cannot swallow and may aspirate feedings. We began to feed them very frequently—in some nurseries every hour or every 2 or 3 hr—and they were awakened for their feeding. As a matter of fact, the nurses whom we get to work in a premature nursery have been studied, and they appear to like the precision of feedings every 2 or every 3 hr.

We had an opportunity in Denver to study babies on self-regulatory feeding (Horton *et al.,* 1952). We fed them whenever they awoke and wanted to be fed. We found that they ate only four or five times a day and were all gaining satisfactorily. We had a premature baby sleep 15 hr between feedings, another 11 hr between feedings, and still another 9 hr between feedings. If one wants to get into prolonged recording, one must get the baby out of the hands of the compulsive nurse whom we have trained to feed babies every 2 or every 3 hr.

Dr. Parmelee: I can respond to this briefly. To some extent, there is a surprising independence of the cycling from the feedings. If we continue recording long after the infant's usual feeding time, frequently he will continue his sleep cycles as usual.

I do want to comment that it seems incorrect to me to talk about adult animals who have sustained brain lesions as if they were identical to prematures or newborns. While there are a lot of similarities, there are a lot of dissimilarities, because the areas below the lesion are adult. Part of what I wanted to illustrate in my presentation was that individual parameters, such as control of respiration, movement, or heart rate, constantly change with maturation, and reflect changes within the brain stem as much as higher cerebral centers. The changes in heart rate control may relate to crib death too, in that the heart rate, for example, in the 24-week fetus is very stable and unresponsive to movement or stimulation; then it gradually adapts and becomes more responsive to movement, and more unstable. At term we find it a very good measure of state, not in terms of rate, but in variability, because we see the longest as well as shortest P-R intervals in active sleep. In many ways, active sleep seems to be an anarchic state. Thus, with maturation, you see periods of stability, then adaptation to environmental stimulation, then instability, and finally stability with adaptability to environmental inputs. It may be that it is during the unstable heart rate control periods during maturation or active sleep that crib deaths occur.

I wish to restate that in contrast to active sleep, quiet sleep is a highly controlled state, highly monitored, if you want to look at it that way. Heart rate and respirations are held steady and body and eye movements are inhibited. With maturation, the ability of the nervous system to sustain this control increases, both in terms of the individual parameters and the concordance of the parameters with each other.

Dr. Roffwarg: I would like to make an apology to Dr. Sterman. He apparently remembers my data better than I do. We did show peaks of heart rate in REMS in neonates, but when we took out of the count muscle twitches and body movements, the REM heart rate tended to even out with the NREM. Heart rate seems to follow body movement.

REFERENCES

Horton, F. H., Lubchenco, L. O., and Gordon, H. H. (1952). Self-regulatory feeding in a premature nursery. *Yale J. Biol. Med.* **24**, 263.

Neal, M. V. (1968). Vestibular stimulation and developmental behavior of the small premature infant. *Nurs. Res. Rep.* **3**, 1-5.

Prescott, J. W. (1970). A developmental psychophysiological theory of autistic-depressive and violent-aggressive behaviors. *Psychophysiology* **6**, 628-629 (abstr.).

Scheibel, M. E., and Scheibel, A. B. (1965). Periodic sensory nonresponsiveness in reticular neurons. *Arch. Ital. Biol.* **103**, 300-316.

DEVELOPMENT OF REFLEX PATTERNS IN SLEEP

12

The Somatosensory Cerebral Evoked Potentials of the Sleeping Human Newborn*

John E. Desmedt and J. Debecker

Electroencephalographic studies, combined with recordings of rapid eye movements (REM) and muscle tone, have disclosed characteristic features of the spontaneous brain activity and sleep patterns in human newborns and premature babies (Roffwarg, *et al.*, 1966; Dreyfus-Brisac, 1967; Parmelee *et al.*, 1967; Ellingson, 1967; Prechtl *et al.*, 1968). The neurophysiological approach to the maturation of brain mechanisms in human babies and infants has more recently been extended by studies of the cerebral potentials evoked by sensory stimulation. The present report deals with the somatosensory responses elicited by mild electric pulses delivered to one or more fingers of the hand and recorded from the scalp overlying the contralateral projection in the parietal cortex. With careful positioning of the recording electrodes and a number of precautions, very consistent evoked potentials (EP) are readily demonstrated by averaging, say,

*Supported by grants from NINDS, from ONR, and from the Belgian Fonds de la Recherche Scientifique Médicale.

16-256 responses with a digital computer (the response of 0.5-10 μV must be extracted from the background noise and EEG activity which may be 10-100 μV). These procedures are mild and well tolerated by the newborns who readily go into their sleep cycles with such electrodes on (Desmedt *et al.*, 1967; Desmedt and Manil, 1970).

The normal newborn is a good subject for sleep studies. He presents sequences of well-identified REM sleep (REMS) and slow wave sleep (SWS) during the day and spends more time in sleep than the adults. The incidence of REMS and SWS stages is about equal. For EP studies we prefer the somatosensory modality, in spite of the fact that these responses occur over a more restricted scalp region and are of smaller amplitude than the visual (VER) or auditory evoked responses (AER). Somatosensory potentials, however, present distinct advantages as a physiological probe for brain studies in the intact human subject (Desmedt, 1971). The sensory stimulus can be specified consistently by the amount of stimulus current (in mA) flowing through the finger electrodes throughout the session. A brief pulse of current up to three or four times threshold is not painful and does not interfere with the sleep cycles. The corticipetal volley thus elicited involve only skin and joint afferents from a well-defined area (Dawson, 1956) and it can be recorded, if needed for further checking, along the appropriate peripheral nerve. The cortical response has a consistent waveform which includes both primary short-latency components and slower, more widely distributed, secondary components (Hirsch *et al.*, 1961; Goff *et al.*, 1966; Debecker and Desmedt, 1964; Giblin, 1964; Domino *et al.*, 1965; Halliday, 1967; Desmedt, 1971).

IMMATURITY OF THE HUMAN BRAIN AT BIRTH

This is correlated with peculiar features of the somatosensory ER. Figure 1 compares rather typical waveforms elicited by a contralateral finger stimulus in a newborn in REMS and in waking adult. We have evidence showing that the newborn responses are very similar in REMS and in the waking state (Desmedt and Manil, 1970) and it is, of course, easier to obtain good records when the newborn is asleep in REMS rather than awake. The newborn response begins with a prominent surface-negative component N-1 of total duration of 10-30 msec, followed by a surface-positive P-1 component of about 100 msec and a slower negative N-2. The total duration of the response for stimuli twice threshold or more is about 0.5-1 sec. The adult response is quite different, and the early negative and positive components have a much faster time course. The negative component 1 of the adult does not exceed 5 msec duration and it is less developed than the newborn N-1. The positive components 2 and 3 (the latter is poorly differentiated in this instance) of the adult also disclose a rather fast time course. The question of possible homologies between the early components in

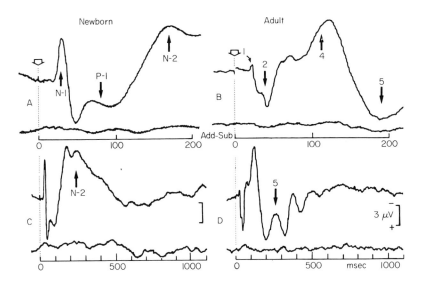

Fig. 1. Comparison of average cerebral responses to a finger stimulus in a normal newborn in REMS state (A,C) and in a conscious adult man aged 31 (B,D) at two different sweep speeds. The nomenclature of components is indicated and it differs for the newborn and the adult. An Add-Sub control of the same data samples is included for each trace. In the Add-Sub control the averaging is performed with alternate addition and subtraction instead of the usual addition mode: this procedure thus eliminates the time-locked responses and permits evaluation of the "noise" contributed by nonstimulus-locked background activities.

the adult and newborn should remain open until more evidence has been collected. In any case, the very consistent prominence of the early negative component N-1 in the newborn response can presumably be ascribed to the earlier maturation of apical dendrites of the cortical pyramidal neurons, in line with the kitten studies (Scherrer and Oeconomos, 1954; Purpura *et al.*, 1964). N-1 undergoes progressive changes leading into the adult pattern as the brain matures after birth. Current longitudinal studies in infants should soon provide quantitative data on the normal processes of brain maturation which will serve as a baseline for similar studies in perinatal pathology (Desmedt *et al.*, 1971).

EVOKED POTENTIALS IN REMS AND SWS

A detailed study of the somatosensory EP's has been performed in over 45 normal neonates ages 1-6 days. Periods of transition between one stage of sleep to another, and periods of atypical sleep not fulfilling all the conventional polygraphic criteria, have not been included in this report. Thus all responses illustrated were recorded during characteristic states of either REMS or SWS (see Desmedt and Manil, 1970). We observed a consistent difference in heart rate

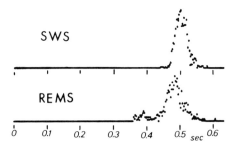

Fig. 2. Histograms of 1000 consecutive intervals between QRS deflections of the EKG in typical SWS and REMS runs in a newborn. Note the increased dispersion of intervals in the REMS state.

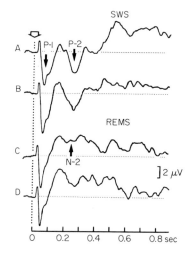

Fig. 3. Male newborn aged 6 days. Apgar index 10 at birth. Recordings from the parietal hand projection on the scalp, with reference electrode at the inion. A stimulus is delivered to three fingers of the contralateral hand. A,B, runs in SWS. C,D, runs in REMS during the same session. The most important changes related to the different sleep states involve the late components P-2 and N-2 of the evoked potential.

between the two sleep states. Histograms of 1000 consecutive intervals between heart beats were computed off-line by the CAT Mnemotron in nine pairs of runs carried out in different babies. The intervals fluctuate consistently more in REMS than in SWS, as indicated by the more dispersed histogram of Fig. 2. The mean intervals for the nine pairs of runs averaged 522 ± 27 msec in the SWS runs and 497 ± 43 msec in the corresponding REMS runs. The difference is highly significant ($P < 0.001$).

Figure 3 presents average potentials evoked by a finger stimulus and recorded from the contralateral scalp region overlying the parietal hand focus. The records correspond to runs recorded while the newborn went through SWS (A and B) and REMS (C and D) states, during the afternoon between two feeds. The most obvious difference between the two waveforms is related to the long-latency components. In SWS, but not in REMS, a characteristic surface-positive component P-2 with a peak latency of about 0.2-0.3 sec has been recorded. This component P-2 is quite distinct from the component P-1 of shorter latency which is recorded in both sleep stages at the hand focus. Furthermore, the surface-negative N-2 component is more consistently developed and occurs with a shorter latency in REMS.

The earliest component N-1 is also influenced by the states of sleep and its changes are consistent, though less important than those involving the surface-positive component P-2. The latency of N-1 is not affected by the sleep states. The duration of N-1 increases from a mean of ~15 to ~20 msec as the neonate goes from REMS to SWS (Desmedt and Manil, 1970).

COMPARISON WITH VERTEX RESPONSES

The parietal hand focus on the scalp is only about 50 mm apart from the midline vertex (Cz) conventional EEG recording site. However, the waveforms are quite different in their early components. A surface-negative N-1 is not present at the vertex and the same is true for the P-1 component. In fact, the most consistent component evoked at the vertex by the finger stimulus is a positive component with latency to onset and to peak similar to those of P-2 seen more laterally. Figure 4 illustrates pairs of responses simultaneously recorded from the hand focus and from the vertex in a newborn. In SWS runs, there is an obvious similarity in the components appearing more than 200 msec after the stimulus at either sites. We can identify in all four records (A and B) components P-2 and P-3, with a more or less developed N-2 between them. By contrast, such a congruence is no longer observed in the REMS runs of the same newborn, in C and D. Here the vertex response shows a component with latency similar to P-2 while no P-2 appears in the response simultaneously recorded at the hand focus. At the latter point a prolonged negative N-2 follows the early N-1-P-1 components.

The similarity of the component with P-2 features at the two recording sites in SWS states and the fact that such P-2 persists at the vertex in REMS could be explained if this component was in fact generated at or near the vertex region. This hypothesis would also account for the appearance of a P-2 component at the ipsilateral hand projection in SWS (Desmedt and Debecker, 1971).

AMPLITUDE OF EVOKED POTENTIALS
IN SLEEP STATES

In the cat, the early primary components of the cerebral somatosensory response were found to be larger in REMS than in SWS, while late nonspecific components were enhanced in SWS (Okuma and Fujimori, 1963; Favale *et al.*,

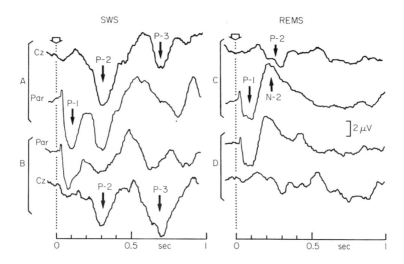

Fig. 4. Female newborn aged 4 days. Apgar index 9 at birth. A stimulus is delivered to three fingers. Average evoked potentials recorded at the midline vertex (Cz) and at the contralateral parietal hand projection (Par) are compared in SWS runs (A-B) and in REMS runs (C-D). The finger stimuli are delivered in B-D at regular intervals of 8 sec, and in A-C at random intervals (mean value = 5.7 sec).

1965; Allison *et al.*, 1966). Our data on the human newborn are not in line with the first of these conclusions (Desmedt and Manil, 1970), and this may well relate to a genuine species difference. Indeed, Goff *et al.* (1966) found in the adult man that the early positive component evoked by nerve stimulation smaller in REMS than in SWS. The histograms of Fig. 5 illustrate voltage components for pairs of runs carried out in either sleep states during the same session in a number of human newborns. No very significant difference is seen in the voltage of the early negative N-1 (A and B) nor in the early positive P-1 (C and D) recorded at the hand focus. If anything, the tendency would be for slightly larger components to occur more frequently in SWS, a trend which would be opposite to that in the cat. These data make it clear that the neural mechanisms of the corticipetal pathways are not affected in the same way by the two main sleep states in adult cat and in human newborns. Conclusions seemingly valid for the former should thus not be extrapolated to the latter.

Since the longer latency positive component P-2 does not usually appear at the hand projection in REMS, its changes in amplitude in the two sleep states can only be appreciated on recordings from the midline vertex (see above). It is interesting that, at the vertex, P-2 is consistently larger in SWS than in REMS ($p < 0.001$) (Fig. 5E, F). This is in line with the current view that such late components not confined to the specific projection area tend to increase in SWS, which appears true both in cat and in man.

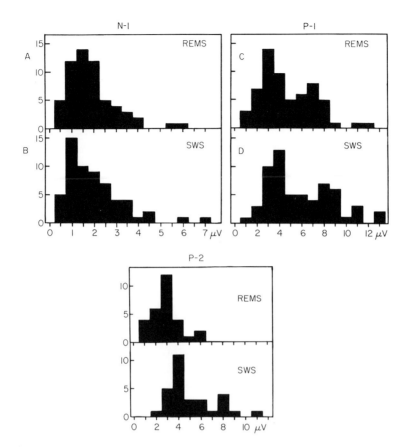

Fig. 5. Histograms of voltage of various components of the somatosensory evoked potential in the normal sleeping newborn. Thirty to sixty pairs of runs in either SWS or REMS are compared. A-B, voltage of component N-1 at the parietal hand projection contralateral to the finger stimulus (2-4 times threshold). C-D, voltage of component P-1 at the same projection, E-F, voltage of component P-2 at the midline vertex.

THE EFFECT OF INTERVALS BETWEEN STIMULI

When the successive finger stimuli are delivered at regular intervals of 8 sec or more, little, if any, distortion of the ER seems to occur (Desmedt and Manil, 1970). Shorter intervals were tested by programming different runs of 2-5 min at any chosen interval condition (16-2 sec) in alternate sequences during either REMS or SWS states. For any newborn tested, the runs carried out at a given interval in a given sleep state (not necessarily the same episode of the session) were pooled in subsequent averaging of the FM-taped data. Figure 6 compares rather typical results for runs at 10 and 5 sec. The responses at 10 sec can be

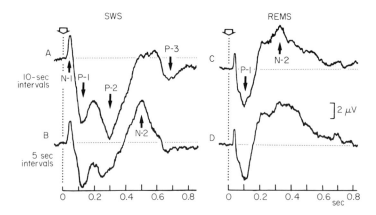

Fig. 6. Female newborn aged 5 days. Apgar index 9 at birth. Somatosensory potentials evoked by stimulation of three contralateral fingers in either SWS (A-B) or REMS (C-D) runs of the same session. The stimuli are delivered at regular intervals of 10 sec in A-C, and at regular intervals of 5 sec in B-D.

considered as a baseline condition, since no difference with respect to runs at, say, 16 sec was found in other sessions. The responses recorded at 5-sec intervals differ consistently, especially in the SWS runs. In B, components N-1 and P-1 are in fact not much different, but component P-2 is markedly reduced while the later component N-2 is increased. In other tests carried out at intervals of 2-3 sec the changes are similar and even more marked. It should be stressed, however, that, provided the intervals are no smaller than about 2 sec, the responses still present features characteristic of SWS, although the full-blown pattern of SWS EP's requires larger intervals of 8-10 sec. In Fig. 6C, D the EP's recorded in REM runs do not present marked differences at the two rates, but component N-2 appears slightly increased at 5 sec as compared to 10 sec.

The above effects on EP's no doubt occur because the individual responses averaged are progressively distorted through sequential interactions which either facilitate or depress certain response subcomponents. The two main sleep states differ consistently in this respect, because the critical interval for obvious interaction effects appear larger in SWS than in REMS. Further studies on the physiological mechanisms involved in each component of the EP are needed for useful discussions of the intervals-sleep states parameters. As a practical suggestion, it would appear that genuine comparison of evoked waveforms in the sleep states should use intervals of at least 5 sec between successive stimuli. The contradictions and inconsistencies of the literature probably result, in part, from the fact that many previous studies were carried out with rates of stimulation of 1/sec or even faster, which severely distort the waveforms.

A potentially useful observation is that the effects of sequential interaction can be reduced by delivering the finger stimuli at random intervals at the same mean frequency. A random interval generator based on a β-ray emitter has been designed (Carmeliet *et al.*, 1971) which delivers random intervals above a chosen minimum value (say, 4 sec) and with adjustable dispersion. Preliminary experiments suggest that random intervals with a mean value of 5-6 sec may produce little distortion of the responses (Fig. 4A, C) as compared to regular intervals of 8-12 sec (Fig. 4B, D). Indeed, component P-2 appears larger for the random intervals in the SWS runs (A) and this offers a suggestive contrast with the observation for regular intervals at 5 sec in Fig. 6B. The effects on later components are somewhat ambiguous, partly because of the well-known variability of these components. It is certainly more difficult to reach clear-cut conclusions about the influence of the interval parameter when considering late components and these rather long (regular or random) intervals. Nevertheless, the impression is gained that randomness in the sequences of intervals may minimize distortions of EP's, presumably by discouraging cumulative facilitation or depression of subcomponents in the successive responses averaged.

CONCLUSIONS AND SUMMARY

Average cerebral potentials evoked by sensory stimulation represent a useful physiological probe for quantitative studies of brain maturation and sleep in man. They also offer unique opportunities for studies on patients with disorders of the brain and of the sensory pathways. The present report describes recent results on the somatosensory EP's recorded in normal sleeping human newborns. The methods used are now well standardized, reliable, and mild. They do not seem to interfere with the normal sleep cycles of the neonate. The waveform of the average potentials evoked by finger stimuli present characteristic features which differ in adult man and in the newborn (Fig. 1). In the latter, clear-cut differences are seen between the responses recorded in either SWS or REMS states (Figs. 3, 4, and 6). These features include both changes in duration and/or voltage of subcomponents and the emergence of new subcomponents in the average response.

Late components, not restricted to the hand projection, tend to increase in SWS states. In contrast to evidence described for the cat, we found that in the human newborn, the early "primary" components of the ER are not larger in REMS (Fig. 5), which hints at a genuine species difference. Sequential interaction between the responses averaged was found to distort the evoked waveforms when the intervals between finger stimuli were reduced below about 8 sec, especially in SWS states. The effect of randomization of the intervals was tested in preliminary experiments. The necessity to use appropriate long intervals between stimuli in sleep and EP studies is emphasized.

REFERENCES

Allison, T., Goff, W. R., and Sterman, M. B. (1966). Cerebral somatosensory responses evoked during sleep in the cat. *Electroencephalogr. Clin. Neurophysiol.* 21, 461-468.

Carmeliet, J., Debecker, J., and Desmedt, J. E. (1971). A random interval generator using beta ray emission. *Electroencephalogr. Clin. Neurophysiol.* 30, 354-356.

Dawson, G. D. (1956). The relative excitability and conduction velocity of sensory and motor nerve fibres in man. *J. Physiol. (London)* 131, 436-451.

Debecker, J., and Desmedt, J. E. (1964). Les potentiels évoqués cérébraux et les potentiels de nerf sensible chez l'homme et l'utilisation de l'ordinateur numérique Mnemotron 400-B. *Acta Neurol. Psychiat. Belg.* 64, 1212-1248.

Desmedt, J. E. (1971). Somatosensory cerebral evoked potentials in man. Report, San Diego International Congress. *Electroencephalogr. Clin. Neurophysiol., Suppl.* (in press).

Desmedt, J. E., and Debecker, J. (1972). In preparation.

Desmedt, J. E., and Manil, J. (1970). Somatosensory evoked potentials of the normal human neonate in REM sleep, in slow wave sleep and in waking. *Electroencephalogr. Clin. Neurophysiol.* 29, 113-126.

Desmedt, J. E., Manil, J., Chorazyna, H., and Debecker, J. (1967). Potentiel évoqué cérébral et conduction corticipète pour une volée d'influx somesthèsique chez le nouveau-né *C. R. Soc. Biol.* 161, 205-209.

Desmedt, J. E., Noël, P., and Debecker, J. (1971). La voie somesthésique chez le nouveau-né et chez l'adulte: vitesses de conduction corticipète à partir des doigts. Rev. Neurol. 123, 350.

Domino, E. F., Matsuoka, S., Waltz, J., and Cooper, I. S. (1965). Effects on cryogenic thalamic lesions of the somesthetic evoked response in man. *Electroencephalogr. Clin. Neurophysiol.* 19, 127-138.

Dreyfus-Brisac, C. (1967). Ontogénèse du sommeil chez le prématuré humain: Etude polygraphique. *In* "Regional Development of the Brain in Early Life" (A. Minkowski, ed.), pp. 437-457. Blackwell, Oxford.

Ellingson, R. J. (1967). Methods of recording cortical evoked responses in the human infant. *In* "Regional Development of the Brain in Early Life" (A. Minkowski, ed.), pp. 413-435. Blackwell, Oxford.

Favale, E., Loeb, C., Manfredi, M., and Sacco, G. (1965). Somatic afferent transmission and cortical responsiveness during natural sleep and arousal in the cat. *Electroencephalogr. Clin. Neurophysiol.* 18, 354-368.

Giblin, D. R. (1964). Somatosensory evoked potentials in healthy subjects and in patients with lesions of the nervous system. *Ann. N.Y. Acad. Sci.* 112, 93-142.

Goff, W. R., Allison, T., Shapiro, A., and Rosner, B. S. (1966). Cerebral somatosensory responses evoked during sleep in man. *Electroencephalogr. Clin. Neurophysiol.* 21, 1-9.

Halliday, A. M. (1967). Changes in the form of cerebral evoked response in man associated with various lesions of the nervous system. *Electroencephalogr. Clin. Neurophysiol., Suppl.* 25, 178-192.

Hirsch, J. F., Pertuiset, B., Calvet, J., Buisson-Ferey, J., Fischgold, H., and Scherrer, J. (1961). Etude des réponses électrocorticales obtenues chez l'homme par des stimulations somesthésiques et visuelles. *Electroencephalogr. Clin. Neurophysiol.* 13, 411-424.

Okuma, T., and Fujimori, M. (1963). Electrographic and evoked potential studies during sleep in the cat. *Folia Psychiat. Neurol. Jap.* 17, 25-50.

Parmelee, A. H., Jr., Wenner, W. H., Akiyama, Y., Stern, E., and Flescher, J. (1967). Electroencephalography and brain maturation. *In* "Regional Development of the Brain in Early Life" (A. Minkowski, ed.), pp. 459-480. Blackwell, Oxford.

Prechtl, H. F. R., Akiyama, Y., Zinkin, P., and Grant, D. K. (1968). Polygraphic studies of the full-term newborn. I. Technical aspects and qualitative analysis. *In* "Studies in Infancy" (M. C. Bax and R. C. MacKeith, eds.), pp. 1-21. Heineman, London.

Purpura, D. P., Shofer, R. J., Housepian, E. M., and Noback, C. R. (1964). Comparative ontogenesis of structure-function relations in cerebral and cerebellar cortex. *Progr. Brain Res.* 4, 187-221.

Roffwarg, H. P., Muzio, J. N. and Dement, W. C. (1966). Ontogenetic development of the human sleep-dream cycle. *Science* 152, 604-619.

Scherrer, J., and Oeconomos, D. (1954). Réponses corticales somesthésiques du mammifère nouveau-né comparées à celles de l'animal adulte. *Etud. Neo-Natales* 3, 199-216.

INVITED DISCUSSION: MORTIMER G. ROSEN

After reading Dr. Desmedt's stimulating study, I am considering the use of this model in some of the work we are attempting to do in the sheep fetus. Most of my discussion will attempt to bridge the gap between the developmental situation and the neonatal ER's.

In our laboratory at the University of Rochester School of Medicine and Dentistry in the Department of Obstetrics-Gynecology, we are attempting to study how developing fetal systems *in utero* relate to development of those same systems after birth. For example, the brain wave and the ER do not suddenly turn on after birth. Rather, these electrical reflections of the developing CNS are present in the later fetal periods and may be shown to mature and display changing patterns. The following figures will be presented as examples of the kinds of models we are using.

Guinea Pig Studies

As we skim the surface of seven years of progress, we may look at several fetal models, e.g., the guinea pig (Rosen and McLaughlin, 1966), sheep (Rosen, 1971), and human fetus (Rosen and Scibetta, 1969). In Fig. 7, we see a guinea pig maternal-fetal preparation. One can monitor the maternal brain (6 and 7) and at the same time the fetal brain (1 and 2). The amphenol socket is sewn in the skin, high on the back of the mother, so as to avoid muscle and movement artifact. The guinea pig fetus can be monitored as long as 16 days, if one is lucky. The average guinea pig gestation period is 65 days. Occasionally, the trauma of surgery induces almost immediate abortion. The average length of time for monitoring runs between 4 and 6 days, which is quite adequate for continuing fetal studies.

If possible, it is important to monitor the fetus at times other than immediately after surgery. The surgical stress or the presence of maternally administered drugs for anesthesia alters the findings of the experimental situation. For example, in Fig. 8, line A, at 42 days gestation, we are able to see fairly consistent EEG activity. However, immediately after surgery, this tracing appears almost flat or equipotential. In a 21-g fetus at 43 days, the EEG (Fig. 8, line B) activity is more apparent with some "bursty" activity still spaced on long periods of electrical silences. By day 45 (Fig. 8, line C), the activity is more continuous, and by day 49 (Fig. 8, line D), the EEG is continuous with faster frequencies apparent. Between this latter period and day 52 (Fig. 8, line E), we see for the first time changing patterns spontaneously occurring when the mother is not moving or stimulated by her environment.

It is near this time (52-55 days) that one first sees an *in utero* fetal AER (Rose, 1971; Scibetta and Rosen, 1969). Figure 9 demonstrates the fetal AER to an externally located sound in a mature fetus. In line D, we note the same fetus after birth by caesarean section with the electrodes in the same locations. A small amount of barbiturate (5 mg/kg)

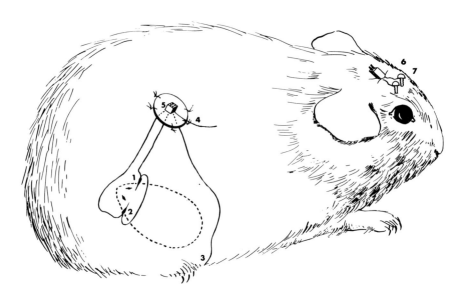

Fig. 7. Schematic drawing for fetal studies after surgery has been completed. Note fetal head EEG electrodes at 1 and 2; EKG electrode at 3; ground electrode at 4; amphenol female jack at 5; and maternal EEG electrodes at 6 and 7. (From Rosen, 1971.)

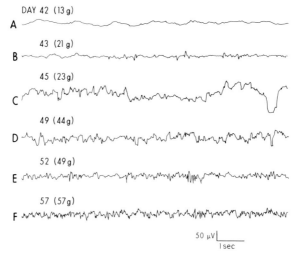

Fig. 8. Guinea pig. Line A, 42-day fetus with low voltage slow 1/sec waves and discontinuous activity. Line B, 43-day fetus with increase in voltage and presence of more activity. Line C, 45-day fetus with bursty slow waves and shorter periods of flattening. Line D, 49-day fetus with almost continuous activity and fast and slow frequencies. Lines E and F, 52- and 57-day fetuses with mature activity and pattern formation. (From Rosen, 1971.)

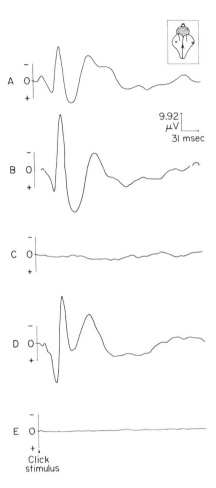

Fig. 9. Auditory evoked response (AER) protocol, fetus 5. Line A, *in utero* AER. Line B, *in utero* AER after pentobarbital (5 mg/kg i.m.). Line C, *in utero* control (no sound). Line D, AER after delivery. Line E, evoked run on dead animal. Insert (upper right corner), electrode location in fetal brain. (From Scibetta and Rosen, 1969.)

administered to the mother tends to increase the amplitude of response. Larger amounts of barbiturate suppress it.

This procedure has been published and adequate controls have been taken. We do not obtain such waveforms with needle electrodes on the skin, in the uterus over the fetal vertex, or in the dead fetus.

Figure 10 shows a guinea pig fetal AER on 3 consecutive days. One of the earliest ER's we were able to obtain was at day 55. The AER sound stimulus was 127 dB in air at 6 in. from a recording device. The duration of the "click" stimulus was 35 msec.

We have considered whether it is possible that this is a vibratory response. However, after

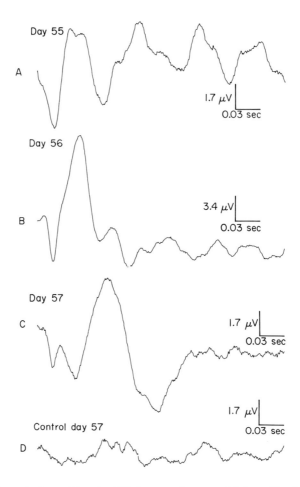

Fig. 10. Guinea pig fetus. Line A, AER *in utero*, fetus age 55 days. Line B, AER same fetus, age 56 days. Line C, AER same fetus, age 57 days (animal died on following day). Line D, control series (200 intervals without stimuli). (From Rosen, 1971.)

delivery of the term fetus, the AER stimulus is delivered in air, and the response does not change in wave shape or latency. Amplitude does increase after birth, but the most plausible explanation for this is the increased energy of sound now delivered to the neonatal ear.

The VER (Fox *et al.*, 1969) in three different fetuses is seen in Fig. 11 along with the AER in that same animal fetus. The VER is less consistent and may relate to the location of the fetus with respect to a unidirectional light source. At times, an absent response could be obtained by repositioning the mother in relation to the light.

Sheep Studies

Let us now move up the phylogenetic scale from guinea pig to sheep fetus (Rosen, 1971). This particular study (Fig. 12) lasted 30 days. The data on Fig. 12 were recorded on 5

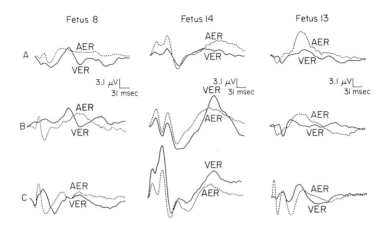

Fig. 11. Dotted lines represent AER; solid lines represent VER. Same guinea pig used throughout experiment. Line A, comparison of *in utero* evoked responses. Line B, *in utero* responses following pentobarbital (5 mg/kg). Line C, neonatal evoked responses with electrodes in same place. (From Fox *et al.*, 1969.)

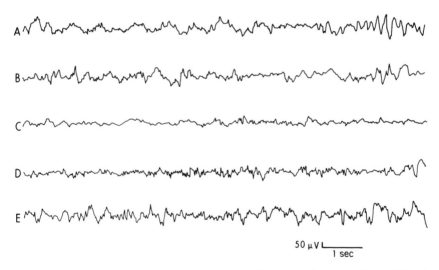

Fig. 12. Fetal sheep EEG following surgery; same fetus throughout experiment. Line A, day following surgery. Line B, day 2. Line C, day 5. Line D, day 7. Line E, day 10. (From Rosen, 1971.)

different days. At delivery, this fetus weighed 1500 g at an estimated 110 days of gestation. The figure demonstrates different EEG patterns in the same fetus, uninfluenced by drugs or surgery.

The sheep fetus has a gestational period of 150 days. It is remarkable in that fetal manipulation *in utero* does not easily induce labor. This remarkable tolerance to manipulation allows one to show developmental brain patterns far more easily than in the guinea pig.

Human Fetal Studies

We have performed human fetal studies during childbirth (Rosen, 1971; Rosen and Scibetta, 1969, 1970; Rosen *et al.*, 1970). Figure 13 (lower) shows a picture of a suction cup electrode. Two of these electrodes are applied to the fetal scalp through the partially dilated uterine cervix after amniotic membranes are ruptured. The needle point in the cup center must be kept isolated from the highly conductive amniotic fluid environment. The disc margins guard the needle from more than superficial skin penetration.

The sound transducer (Fig. 13, upper) is placed adjacent to the fetal scalp; thus, in the human fetus as in the neonate, we obtain both EEG and AER.

We have monitored both mature and premature fetuses. Figure 14, line A, documents the

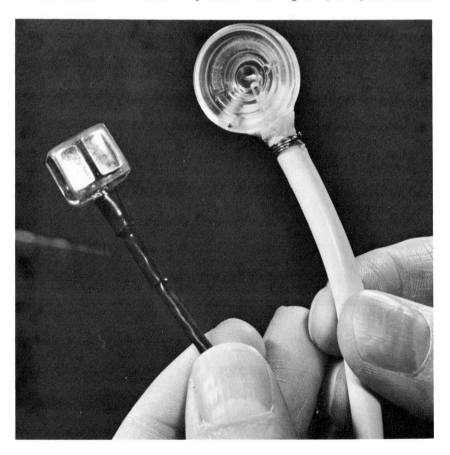

Fig. 13. Lower—Lucite suction cup electrode with central needle. Upper—sound transducer.

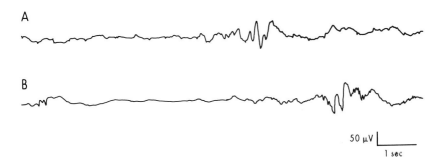

Fig. 14. Line A, premature 1300-g fetus with sporadic EEG activity. Spaced on flat intervals without apparent EEG. Line B, another 1300-g neonate studied in the nursery several days after birth. (From Rosen *et al.,* 1970.)

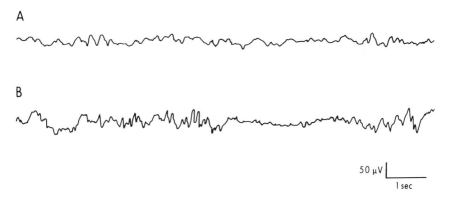

Fig. 15. Line A, recording of mature fetus; at this time activity was continuous, with wave amplitudes of 50 μV/cm and wave frequencies between 1½ and 7 Hz. Line B, burst suppression (*tracé alternant*) pattern occurred spontaneously in same unmedicated fetus. In addition, pattern frequencies of faster waves now run 15 Hz. (From Rosen *et al.,* 1970.)

EEG of a 1300-g fetus which mimics that of a premature infant (line B) after birth. The mature fetus at term displays continuous activity (Fig. 15, line A) and patterns similar to burst suppression (*tracé alternant)* (Fig. 15, line B). This fetus is unmedicated.

It is important to make the distinction between EEG recordings before and after maternally administered drugs. For example, meperidine, administered to a mother, rapidly crosses the placenta and is seen in the fetal EEG recording (Fig. 16, lines A-E).

Figure 17 displays our recording protocol, which may be of interest. The lines are appropriately labeled and will not be described further. It is almost impossible to scan visually hours of chart recording with accuracy. Our data are converted to an on-line digital recording form which is then evaluated in EEG programs and which is correlated with fetal heart rate and *in utero* pressure.

Figure 18 shows three *in utero* fetal AER's and compares them with the same responses after birth. The time scale is 1.25 sec. The intensity of the sound is 32 dB in air, but the transducer is placed against the fetal scalp; therefore, we cannot estimate the energy reaching the fetus. Polarity is almost meaningless, since both electrodes are often over recording areas of the brain. As in the guinea pig, we may say that in the normal situation the fetus responds to sound with an AER similar but lower in amplitude to the response obtained after birth.

Summary

We have demonstrated the fetal EEG and ER in several species. The environment reflects itself on the maturing brain *in utero*, at least as a sound stimulus. EEG pattern formation occurs prior to birth and is closely related to fetal maturity.

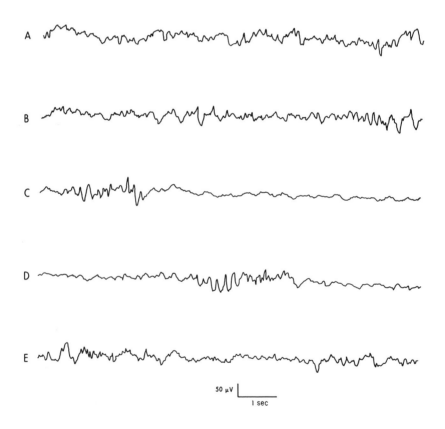

50 μV

1 sec

Fig. 16. Line A, fetal EEG prior to the administration of 50 mg of meperidine intravenously to the mother. Line B, 1 min after administration of meperidine. Lines C and D, 20 min after administration of meperidine. 20 sec of *tracé alternant.* Line E, 60 min after administration of meperidine. *Tracé alternant* not as apparent. Faster activity. (From Steinbrecher, 1970.)

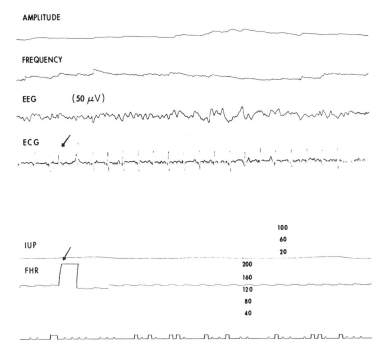

Fig. 17. Protocol for computer analysis. Line 1, amplitude: conversion of EEG amplitude to a more simplified analog. Line 2, frequency: conversion of EEG wave frequencies to a more simplified analog. Line 3, fetal EEG. Line 4, fetal EEG; arrows indicate fetal extrasystole. Line 5, IUP: intrauterine pressure during labor in mmHg. Line 6, FHR; fetal heart rate, converted from fetal heart beat. Line 7, time marker.

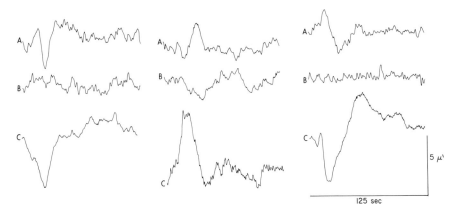

Fig. 18. Human fetal AER; three different fetuses. Line A, fetal AER. Line B, control interval for each fetus. Line C, neonatal AER for each fetus. (From Scibetta *et al.,* 1971.)

REFERENCES

Fox, H., Scibetta, J. J., and Rosen, M. G. (1969). Unpublished material.

Rosen, M. G. (1971). Developmental fetal EEG studies in the guinea pig, lamb, and human fetus. *In* "Brain Development and Behavior" (M. B. Sterman, D. J. McGinty, and A. M. Adinolfi, eds.), pp. 185-202. Academic Press, New York.

Rosen, M. G., and McLaughlin, A. (1966). Fetal and maternal electroencephalography in the guinea pig. *Exp. Neurol.* **16**, 181-190.

Rosen, M. G., and Scibetta, J. J. (1969). The human fetal electroencephalogram. I. An electrode for continuous recording during labor. *Amer. J. Obstet. Gynecol.* **104**, 1057-1060.

Rosen, M. G., and Scibetta, J. J. (1970). The human fetal electroencephalogram. 2. Characterizing the EEG during labor. *Neuropaediatrie* **2**, 17-26.

Rosen, M. G., Scibetta, J. J., and Hochberg, C. J. (1970). Human fetal electroencephalogram. III. Pattern changes in presence of fetal heart rate alterations and after use of maternal medications. *Obstet. Gynecol.* **36**, 132-140.

Scibetta, J. J., and Rosen, M. G. (1969). Response evoked by sound in the fetal guinea pig. *Obstet. Gynecol.* **33**, 830-836.

Scibetta, J. J., *et al.* (1971). *Am. J. Obs. Gyn.* **109**, 82-85.

Steinbrecher, M. (1970). Human fetal EEG monitoring during labor and delivery. *Amer. J. EEG Technol.* **10**, 7-11.

GENERAL DISCUSSION

Dr. Ellingson: We have recorded somesthetic responses from newborns too, and have observed, as did Dr. Desmedt, that the later components of such responses can be demonstrated at the vertex and display a wider field of activity. We have also recorded from transverse rows of linked bipolar electrode pairs to a number of subjects. Such recordings confirm his observation that the earlier components of the response show phase reversals laterally, approximately over the hand area of the somesthetic cortex. The later components of the response show phase reversals at the vertex.

Dr. Lindsley: Dr. Desmedt, you said that you found no focus of activity for N-1, P-1 on the ipsilateral side, but that you did on the contralateral side. At what age was this? Was it in a newborn?

Dr. Desmedt: Yes, newborn, less than 5 days.

Dr. Lindsley: The ipsilateral activity will come in later, will it not?

Dr. Desmedt: Yes, but I am not able to tell you exactly at what age.

Dr. Lindsley: Another question I have is related to P-2, P-3, which I think you said were absent during REMS. How do you interpret that? Is it an instance of absence of activity in the reticular activating system?

Dr. Desmedt: The view that we could present is that these positive components would be generated at the vertex rather than laterally in the parietal area. One way of looking at this would be to say that in REMS or in wakefulness, you have electrogenesis, which would be less sensitive and of less intensity and would restrict itself more to the vertex, in which case you would record much less of it at the hand focus. What I meant to say was that these components were still recordable at the vertex, but they were smaller and had different shapes.

One can consider that the potential recorded at the parietal focus is a combination of components which are perhaps generated in different places. You have the most restricted generation for the early negative component and then you have the later component which involves more cortex and cortex which is more deeply situated.

REMS, as opposed to SWS, changes the phases between these different components and you end up with different waveforms when you record at the parietal focus. The waveform, however, is not generated entirely locally under your electrodes, but involves different regions of the cortex.

Dr. Prescott: Dr. Rosen, what were the frequency and intensity characteristics of the stimulus you used?

Dr. Rosen: In the guinea pig, this was 127 dB in air sound stimulus; it was a loud click sound stimulus. We have also used a tone stimulus, but it is not a pure tone stimulus.

Dr. Prescott: Is it possible that the response is not an acoustic response but a sound pressure response due to vibration or resonance induced by your very high level stimulation?

Dr. Rosen: If it is a sound pressure response, I would have expected to have seen some of this in the electrodes on the skin itself closest to the speaker, others at the needle electrode, and less of it *in utero,* and we did not see that when we attempted to control the situation.

Dr. Weitzman: Dr. Rosen, what was your reference electrode to that AER?

Dr. Rosen: The electrodes are placed across the head. We can duplicate it in the neonate with the same positions. We can see where the electrodes were.

Dr. Akiyama: I would like to ask about the infant of the mother who received Demerol that you recorded intrauterinely. You said the EEG patterns looked like the *tracé alternant* pattern which went on for about 2 hr. Do they look like a full-term infant type of discontinuous activity or more like a premature infant type? And how long did this persist after the infant had been born?

Dr. Rosen: See Fig. 10 of this chapter. Line A shows the fetal trace prior to the mother's being medicated. Line B is 1 min after an intravenous injection of 50 mg of Demerol had been given to the mother. Lines C and D in this case are at 23 min. Between these two times, and actually on the running trace, can be seen a burst suppression-like pattern within 5 min. The first thing seen is an increase in the slow wave pattern. It is very transient and quickly changes to a burst suppression pattern.

At the end of an hour (line E), there are marked burst suppression patterns. After 2 hr, there still exists some of this activity, but it is disappearing. At least visually it becomes a little more difficult to see 2 hr after the intravenous injection. We are now submitting these data to computer analysis.

I am not certain whether this looks more like the premature or the full-term infant. This is drug-induced and somewhat different. I am not trying to say that a drug-induced pattern is *tracé alternant.* I would say it is burst suppression in appearance and it is fixed. Once that starts, there are no changes in pattern.

Dr. Ellingson: To me, that does not particularly resemble either a natural *tracé alternant* nor the EEG pattern of an early (24-27 week) premature.

Dr. Rosen: This is drug-induced. The burst suppression that I referred to before was not drug-induced; the mother was unmedicated.

Dr. Roffwarg: When you are recording from the scalp of the fetus, the human fetus during labor, and when you get fetal kicking, do you get artifacts in your recording so that you cannot read the EEG? Or can you still see it?

Dr. Rosen: I have been unable to identify fetal kicking. There is so much else going on, such as maternal kicking. I do not think I could identify it.

Dr. Roffwarg: What about during maternal kicking?

Dr. Rosen: On good tracings, such as those you have seen, less than 10% of my recording time is artifact. It is easier on a good quality recording to monitor the fetus *in utero* than the neonate in your nursery because there is less movement artifact. He does not cry or move his head, and we get very little maternal problems. On a poor quality trace, it is different.

Dr. Roffwarg: He may not get into REMS either under those circumstances. We were discussing the fact that fetal brain waves seem to change, but if we damped the fetal activity to the point that he is not kicking and moving, he may be under influences which would probably make this 3 or 4 hr that one is recording not very typical for sleep-waking patterns. One might learn more from chronic recordings in animals where one does not have the problem of labor.

Dr. Weitzman: I would like to make a comment and ask Dr. Rosen a question. If one is sure one is defining stages as best as one can, these waves fall into a time sequence regarding latency and polarity relationships. There is a consistent pattern which at first glance may be very confusing.

Dr. Leonard Graziani and I have been doing studies on VER in noxious states and have shown that there can be a marked decrease in amplitude of waves. Indeed, one can lose the waves during anoxia and when the baby recovers from this, the wave components will come back. During the period of time of delivery one could presume there may be periods of anoxia. Have you seen any marked depression of response which would return after delivery?

Dr. Metcalf: I would like to ask Dr. Rosen if he has had experience with drugs under these circumstances.

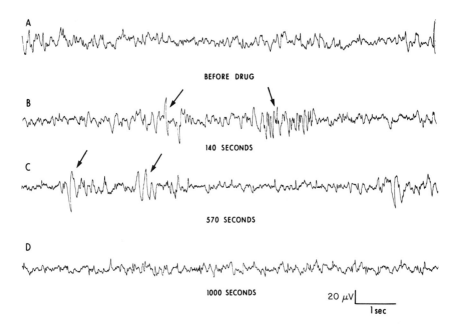

Fig. 19. Carbocaine paracervical block. Line A, fetal EEG prior to Carbocaine injection. Line B, 50 µV bursty, faster patterns after injection (arrows). Line C, persistence of similar waveforms 570 sec after injection. Line D, little evidence of drug effect at 1000 sec. (From Rosen *et al.,* 1970.)

Dr. Rosen: I would like to show Fig. 19 in response to Dr. Metcalf's question. This is Carbocaine given in a paracervical injection and the transfer, whether directly through the uterus or bloodstream, is relatively transient. It crosses the fetal brain easily and quickly. Line A is recorded before the drug and line B is 140 sec after the injection. In line C, it seems to be disappearing at 570 sec and at 1000 sec, I am not sure I can see the burst any more.

Figure 20 is in reference to Dr. Weitzman's question. Line A is the fetal EEG with the fetal heart rate at 140. As you know, fetal distress is defined in association with the onset of uterine contractions. The late onset of fetal heart rate deceleration is apparently associated at least with fetal distress and changes in pH.

In line B, the heart beat is down to 122. We begin to see a small change. At 110, we see a great deal of change. We have discontinuous bursts of activity on long equipotential periods. With a fetal heart beat of 90, there is an almost total flat line. At 70, it is very much similar. There is no question of a difference between these stages. As the fetal distress clears, we go through this in the reverse way and suddenly we are back at what visually appears to be a normal EEG pattern.

There is some information that we have now on 1 year followup that would seem to suggest that we had best look very early in labor, and even prior to labor, for some of the problems these children are developing. This is one problem we see. The other, abnormal waveforms, we have not published yet.

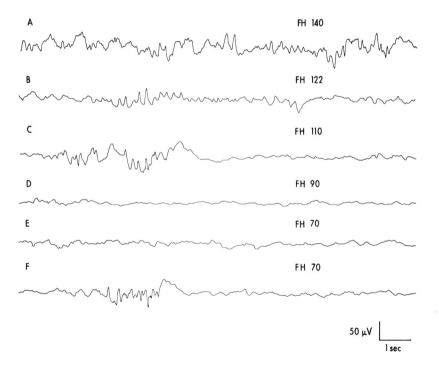

Fig. 20. Human fetus. Line A, fetal heart rate at 140 with EEG pattern preceding fetal distress. Line B through F, see text for explanation.

13

Patterns of Reflex Excitability during the Ontogenesis of Sleep and Wakefulness *

Michael H. Chase

INTRODUCTION

The investigation of somatic reflexes during *ontogeny* is at least as old as Harvey's observations on the development of motor activity in the hen embryo, which was published in 1651 (Harvey, 1651). The analysis of reflex activity during sleep postdates this investigation, for it was not until 1913, in a review by Pieron, that a total of 14 studies could be annotated. Widely conflicting results were reported, due most probably to the belief that sleep was a homogeneous behavior rather than being comprised of two distinct phases, which were

*Supported by the Veterans Administration and by a grant from NIMH (MH-10083). Bibliographic assistance was received from the Brain Information Service which is part of the Neurological Information Network of NINDS and is supported under Contract NIH-NINDS-70-2063.

described in 1958 (Dement, 1958). This discovery resulted in a plethora of studies in adult animals comparing reflexive activity during the two sleep states (quiet and active sleep) with wakefulness. Since it has only recently been recognized that there is a progressive maturation of sleep and waking states, the analysis of the development of reflex activity in neonatal animals during sleep and wakefulness represents a new and relatively unexplored area.

Underlying the development of state-dependent reflex responses is the maturation of the component parts of the reflex arc. Certain reflexes in young animals are truly immature on the basis of their intrinsic anatomy and physiology. Their activity is a function not only of suprasegmental influences, but also of the interaction between descending effects and the unique response pattern of an immature segmental system. The following examples probably reflect actual "immaturity" within the reflex arc: (1) primary sensory terminals have different functional properties than they have in the adult (Skoglund, 1960b); (2) posttetanic potentiation of spinal monosynaptic reflexes is absent in young kittens (Eccles and Willis, 1965; Skoglund, 1960d); (3) in contrast to the adult pattern of response, excitation of flexors and extensors can be elicited from widespread cutaneous areas in neonatal animals; extensors are inhibited only from circumscribed portions while flexors cannot be inhibited at all (Vlach, 1968; Ekholm, 1967a, b); (4) an exteroceptive stimulus, such as pinching the skin, leads to mass reflexes or bilateral flexion with extensor thrusts; in the adult it results in localized patterns of crossed extension (Langworthy, 1924; Pollock and Davis, 1930; Skoglund, 1960c); (5) there is a predominance of flexor rather than extensor tone in the newborn during sleep as well as wakefulness (Vlach, 1968; Skoglund, 1966; Wagner, 1938; Schulte and Schwenzel, 1965); and (6) when kittens are decerebrated by midcollicular transection, flexor rather than extensor rigidity is observed (Langworthy, 1924; Skoglund, 1960c; Pollock and Davis, 1931; Weed, 1917). The above phenomena reach an adult pattern of response after 2-3 weeks of postnatal life.

Many reflexes, on the other hand, are mature in the early neonatal period in the sense that their component parts have ceased developing. Their patterns of excitability and response are different from the adult, not because these reflexes are necessarily "immature," but because they exist in an "immature" organism. The descending suprasegmental control, in this case, would be the primary causal event leading to a pattern of reactivity distinct from that found in the adult. For example, the Babinski response is a reflex which appears mature in the neonate and ostensibly disappears during development, only to reappear when the balance of suprasegmental influences is disrupted due to lesions within the central nervous system. Similarly, the grasp reflex is gradually replaced (in the infant) by volitional grasping with conspicuous involvement of the thumb

(Ausubel, 1966; Bieber, 1940). This reflex,. as well as the sucking reflex, reappears in the adult after circumscribed forebrain damage (Ausubel, 1966; Bieber, 1940).

The presence of these responses in the neonate and adult most probably reflects the relative development of (or damage to) suprasegmental structures which influence the reflex arc, but which do not form a basic link in it. Thus, the combination of developmental changes in reflex activity and sleep and wakefulness results in complex interactions as the mechanisms underlying each system mature at their own rate and reach an adult configuration at different periods in the organism's development. Small wonder then that the present investigation indicates a dynamic pattern of reflex modulation in the maturing kitten during the period when the systems which control sleep and wakefulness are in the process of developing. Rather than a smooth transition from an "immature" to a "mature" pattern of excitability, indicative of a gradual uni-directional pattern of change, it appears that during the postnatal period basic reflex responses and their variation in amplitude during states of sleep and wakefulness are qualitatively different from the pattern observed in the adult.

In order to clarify the variations in brain stem reflex amplitude during sleep and wakefulness, which occur in the young kitten and reflect the activity of either segmental or suprasegmental systems, it is essential to bear in mind the pattern of reflex activity which takes place in the intact adult animal. The fluctuations in amplitude of numerous spinal cord reflexes have been examined during sleep and waking states in the adult cat (Pompeiano, 1967); a similar pattern of reactivity occurs for homonymous and heteronymous monosynaptic, polysynaptic, and flexion reflexes. This pattern consists of little or no decrease in amplitude during quiet sleep compared with wakefulness and marked depression during active sleep. Brain stem somatic reflexes show a different pattern of modulation during comparable sleep and waking states (Chase, 1971; Chase *et al.*, 1968). The mean amplitude of the masseteric reflex (jaw closing) is reduced during quiet sleep compared with wakefulness, and during active sleep compared with quiet sleep (Figs. 1-3). The digastric reflex (jaw opening) is smaller during wakefulness compared with quiet sleep (Figs. 1 and 4); during active sleep its amplitude is lower than during wakefulness (Figs. 1 and 4). Thus, in a progression from wakefulness to quiet sleep to active sleep, the masseteric reflex becomes gradually smaller (Figs. 2 and 3), while the digastric reflex first increases (during quiet sleep) and then decreases (during active sleep) below the level of the waking state (Fig. 4). Superimposed upon this basic pattern is a striking reduction in the amplitude of the digastric reflex when the cat is aroused, even below the mean level of active sleep (Fig. 5). The masseteric reflex usually increases in amplitude during arousal, but occasionally may be reduced

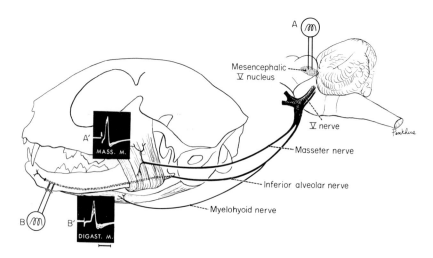

Fig. 1. Adult cat: Reflex stimulation and recording paradigm. Masseteric reflex: an electrical pulse delivered to the mesencephalic nucleus of the fifth nerve (A) excites cells whose fibers originate in proprioceptors within the masseter muscle. Discharge from these sensory cells induce, monosynaptically, activity in the motor nucleus of the fifth nerve and contraction of the masseter muscle (A′), resulting in jaw closing. Digastric reflex: stimulation of the inferior alveolar nerve (B), as it runs within the mandibular canal, yields polysynaptic excitation of cells in the motor fifth nucleus, resulting in contraction of the anterior belly of the digastric muscle (B′) and jaw opening. Calibration line: 10 msec and 200 μV.

for brief periods below the mean level for this state. During the bursts of rapid eye movements (REM) which accompany active sleep, both the masseteric and digastric reflexes are reduced to a greater extent than during those periods of active sleep which lack ocular movements.

BRAIN STEM REFLEX ACTIVITY
IN THE KITTEN

The preceding studies in the adult cat provided the background for the present investigation of brain stem somatic reflex activity during sleep and wakefulness in the kitten. As in the adult, the masseteric reflex was induced by stimulation of the mesencephalic nucleus of the fifth nerve, recorded electromyographically as a stimulus time-locked contraction of the masseter muscle, and observed as closure of the jaw (Fig. 1). Stimulation of the inferior dental nerve initiated the digastric reflex which resulted in contraction of the anterior belly of the digastric muscle and opening of the jaw (Fig. 1).

The masseteric and digastric reflexes were monitored in a series of 16 kittens

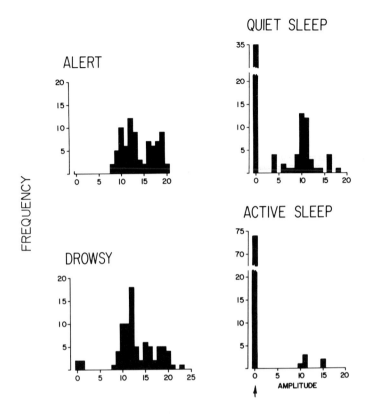

Fig. 2. Adult cat: Frequency histograms of the amplitudes of 80 consecutive masseteric reflex responses. These potentials were obtained during the alert, drowsy, quiet sleep, and active sleep states. The amplitude of the motor responses are plotted on an arbitrary scale as a function of the frequency of their occurrence. High amplitude potentials are reduced and then almost totally abolished as the animal progresses from wakefulness, through drowsiness and quiet sleep, into active sleep. (From Chase *et al.*, 1968.)

which were between 1 and 8 weeks of age. Each kitten was initially anesthetized with sodium pentobarbital and electrodes were implanted to induce and record both reflexes. Other electrodes were placed to monitor eye movements, neck tone, and the electrical activity of the cerebral cortex. Insulated wires from all electrodes were soldered to a Winchester plug which was permanently affixed to the calvarium with dental cement. After recovery from anesthetization and surgery, each kitten was placed in an environmental chamber on at least four separate occasions where they were kept, each time, for the duration of approximately four complete sleep cycles. During these periods, either the masseteric or digastric reflex was continuously evoked and recorded on an ink writing polygraph along with ocular, neck, and cerebral cortical activity (Chase,

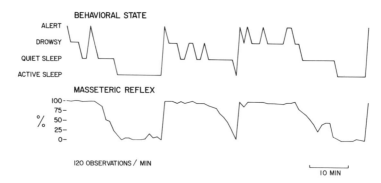

Fig. 3. Adult cat: This figure shows the percent occurrence of the masseteric reflex during consecutive sleep cycles. In this analysis the reflex responses were counted as either present or absent. Note the gradual decrease in the percent response during the periods of quiet sleep preceding active sleep. (From Chase *et al.*, 1968.)

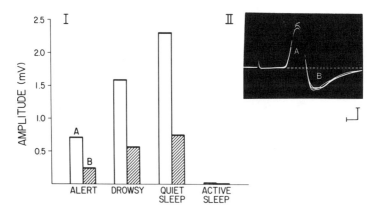

Fig. 4. Adult cat: Mean amplitude of 50 consecutive digastric reflex responses during states of sleep and wakefulness. Each wave of the reflex (IIA, B) was measured separately as the extent of its excursion from the baseline level (II, dotted line). As the animal changed state, the amplitude of both waves varied in a parallel fashion. An increase in amplitude occurred when the drowsy state was compared with the alert state (actually quiet alert), and when quiet sleep was compared with the drowsy state. During active sleep, the reflex response decreased below the level obtained during the quiet alert state. Inferior dental nerve: 1.5 V, 0.1 msec, 1/sec. Calibration (II): 200 μV, 2 msec. (From Chase, 1971.)

1971). In all instances, the level of reflex excitation was chosen so that it (1) yielded responses during the behavioral state when the reflex was smallest, and (2) was not of supramaximal value during the state when the reflex was greatest.

In neonatal kittens, the amplitude of both the masseteric and digastric reflex was greatest during active sleep. During wakefulness, a striking reduction in response occurred below the level obtained during any other state. A

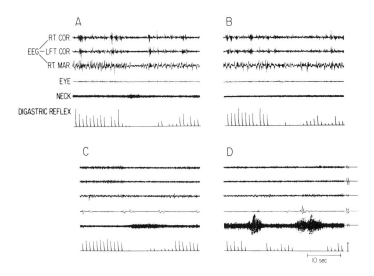

Fig. 5. Adult cat: Reflex suppression during arousal. Cerebral cortical desynchronization (A-C) and/or behavioral arousal (D) was invariably accompanied by a decrease in reflex amplitude. In A and C, a slight increase in neck tone occurred in conjunction with reflex suppression. In B, EEG desynchronization was accompanied by minimum ocular activity, no change in neck tone, and prominent reflex depression. In D, although there was no clearly discernible change in the ongoing desynchronized EEG, the digastric reflex was suppressed during the gross body movements which accompanied the bursts of neck activity. Inferior dental nerve: 0.5 V, 0.1 msec, 1/sec. Calibration: EEG, EOG, EMG, 50 μV; reflex, 500 μV. (From Chase, 1971.)

nonreciprocal increase in amplitude during active sleep and decrease during wakefulness represent the basic pattern of modulation of these jaw reflexes during sleep and wakefulness in the kitten during the first 10 days of life.

In the youngest kittens studied, the amplitude of the masseteric reflex was small during both the awake and quiet sleep states compared with active sleep (Figs. 6 and 7). At this age, periods of arousal during awake behavior were correlated with a reduction in reflex response (Fig. 6). During quiet sleep, there was only a slight increase in amplitude above the level of wakefulness (Figs. 6 and 7). By 2 weeks of age the reflex was consistently present during quiet sleep, still reduced during wakefulness, and of greatest amplitude during active sleep (Fig. 7). The relative degree of suppression during the awake state was less than in the 10-day-old kitten (Fig. 7). Phasic reduction in amplitude accompanied bursts of REM during active sleep in 2-week-old kittens, but not in younger animals (Fig. 6). By 4 weeks the adult pattern of decreasing amplitude during quiet sleep compared with wakefulness and during active sleep compared with quiet sleep was observed (Fig. 7). Phasic facilitation and inhibition during arousal, and phasic inhibition during the REM of active sleep became evident.

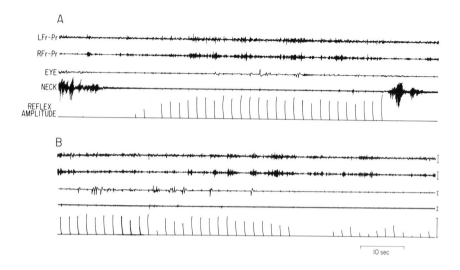

A
LFr-Pr
RFr-Pr
EYE
NECK
REFLEX
AMPLITUDE

B

10 sec

Fig. 6. Relation of reflex amplitude to abrupt changes in state. In the young (10-day-old) kitten, changes in state were accompanied by rapid variations in reflex amplitude. In A, note the correspondence between the increase in reflex amplitude during active sleep and its decrease during arousal. Occasionally, the kitten would pass from active sleep directly to quiet sleep; the reflex amplitude followed closely this change of state. Masseteric reflex: 3 V, 0.5 msec, 0.5/sec. Calibration: EEG, EMG, EOG, 50 μV; reflex, 500 μV.

Thus, 2-4 weeks of age represents a transitional period when it is possible to obtain little or no change in reflex amplitude during consecutive sleep cycles (Figs. 7 and 8). If one pictures the open bar in Fig. 7 as a fulcrum, then 3 weeks of age would be that time when the relative decrease in amplitude of the masseteric reflex during active sleep is equal to the increase during wakefulness (Figs. 7 and 8).

The amplitude of consecutively evoked digastric reflex responses obtained from 10-, 14-, 21-, and 42-day-old kittens are shown in Fig. 7. At 10 and 14 days, the digastric reflex became progressively larger as the kitten changed from the awake state to quiet sleep to active sleep. The adult pattern was achieved by about 3 weeks of age with the reflex being largest during quiet sleep, smallest during active sleep, and of intermediate amplitude during wakefulness. In animals less than 10 days old, it was not always possible to obtain a digastric reflex response except at very high levels of stimulation (prior to this period, the masseteric reflex was consistently obtained). During the waking and quiet sleep states in the 10-day-old kitten, there were only slight differences in digastric reflex amplitude (Fig. 7). When the kitten aroused, it decreased in size according to the degree of arousal, i.e., the greater the extent of arousal, the greater the extent of reflex depression (in a fashion similar to that observed in the adult)

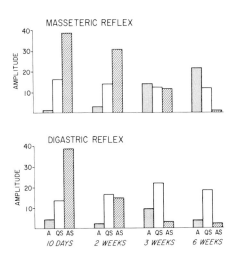

Fig. 7. Kitten: Reflex amplitudes during sleep and wakefulness plotted on an arbitrary but relative scale for each age group. In the 10-day-old kitten both reflexes are of maximum amplitude during active sleep, whereas they are of minimal amplitude during this state in the adult or older kitten. Note that both reflexes are smallest during the alert state in the 10-day-old and 2-week-old kitten. By 6 weeks, during the alert state, the digastric reflex is still of minimal amplitude and the masseteric reflex of maximum amplitude, which is the pattern observed in the adult. Each bar represents the mean amplitude of 100 consecutive reflex determinations for each state (evoked at the rate of 0.5/sec).

(Fig. 5). By 2 weeks of age, the reflex was consistently present during active sleep; however, the reflex was occasionally depressed during active sleep, especially in conjunction with bursts of REM (Fig. 9). By 3 to 4 weeks, digastric reflex modulation was indistinguishable from that reported in the mature cat (Fig. 7) (Chase, 1971).

A number of departures from the adult pattern of sleep and wakefulness were observed, and it was of interest to examine the changes in reflex response which accompanied them. As reported in other studies (Korner, 1968; Roffwarg *et al.*, 1966; Jouvet-Mounier *et al.*, 1970), the young kitten on many occasions passes directly into active sleep from the alert state. In Fig. 6, the reflex followed, quite precisely, an abrupt change of state from wakefulness to active sleep (the duration of quiet sleep was less than 10 sec). At the termination of the active sleep episode, the reflex was depressed as it was during the preceding waking period at the beginning of the record. Quiet sleep rarely followed active sleep, but when it did, the reflex response followed in a state-dependent fashion according to the pattern previously described for that age. Both reflexes were depressed during very brief periods of wakefulness, which frequently occurred during episodes of quiet sleep.

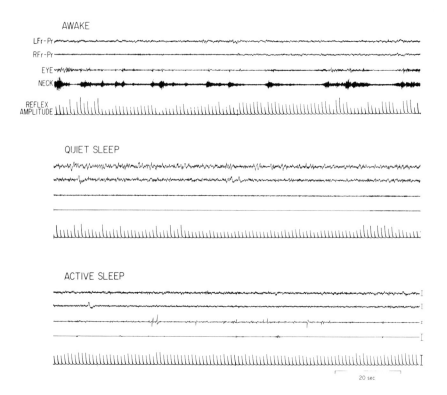

Fig. 8. Kitten: Transitional period of masseteric reflex modulation. At 3 weeks of age, the pattern of reflex response exhibits few state-dependent variations. During wakefulness, a slight increase in amplitude accompanies bursts of neck tone. Little change in amplitude is found when quiet sleep is compared with active sleep. A few days later, during episodes of active sleep, the amplitude becomes clearly lower than that of quiet sleep, and additionally, bursts of rapid eye movements begin to be accompanied by a time-locked reduction in the reflex response. Masseteric reflex: 4 V, 0.5 msec, 1/sec; Calibration: EEG, EOG, EMG, 50 μV; masseteric reflex, 500 μV.

DISCUSSION

The analysis of somatic reflexes during sleep and wakefulness may reveal, as in the present study, not only marked differences in activity between states, but also different patterns when responses in the neonate are compared with those in the adult. The question arises whether state-dependent phenomena in the neonate reflect primarily the activity of immature sleep and waking systems, or whether they represent immature patterns of physiological activity whose maturation is not directly dependent upon the development of sleep and wakefulness. For those reflexes which are mature in the young animal, a change

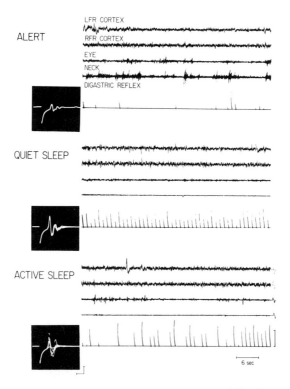

Fig. 9. Kitten (2 weeks old): On-line record of the EEG, EOG, EMG, and digastric reflex during sleep and wakefulness. The polygraphic record of the digastric reflex represents the peak amplitude of its first component. This record was obtained at the same time as the oscilloscopic recordings (5 superimposed traces). Note, in the oscilloscopic records, that both components fluctuated in parallel during sleep and wakefulness. Inferior dental nerve: 1.2 V, 0.01 msec, 1/sec; Calibration (oscilloscopic records): 200 μV, 5 msec; EEG, EOG, EMG, 50 μV; digastric reflex, 500 μV. (From Chase, 1971.)

in response to identical stimuli during maturation most probably reflects the development of suprasegmental systems. As these systems mature, they affect reflex activity directly, and also indirectly, by virtue of their developing interaction. When the component parts of the reflex arc also mature during the postnatal period, an almost bewildering complexity of possible determinants of reflex modulation arise at any given moment during ontogenesis.

Prior to any description of state-dependent reflex activity, one must first accept the concept of an independent variable in the analysis, which is that sleep and wakefulness exist in the neonate. During the course of this conference the following question arose: "Is it appropriate or possible to define states of sleep and wakefulness in the newborn?" I believe that these states can be clearly differentiated in the neonate. Some physiological processes which are associated with them do not appear in their adult configuration, but enough are present so as to make a state-dependent analysis possible. The behavioral pattern during the awake state in the neonate is similar to that of the adult (Jouvet-Mounier *et al.*, 1970; Wolff, 1966; Valatx *et al.*, 1964; Parmelee *et al.*, 1968; Jouvet, 1967) and is perhaps even more clearly differentiated from sleep, since the transitional drowsy periods of long duration which occur in the adult are not present in the young animal. Neonatal behavior during quiet sleep is homologous to adult behavior (Jouvet-Mounier *et al.*, 1970; Wolff, 1966; Valatx *et al.*, 1964; Parmelee *et al.*, 1968; Jouvet, 1967). This state may be separated from active sleep in the newborn by specific physiological criteria, e.g., there are no REM, respiration and cardiac activity are regular, muscle tone is present (in the human), EEG activity is similar to the adult, etc. (Korner, 1968; Jouvet-Mounier *et al.*, 1970; Wolff, 1966; Parmelee *et al.*, 1968; Jouvet, 1967). During active sleep in the neonate there occur REM, hippocampal theta (personal observation), pontogeniculate spikes (personal observation), muscular atonia, irregular respiration and heart rate, pupillary and cardiovascular fluctuations, and myoclonic jerks. In addition, the neonate's behavior during this state is similar to that of the adult when it is in active sleep (Korner, 1968; Jouvet-Mounier *et al.*, 1970; Wolff, 1966; Valatx *et al.*, 1964; Parmelee *et al.*, 1968; Jouvet, 1967; Gupta and Scopes, 1965; Prechtl *et al.*, 1967b); it therefore seems quite justifiable to denote the state as one of active sleep.

It does not seem reasonable to discard the notion of sleep and wakefulness in the newborn on the basis of a variation from the adult pattern of a few epiphenomena, such as reflex inhibition during the alert state which, for the masseteric reflex in the kitten, most likely reflects an immature gamma motoneuron system rather than a fundamentally different state. Therefore, since it is a constellation of physiological phenomena which defines a state as one of sleep or wakefulness, one can either take the position that these states do not exist until all phenomena reach their adult configuration, or that these states exist in the young animal and that the specific systems which determine sleep and wakefulness are in the process of maturing along with others which may be influenced by these states.

The present study indicates that in kittens less than 2 weeks of age both brain stem somatic reflexes and EEG activity during sleep and wakefulness do not show the characteristic changes observed in the adult. Brain stem reflex modulation reaches an adult pattern by 4 weeks of age, which is a period later than the mature configuration of EEG rhythms (Valatx *et al.*, 1964), and yet antecedent to a stable circadian distribution of episodes of sleep and wakefulness, which does not occur until 3 months of age (Fig. 10) (Chase and Sterman, 1967). Thus, during the course of maturation it is clear that the mechanisms which are responsible for determining the level of reflex response, be they of segmental or suprasegmental origin, develop at a different rate from those factors which determine not only the total time spent awake and asleep but also the activity of the EEG during these states.

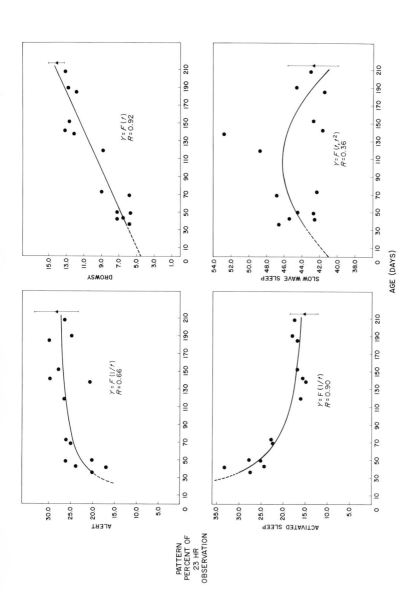

Fig. 10. Kitten: Determined on a cross-sectional basis, curves of best fit were generated for the total percentage values of each state for all animals. The mathematical functions for the alert and active sleep states were the same; however, the alert pattern was a positively accelerating function, while active sleep was negatively accelerating. Asymptotes for both were reached at approximately the same age. The analysis of the quiet sleep pattern showed no systematic trend with age, since the curve of best fit indicated no significant correlation with the data. (From Chase and Sterman, 1967.)

In contrast to the data of this report of reflex activity in the kitten, Prechtl and others found that some reflexes fluctuate in the newborn infant during sleep and wakefulness much as they do in the adult (Prechtl *et al.*, 1967; Hodes and Dement, 1964; Hodes and Gribetz, 1962). The modulation of monosynaptic spinal cord reflexes during quiet sleep, compared with active sleep, is similar in the neonate and adult (Prechtl *et al.*, 1967b), although the amplitude during quiet sleep is greater than during awake behavior (Prechtl, Chapter 14). On the other hand, the tonic myotatic reflex, as well as a number of exteroceptive skin reflexes, increase from quiet to active sleep but are largest during wakefulness (Vlach *et al.*, 1969). Other reflexes reveal different variations or a complete lack of state-dependent modulation (Prechtl *et al.*, 1967a; Lenard *et al.*, 1968). No uniform pattern emerges from an analysis of this infant data, for during each state of sleep and wakefulness some reflexes are larger than during the other states, and while the adult pattern is observed in some instances when comparing two states, the amplitude during the third state is anomalous.

A possible basis for these findings is that at birth the infant, by a number of criteria, is relatively more mature than the kitten. It is only postnatally that the kitten's developmental schedule precedes that of the human infant. For examples, H reflexes appear more mature in newborn infants than in newborn kittens (Skoglund, 1960d; Blom *et al.*, 1964). In the infant, tonic muscle tone is present during quiet sleep, whereas in the kitten it is not until the second or third postnatal week that muscular activity is maintained during this state (Jouvet-Mounier *et al.*, 1970; Valatx *et al.*, 1964; Jouvet, 1967). Additionally, state-dependent EEG patterns can be differentiated in the neonatal infant but not in the neonatal kitten (Jouvet-Mounier *et al.*, 1970; Valatx *et al.*, 1964; Jouvet, 1967). The interaction between the maturing suprasegmental systems which govern reflex excitability during sleep and wakefulness and the developmental changes in the reflex arc most probably represent the major basis for the differences in the state-dependent reflex responses when kittens are compared with infants.

Thus far, no studies have been carried out to determine the presynaptic and postsynaptic factors which contribute to the modulation of brain stem reflexes during sleep and wakefulness. However, at the level of the spinal cord, these synaptic influences have been investigated as have the structures which give rise to them (Pompeiano, 1967). During quiet sleep, there is a depression of γ motoneuron activity; during active sleep, there is a further reduction of their excitability as well as postsynaptic depression of α motoneurons. This depression of α motoneuron activity is likely due to descending reticulospinal inhibitory volleys. The phasic inhibitory and facilitory phenomena which accompany the REM of active sleep are dependent upon the functional integrity of the medial and descending vestibular nuclei.

It has been suggested that the pyramidal system, red nucleus, and midbrain reticular formation participate in the phasic episodes of motor facilitation which take place during active sleep. It is not known whether these mechanisms and systems play a similar role in the determination of brain stem reflex excitability, although the digastric reflex does react to excitation of the preceding structures in a manner consistent with the pattern of reflex variations observed during sleep and wakefulness (Chase, 1971). Therefore, for the time being, it seems judicious to assume that similar factors play a role in brain stem reflex modulation as has been described for spinal cord reflexes.

Reduced reflex amplitude during the awake state, relative to quiet sleep, occurs for the digastric reflex in both the kitten and adult cat, and for the masseteric reflex only in the kitten (present study; Chase, 1971; Chase *et al.*, 1968). These three situations have in common the lack of a functional γ motoneuron system (Ekholm, 1967a; Skoglund, 1960a, c, e); consequently, there is an absence of tonic stretch reflex activity (Skoglund, 1960c, e). γ motoneuron discharge provides for a heightened reflex response during the awake state (accompanied by EEG desynchronization) (Euler and Soderberg, 1956; Hongo *et al.*, 1963). Since these motoneurons are not functional in the young kitten, a response pattern for the masseteric reflex similar to that of the digastric reflex was not unexpected.

The preceding may serve as a model for a system which at one period during development is immature in the sense that its component parts do not function as they do in the adult. The reflex arc once fully developed, including the gamma motoneuron system, remains despite destruction of suprasegmental structures. For example, in the decerebrate animal, arousing stimuli lead to masseteric reflex facilitation as it does in the intact adult cat (see McGinty's discussion in this chapter). However, during active sleep in this preparation there is also reflex facilitation, which in this case probably reflects an imbalance of suprasegmental control. It is therefore proposed that the response of the masseteric reflex during the awake state in the young animal is due to the interaction between an undeveloped reflex arc and suprasegmental influences, and during active sleep in the decerebrate its response is dependent upon suprasegmental influences rather than on the disruption of the component parts of the reflex arc.

Another variation from the adult pattern which occurs in the kitten is reflex facilitation during active sleep. In this regard an anomaly which arises is the heightened reflex state coincident with tonic muscular atonia. This is not the only dissociation of muscular activity and reflex amplitude. In the kitten, during the awake state, a marked decrease in reflex amplitude is observed in conjunction with high levels of EMG activity. In the adult cat, a decrease in amplitude of the digastric reflex occurs during arousal, although the masseteric reflex usually shows a concomitant increase in size (Chase, 1971; Chase *et al.*,

1968). In the adult decerebrate cat, during active sleep, there is atonia of the neck musculature coincident with facilitation of the masseteric and digastric reflexes (see the discussion by McGinty which follows). Therefore, not including the present report, there are ample descriptions of reflex facilitation accompanying muscular atonia. There is other evidence that the level of reflex excitability need not bear any strict relationship to tonic EMG activity, for as Henatsch and Schulte (1958) have shown, an increase in reflex response may occur in the presence of a decrease in α motoneuron discharge.

No information is available which would indicate the probable basis for atonia and heightened reflex activity in the kitten during sleep. Any one of the following general hypotheses seem able to account for these findings: (1) presynaptic inhibitory processes may not function in the young kitten as they do in the adult, or they function exclusively during the awake state (Eccles and Willis, 1963) (Note: there is evidence that inhibitory synaptic processes are more pronounced in kittens and would presumably exert their influence principally during wakefulness (Skoglund, 1960b)); (2) during sleep, the decrease in descending activation of α motoneuron discharge might allow a greater response when initiated by segmental afferents (Henatsch and Schulte, 1958) which may occur in conjunction with the absence of descending inhibition.

A lack of knowledge often provides a firm foundation for the generation of a seemingly endless series of hypotheses which at best can serve only as guidelines for experimentation. It appears advisable simply to wait for future research to clarify the causal processes whose end product is facilitation of reflex activity in the neonatal kitten during active sleep and suppression during arousal.

The principal arguments which are usually proposed to justify ontogenetic research are that "it is easier to examine a simpler system," which is based upon the belief that the immature organism represents one, and that "an examination of a physiological system in an immature animal will aid in the understanding of its activity in the adult." The study of reflex activity in kittens during ontogeny would, therefore, be expected to shed light on the mechanisms responsible for their modulation in the mature cat. The assumption is made that systems in the young animal develop structurally and functionally in a linear fashion and gradually reach maturity. However, a number of reports at this conference indicate that many physiological processes in the neonate are diametrically different from those observed in the adult. It is therefore suggested that the processes which govern the basic sleep and waking states mature at a rate which in many instances does not parallel the development of those physiological systems which exhibit state-dependent variations. It is this interaction of differentially maturing systems which results in unique patterns of reflex activity during sleep and wakefulness, as was reported in the present study.

REFERENCES

Ausubel, D. P. (1966). A critique of Piaget's theory of the ontogenesis of motor behavior. *J. Genet. Psychol.* 109, 119-122.

Bieber, I. (1940). Grasping and sucking. *J. Nerv. Ment. Dis.* 91, 31-36.

Blom, S., Hogbarth, K. E., and Skoglund, S. (1964). Post-tetanic potentiation of H-reflexes in human infants. *Exp. Neurol.* 9, 198-211.

Chase, M. H. (1971). The digastric reflex in the kitten and adult cat: paradoxical amplitude fluctuations during sleep and wakefulness. *Arch. Ital. Biol.* 108, 403–422.

Chase, M. H., and Sterman, M. B. (1967). Maturation of patterns of sleep and wakefulness in the kitten. *Brain Res.* 5, 319-329.

Chase, M. H., McGinty, D. J., and Sterman, M. B. (1968). Cyclic variation in the amplitude of a brain stem reflex during sleep and wakefulness. *Experientia* 24, 47-48.

Dement, W. (1958). The occurrence of low voltage, fast electroencephalogram patterns during behavioral sleep in the cat. *Electroencephalogr. Clin. Neurophysiol.* 10, 291-296.

Eccles, R. M., and Willis, W. D. (1963). Presynaptic inhibition of the monosynaptic reflex pathway in kittens. *J. Physiol. (London)* 165, 403-420.

Eccles, R. M., and Willis, W. D. (1965). The effect of repetitive stimulation upon monosynaptic transmission in kittens. *J. Physiol. (London)* 176, 311-321.

Ekholm, J. (1967a). Postnatal changes in cutaneous reflexes and in the discharge pattern of cutaneous and articular sense organs: A morphological and physiological study in the cat. *Acta Physiol. Scand., Suppl.* 297, 1-130.

Ekholm, J. (1967b). Postnatal development of excitatory and inhibitory skin areas for hindlimb muscles in kittens. *Acta Soc. Med. Upsal.* 72, 20-24.

Euler, C. V., and Soderberg, V. (1956). The relation between gamma motor activity and the electroencephalogram. *Experientia* 12, 278-279.

Gupta, J. M., and Scopes, J. W. (1965). Observations on blood pressure in newborn infants. *Arch. Dis. Childhood* 40, 637-644.

Harvey, W. (1651). "Exercitationes de Generatione Animalium." O. Pulleyn, London.

Henatsch, H. D., and Schulte, F. J. (1958). Reflexerregung und Eigenhemmung tonischer und phasischer Alpha-Motoneurone während chemischer Davererregung der Muskelspindeln. *Pfluegers Arch. Gesamte Physiol. Menschen Tiere* 268, 134-147.

Hodes, R., and Dement, W. C. (1964). Depression of electrically induced reflexes ("H-reflexes") in man during low voltage EEG sleep. *Electroencephalogr. Clin. Neurophysiol.* 17, 617-629.

Hodes, R., and Gribetz, I. (1962). H-reflexes in normal human infants: depression of these electrically induced reflexes (EIR's) in sleep. *Proc. Soc. Exp. Biol. Med.* 110, 577-580.

Hongo, T. M., Kubota, K., and Shimazu, H. (1963). EEG spindle and depression of gamma motor activity. *J. Neurophysiol.* 26, 568-580.

Jouvet, M. (1967). Neurophysiology of the states of sleep. *Physiol. Rev.* 47, 117-177.

Jouvet-Mounier, D., Astic, L., and Lacote, D. (1970). Ontogenesis of the states of sleep in rat, cat, and guinea pig during the first postnatal month. *Develop. Psychobiol.* 2, 216-239.

Korner, A. F. (1968). REM organization in neonates: Theoretical implications for development and the biological function of REM. *Arch. Gen. Psychiat.* 19, 330-340.

Langworthy, O. R. (1924). A correlated study of the development of reflex activity in fetal and young kittens and the myelinization of tracts in the nervous system. *Contrib. Embryol. Carnegie Inst.* 20, 127-172.

Lenard, H. G., von Bernuth, H., and Prechtl, H. F. R. (1968). Reflexes and their relationship to behavioral state in the newborn . *Acta Paediat. Scand.* 57, 177-185.

Parmelee, A. H., Akiyama, Y., Schultz, M. A., Wenner, W. H., Schulte, F. J., and Stern, E. (1968). The electroencephalogram in active and quiet sleep in infants. *In* "Clinical Electroencephalography in Childhood" (P. Kellaway and I. Peterson, eds.), pp. 77-88. Almqvist & Wiksell, Stockholm.

Pieron, H. (1913). *Le problème physiologique du sommeil.* Masson, Paris.

Pollock, L. J., and Davis, L. (1930). The reflex activities of a decerebrate animal. *J. Comp. Neurol.* 50;, 377-411.

Pollock, L. J., and Davis, L. (1931). Studies in decerebration. VI. The effect of deafferentation upon decerebrate rigidity. *Amer. J. Physiol.* 98, 47-49.

Pompeiano, O. (1967). The neurophysiological mechanisms of the postural and motor events during desynchronized sleep. *In* "Sleep and Altered States of Consciousness" (S. S. Kety, E. V. Evarts, and H. L. Williams, eds.), pp. 351-423. Williams & Wilkins, Baltimore, Maryland.

Prechtl, H. F. R., Grant, D., Lenard, H. G., and Hrbek, A. (1967a). The lip-tap reflex in the awake and sleeping newborn infant, a polygraphic study. *Exp. Brain Res.* 3, 184-194.

Prechtl, H. F. R., Vlach, V., Lenard, H. G., and Grant, D. (1967b). Exteroceptive and tendon reflexes in various behavioural states in the newborn infant. *Biol. Neonatorum* 11, 159-175.

Roffwarg, H. P., Muzio, J. N., and Dement, W. C. (1966). Ontogenetic development of the human sleep-dream cycle. *Science* 152, 604-619.

Schulte, F. J., and Schwenzel, W. (1965). Motor control and muscle tone in the newborn period. Electromyographic studies. *Biol. Neonatorum* 8, 198-215.

Skoglund, S. (1960a). The activity of muscle receptors in the kitten. *Acta Physiol Scand.* 50, 203-221.

Skoglund, S. (1960b). Central connections and functions of muscle nerves in the kitten. *Acta Physiol. Scand.* 50, 222-237.

Skoglund, S. (1960c). On the postnatal development of postural mechanisms as revealed by electromyography and myography in decerebrate kittens. *Acta Physiol. Scand.* 49, 299-317.

Skoglund, S. (1960d). The reactions to tetanic stimulation of the two-neuron arc in the kitten. *Acta Physiol. Scand.* 50, 238-253.

Skoglund, S. (1960e). The spinal transmission of proprioceptive reflexes and the postnatal development of conduction velocity in different hindlimb nerves in the kitten. *Acta Physiol. Scand.* 49, 318-329.

Skoglund, S. (1966). Muscle afferents and motor control in the kitten. *In* "Muscle Afferents and Motor Control" (R. Granit, ed.), pp. 245-259. Almqvist & Wiksells, Stockholm.

Valatx, J. L., Jouvet, D., and Jouvet, M. (1964). Evolution électroencéphalographique des différents états de sommeil chez le chaton. *Electroencephalogr. Clin. Neurophysiol.* 17, 218-233.

Vlach, V. (1968). Some exteroceptive skin reflexes in the limbs and trunk in newborns. *In* "Studies in Infancy" (M. C. Bax and R. C. MacKeith, eds.), pp. 41-54. Heinemann, London.

Vlach, V., von Bernuth, H., and Prechtl, H. F. R. (1969). State dependency of exteroceptive skin reflexes in newborn infants. *Develop. Med. Child Neurol.* 11, 353-362.

Wagner, I. F. (1938). The sleeping posture of the neonate. *J. Genet. Psychol.* 52, 235-239.

Weed, L. H. (1917). The reactions of kittens after decerebration. *Amer. J. Physiol.* 43, 131-157.

Wolff, P. H. (1966). The causes, controls, and organization of behavior in the neonate. *Psychol. Issues* 5, Monogr. 17, 1-105.

INVITED DISCUSSION*: DENNIS J. MCGINTY

Development of Forebrain Control of Sleep

The developmental changes in reflex modulation during sleep, which were described by Dr. Chase, provide a useful neurophysiological model for the ontogeny of sleep. In neonatal kittens, reflex conduction is augmented during active sleep compared to quiet sleep (Iwamura *et al.*, 1968). Between 3 and 6 weeks of age, the augmentation gradually changes the reflex inhibition which characterizes the adult cat (Pompeiano, 1967). We were interested in assessing the nature of this developmental change, and, in particular, to test the hypothesis that descending forebrain influences modulate reflex conduction. We tested this hypothesis by studying the effect of the removal of the forebrain above the level of the mesencephalon. In our preparations, we make a brain stem transection and aspirate the forebrain above the transection except for a hypothalamic island. We are frequently able to keep these preparations for several weeks. As Jouvet (1962) has shown, these decerebrate animals continue to show the periodic occurrence of a phenomenon that looks very much like active sleep.

Figure 11 is a continuous record from a chronic decerebrate cat. These are six strips from a continuous recording, showing the pontile EEG recording, eye movements, neck muscle tone. In this record of approximately 45 min, there are three episodes characterized by the disappearance of neck muscle tone and phasic activity of active sleep. This state is called the atonic phase.

I would like to point out that a feature of this atonic state in the midbrain decerebrate animal is a rather high rate of pontile EEG spiking activity and high rate of eye movements, much like that seen in the kitten.

We have recorded the masseteric reflex on decerebrate animals, using the same technique that is utilized in the adult (Chase *et al.*, 1968). Figure 12 compares recordings of reflex amplitude in the kitten, adult cat, and midbrain decerebrate cat. In each record there is a period of quiet sleep (or quiet state in the case of the decerebrate) followed by a period of active sleep.

Figure 12A is a recording from a kitten at 12 days of age. The reflex is augmented during active sleep. In the adult cat (Fig. 12B), on the other hand, we see a striking depression of reflex amplitude.

In an animal with transection of the midbrain (Fig. 12C), we see a restoration of a kitten pattern. That is, at the onset of the atonic phase marked by the disappearance of EEG activity, the masseteric reflex is augmented as it is in the kitten. We have seen this phenomenon after transections of the midbrain, ranging from the level of the red nucleus through the posterior hypothalamus, and, in general, the phenomenon is stable for several weeks after the transection.

If we make the transection at a lower level, that is, at the rostral pontile or caudal midbrain level, instead of reflex augmentation, we observe inhibition of reflex amplitude. That is, reflex modulation looks similar to that which we see in an adult cat. But there is an important difference. In these lower transected animals, there are very few eye movements and little phasic activity. The overall pattern in the atonic phase is not like active sleep in the kitten. However, in the higher transections we do see the pattern of activity that looks like the kitten.

*This research was supported by a grant from the U.S. Public Health Service (MH-10083), and by the Veterans Administration. Bibliographic assistance was received from the UCLA Brain Information Service which is part of the National Institute of Neurological Diseases and Stroke and is supported under Contract No. DHEW PH-43-66-59.

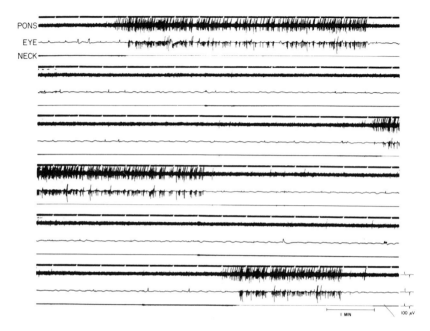

Fig. 11. Polygraphic record of pontile EEG, eye movements, and neck EMG from a chronic midbrain decerebrate cat. During this continuous 45-min sample, three episodes of the atonic phase were observed.

The next problem is to determine the lowest transection level, above the midbrain, which preserves the adult reflex pattern during active sleep. Our results suggest that the thalamic animal continues to show the adult pattern. In the thalamic preparation, we spare the basal forebrain and preoptic area of the hypothalamus as well as the thalamus. Our current hypothesis is that this depression of activity originates in that general part of the brain.

These results suggest that some of the somatic changes that characterize sleep have their origins in the rostral diencephalon. I would like to extend this point of view to more general properties of sleep.

Forebrain influences in the control of sleep are well established. Lesions of the basal forebrain area bring about the abolition or suppression of sleep (Nauta, 1946; McGinty and Sterman, 1968), while either electrical or chemical stimulation of the same area can cause the initiation of sleep (Sterman and Clemente, 1962; Hernández-Peón *et al.*, 1963). The lesions suppress both quiet sleep and active sleep. This is a surprising result, since active sleep can occur following complete ablation of the forebrain. The lesions appear to release a descending influence which suppresses the initiation of active sleep. When such lesions produce a partial suppression of quiet sleep, active sleep is reduced proportionately. A similar result was obtained by Jouvet (1967) following suppression of quiet sleep after lesions of the raphe nuclei of the brain stem.

One of the forebrain functions in the control of sleep is suggested by observation of cats with basal forebrain lesions. Moderate-sized lesions producing a partial suppression of sleep also alter the postural characteristics of sleep. This result is indicated in Fig. 13. The residual sleep seen 2 weeks after this lesion occurs almost exclusively while the cat is standing up. These animals walk around the cage or across the room until they come to a wall or

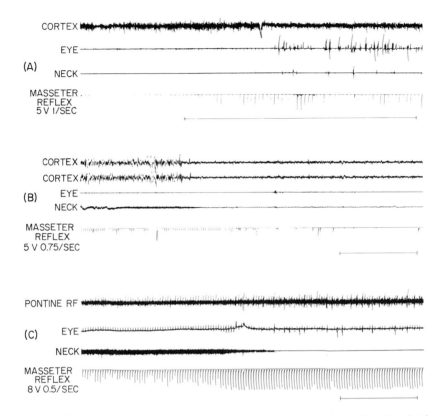

Fig. 12. Modulation of the monosynaptic masseteric reflex during active sleep in the 12-day-old kitten (A), adult cat (B), and after midbrain transection (C). The onset of active sleep is indicated by eye movements, twitches, neck muscle atonia, or EEG desynchronization. Reflex transmission is facilitated in the kitten but inhibited in the adult. Removal of the forebrain restores the modulation pattern of the kitten.

obstruction where they stop. Generally when they are motionless against the obstacle, the EEG shows the characteristics of SWS, including slow waves and spindle bursts. We have not yet looked at reflex modulation in animals with lesions, but these behavioral observations suggest that suppression or inhibition influences on the motor system that originates in the forebrain are required for the initiation of sleep postures in the adult.

Basic motor mechanisms for suppression of postural reflexes probably reside in the lower brain stem. Thus, as mentioned above, reflex inhibition can be observed during the atonic state in the pontile cat. However, in the adult, sleep and wakefulness may reflect the balance of rostral brain stem excitatory and forebrain inhibitory influences (McGinty *et al.*, 1971).

As several of the contributors to this symposium have pointed out, the neonate, particularly in species such as the cat and rat which are relatively immature at birth, exhibits primarily active sleep (Jouvet-Mounier, 1968). During development, quiet sleep gradually increases in amount and becomes the predominate phase of sleep. The emergence of quiet sleep may depend on the maturation of forebrain influences. The sleep state of the neonate, and probably most of the manifestations of active sleep in the adult, are controlled by the

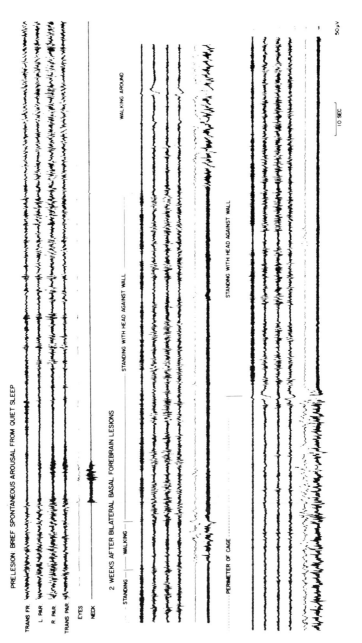

Fig. 13. EEG synchronization is observed during normally waking postures after lesions of the basal forebrain area. Although such lesions suppress sleep, residual sleeplike states may occur without postural relaxation.

brain stem. During development, the brain stem sleep mechanisms come under the control of forebrain mechanisms. This process may be described as the *encephalization of the neural control of sleep* (McGinty, 1971).

The concept of encephalization provides an explanation for the finding of neural substrates for sleep at several levels of the neuraxis (Batini *et al.*, 1959; Jouvet, 1967; McGinty and Sterman, 1968). Each region may contain elements in a chain of neural mechanisms associated with the complex sleep process. Interruption of the chain at any level can produce a disorganization of the sequence of steps or processes which contribute to sleep. For example, a lesion may disrupt the inhibition of antigravity postural reflexes, depression of autonomic activity, filtering of sensory input to reduce arousal, hypothetical neuroendocrine receptors involved in the regulation of sleep, integration sites for the voluntary postural preparations for sleep, or mechanisms that suppress alternate drives. During development, these different aspects of sleep may mature gradually. We must begin to measure the properties of sleep at each age. We have not developed procedures of distinguishing these possibilities; previous studies have leaned heavily on the net effect, the amount of polygraphically defined sleep.

The nature of the physiological requirement for sleep continues to elude scientific explanation. Sleep deprivation experiments suggest that the brain suffers some kind of "fatigue." Sleep deprivation in humans reliably produces a number of disturbances in behavior, notably lapses in attention, irritability, feelings of fatigue, disorientation, impaired short-term memory, and slower cognitive operation (although some of these deficits may be caused by the intrusion of brief moments of drowsiness). A small but significant proportion of subjects exhibit definite psychotic episodes (Johnson, 1969). Moreover, prolonged deprivation has been reported to produce visual and occasionally auditory illusions in man (Naitoh, 1969). Such deprivation has been reported to result in death in experimental animals (summarized in Kleitman, 1963). However, except for a single report of deficits in ATP metabolism in red cells (Lucy *et al.*, 1960), no proposals have been advanced to account for these phenomena. Thus, practically nothing is known about what is fatigued and what is restored during sleep. The term "fatigue" may refer to any physiological process where some limited rate of synthesis, transport, metabolism, or other mechanism results in a degradation of the performance of the nervous system.

Immature animals sleep more than adults. For example, the human neonate sleeps ~16 hr daily, compared to the adult's 7½ hr of sleep. A number of suggestions could be made to account for this increased sleep. (1) It is generally suggested that the immature nervous system is undergoing changes as a result of both growth and experience. Indeed, these two factors seem to be interrelated in some neural pathways. (2) Immature neural mechanisms seems to be more fatigable. Metabolic mechanisms supporting the biochemical processes underlying neuronal firing or synaptic transmission are simply less rapid in the immature nervous system. (3) Increased sleep may reflect the incomplete development of a neural mechanism mediating wakeful behaviors that antagonize sleep. (4) The higher metabolic rate of immature animals may result in greater sleep drive. This list is surely incomplete, but two general types of factors seem to emerge. The first two possibilities are related to the special functional activities of the immature brain. The second two possibilities are the result of the immaturity of the brain without regard to the ongoing experience of the organism.

Experiments were designed to test the hypothesis that functional activity of the brain associated with immaturity produces an increased drive for sleep and to separate this from the factors of immaturity per se. It was decided to study the amount of sleep in animals where the environmental stimulation was drastically reduced.

It has been shown that animals reared in an inpoverished environment exhibit retarded behavioral development. In studies where specific forms of sensory stimulation are reduced, normal neural development is retarded. Thus, this treatment appears to reduce the functional activity of the forebrain, especially that activity associated with the response to varied experience; *at the same time the immaturity of the organism is prolonged.*

Half of the kittens from three litters were placed at weaning into individual completely enclosed cages, while their littermates were reared in a normal group with frequent handling and complex stimulation. All animals were surgically prepared with chronically implanted electrodes for recording EEG, neck muscle, and eye movement activity. Then, 22-hr continuous recordings were obtained to measure sleep during the period of isolation, at about 12 weeks of age. When the kittens were 23 weeks of age they were taken out of isolation and returned to the normal environment. During this period, these kittens undergo very rapid changes in behavior as a consequence of their exposure to novel environment. The sleep patterns of these animals were studied again 2-4 days after they were placed in a normal environment.

The results of the experiment are shown in Fig. 14. Animals living in an isolated impoverished environment sleep much less than their normally raised littermates. Indeed, such animals sleep less than adult animals. The depression of sleep is observed in both quiet sleep and active sleep.

A striking reversal of this result was seen when the isolated animals were placed in a novel environment. Following this period of intense novel stimulation, these animals were sleeping much more than their normal littermates. Indeed, they slept as much as kittens who were several months younger.

The depression of sleep in isolated animals is consistent with observations of a high level of behavioral arousal in such animals. Analysis of the EEG frequency spectrum and evoked potentials in dogs also indicated a high arousal level in response to exposure to the novel environment (Melzack and Burns, 1965). The present data support these findings, but stress that the arousal of isolated animals is reflected tonically by reduced sleep within the familiar home cage.

The study of isolation-reared animals provided strong suggestive evidence that environmental stimulation was necessary for the elevated sleep drive of immature animals. However, isolation-reared animals are different from the normal animals in a variety of ways. The differences reflect the effect of social stimulation, changes of appetite, in sensory sensitivities, as well as in plastic changes in the nervous system. Therefore, it was decided to do a second kind of experiment where more precise control of the effects of environmental stimulation was possible. Specifically, the amount of sleep was studied following specific "doses" or periods of exposure to novel environmental stimulation. For this purpose, sleep was studied in isolation-reared animals following 4½-hr periods of exposure to a novel stimulating environment. As a control procedure, sleep was measured in the same animals following 4½-hr of sleep deprivation in the animals' home cage. The sleep deprivation control was necessary because animals did not sleep in the novel environment. An additional procedure, employed to control for the "stress" of exposure to novel stimulation, was the restraint of the kittens in a small cubicle. Restraint is known to produce classic stress responses in rats (Brodie, 1962). The results are shown in Fig. 15. Following 4½-hr of novel stimulation, isolation-reared animals exhibited increased sleep when compared with the equivalent amount of sleep deprivation or restraint. Sleep deprivation and exposure to environmental stimulation were not differentially effective in modifying sleep in normal animals. Of course, the environmental stimulation was not novel for the normal kittens. Thus, in this experiment, facilitation of sleep was specifically tied to exposure to a novel stimulating environment.

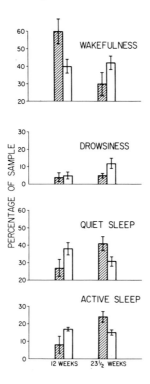

Fig. 14. Comparison of the amount of quiet sleep and active sleep in kittens reared in an isolated impoverished environment and normally reared littermates. (▨) Isolated; (☐) control. Kittens exhibited reduced sleep during isolation, but augmented sleep following 2-4 days exposure to the normal environment. The reduction in sleep in control kittens is the normal developmental change. (From McGinty, 1971.)

Taken together, these experiments provide strong support for the hypothesis that sleep is facilitated by exposure to a novel stimulating environment. Furthermore, the elevated amounts of sleep found in immature animals appear to depend upon the effects of the environment. It seems reasonable to hypothesize that a novel stimulating environment is critical because of the complex neural responses to "experience" that it produces in the animal.

Sleep was reduced about 40% by prolonged isolation in an impoverished environment and increased about 25% by novel stimulation. The neural response associated with "experience" accounts for a significant fraction of the requirement for sleep. Although "experience" cannot be completely eliminated experimentally, it appears the neural activity occurring in the absence of specific "experience" may account for a major part of the sleep need. These data suggest that the fatigue associated with "experience" is superimposed on a spontaneous rate of fatigue. This account is consistent with the concept of the spontaneously active nervous system which is repatterned by functional inputs.

In the immature animal, elevated sleep may reflect increased experience or fatigability or both. The fatigability of the immature nervous system has been noted by several investigators (Scheibel and Scheibel, 1964; Purpura, 1961; Ellingson and Wilcott, 1960). Further studies will be required to clarify this problem.

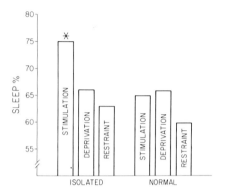

Fig. 15. The percentage of sleep in 18 hour recordings following 4½-hr exposure to a complex environment or control conditions in isolation-reared and normal kittens. The intense novel stimulation provided to the isolated kittens augmented the subsequent sleep more than sleep deprivation or stress caused by restraint. The sleep of normal kittens was not differentially changed by the exposure to the familiar complex environment. The asterisk indicates statistical significance (t test, $p < 0.05$). (From McGinty, 1971.)

These experiments are among the first to test directly the hypothesis that sleep is facilitated following neural activity associated with the experience of the animal. However, there is a good deal of indirect evidence relating sleep to complex or "cognitive" brain functions. Feinberg has correlated the amount of active sleep to functional capacities in several clinical populations in man. In retarded children, the amount of REM activity associated with active sleep is positively correlated with the IQ (Feinberg, 1968). At the other extreme, depression of sleep in the aged can be associated with the appearance of other signs of senility (Feinberg *et al.*, 1967). A depression of sleep is also observed during the disorganization of behavior associated with periods of acute illness in depressed and schizophrenic patients (Snyder, 1969).

I have reviewed some suggestive evidence that the control or regulation of sleep in the adult is directed by forebrain neural mechanisms. Forebrain regulation is superimposed on basic excitatory and inhibitory processes organized in the brain stem during ontogenetic development. Studies of sleep drive suggest that forebrain functions may be particularly dependent on the restorative properties of sleep. The neural regulation of sleep may have evolved concomitantly with the phylogenesis of complex forebrain functions.

REFERENCES

Batini, C., Moruzzi, G., Palestini, M., Rossi, G. F., and Zanchetti, A. (1959). Effects of complete pontine transections on the sleep-wakefulness rhythm: the midpontine pretrigeminal preparation. *Arch. Ital. Biol.* 97, 1-12.

Brodie, D. A. (1962). Ulceration of the stomach produced by restraint in rats. *Gastroenterology* 43, 107-109.

Chase, M. H., McGinty, D. J., and Sterman, M. B. (1968). Cyclic variation in the amplitude of a brain stem reflex during sleep and wakefulness. *Experientia* **24**, 47-48.

Ellingson, R. J., and Wilcott, R. C. (1960). Development of evoked responses in visual and auditory cortices of kittens. *J. Neurophysiol.* **23**, 363-375.

Feinberg, I. (1968). Eye movement activity during sleep and intellectual function in mental retardation. *Science* **159**, 1256.

Feinberg, I., Koresko, R. L., and Heller, N. (1967). EEG sleep patterns as a function of normal and pathological aging in man. *J. Psychiat. Res.* **5**, 107-144.

Hernández-Peón, R., Chávez-Ibarra, G., Morgane, P. J., and Timo-Iaria, C. (1963). Limbic cholinergic pathways involved in sleep and emotional behavior. *Exp. Neurol.* **8**, 93-111.

Iwamura, Y., Isuda, K., Kudo, N., and Kohama, K. (1968). Monosynaptic reflex during natural sleep in the kitten. *Brain Res.* **11**, 456-459.

Johnson, L. C. (1969). Physiological and psychological changes following total sleep deprivation. *In* "Sleep: Physiology and Pathology" (A. Kales, ed.), pp. 206-220. Lippincott, Philadelphia.

Jouvet, M. (1962). Recherches sur les structures nerveuses et les mécanismes responsables des differentes phases du sommeil physiologique. *Arch Ital. Biol.* **100**, 125-206.

Jouvet, M. (1967). Mechanisms of the states of sleep: A neuropharmacological approach. *In* "Sleep and Altered States of Consciousness" (S. S. Kety, E. V. Evarts, and H. L. Williams, eds.), pp. 86-126. Williams & Wilkins, Baltimore, Maryland.

Jouvet-Mounier, D. (1968). Ontogénèse des états de vigilance chez quelques mammifères. Doctoral Dissertation, J. Tixier & Fils, Lyon.

Kleitman, H. (1963). "Sleep and Wakefulness," rev. ed. Univ. of Chicago Press, Chicago.

Lucy, E. D., Frohman, C. E., Grisell, J. L., Lenzo, J. E., and Gottlieb, J. S. (1960). Sleep deprivation: Effects on behavior, thinking, motor performance, and biological energy transfer systems. *Psychosom. Med.* **22**, 182-192.

McGinty, D. J. (1971). Encephalization and the neural control of sleep. *In* "Brain Development and Behavior" (M. B. Sterman, D. J. McGinty, and A. M. Adinolfi, eds.), pp. 335-357. Academic Press, New York.

McGinty, D. J., and Sterman, M. B. (1968). Sleep suppression after basal forebrain lesions in the cat. *Science* **160**, 1253-1255.

McGinty, D. J., Sterman, M. B., and Iwamura, Y. (1971). Activity and atonia in the decerebrate cat. *Psychophysiology* **7**, 309.

Melzack, R., and Burns, S. K. (1965). Neurophysiological effects of early sensory restriction. *Exp. Neurol.* **13**, 163-175.

Naitoh, P. (1969). "Sleep Loss and its Effects on Performance," Rep. No. 68-3. Dept. of the Navy.

Nauta, W. J. H. (1946). Hypothalamic regulation of sleep in rats: An experimental study. *J. Neurophysiol.* **9**, 285-316.

Pompeiano, O. (1967). The neurophysiological mechanisms of the postural and motor events during desynchronized sleep. *In* "Sleep and Altered States of Consciousness" (S. S. Kety, E. V. Evarts, and H. L. Williams, eds.), pp. 351- 423. Williams & Wilkins, Baltimore, Maryland.

Purpura, D. (1961). Analysis of axodendritic synaptic organizations in immature cerebral cortex. *Ann. N.Y. Acad. Sci.* **94**, 604-654.

Scheibel, M., and Scheibel, A. (1964). Some structural and functional substrates of development in young cats. *Progr. Brain Res.* **9**, 6-25.

Snyder, F. (1969). Sleep disturbance in relation to acute psychosis. *In* "Sleep: Physiology and Pathology" (A. Kales, ed.), pp. 170-182. Lippincott, Philadelphia.

Sterman, M. B., and Clemente, C. D. (1962). Forebrain inhibitory mechanisms: sleep patterns induced by basal forebrain stimulation in the behaving cat. *Exp. Neurol.* **6**, 103-117.

DEVELOPMENT OF EARLY MOTOR ACTIVITY
IN THE MONKEY*

The newborn monkey, like other placental mammals, develops its ability to move very early in embryonic life. Although its motor capability is far from complete, it can soon crawl, climb, move its head and eyes, and vocalize. From this baseline of motor capability, arbitrarily marked by the event of birth, one can follow the development, over a period of less than a year, of the precise, graceful, and marvelously rapid and skillful movements of the juvenile.

In the same manner, one can follow the progressive development of movement from a more significant baseline—the time of onset of the very first muscular movement. This can be done either after removal of the embryo from the uterus, or with the embryo remaining within the intact amniotic cavity. The photographs of spontaneous movements, made through the muscular wall of the uterus, are perhaps the first to be reported.

By beginning with the baseline of onset of the very first movements, one has the additional opportunity of relating the crucial beginnings of development of nerve cell interconnections, or synaptic development, with the onset and progressive development of its behavioral expression.

In the spinal region, the behavioral expression of synaptic development is muscular movement. At first, the movement is reflexly initiated. Later, the spinal mechanism for reflex responses is used for "spontaneous" movements within the amniotic cavity.

The specimens have been selected to exhibit the maximal degree of activity at each stage of development. It is only in this way that the maximal motor capability of a particular stage can be assessed, since in other specimens a variety of factors may reduce the activity of the embryo at the time of observation.

The following results were obtained: A series of 13 macaque fetuses of estimated ovulation ages 42-51 days (17-41 mm) was subjected to behavioral analysis with umbilical cord intact (in and out of the amnion), and to light and electron microscopic analysis of the cervical spinal cord. This period is a critical one in terms of onset and early development of spontaneous activity and of cutaneous reflexes. Behavioral criteria, reinforced by well-defined microscopic characteristics, suggested a grouping of specimens into three major stages, namely, a prereflex group (stage 1: 17-22 mm); a group in the period of onset of primitive spontaneous activity and of precocious local cutaneous reflexes in the

*Summary of film presentation by David Bodian.

trigeminal-cervical region (stage 2: 24-28 mm); and a group characterized by the development of more vigorous activity, spontaneous and otherwise, and of long intersegmental and crossed reflexes (stage 3: 32-41 mm). The evidence suggests that junctional differentiation and occurrence of a cluster of agranular spheroid synaptic vesicles characterize the primitive synaptic knobs which appear on motoneuron dendrites coincident with earliest reflexes. Onset of active, long intersegmental reflexes in stage 3 is coincident with development of axosomatic synaptic knobs, and of F-type (flattened) synaptic vesicles in a rapidly increasing fraction of all synaptic bulbs in the motoneuron neuropil. Total volume of all synaptic bulbs increases gradually as a fraction of the volume of the motoneuron neuropil until birth, but a steep increase in proportionate number of F-type synaptic knobs occurs in stage 3.

SELECTED BIBLIOGRAPHY

Bodian, D. (1966a). Development of fine structure of spinal cord in monkey fetuses. I. The motoneuron neuropil at the time of onset of reflex activity. *Bull. Johns Hopkins Hosp.* 119, 129-149.

Bodian, D. (1966b). Synaptic types on spinal motoneurons: an electron microscopic study. *Bull. Johns Hopkins Hospital* 119, 16-45.

Bodian, D. (1970). A model of synaptic and behavioral ontogeny. *In* "The Neurosciences: Second Study Program" (F. O. Schmitt, ed.), pp. 129-140. Rockefeller Univ. Press, New York.

Bodian, D., Melby, E. C., Jr., and Taylor, N. (1968). Development of fine structure of spinal cord in monkey fetuses. II. Pre-reflex period to period of long intersegmental reflexes. *J. Comp. Neurol.* 133, 113-166.

GENERAL DISCUSSION

Dr. Prescott: The findings of Dr. McGinty on the effects of isolation-rearing upon sleep behavior is an extremely significant contribution which again highlights the importance of neonatal and postnatal life experiences in influencing the developing brain and behavior. With respect to the effects of isolation rearing of mammals upon later behavior, it appears quite consistent across mammalian phylogenesis that hyperactivity, hyperreactivity, and increased CNS excitability are invariably the consequences of such early deprivation, particularly, if the somatosensory system is involved. Further, it is questionable whether such effects can be obtained with deprivation in the other sensory modalities provided sufficient somatosensory stimulation is present during early development (Prescott, 1967, 1970, 1971). Further, the effects of somatosensory stimulation in reducing emotionality, rage, and aggressive behaviors, arousal levels, and adrenocortical response to stress are sufficiently known so that additional emphasis is not required. In this context, the effects of sensory deprivation and stimulation upon stimulus seeking behaviors and their reduction, particularly emotionality and arousal levels, could provide the theoretical framework to account for the results reported by Dr. McGinty. Briefly, the isolation-reared animal is characterized by hyperactivity, increased emotionality, and central neural excitability.

Therefore, these animals should sleep less, as has been reported. However, if these animals are stimulated, particularly with somatosensory stimuli, as was done in the enriched environment, the state of hyperneural excitability and associated behaviors would be reduced and would be reflected in increased sleeping time as reported.

With respect to identifying specific physiological mechanisms that mediate these effects, it has been suggested elsewhere (Prescott, 1971) that Cannon's law of denervation supersensitivity may be the explanatory neurophysiological principle underlying these phenomena. This is to say that isolation-rearing represents a special case of functional somatosensory deafferentation where denervation supersensitivity would characterize the relevant neural structures that have been deprived of their afferent input. If this be the case, then confirmation of these effects should be possible by systematic neuroelectric, neurochemical, and neuromorphological studies. In passing, it may be worth mentioning that a neurofunctional system involving the cerebellum, frontal orbital cortex, reticular, and limbic system structures has been postulated to account for the effects of isolation-rearing (Prescott, 1971).

A final comment on another finding reported by Dr. McGinty appears relevant, as it may have unusual implications for the utilization of sleep EEG characteristics as a diagnostic measure of the effectiveness and durability of certain therapeutic procedures. Specifically, his report that exposure of isolated animals to a stimulated environment resulted in sleep facilitation and EEG changes during the first 18 hr of recording, but that the effects of this manipulation were not observable during the second block of 18 hr of recording and observation, suggest that sleep EEG characteristics may well prove to be a useful monitor of the effectiveness and duration of "therapeutic intervention" as represented by increased sensory stimulation. If sustained by further research, Dr. McGinty's results should have more than passing interest to many applied problems in clinical pediatrics and neural-behavioral development.

Dr. Morgane: I would like to make one remark pertaining to Dr. McGinty's paper. We, too, have seen cats with raphe lesions who walk around idly, go up against walls, and maintain a stance for many hours. There is almost a catatonic-like posture and the animal tends to show slow waves and spindles in the EEG while standing up. This seems to be similar to your findings.

Dr. Metcalf: Dr. McGinty, did you have an opportunity to examine the partitioning of SWS and PS in your stimulated isolated kittens?

Dr. McGinty: Yes. In the isolated kittens, both slow sleep and active sleep were reduced. The two states of sleep were reduced proportionately. When the kittens were stimulated, both active sleep and SWS were increased, although the changes were not great, and the increase in active sleep was not significant. Only the increase in overall sleep was statistically significant.

Dr. Metcalf: That is different, in a sense, from what we would expect in our experiments with altering visual input in the human being. It is very interesting.

Dr. Rose: Dr. McGinty, in your study in which animals were isolated and placed in a different environment, did you obtain EEG recordings both in the new environment as well as the original isolation environment?

Dr. McGinty: The sleep recordings were always done in the home cages of the animals. In the studies of animals exposed to the environment for a few hours a day, they were returned to their home cage for the 24-hr period of the sleep pattern recording.

Dr. Rose: The reason I mentioned this is that in a study by Scherrer and Fourment (1964) dealing with isolation and visual deprivation, the resultant EEG tracings, obtained while the animal was in the rearing environment as opposed to a novel environment, were considerably different. Kittens were reared isolated in the dark from 4 to 12 months. When spontaneous electrocortical recordings were obtained under rearing conditions, the records were comparable to those of the controls. However, intense and long-lasting arousal was observed in initial recordings carried out in a dark but novel environment.

Dr. Roberts: To stay awake really may require an effort. This suggests that inhibitory mechanisms may have to be much more active during the time that an animal is awake than when he is asleep, in order to maintain the coordination of adaptive function. The exhaustion of inhibitory mechanisms during sleep deprivation would be consistent with the loss of coordinated behavior when an animal is kept awake continually. The monaminergic and GABA systems all may be involved in active waking behavior. There may be a differential exhaustion of one of the pertinent systems, which might require a period of metabolic buildup, and this kind of phenomenon be involved in sleep mechanisms. It might be more meaningful to study the balance and interaction of the systems rather than to try to think in terms of one or the other alone.

Dr. Purpura: Dr. Chase, you had an opportunity in this study on the masseteric reflex to examine the question of electrotonic coupling in the mesencephalic nucleus of the trigeminal. You did not use the pathway at all, did you?

Dr. Chase: No, I did not.

Dr. Purpura: These are the only neurons in the mammalian nervous system where there is physiological evidence for electronic coupling between the neurons, according to R. Llinás (personal communication). A stimulus to this whole system, of course, is not as good as putting the afferent pathway to work. Did you grade this response with a graded stimulus?

Dr. Chase: There appeared to be better gradation of response in the adult. In the kitten, both the masseteric and digastric responses were, to a great extent, either recordable or not. When present, they reached their maximum amplitude at a level of excitation which was barely above the threshold value. Thus, it was rather difficult to get a midline amplitude that could be augmented or reduced in a state-dependent fashion during the sleep states.

Dr. Purpura: Let me suggest, if you use the afferent pathway, you might have an important clue on intercellular interaction. The next thing I want to ask is, if you stimulate the basal forebrain region in the young animal, when is the first time you see the appearance of synchronization?

Dr. Chase: This is an important question, and we are currently pursuing it, but thus far we have no information to communicate.

Dr. Sterman: Dr. Clemente and I tried this once in acute kitten preparations. Although it was very difficult, we did get some effects at about 1 month.

Dr. Clemente: Those experiments were not complete, however.

Dr. Purpura: You can get it a lot earlier from thalamic stimulation.

Dr. Clemente: We had difficulties in keeping our kitten alive through an extended acute experiment.

Dr. Purpura: Is there a site that one might stimulate in the acute experiment where one might be able to induce the adult pattern of response in the young kitten? The pathways must be there and probably could be activated electrically.

Dr. Clemente: In other words, excite connected circuits that are as yet not functional.

Dr. Purpura: There is no pathway in the brain that cannot be stimulated to work even though it may not be working spontaneously. Could the pathway coming from the cortex be stimulated in order to show a depression of the facilitated masseteric or digastric reflex in a kitten?

Dr. Chase: We have done that experiment in the adult cat.

Dr. Purpura: I know. That is what I am asking about the kitten. You want to know where the pathway arises.

Dr. Chase: We have just begun to examine the excitability of the reticular formation and cortex in the kitten during sleep and wakefulness. As the animal matures, we are especially interested in determining the interaction between these suprasegmental systems and the reflex responses at a period when the reflex activity exhibits paradoxical patterns of modulation during sleep and wakefulness.

Dr. Desmedt: I want to direct a question to Dr. Chase. You are aware, of course, that others have also been studying these reflexes. Hugelin and Dumont's experience in Paris has been that depression of the digastric reflex to reticular stimulation might be related to presynaptic inhibition of the primary afferents (Hugelin, 1955, 1961; Hugelin and Dumont, 1961). They argued that there would be two effects involved, namely, facilitation of the motoneurons on the one hand and presynaptic inhibition of the primary afferents on the other.

You didn't mention this, and I wondered whether you would accept this idea to explain your own results? In other words, whether you might perhaps consider that in the kitten the presynaptic inhibition of primary afferents would not be operative, and therefore, you would have facilitation of the reflex as you do in activated sleep.

Dr. Chase: The hypothesis which I presented is not at all contradictory to their results. What they propose is that there is a direct pathway to digastric motoneurons from the reticular formation which leads to postsynaptic excitation (Hugelin, 1955, 1961; Hugelin and Dumont, 1961). Additionally, there is evidence of an indirect pathway to terminals which result in presynaptic inhibition. Stimulation of the reticular formation at moderate levels leads to inhibition of the digastric reflex. But if one stimulates the reticular formation at extremely high levels of excitation, then reflex facilitation rather than inhibition takes place. In other words, the excitatory effect upon the motoneuron overrides the inhibition of presynaptic origin. Therefore, I proposed that in the young animal, the level of reticular activity might be relatively higher than that in the adult, due to the absence of forebrain inhibitory circuitry. During the alert state in the kitten, there may be a presynaptic effect which would be one of inhibition, and during the active sleep state, due to the high intensity of tonic reticular discharge, one might see the facilitation which is found following reticular stimulation at high levels of excitation.

Dr. Roberts: Is presynaptic inhibition still accepted?

Dr. Purpura: It is in different systems. Whether it exists above the level of the spinal cord is another problem that is still being actively investigated.

Dr. Roberts: It is proved in the spinal cord.

Dr. Purpura: There is good evidence for it in some areas of the dorsal horn.

REFERENCES

Hugelin, A. (1955). Analyse de l'inhibition d'un réflexe nociceptif (réflexe linguo-maxillaire) lors de l'activation du système reticulo-spinal dit "facilitateur." *C. R. Soc. Biol.* **149**, 1893-1898.

Hugelin, A. (1961). Intégrations motrices et vigilance chez l'encéphale isolé. II. Controle reticulaire de voies finales communes d'ouverture et de fermeture de la gueule. *Arch. Ital. Biol.* **99**, 244-269.

Hugelin, A., and Dumont, S. (1961). Intégrations motrices et vigilance chez l'encéphale isolé. I. Inhibition réticulaire du réflexe d'ouverture de la gueule. *Arch. Ital. Biol.* **99**, 219-243.

Prescott, J. W. (1967). Invited commentary. *In* "Psychological Stress" (M. H. Appley and R. Trumbull, eds.), pp. 113-120. Appleton, New York.

Prescott, J. W. (1970). A developmental psychophysiological theory of autistic-depressive and violent-aggressive behaviors. *Psychophysiology* **6**, 628-629 (abstr.).

Prescott, J. W. (1971). Early somatosensory deprivation as an ontogenetic process in the abnormal development of the brain and behavior. *In* "Medical Primatology" (I. E. Goldsmith and J. Moor-Jankowski, eds.), Karger, Basel (in press).

Scherrer, J., and Fourment, A. (1964). Electrocortical effects of sensory deprivation during development. *In* "The Developing Brain" (W. A. Himwich and H. E. Himwich, eds.), pp. 103-112. Elsevier, Amsterdam.

14

Patterns of Reflex Behavior
Related to Sleep in the Human Infant*

H. F. R. Prechtl

The relationship between behavioral state and responses to sensory stimulation has been approached in three different ways.

1. Reflexes and responses were found to vary with changes in state, such as wakefulness and sleep.

2. Response intensities have been used as an indicator of depth of sleep and of the level of arousal, respectively.

3. Control of state was introduced in the reflex and response examination for standardization of the procedure.

For a long time it was generally agreed that reflexes and responses to sensory stimulation vary inconsistently when studied in young infants. This unpredictable behavior of the infant prevented, until recently, the introduction of a clinical neurological examination technique for early detection of brain damage.

*My thanks to Dr. Akiyama for his kind help in the preparation of the manuscript.

Research has focused on the infant's capacity to respond to various stimuli rather than on systematic changes of the response intensity in relation to changes in the state of the organism.

This situation has drastically changed in the last 10 years due to the awareness of the importance of state. Simultaneously, with the advent of the new interest in sleep, the apparent state dependency of many responses has been explored. The practical application of this cognizance led to a standardized neurological examination method (Prechtl and Beintema, 1964) in which tests have to be carried out in an optimal state for each particular response. While here the state was used as an aid to study responses, in a new series of investigations responses were used to explore state. In order to understand better the physiological properties and the neurological organization of states a systematic investigation of this problem was carried out in a series of studies which will be reported here.

THE DEFINITION OF STATE

Whenever behavior is categorized into states, this is subjective and arbitrary because it is based on intuition and experience. Depending on the choice of the indicators used as criteria a variety of scales of categories have been designed. The EEG as a criterion led to the distinction between slow wave sleep (SWS) and low-amplitude high-frequency sleep, the observation of rapid eye movements (REM) has led to the distinction of REM sleep (REMS) and non-REM sleep (NREMS), the regularity vs irregularity of the respiration led to the distinction between regular sleep and irregular sleep. Often a continuum of this scale of states was implied saying that in the cat, REMS is deep sleep while SWS has been considered as light sleep. The reverse order, however, was implied by investigators working with humans. In order to avoid such problems of interpretation behavioral states can be considered as qualitatively different, distinct, and mutually exclusive conditions of the organism or the nervous sytem. Easily observable variables, such as regularity of respiration, opening or closing of the eyes, movements of head and limbs, and vocalization were selected as criteria to design a five-point scale (Prechtl and Beintema, 1964).

> State 1: regular respiration, eyes closed, no movements.
> State 2: irregular respiration, eyes closed, small movements.
> State 3: eyes open, alert but inactive.
> State 4: eyes open, gross movements, no crying.
> State 5: eyes open or closed, active and crying.

These states are expressions of the condition of an overall neural activity. What we can observe are a number of phenomena which are employed as indicators. The nervous system is treated as a black box. Since the behavioral states change from one to another in an organized way, programming of the sequence of states

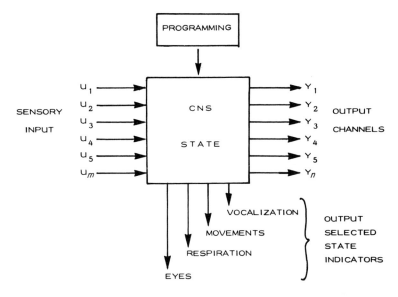

Fig. 1. Schematic diagram of input-output channels of the central nervous system, the hypothetical programming system for state and the selected output variables, which are employed as indicators of state.

must be assumed. We do not know whether this "programmer" is inside or outside the nervous system. However, a consequence of this model is the assumption that the input-output relation of the black box will be altered by changes in the state. Schematically, this is illustrated in Fig. 1.

STATEMENT OF THE PROBLEM

According to the model shown in Fig. 1, the intensity in the output channels y_1 through y_n will be determined by the ongoing state whenever the corresponding input channels are stimulated. Although the state itself is determined by a programming system, there is also a modification of the state possible through the input channels. There are a number of stimuli which may disrupt a steady state, but this is commonly shortlasting.

By exploring systematically the infant's responsiveness to stimulation through various input channels (that is, sensory modalities), we can obtain clues about the neural organization in the different states. While the state is continuously monitored by polygraphic recordings, stimuli are presented in more or less regular intervals of suitable length and the responses assessed from the record or by observation.

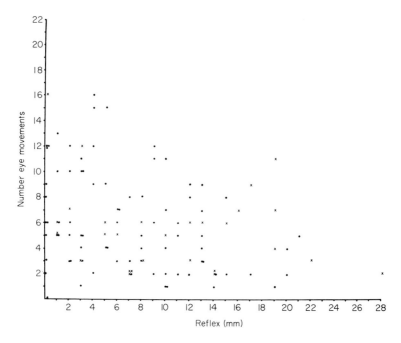

Fig. 2. Correlation between number of eye movements—counted from 10 sec before to 10 sec after stimulation—and size of lip-jerk reflex in millimeters of pen deflection of EMG. Dots represent responses consisting of lip-jerk only, crosses, lip-jerk followed by lip-protrusion reflex (r = −0.69). (From Prechtl *et al.*, 1967a. Courtesy of Springer Verlag.)

PROPRIOCEPTIVE AND VESTIBULAR REFLEXES

In the quiet awake baby (state 3) the phasic muscle stretch reflexes (tendon reflexes) are well expressed, but they are not clonic. As soon as the infant falls asleep and enters a state 2 (irregular sleep), these reflexes become tonically depressed (knee jerk, biceps jerk, lip tap reflex). Simultaneously, with the occurrence of many REM, the reflexes are phasically abolished (there exists a negative correlation between the number of eye movements and the size of the EMG discharge associated with the reflex (Prechtl and Lenard, 1967) (Fig. 2). In contrast to the diminution of these reflexes during state 2, they are enhanced in state 1 (regular sleep). Not only is their size increased, but there is also a tendency to clonic discharge (Prechtl *et al.*, 1967a, b). Ankle clonus, sometimes sustained, is also found during state 1, but is absent in other states in normal newborns (Lenard *et al.*, 1968).

The tonic myotatic reflex, for example, elicited by slow stretching of the tibial anterior muscle (plantar flexion of the foot) is also consistently present in awake and quiet newborns (Fig. 3). In striking contrast to the phasic stretch reflex, the tonic stretch reflex is nearly abolished in state 1 (absent in 82%) and weak (absent in 61%) in state 2 (Vlach *et al.*, 1972).

The third type of proprioceptive responses which should be mentioned here is the Moro response. There are two ways of eliciting this response: the one is to lower the baby's head abruptly while the trunk is supported, and the second is to tap the surface on which the baby is lying near the baby's head. The response consists in both cases of a rapid extension and abduction of the arms. The receptors involved are the vestibuli or the neck joint receptors or both.

In the awake baby the response is consistently elicitable, and also during state 1 (Fig. 4). In state 2, however, the Moro response fails to occur in 60%, or is markedly diminished in amplitude, and its latency is about three times longer than during state 1 (Lenard *et al.*, 1968; von Bernuth, 1972). There is no difference between the head-drop Moro and the elicitation by tap in respect to their state dependency.

As a further example, we have studied the input-output relation of the vestibuloocular reflex (von Bernuth and Prechtl, 1969). If an infant is stimulated by side-to-side rocking along his longitudinal axis, the eyes move compensatory to the movement of the head in the opposite direction. This has also been called the doll's eye phenomenon. Again, this response is best expressed in the awake state. It is nearly fully depressed in state 1 but, surprisingly, well expressed during state 2. REM, when they occur, are superimposed on the oscillating eye movements (Fig. 5).

None of the mentioned proprioceptive and vestibular stimuli show any noticeable effect on the duration of the behavioral states, when the duration of the states with and without stimulation are compared in the same infant.

EXTEROCEPTIVE SKIN REFLEXES

A large number of different stimuli to the skin have been applied, such as touch, mild pressure, and mild scratch. The responses are always tonic in nature, have a gradual onset, and outlast the stimulus. However, their pattern of dependency of state is different and can be classified into three groups.

(1) The rooting response, elicited by tactile stimulation of the perioral region is absent in both sleep states and can only be evoked in states 3 and 4 (Prechtl, 1958; Lenard *et al.*, 1968).

(2) The next group consists of all those responses which are absent in state 1, of weak or moderate intensity in state 2, and clearly expressed in state 3. To them belong the palmar and plantar grasp reflex, the Babkin reflex, the palmomental reflex, and all those which can be elicited by gently stroking the skin above a certain muscle, such as the finger, toe, tibial (Fig. 6), fibular, axillary, and lip protrusion reflexes (Vlach *et al.*, 1969; Prechtl *et al.*, 1967a, b).

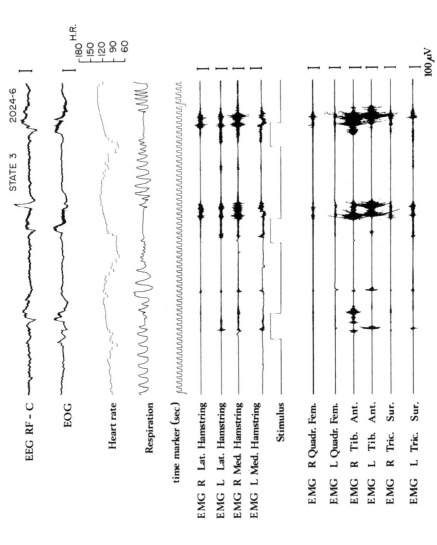

Fig. 3. Polygram of 6-day-old newborn with bilateral elicitation of tonic myotatic reflex in the tibial anterior muscles by plantar flexion of the feet. Awake state.

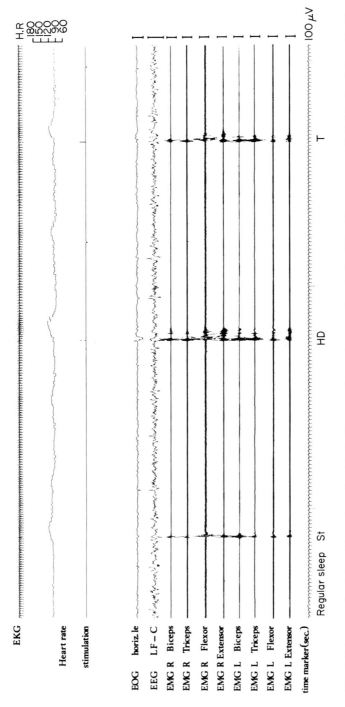

Fig. 4 Polygram of a 5-day-old newborn in state 1. St. = spontaneously occurring startle; HD = Moro response elicited by head drop; T = Moro response elicited by tap on the surface. Note difference between startle and Moro response, the first without tonic after discharge. (From von Bernuth, 1972.)

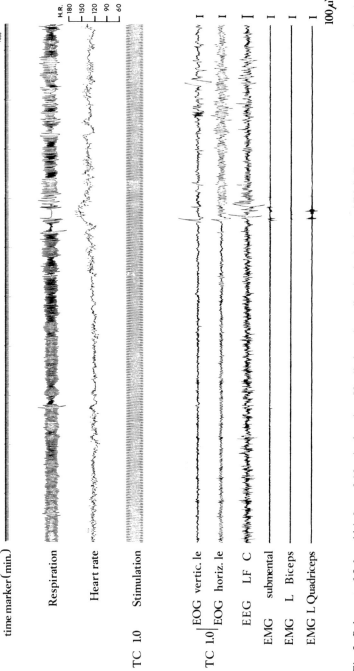

Fig. 5. Polygram of 8-day-old infant of 10 min duration. Vestibuloocular reflex in the horizontal EOG. Transition of state 1 into state 2 indicated by movement (EMG activity), the response is suddenly increased. Time marker in seconds and large downward deflection in minutes. Stimulus was 38° rocking over longitudinal axis and at a rate of 0.75/sec. (From von Bernuth and Prechtl, 1969. Courtesy of Hippokrates Verlag GMBH.)

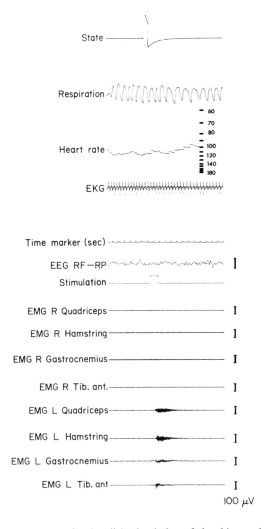

Fig. 6. Response to exteroceptive (tactile) stimulation of the skin overlying the front of the left ankle joint. Tonic activity occurs in the stimulated leg. (From Prechtl *et al.*, 1967b. Courtesy of S. Karger; Basel, New York.)

(3) Reflexes which did not show any state dependency but are equally present in all states. To this group belong the Babinski, abdominal skin, thigh, pubic, and inguinal reflexes. All of them are nociceptive in nature, and all of them disturb the steady pattern of state 1, frequently eliciting a startle. Wolff (1966), applying a tickling stimulus to the nasolabial fold, found no difference in the responses in relation to state.

ACOUSTIC ORIENTING RESPONSE

Movements elicited by a presentation of a tone (square waves of 125 and 250 Hz have been found to be most effective) (Hutt *et al.*, 1968a) of about 25 dB above ambient noise level, can be considered as an important component of the orienting response. They were most pronounced in the awake infant (Fig. 7), somewhat diminished during state 2, and markedly depressed in state 1 (Hutt *et al.*, 1968b). Similar findings were obtained by Wolff (1966) and Korner (1968). Thus, the auditory input-output relation behaves similarly to the vestibulo-ocular response.

DISCUSSION

The purpose of our investigations of the input-output relations in the different states was to investigate the functional organization of the nervous system in the various behavioral states. Our previous studies on unstimulated infants, recorded polygraphically for many hours, served as baseline data for comparison with the results in the stimulated infants (Prechtl, 1968; Prechtl *et al.*, 1968, 1969). As mentioned before, different sensory modalities showed distinct and state-specific input-output relations, which are summarized in Table I.

In state 1, the vestibuloocular reflex and the tonic myotatic reflex, all exteroceptive skin reflexes in which tactile and pressure receptors are involved, as well as the auditory orienting response are clearly diminished or abolished. In striking contrast to these responses, all monosynaptic phasic stretch reflexes (tendon reflexes) and, surprisingly, also the Moro-responses are enhanced and often even more brisk than in the awake state. None of the stimuli and responses have any lasting effect on the state.

It is not clear whether the increase of the reflexes is due to a depolarizing pressure on the spinal α neurons or to γ_1 driving, which makes the primary spindle endings especially sensitive to sudden stretch. Since an infant in state 1 has tonic activity in the submental and limb muscles, α and γ_1 neurons may be active. The secondary endings of the muscle spindle seem to be inactive because the tonic myotatic response is absent.

The Moro response, again a phasic phenomenon, is present. The vibration-sensitive components of the labyrinths localized in the utriculus and sacculus are very likely the receptors for the elicitation of the Moro response. Despite the gross motor output, the elicitation of the Moro response does not disturb the ongoing state 1.

Findings obtained from adult cats (Pompeiano, 1967a, b; Baldissera *et al.*, 1966; Kubota *et al.*, 1965) showed a similar relationship as far as the monosynaptic spinal reflexes are concerned, although a decrease of 15% was found in the amplitude in relation to the awake state, but no increase as in the

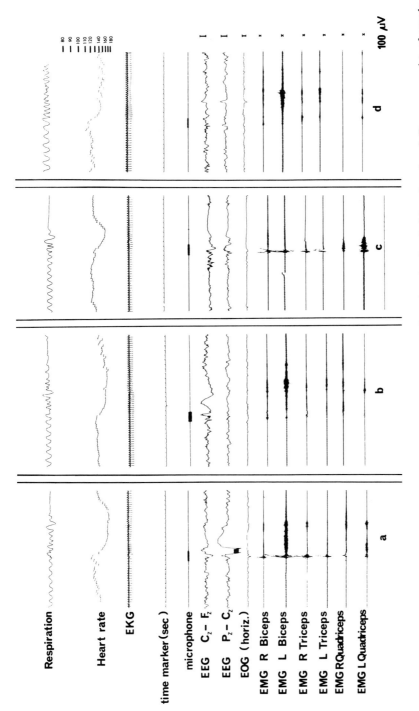

Fig. 7. Elicitation of the auditory orienting response by sound stimulation of 2 sec duration (marked by microphone). Response consists of muscle activity, tachycardia, irregularity of respiration, and sometimes eye movements. (From Hutt *et al.*, 1968b).

TABLE 1 *Effects of State on the Intensity of Responses to Sensory Stimulation in Different Modalities*

	State 1	State 2	State 3
Proprioceptive reflexes			
Knee jerk	+++	±	++
Biceps jerk	+++	±	++
Lip jerk	+++	±	++
Ankle clonus	+++	−	−
Moro tap	+++	−	++
Moro head drop	+++	−	++
Vestibuloocular	−	++	+++
Tonic myotatic	−	++	+++
Exteroceptive skin reflexes			
Tactile			
Rooting	−	−	++
Palmar grasp	−	+	++
Plantar grasp	−	++	++
Lip protrusion	−	+++	++
Finger reflex	−	+	++
Toe reflex	−	++	++
Tibial reflex	±	++	++
Fibular reflex	±	++	++
Axillary reflex	±	++	++
Pressure			
Babkin	−	+	++
Palmomental	−	++	++
Nociceptive			
Babinski reflex	++	+++	+++
Abdominal reflex	++	+++	+++
Thigh	++	+++	+++
Pubic	++	+++	+++
Inguinal	+++	+++	+++
Auditory response			
Auditory orienting	±	++	+++

infant. The stimulation of the primary spindle afferents (1a) did not have an arousing effect on the EEG (Pompeiano and Swett, 1962). The same is found for stimulation of the VIIIth nerve by electric pulses (Lenzi et al., 1968). It is still completely unknown how the Golgi afferents behave in state 1. If they were depressed, the α neurons may be released from their inhibitory influence. However, there could be also a tonic facilitating barrage from supraspinal structures on the α and γ neurons. A strong γ control of the intercostal muscles and the diaphragm is also in favor with regularity of the respiration found in state 1.

Although the baby has a spontaneous and steady tonic activity in muscles (antigravity?), only phasic phenomena can be easily elicited. All tonic responses are diminished with the exception of nociceptive reflexes. This seems to be in contradiction with findings in the adult cat, in which polysynaptic skin reflexes are only slightly depressed in the comparable state (Pompeiano, 1967a). This also holds true for the tonic eye deviation following (electrical) stimulation of the vestibular nerve (Hodes and Suzuki, 1965), while in the infant the vestibuloocular reflex is diminished.

Strikingly different from the conditions in state 1 is the pattern found in state 2. As soon as the respiration of the infant becomes irregular, even before REM occur and the EEG flattens, the tendon reflexes disappear and so does the Moro response. If many REM occur, both reflexes are abolished for a short time. On the other hand, polysynaptic skin reflexes, the tonic myotatic reflex, the auditory orienting response, and the vestibuloocular response can be elicited. A relationship to the occurrence of REM is not found.

The tendon reflexes of the baby behave in the same manner as in the adult cat (Pompeiano, 1967a, b; Baldissera *et al.*, 1966). There seems to be a tonic postsynaptic inhibition of the α neurons and, additionally, a phasic presynaptic inhibition of the Ia afferents during REM. Evidence for a postsynaptic inhibition can be drawn from the studies on the H reflex, which diminishes or disappears during REMS in the human newborn (Mayer and Mosser, 1969) as well as in adults (Hodes and Dement, 1964). In the cat, a presynaptic inhibition was also found for the trigeminal afferents, in the nucleus cuneatus, and in the lateral geniculate body (Pompeiano, 1967b), and the role of the vestibular nuclei in this phenomenon was demonstrated. It may very well be that these inhibitory mechanisms are not yet operational in the infant. As long as we do not yet know how the reflexes in human adults behave during REMS the possibility of species differences should still be considered.

More recently, the effect of the activity of the vestibular nuclei on the autonomic system has been demonstrated (Morrison and Pompeiano, 1970). The phasic increase in heart rate during REM bursts in the cat is abolished after bilateral destruction of the medial descending part of the vestibular nuclei. In the infant, we found the occurrence of REM connected with an increased respiratory irregularity and rate, but this was less so in the heart rate (Prechtl and Lenard, 1967). It seems very likely that the firing of the vestibular nuclear cells, generating the REM, impinge also on the medullary respiratory "center" and on the hypothalamus.

It has also been shown, that the twitches in REMS are linked with REM, probably via activity in the corticospinal system, which is mediated from the vestibular nuclei (Morrison and Pompeiano, 1966). A temporal coincidence of REM and the twitches in the distal limb musculature is also observed in the baby (Prechtl and Lenard, 1967).

A very important question, which has not yet been raised so far by the Italian group, is, how the irregular firing of the medial vestibular nuclei in REMS is brought about. Perhaps a possible link to the biochemical changes, characteristic for the two sleep states, should be explored.

So far, only two responses have been shown to be absent in both sleep states. In the infant, rooting to tactile stimulation in the perioral region can only be elicited during wakefulness. In the adult, optokinetic nystagmus disappears during sleep (the eyes are artificially kept open) (Gardner and Weitzman, 1967).

The puzzling problem remains of why a variety of responses have such different input-output relations in state 2 in the adult cat as compared to those in the baby. It is still unknown whether this is due to developmental differences or to dissimilarities in species. Studies in the adult human and in the newborn kitten may help to answer this question.

REFERENCES

Baldissera, F., Broggi, G., and Mancia, M. (1966). Monosynaptic and polysynaptic spinal reflexes during physiological sleep and wakefulness. *Arch. Ital. Biol.* **104**, 112-133.

Gardner, R., and Weitzman, E. D. (1967). Examination for optokinetic nystagmus in sleep and waking. *Arch. Neurol.* **16**, 415-420.

Hodes, R., and Dement, W. C. (1964). Depression of electrically induced reflexes ("H-reflexes") in man during low voltage EEG sleep. *Electroencephalogr. Clin. Neurophysiol.* **17**, 617-629.

Hodes, R., and Suzuki, J. I. (1965). Comparative thresholds of cortex, vestibular system and reticular formation in wakefulness, sleep and rapid eye movement periods. *Electroencephalogr. Clin. Neurophysiol.* **18**, 239-248.

Hutt, C., von Bernuth, H., Lenard, H. G., Hutt, S. J., and Prechtl, H. F. R. (1968a). Habituation in relation to state in the human neonate. *Nature (London)* **220**, 618-620.

Hutt, S. J., Hutt, C., Lenard, H. G., von Bernuth, H., and Muntjewerff, W. F. (1968b). Auditory responsivity in the human neonate. *Nature (London)* **218**, 888-890.

Korner, A. F. (1968). REM organization in neonates. *Arch. Gen. Psychiat.* **19**, 330-340.

Kubota, K., Iwamura, Y., and Niimi, Y. (1965). Monosynaptic reflex and natural sleep in the cat. *J. Neurophysiol.* **28**, 125-138.

Lenard, H. G., von Bernuth, H., and Prechtl, H. F. R. (1968). Reflexes and their relationships to behavioural state in the newborn. *Acta Paediat. Scand.* **3**, 177-185.

Lenzi, G. L., Pompeiano, O., and Satoh, T. (1968). Input-output relation of the vestibular system during sleep and wakefulness. *Pfluegers Arch. Gesamte Physiol. Menschen Tiere,* **299**, 326-333.

Mayer, R. F., and Mosser, R. S. (1969). Excitability of motoneurons in infants. *Neurology* **19**, 932-945.

Morrison, A. R., and Pompeiano, O. (1966). Vestibular influences during sleep. II. Effects of vestibular lesions on the pyramidal discharge during desynchronized sleep. *Arch. Ital. Biol.* **104**, 214-230.

Morrison, A. R., and Pompeiano, O. (1970). Vestibular influences during sleep. VI. Vestibular control of autonomic functions during the rapid eye movements of desynchronized sleep. *Arch. Ital. Biol.* **108**, 154-180.

Pompeiano, O. (1967a). The neurophysiological mechanisms of the postural and motor events during desynchronized sleep. *In* "Sleep and Altered States of Consciousness" (S. S. Kety, E. V. Evarts, and H. L. Williams, eds.), pp. 351-423. Williams & Wilkins, Baltimore, Maryland.

Pompeiano, O. (1967b). Sensory inhibition during motor activity in sleep. *In* "Neurophysiological Basis of Normal and Abnormal Motor Activities" (M. D. Yahr and D. P. Purpura, eds.), pp. 323-378. Raven Press, New York.

Pompeiano, O., and Swett, J. E. (1962). Identification of cutaneous and muscular afferent fibers producing EEG synchronization or arousal in normal cats. *Arch. Ital. Biol.* **100**, 343-380.

Prechtl, H. F. R. (1958). The directed head turning response and allied movements of the human baby. *Behaviour* **13**, 212-242.

Prechtl, H. F. R. (1968). Polygraphic studies of the full-term newborn infant. II. Computer analysis of recorded data. *In* "Studies in Infancy" (M. C. Bax and R. C. MacKeith, eds.), pp. 22-40. Heinemann, London.

Prechtl, H. F. R., and Beintema, D. J. (1964). "The Neurological Examination of the Full-term Newborn Infant, Clinics in Developmental Medicine No. 12." Heineman, London.

Prechtl, H. F. R., and Lenard, H. G. (1967). A study of eye movements in sleeping newborn infants. *Brain Res.* **5**, 477-493.

Prechtl, H. F. R., Kerr Grant, D., Lenard, H. G., and Hrbek, A. (1967a). The lip-tap reflex in the awake and sleeping newborn infant. A polygraphic study. *Exp. Brain Res.* **3**, 184-194.

Prechtl, H. F. R., Vlach, V., Lenard, H. G., and Kerr Grant, D. (1967b). Exteroceptive and tendon reflexes in various behavioural states in the newborn infant. *Biol. Neonatorum* **11**, 159-175.

Prechtl, H. F. R., Akiyama, Y., Zinkin, P., and Kerr Grant, D. (1968). Polygraphic studies of the full-term newborn infant. I. Technical aspects and qualitative analysis. *In* "Studies in Infancy" (M. C. Bax and R. C. MacKeith, eds.), pp. 1-21. Heinemann, London.

Prechtl, H. F. R., Weinmann, H., and Akiyama, Y. (1969). Organization of physiological parameters in normal and neurologically abnormal infants: comprehensive computer analysis of polygraphic data. *Neuropaediatrie* **1**, 101-129.

Vlach, V., von Bernuth, H., and Prechtl, H. F. R. (1969). State dependency of exteroceptive skin reflexes in newborn infants. *Develop. Med. Child Neurol.* **11**, 353-362.

Vlach, V., Akiyama, Y., Casaer, P., and Prechtl, H. F. R. (1972). State dependency of a tonic myotatic reflex in the newborn (in press).

von Bernuth, H. (1972). Investigations on the Moro response in the neonate (in press).

von Bernuth, H., and Prechtl, H. F. R. (1969). Vestibulo-ocular response and its state dependency in newborn infants. *Neuropaediatrie* **1**, 11-24.

Wolff, P. H. (1966). The causes, controls and organizations of behavior in the neonate. *Psychol. Issues* **5**, (Monogr. 17), 1-105.

INVITED DISCUSSION: F. J. SCHULTE

Excitation and Inhibition in Spinal Motoneurons of Preterm and Full-Term Newborn Infants

The simplest test of synaptic transmission in the infantile spinal cord is the monosynaptic stretch reflex elicited by a tendon tap or an electrical stimulus to the sensorimotor nerve. In all infants tested from 25 weeks conceptional age up to term we never failed to evoke the monosynaptic reflex muscle action potential, although in some preterm infants the corresponding muscle contraction could not be seen. Its absence might have been due either to a low degree of synchronization of spinal motoneurons, or to a lack of muscle power, or both. In the youngest preterm infant of 25 weeks conceptional age, the low degree of motoneuron synchronization could be demonstrated electromyographically. The bioelectric reflex muscle activity evoked by a tendon tap consisted of a short train of impulses rather than of one compound muscle action potential as normally seen in older infants, children, and adults (Fig. 8). Various reasons could account for this asynchronization.

1. A wide variation of a comparatively low impulse conduction velocity in afferent and efferent nerve fibers would result in asynchronous activation of both spinal motoneurons and muscle fibers.

2. It is reasonable to assume that in very immature preterm infants the muscle stretch receptor activity evoked by a tendon tap is monosynaptically transmitted only to some spinal motoneurons and that, in addition, other motoneurons are activated after polysynaptic delays. Such a buildup of motoneuron depolarization pressure in excitatory spinal interneurons is by no means restricted to very immature preterm infants. However, in adults, both human and animal, the first synchronous reflex burst of spinal motoneurons creates strong inhibitory influences on themselves and on surrounding motoneurons, thus eliminating the possibility of immediate repetitive firing.

In older infants, children, and adults, nerve cell inhibition following the discharge of spinal motoneurons is guaranteed by several mechanisms (Fig. 9).

1. Each spike potential is followed by membrane hyperpolarization, due to a postexcitatory increase of membrane permeability to potassium. This membrane potential shift is called positive after-potential.

2. Each motoneuron action potential, before leaving the grey matter of the spinal cord, activates interneurons, called Renshaw cells, which in turn inhibit the surrounding motoneurons. This pathway represents an intraspinal inhibitory feedback mechanism.

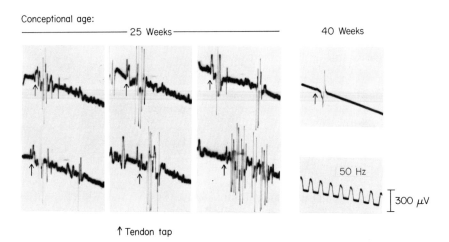

T Reflex (gastrocnemius)

Conceptional age:
——————————————— 25 Weeks ——————————————— 40 Weeks

↑ Tendon tap

Fig. 8. The monosynaptic stretch reflex elicited by a tendon tap in a preterm infant of 25 weeks conceptional age. (From Schulte *et al.*, 1969.)

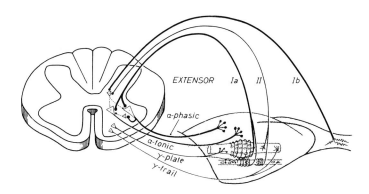

Fig. 9. Important pathways in the spinal motor system for extensor muscles. (–) Excitatory connections; (– –) inhibitory connections; α-phasic: phasic α-motoneurons activate the skeletal muscles and generally cause fast movements by means of short bursts of action potentials; α-tonic: tonic α-motoneurons which activate the skeletal muscle for longer periods of contraction by means of a series of repetitive action potentials (while still within the gray matter, axon collaterals of the α-motoneurons activate Renshaw cells which act as inhibitors on the α-motoneurons; γ plate, γ trail: fusimotoneurons innervating muscle fibers within the muscle spindles (intrafusal muscle fibers). Ia, II, Ib: Sensory afferent nerve fibers of muscle receptors activated by stretch. Ia: Primary sensory muscle spindle ending of spiral formation located in the equatorial zone of the intrafusal muscle fibers. The impulses of these nerve fibers activate the motoneurons of the same muscle monosynaptically. II: Secondary sensory muscle spindle endings of spiral or semispiral formations. The impulses of the secondary muscle spindle fibers via interneurons activate the motoneurons of flexors but inhibit the motoneurons of extensors. Ib: Sensory nerve fibers from Golgi tendon organs which inhibit the motoneurons of the same muscle via interneurons. (From Schulte, 1968.)

3. The reflex muscle twitch activates Golgi tendon organs, the afferent impulses of which inhibit spinal motoneurons via interneurons. This pathway represents a musculospinal inhibitory feedback mechanism.

4. Muscle spindle afferents are silenced by the reflex shortening of the muscle, thus part of the continuous afferent drive of spinal motoneurons from peripheral sources is eliminated for the short time while the muscle is contracting.

The sum of spinal inhibitory mechanisms, activated by a synchronous burst of motoneuron discharges, can be demonstrated electromyographically. Each reflex compound action potential is followed by the *Innervationsstille* (Hoffman, 1922, 1934) or silent period in the ongoing background activity (Fig. 10). In newborn infants, as well as in adults, the duration of this silent period depends on the amount of background activity, that is, the supraspinal depolarization pressure on spinal motoneurons (Schulte and Schwenzel, 1965). The duration of the silent period decreases with increasing background activity: this shows that spinal inhibitory mechanisms can, in part, be outweighed by supraspinal excitatory drive (Paillard, 1955). The duration of the silent period—measuring the amount of inhibitory influences on spinal motoneurons subsequent to the monosynaptic stretch reflex—increases with conceptional age (Fig. 11). However, the minimum duration of the silent period after the monosynaptic reflex during the strongest supraspinal motoneuron excitation is almost equally maintained through all ages, including immature preterm infants. This result is consistent with the hypothesis that a minimum of postexcitatory

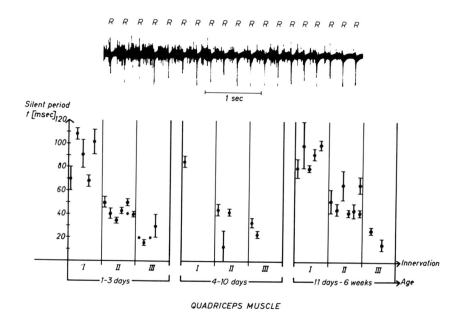

Fig. 10. Each reflex action potential evoked by tendon tap is followed by a silent period, the duration of which decreases with increasing background activity, the amount of which is indicated by I-III: I (weak), sparse activity, only single-action potentials; II (moderate), background activity with one action potential immediately followed and sometimes even superimposed by another; III (strong), maximum activity with the action potentials superimposed on each other. The silent period is measured from the end of the reflex action potential to the recurrence of the background activity. Possible age-dependent changes in the duration of the silent period were not statistically evaluated for the time after birth at term. (From Joppich and Schulte, 1968.)

inhibition, possibly due to basic membrane phenomena, is well developed in preterm infants of 30 weeks conceptional age. However, surplus inhibition, due to more complex computational synaptic mechanisms in the spinal cord, proceeds with conceptional age.

REFERENCES

Hoffman, P. (1922). "Untersuchungen über Eigenreflexe (Sehnenreflexe) Menschlicher Muskeln." Springer-Verlag, Berlin and New York.
Hoffman, P. (1934). Die physiologischen eigenschaften der eigenreflexe. _Ergeb. Physiol. Exp. Pharmakol._ **36**, 15-108.
Joppich, G., and Schulte, F. J. (1968). "Neurologie des Neugeborenen." Springer-Verlag, Berlin and New York.
Paillard, J. (1955). "Réflexes et régulations d'origine proprioceptive chez l'homme." Arnette, Paris.
Schulte, F. J. (1968). Die elektromyographie. _In_ "Neurochirurgie des Gehirns und Rückenmarks im Kindes- und Jugendalter" (K. A. Bushe and P. Glees, eds.), pp. 170-191. Hippokrates Verlag, Stuttgart.

Schulte, F. J., and Schwenzel, W. (1965). Motor control and muscle tone in the newborn period. Electromyographic studies. *Biol. Neonatorum* 8, 198-215.

Schulte, F. J., Linke, I., Michaelis, R., and Nolte, R. (1969). Excitation, inhibition and impulse conduction in spinal motoneurones of preterm, term and small-for-dates newborn infants. *In* "Brain and Early Behaviour: Development in the Fetus and Infant" (R. Robinson, ed.), pp. 87-114. Academic Press, New York.

INVITED DISCUSSION: ELLIOT D. WEITZMAN

I would like to show some of our own results which relate to a number of studies in this volume. This work was done in collaboration with Dr. Leonard Graziani (Weitzman and Graziani, 1968). The first few figures will demonstrate the EEG patterns and some autonomic measurements recorded in a premature infant. Figure 12 shows a 28.5-week postconceptional age (PCA) infant. Recording is made monopolar on the scalp with the ears as reference. The flat EEG periods alternate with intermittent burst activity.

Figure 13 shows an older infant, in which, by 36 weeks one can begin to differentiate between the intermittent burst EEG pattern similar to that which was present at a younger age and a more continuous EEG activity, irregularity of respiration and eye movements.

Figure 14 is an older infant, about term. Again, during the quiet sleep phase, there is the alternating type EEG activity, whereas during the active sleep phase the EEG is lower voltage and more homogeneous in its activity. There are periods of irregular respiration, eye movements, and arm and leg movements. As quiet sleep increases with decreasing frequency of body movements, this is associated with an EEG pattern similar to the EEG pattern present in the younger infant when there are many muscular movements.

We obtained evoked responses during these maturation periods. We used a speaker placed above the head of the infant in an isolette with a maximum impact noise of approximately 113 dB. If one measured with a noise analyzer, it was approximately 95 dB.

If we measure impact noise in the incubator in a full-term infant with a lusty cry, the value will, on occasion, go up to 120 dB. So, an infant's own cry measured by peak impact noise can be as high, if not higher, than the stimulus we have applied.

Figure 15 shows some of the responses obtained on a 25- and 26-week PCA infant. We recorded the response from 10 electrode positions on the scalp and found that the earliest clear response was a large negative wave occurring widely from all areas. In some cases, the lateral response was larger than the vertex and anterior scalp response. A large positive response frequently followed the negative wave with a latency going out to 1 sec and longer.

As maturation continued (Fig. 16), one could see the differentiation of this negative response—the latency became shorter for the posterior midline electrodes as compared to the anterior ones.

Figure 17 shows the sequence of evoked response events in which one can see a shift of the latency in the midline electrodes, especially at the vertex region without a shift of latency in the more lateral regions. In addition, an earlier positive response is present, particularly in the more frontal midline region. The more anterior electrode had a lower amplitude response than the most posterior responses in the lateral area.

The reference electrodes were applied to both ears. The negativity or positivity of the response is as recorded at the electrode site on the scalp.

Figure 18 shows the similarity of pattern we obtained on identical twins. The first recording was made at 31½ weeks and then every 2 weeks to the time the infants left the premature unit and then 5 weeks and 4½ months later. These were all taken during a quiet sleep period or a sleep period in which there was high voltage or slow wave intermittent

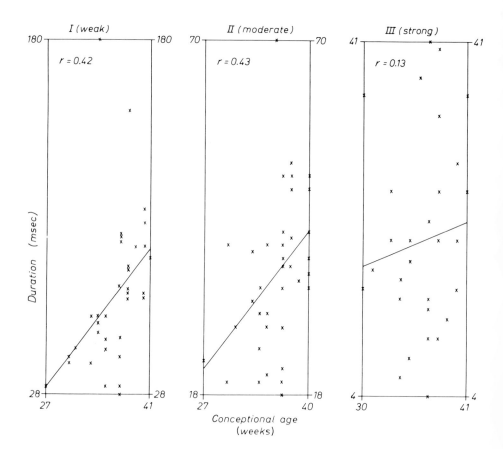

Fig. 11. The duration of the postreflex silent period, being dependent upon background muscle activity (weak, moderate, strong), increases slightly with conceptional age, the Pearson correlation coefficient (r) being 0.42 during weak, 0.43 during moderate, and 0.13 during strong, background activity. However, the duration of the silent period subsequent to a monosynaptic reflex elicited during strong muscle (quadriceps) contraction shows only slight variation with age. (From Schulte *et al.,* 1969.)

burst pattern, and I particularly chose responses which were similar in appearance to show the degree of similarity that can be present. One infant was recorded the day before the other.

Figure 19 shows the presence of a muscle response to the click. When we changed the analysis length to 125 msec, we found a consistent response very early, at approximately 15 msec. This response was augmented when the baby was awake and crying, disappeared, or was barely detectable, during quiet sleep periods, and was intermediate in amplitude during an active sleep phase. We concluded that the ear electrode was the source of this early response and was probably a muscle response to the auditory stimulus.

Figure 20 is a composite summary of all the latency data from all the babies of all the components of the responses. We found a progressive decrease in latency for wave N-1 and

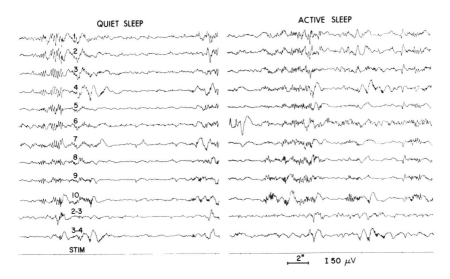

Fig. 12. Examples of EEG activity obtained from a 1010-g premature infant at 28.5 weeks (PCA).

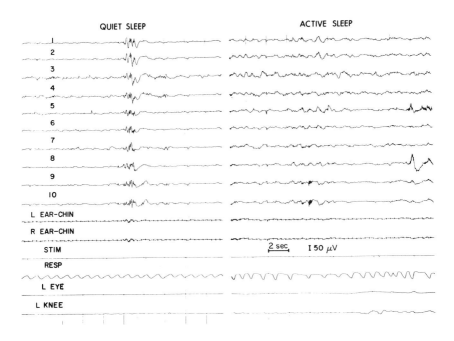

Fig. 13. Examples of EEG activity obtained from a 1730-g infant at 36 weeks (PCA) for quiet and active sleep periods.

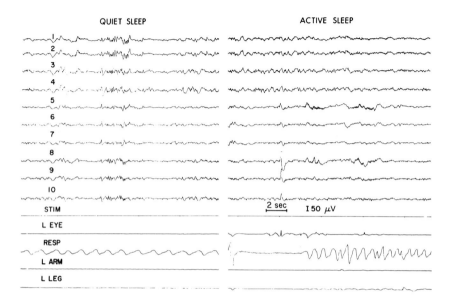

Fig. 14. Examples of EEG activity obtained from a 2010-g infant at 42 weeks (PCA) for quiet and active sleep periods.

P-2 as a function of maturation at all electrode sites. Component N-2, however, did not follow this pattern but maintained a more constant latency as a function of age. For the medial electrodes, however, a difference in latency for this N-2 wave similar to that found for the N-2 and P-2 components exists in the anteroposterior direction. However, this anteroposterior difference cannot be recognized from the lateral electrode recordings.

Our previous studies, and those of other investigators, have indicated that a decrease in latency of certain components of the auditory evoked response (AER) occurs during REMS as compared to NREMS in the adult, and active vs quiet sleep in the full-term infant. We have extended this method of analysis to the premature infant. The EEG record was classified during each summed evoked response period (400 sec) into one of three patterns: I (intermittent), C (continuous) or I/C. Pattern I consisted of bursts of high-voltage waves alternating with low-voltage activity. These alternations had a periodicity of 5-15 sec. Pattern C consisted of a record of low to moderate voltage activity with minimal or no evidence of the intermittent, high-voltage burst pattern. Pattern I/C was a mixture of I and C, and in most instances represented a transitional time period between the two physiological EEG states. This visual EEG classification was done without knowledge of the evoked response wave latency values. It was found that for the infants 34-35 weeks and older, this classification was possible. However, between 30 and 34 weeks, although these two EEG patterns could be recognized, the C pattern was rarely sustained for 400 sec. As indicated before, below 29 weeks, the record was almost continuously a high-voltage burst pattern.

The mean latency values of waves N-1, P-2, and N-2 only in the I and C state were compared with the mean latency values of all the evoked responses for babies 34 weeks ECA and older (Fig. 21). A consistently greater latency was found in the I state for electrodes 1, 2, 3, 4 and electrode pair 5-8 for waves N-1 and P-2 across age groups as compared with the

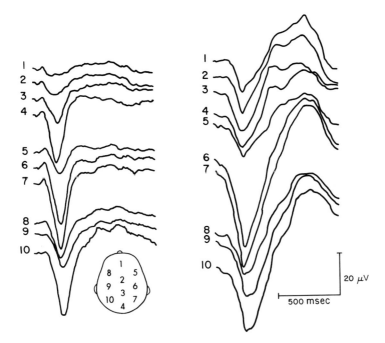

Fig. 15. Auditory evoked responses from two infants, 25 and 26 weeks (PCA) (670 and 880 g). Electrode positions are as numbered on the scalp; the reference electrodes are both ears. Negative polarity is down. Responses from each infant are obtained simultaneously by the algebraic summation of 100 clicks, each click applied every 4 sec. (From Weitzman and Graziani, 1968. Courtesy of John Wiley & Sons, Inc.)

C state. Electrode pair 6-9 did not show a consistent difference for wave N-1, but did so for P-2. However, latency values of the posterolateral electrode pair (7-10) did not show a consistent difference between I and C state for N-1 and P-2. The wave N-2 values were not consistently different for the I and C states for any of the 10 electrodes.

In summary, we found that the AER in the premature infant is a complex one. The wave patterns are a function of maturational age, a function of sleep state, a function of topography, and other factors not yet defined.

REFERENCE

Weitzman, E. D., and Graziani, L. J. (1968). Maturation and topography of the auditory evoked response of the prematurely born infant. *Develop. Psychobiol.* 1, 79-89.

GENERAL DISCUSSION

Dr. Morgane: I would take exception to Dr. Shulte's comments about myelination. Myelin is not just a sort of insulator on neural cables concomitantly associated with an increased conduction velocity in neurons. It should not, perhaps, be dismissed so casually. I would agree that synaptogenesis is more important than what is going along the axon stalk,

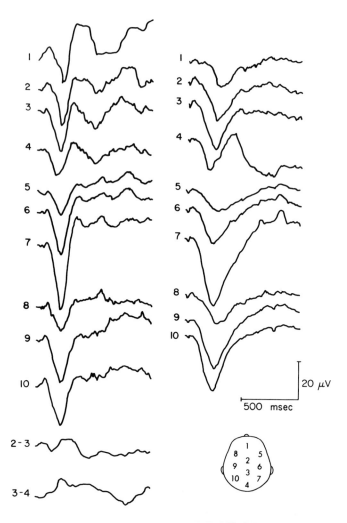

Fig. 16. Auditory evoked responses from two infants, ages 29.5 weeks (male, 1100 g) and 30 weeks (female, 1300 g). Stimulus and recording conditions as described in legend, Fig. 15.

but until more is known about myelogenesis I do not think it is "out-dated." Nevertheless, it still has its uses, since its development parallels the ontogeny of many mechanisms in the brain and is a valuable index of regional maturation correlating well with development of function in neural systems.

Dr. Purpura: Dr. Weitzman, the N-1 response over the vertex cannot be the same as the N-1 response over the lateral areas. You are calling it N-1 but it is not the same.

Dr. Weitzman: It is the same in terms of its comparative latency and shape. For the 26- to 29-week-old infant, their appearances are almost identical, and the responses are recorded

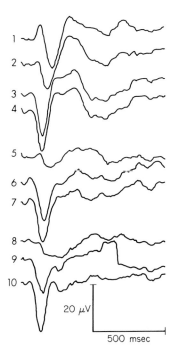

Fig. 17. Auditory evoked responses from one infant, age 37 weeks, 1940 g.

from all electrodes. As maturation occurs, the latency of the N-1 response decreases more at the vertex than laterally and anteriorly. I do not know how to interpret this, but one possibility is that there is a difference in regional cortical maturation.

Dr. Purpura: It is not going to be in the cortex. If you shift latency, it must be an entirely different response if they are differentially affected in terms of latency. If there is anything that reflects the operation of at least two different systems, it is when latency changes. This is more important than polarity reversals. If you have a latency change, that means a new pathway or a new system may be in operation.

Dr. Weitzman: Yes, there may be a new system developing. For example, there may be a different synaptic organization occurring in certain regions of the cortex, which may be dependent on other pathway innervation.

Dr. Purpura: There may be confusion in calling them both N-1 when they seem to be representing entirely different kinds of systems. Look at how much latency change is occurring in that N-1 period.

Dr. Weitzman: Quite a significant amount. Approximately 75 msec for the N-1 and P-2 waves between our midline electrode 1 and 4 at 36-38 weeks (PCA).

Dr. Purpura: The changes in latency must reflect different transit times in different subcortical-cortical projection systems. This follows from the fact that there are not very great differences in the maturational status of different cortical areas in the human neonate.

Dr. Ellingson: I do not think that anybody believes that the vertex response is a primary response mediated directly by the afferent auditory pathways. The anatomical substrate of this large vertex response remains a mystery.

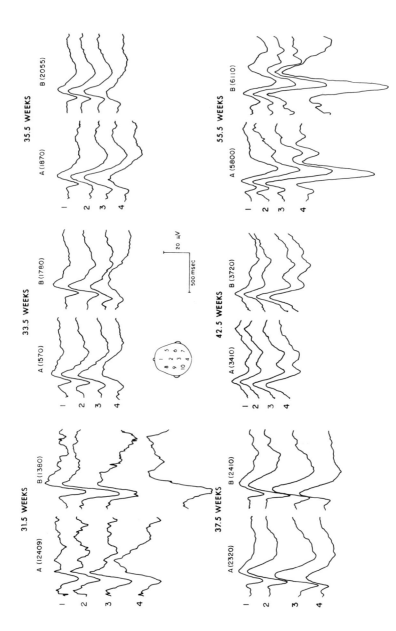

Fig. 18. Comparison of auditory evoked response patterns of a pair of identical twins (A and B) during maturation. Twin B's responses were recorded 1 day after A for each estimated conceptional age. (From Weitzman and Graziani, 1968. Courtesy of John Wiley & Sons, Inc.)

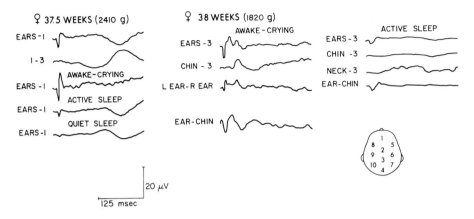

Fig. 19. Short latency evoked responses to auditory stimulation. (From Weitzman and Graziani, 1968. Courtesy of John Wiley & Sons, Inc.)

Dr. Purpura: I am objecting to saying it is like the N-1 over the somatosensory region.

Dr. Weitzman: No. N-1 is a term which arose because we had to label them, and we compared the waves to the adult pattern. If one looks at the progressive decrease in latency of N-1 it approaches fairly closely the N-1 latency wave of the adult when you record in a similar manner. We do not know what or where the generator is, of course, but in purely descriptive terms as a function of maturation one can see a continuity of this wave to the adult.

Dr. Purpura: Is there any evidence that it is in the cortex at all?

Dr. Ellingson: Not that I know of. I suspect that it is not. This is a fascinating problem. If you record from bipolar arrays of electrodes in various planes, it can be demonstrated that all phases of the response show phase reversals at, or just anterior to, the vertex. I do not know where the response originates in the brain. If someone can find out, it will be a significant contribution.

Dr. Sterman: Several years ago, Dr. Goff, Dr. Allison and I (Goff *et al.*, 1966) reported what we termed a *midline late response* at the vertex in the adult cat. It was a positive potential of about 125 msec latency that appeared over the posterior midline only during quiet sleep. At that time we were trying very hard to relate this to the human vertex response. Recently, Dr. Allison told me that he did some transcortical recordings and is now convinced that this response is not coming from cortex at all. They have ruled out the corpus callosum, so the only reasonable source is the thalamus.

Dr. Purpura: A similar problem has been encountered in the analysis of the recruiting responses. Thus, the surface negativity has a turnover in the depths of the cortex at about 1.00 mm in the cat. Below this, it is positive, but further probing of a microelectrode does not reveal attenuation of the positivity in the white matter. The positive wave is recorded all the way down to the thalamus. Unit discharges are extracellularly recorded in the period between the positive waves of the thalamically recorded recruiting responses. Finally, when a microelectrode is put inside thalamic neurons, the extracellular positive waves are found to be synchronized IPSP's. It is remarkable indeed that the IPSP's generated in large populations of thalamic neurons can be reflected all over the thalamus and thalamocortical radiations and subcortical white matter as large positive waves.

Dr. Weitzman: If we have a single dipole generator, how can there be a latency shift across scalp regions?

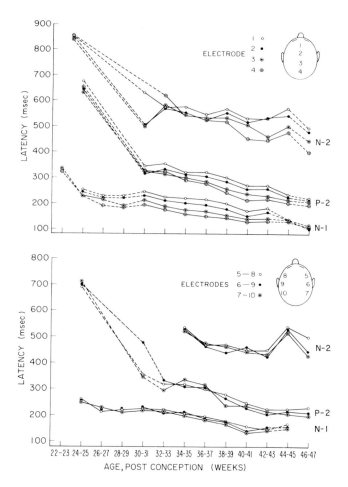

Fig. 20. Graphed summary of change of peak latency value (msec) of 3 waves (N-1, P-2, N-2) for all electrodes (1-10) as a function of conceptual age. Each point was obtained by first determining the mean value of the peak latency for each wave of all evoked responses obtained during a recording session for a baby. Then, a mean of these means was obtained as a function of the estimated conceptual age groups. Age groups were combined into 2-week periods. The values for electrodes 5 and 8, 6 and 9, and 7 and 10 are combined, since no difference in latency was found for the right and left homologous electrode sites. (From Weitzman and Graziani, 1968. Courtesy of John Wiley & Sons, Inc.)

Dr. Purpura: When you are looking at an evoked potential, there is always the problem of defining the takeoff point of a particular response. You know, if another component algebraically summates with that negativity, then your peak point is lost. Latencies of evoked potentials are extremely tricky to evaluate.

Dr. Weitzman: You have to have another dipole, then a multiple dipole system.

Dr. Purpura: That is the problem. What we do not have is depth recording in infants, thank goodness.

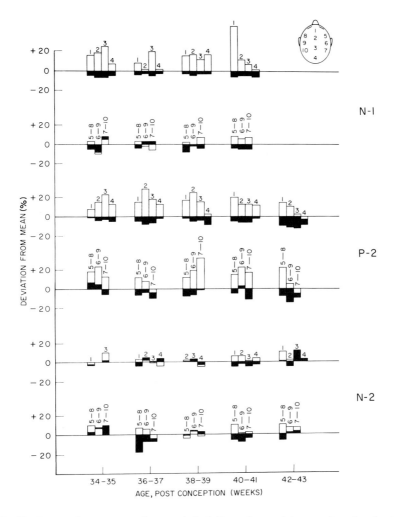

Fig. 21. Bar graph summary of percent deviation of wave latency values for the two defined EEG states, I and C. The 0% is the mean value of all waves as graphed in Fig. 20. The bars represent the percent deviation (positive or negative) for only the I and C EEG patterns (☐) intermittent; (■) continuous. (From Weitzman and Graziani, 1968. Courtesy of John Wiley & Sons, Inc.)

Dr. Sterman: After seeing the distinctive pathways that Dr. Scheibel showed us in the immature brain and Dr. Purpura's evidence that different portions of the cell may be utilized, how can one interpret cortical evoked potentials in the newborn? I would like to hear more discussion about this dynamic state when the neuron is developing different input-output apparatus and connections are changing rather rapidly. What kind of interpretations can one make about sensory pathways and responses?

Dr. Purpura: In responding to Dr. Sterman, I would suggest that the problem of latency shift is not going to be explained by considering factors of cortical organization alone. The field is too big, the distribution too wide, to allow for explanations in terms of cortical synaptogenesis alone. Perhaps what is needed is a laminar analysis of the responses.

Dr. Metcalf: I was struck by the great similarity of the twins I saw in the close grouping of all of your data on your last slides.

Dr. Weitzman: Those were mean values.

Dr. Metcalf: Where do twins fall among nontwins, therefore?

Dr. Weitzman: You mean how variable were the other twins?

Dr. Metcalf: Right.

Dr. Weitzman: Those were identical twins. I don't think we have enough data to make the comparison of identical twins and we have not analyzed for it.

Dr. Metcalf: I believe electrophysiological work with twins is conceptually tricky. One must pay strict attention to sampling problems, not only in terms of subjects, but also data selection. In my experience, this has not been done by most workers.

I wanted to ask Dr. Akiyama about the Moro response. Do you think there is any relationship between Moro responses and sleep, and spontaneous motor discharges in sleep and Moro-like or startle-like response in sleep?

Dr. Akiyama: On the polygram, they look different because you do not see the tonic phase in the spontaneous body jerk or startle—if you want to call them that. So I think there is probably a difference, but the amount of motor activity in the initial portion of the EMG response seems similar.

REFERENCE

Goff, W. R., Sterman, M. B., and Allison, T. (1966). Cortical midline late responses during sleep in the cat. *Brain Res.* 1, 311-314.

DEVELOPMENTAL ASPECTS OF NORMAL AND ABNORMAL SLEEP BEHAVIOR

15

Sleep Deprivation and the Organization of the Behavioral States *

William C. Dement

There seems to be very little question that one of the things newborn mammals do best is sleep. Although the total daily amount of neonatal sleep is likely to vary substantially, depending upon the species under observation,† we are probably correct in assuming that most neonates spend a good deal more of their time asleep than awake. Since the prevailing belief now appears to be that active processes subserve each of the three major states of vigilance (wakefulness, rapid eye movement sleep (REMS), non-REM sleep (NREMS)), the task of the developmental biologist in understanding how existence is compartmentalized is formidable.

*Supported by grants from NIMH (MH-13860), from NASA (NGR 05-020-168), and by a Research Scientist Award from NIMH (MH-5804)

† For example, Daniele Jouvet-Mounier and her colleagues (1970) extrapolating from 12-hr recordings have shown that the newborn guinea pig sleeps about 8 hr/day, while total sleep in the newborn rat accounts for about 17 hr out of 24.

There are at least two basic questions involved in a consideration of the maturation of brain mechanisms pertaining to the sleep side of the problem. First, what, if any, crucial role does sleep play in the developing organism? Second, what are the mechanisms underlying the unique distribution of its two major phases and their relation to wakefulness at different developmental stages, and particularly in the neonate?

It is difficult to define precise approaches to these problems because the descriptive information that would enable us to establish norms for total amounts of sleep and individual differences is relatively sparse. Comprehensive 24-hr studies over several consecutive days are notably lacking in human neonates, and 24-hr recordings over a single day are rare. Faced with this situation, most investigators are forced to generalize from small subject samples and extrapolate to the whole day from shorter recording periods. Obviously, such procedures could be misleading.

In the human adult, we know from polygraphic observations that presumably normal habitual daily sleep times can vary from less than 3 hr (Jones and Oswald, 1968) to more than 12 hr (Verdone, 1968), although, admittedly, individuals whose sleep "requirements" lie at these extremes are not common. However, there is no reason to suppose that a similarly thorough polygraphic documentation of sleep in newborn infants would not turn up comparable individual variation. By the same token, although admirable beginnings have been made, we need more information derived from consecutive 24-hr recordings in newborn experimental animals. When the results from such work are put together, we may expect to have a much clearer idea of the problem as well as, hopefully, some new approaches.

In this chapter, I will devote the major share of my attention to the first of the two basic questions mentioned earlier, in essence, the functional problem from a developmental point of view, and only secondarily, but nonetheless necessarily, the problem of the mechanisms that underlie the unique distribution of behavioral states at any particular age and during any particular experimental manipulation.

When we consider an experimental approach to the possibility that REMS and/or NREMS might perform an important function in either the adult or the developing organism, we usually fall back on the technique of sleep deprivation as the method of assessing such a function. In recent years, I have become very concerned about the ability of total, partial, and particularly selective sleep deprivation to give us clear-cut answers. This concern arises from two sources. The first is the general development of new concepts of sleep in which we think in terms of biochemical-neurophysiological processes rather than totally unique states of being. In other words, sleep states appear to consist of a temporal conglomeration of mechanisms or operating systems whose simultaneous activity may have some special value for the organism, but which can also operate in a totally independent fashion in certain circumstances. The second source of concern is the possibility that sleep deprivation or selective sleep deprivation are really techniques that cause a redistribution of behavioral states rather than an elimination. For example, we might reduce the nocturnal NREMS time by 4 hr using vigorous stimulation only to find that the lost sleep was merely shifted to the 16-hr wake period where it occurred as a large number of brief periods of drowsiness or microsleeps. This possibility seems even more likely in experimental animals and neonates than in human adults.

INDEPENDENT PROCESSES IN THE STATES OF VIGILANCE

In this section, I will attempt to define the states of sleep and wakefulness in terms of a temporal confluence of a number of more or less independent processes, but such characterizations will not consist entirely of a recitation of their well-known physiological attributes; rather, some attempt will be made to focus on the functional consequences of these attributes.

NREMS

I believe that important and defining differences between wakefulness and sleep are indeed hard to come by. What *is* the essential difference between being awake and being asleep? It is certainly not the cessation of motility, although the sleeping organism is almost always quiescent. However, the cat, the dog, and a host of mammals are able to be totally motionless for short intervals at least while fully awake. It does not appear to be a drastic diminution in blood pressure, heart rate, cerebral blood flow, or even the discharge of individual neurons that most closely captures the essence of falling asleep. Studies of these and other variables have suggested that very little change occurs in going from the last moments of wakefulness to the first moments of sleep. It is, of course, possible that more sophisticated analyses of things like contingency patterns in multiple-unit firing patterns (Noda and Adey, 1970) will show dramatic and revealing correlations with the process of falling asleep, but such information is not currently available.

In my opinion, the essential attribute of NREMS, which could be stated in several ways and must involve more than one neural system, is simply a loss of awareness. Wakefulness ends and sleep begins at that precise moment when a meaningful stimulus cannot elicit its accustomed response. This by no means entails the elimination of all responses as is obvious. For example, waking up is a response. Furthermore, evoked potentials (EP) clearly show that sensory stimuli affect the central nervous system (CNS) during sleep.

In humans, the moment of sleep is characterized by a cessation of the process

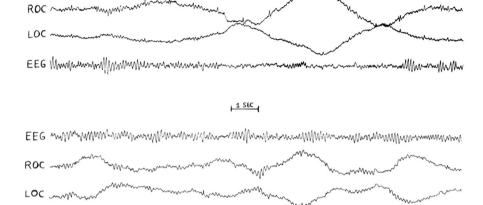

Fig. 1. Slow eye movements at the onset of sleep. Deprivations: ROC, right outer canthus electrode referred to the opposite ear lobe; LOC, left outer canthus electrode referred to the opposite ear lobe (when the pens move in opposite directions, the eyes are moving in the same direction); EEG, brain waves from monopolar scalp electrode. The sample at the top shows large swings of the eyeballs accompanied by an EEG change from waking α rhythm to NREM stage 1 and back to waking α at the end. The bottom sample shows eye movements that are a little smaller occurring before any change in the EEG is apparent. (From Dement, 1970. Reprinted with permission of the publisher.)

of perceiving noises, touches, lights, etc. There is often a loss of awareness of time, place, and even person. For some, this is experienced as total oblivion. For others, it is a lapsing into hypnagogic reveries. The absolutely essential component, however, is simply a loss of awareness of the environment.

It is my opinion that the change from wakefulness to sleep—the moment of sleep—is quite abrupt, and while there may be important predisposing changes leading up to it, and consequences of its occurrence leading away from it, the point itself is relatively easy to distinguish and can be easily localized within a second or two. Rechtschaffen and Foulkes' experiment (Rechtschaffen and Dement, 1965) with taped-open eyelids and visual stimuli seems relatively conclusive in this regard, as does our own study involving click stimuli, mental content, and the breakdown of visual fixation at the onset of sleep (Dement, 1965a).

The transition point between sleep and wakefulness is frequently, though not necessarily, associated with an attenuation of α rhythm (Fig. 1). It is *never* associated with the appearance of full-blown sleep spindles in the EEG, although the possibility cannot be ruled out that the neural processes which generate spindles begin operating immediately but at intensities insufficient to produce visually detectable waveforms. In spite of such qualifications, it is probably safe to say that the sudden and massive shutdown of perceptual activities characterizing the moment of sleep is *not* signaled by some equally dramatic event in the scalp EEG.

Another point is that the mechanisms mediating this incredible functional alteration seem to include some involvement with processes subserving short-term memory. It seems reasonably clear from the work of Portnoff *et al.* (1966) and the unpublished results of Kamiya and his colleagues, that sleep erases short-term memories, or that short-term memory mechanisms do not operate in NREMS. Thus, with neither perceptual processes nor memory processes operating, the organism has no will, no motivation, and in fact, about the only meaningful response to either external or internal stimuli left in its repertoire is arousal.

Once established, the state of sleep tends to be self-perpetuating. Although they are highly characteristic of NREMS, the appearance of sleep spindles and slow waves may only represent an additional recruitment and consolidation of processes initiated somewhat earlier. They may, however, have some significance in representing the activity of processes that operate to maintain sleep over lengthy periods of time. In the young child, NREMS is reversible for some minutes, and then, more or less in relation to the development of stage 4 EEG patterns, even the nonspecific response of arousal to external stimuli ceases to be obtainable. Indeed, the young child appears to be a genuine exception to the principle that sleep is, by definition, reversible. Is it possible that the neural mechanisms subserving arousal are totally shut down at this time, in particular, the synthesis of arousal transmitters? Such a shut-down would explain the inability of some children to achieve complete arousal during episodes of sleep-walking, sleep-talking, and NREM nightmares (Broughton, 1968; Kales *et al.*, 1966).

Wakefulness

With regard to the foregoing, wakefulness is best characterized as the absence of sleep. It is a state in which environmental stimuli are perceived and responses are elaborated. Short-term memory processes are operating at optimal levels. Motivation and "will" are present, decisions can be made, etc. Motility ensues if it is an appropriate response to the environmental impingement. EEG correlates of wakefulness are highly characteristic and consistent, but may not be necessary.

Lest the foregoing oversimplifications go totally unchallenged, I would like to mention some other rather surprising possible characteristics of NREMS vs. wakefulness that have been suggested from as yet unpublished experiments conducted by Dr. Appletree Rodden and his colleagues and Dr. Takeo Deguchi and his colleagues at Stanford University. They were performed as part of a major collaborative effort between the Sleep Laboratory, the Biochemistry Laboratory of Dr. Jack Barchas, and the Nuclear Medicine Laboratory of Dr.

Joseph DeGrazia which aims at an extensive characterization of the biochemical correlates of sleep. In short, there appears to be a strong possibility of certain peripheral metabolic changes occurring specifically as a function of state. These include changes in the rate of whole-body tryptophan metabolism in human adults, changes in activity of liver tryptophan pyrrolase and tyrosine hydroxylase in the rat, and alternation in protein metabolism in the rat. A number of controls have ruled out nonsleep associated effects. The point of mentioning this somewhat tangential information is that specific correlates of the states of vigilance may exist in the liver and kidney as well as the brain. If this possibility is confirmed by additional experimentation, we might have to modify some of our current thinking about the adaptive significance and biological purposes of sleep.

REMS

This state appears to entail the simultaneous occurrence of at least three distinct processes.

Tonic Inhibition

Perhaps the most essential and characteristic process of REMS is an actively induced, tonic motor inhibition. The most widely used and convenient indicator of this inhibitory process is a continuous recording of the electromyogram (EMG). EMG suppression (Fig. 2) is highly correlated with other attributes of REMS and with other indicators of active motor inhibition (Hodes and Dement, 1964; Pompeiano, 1969). According to Pompeiano (1969), there is a tonic hyperpolarization of α motor neurons, and if the cataplectic attack in narcoleptic patients is representative of the effectiveness of this inhibitory process (Dement and Rechtschaffen, 1968), REMS is a time of profound motor paralysis in which tendon reflexes cannot be elicited and in which voluntary movement is impossible. In cats, the presence of motor paralysis is also confirmed by an extreme flaccidity.

Phasic Activity

The second process has been called phasic activity. Some center or system inside the brain spontaneously begins to emit bursts of activity. These bursts of discharge apparently give rise to a whole series of temporally related short-lasting events which include the REMs themselves, cardiovascular irregularities, respiratory changes, muscular twitching, as well as other things such as sudden changes in pupil diameter, fluctuations in penile tumescence, and finally, unique bursts of high amplitude, monophasic, sharp waves in the electrical recordings from the pons, oculomotor nuclei, lateral geniculate nuclei, and visual cortices of the cat (Brooks and Bizzi, 1963; Mouret et al., 1963; Michel et al., 1964). A flurry of phasic activity during REMS is illustrated in Fig. 3.

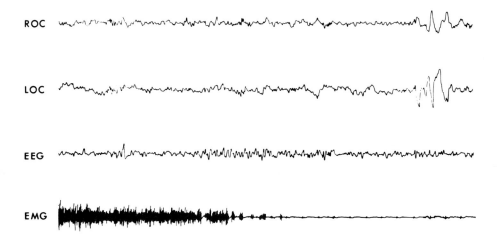

Fig. 2. The onset of REMS. Electrode placements: ROC, right outer canthus referred to ears; LOC, left outer canthus referred to ears; EEG, left parietal electrode referred to left occipital electrode; EMG, bipolar electrodes placed on anterior neck muscles. Note that the tonic EMG potentials that were present all during NREMS disappear rather abruptly. A few seconds later, the first REM potentials appear (at the left of the figure in ROC and LOC). (From Dement, 1965a.)

It seems likely that the aforementioned monophasic sharp waves, hereafter referred to as PGO (pontine-geniculate-occipital) spikes, may represent a kind of characteristic low threshold response to the phasic event generator, and are therefore, highly correlated with the occurrence of other phasic activity. However, the PGO spike should not be mistaken for the putative primary phasic event any more than one would consider the eye movement or muscle twitch in this category. Nonetheless, the PGO spike is very important because it is so consistent in its occurrence, so convenient to record, and may be clearly seen when no other phasic activity is evident.

REM periods in cats with adequate placements of the implanted recording electrodes are *always* associated with the occurrence of PGO spikes. The spike activity in the cerebral cortex is best recorded from special transcortical electrodes which record the potential difference between cortical surface and white matter (Brooks, 1967). Results with this technique have shown that cortical spiking is widely distributed with perhaps two-thirds of the cat's neocortex participating in the generation of the potential changes. PGO spikes do not seem to be nearly so conspicuous and characteristic in other species, and indeed, in spite of many attempts have not been unequivocally documented in the laboratory rat. We have tried on numerous occasions in our own laboratory to record spikes in the geniculate bodies of this rodent without success. However, the fact that other phasic activities, e.g., muscle twitches, eye movements, etc., are always associated with REM periods in the rat strongly suggests the

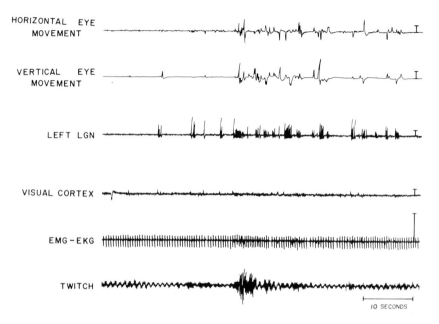

Fig. 3. A "flurry" of phasic events. Toward the middle of the tracing, a typical multisystem flurry of activity begins. In addition to the bursts of eye movements and PGO spikes, there are also a transient acceleration of heart rate and an upsurge of activity in the actogram (twitches). In all likelihood, additional measurements would have shown respiratory changes, plethysmographic changes, etc. had it been possible to make them. LGN, lateral geniculate nucleus; EMG electromyogram; EKG, electrocardiogram. Calibrations: 50 μV, 10 sec. (From Dement *et al.*, 1969a.)

presence of basic neural events analogous to those which trigger the feline PGO spike, even though a similar electrical response may not be observable. Clear-cut PGO spikes have been described in the squirrel monkey and the rhesus monkey. PGO spikes have not been described in the human. At the moment, we may assume that this lack is due mainly to the restricted use of implanted electrodes. It is possible that the sawtooth waves seen in the scalp EEG of the human before and during REM periods represent a discharge analogous to PGO spikes (Fig. 4). The vertex localization of sawtooth waves does not rule out this possibility in view of the recent realization that spike discharge is probably not limited to the primary visual areas in the cat.

Although absolutely characteristic of REM periods in the cat, it is also true that phasic activity in the form of PGO spikes may be present in more than 50% of the total amount of NREMS in certain cats (Fig. 5). In addition, intervals of NREMS in which there are no PGO spikes at all are relatively brief, for the most part no longer than 2 or 3 min. The amplitudes of PGO spikes are usually much

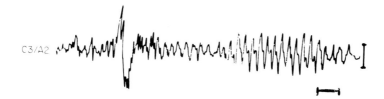

Fig. 4. A tracing during a stage 2 REMS transition which illustrates a typical K complex and a burst of sawtooth waves. The sawtooth waves may be a human analog of the cortical component of the PGO spike in the cat.

greater in NREMS and nearly all spikes occur singly, while in REM periods they tend to occur in clusters of three or more (Fig. 6). We have found that the mean discharge rate of PGO spikes during REM periods varies from cat to cat, ranging from around 40/min to more than 100. The discharge rates during short epochs of NREMS are highly variable, although always well below the rates seen during REM periods. The total number of PGO spikes per day in the cat has been estimated to vary between 10,000 and 20,000. Somewhere around 15% of the total typically occur in NREMS. Several investigators have pointed out the unvarying sequence of events in which the onset of REM periods is heralded by the onset of PGO spike activity about 30 sec earlier (Fig. 7). This unvarying sequence has led to the plausible suggestion that the spikes, or whatever more basic neural process they reflect, are an important part of the mechanism that actually triggers the REM periods.

I have highlighted a description of PGO spikes because they are a very interesting aspect of sleep. Moreover, the fact that they occur in both REMS and NREMS is one piece of evidence suggesting that the qualitative distinction between these two states of sleep may be more apparent than real.

In addition to the previously mentioned tonic inhibition of motor activity, it has also been demonstrated that a phasic inhibitory influence on motor discharge in the cat typically occurs in association with spike bursts during REMS (Pompeiano, 1969). This phasic inhibition *within* REM periods cannot be seen in the EMG which is already totally suppressed. However, it is occasionally manifested in the cat during NREMS as a brief transitory EMG suppression.

Such information has made it possible to infer the presence of phasic activity and possibly, of PGO spike discharge in human NREMS. Pivik and Dement (1970; Pivik *et al.*, 1969) have recently described a phasic suppression of the tonic EMG activity during NREMS in human subjects, which is quite similar to that seen in cats in association with PGO spikes occurring in NREMS (Fig. 8). The confirmation of an active, phasic, inhibitory process in humans was provided by showing that the electrically elicited monosynaptic reflex of peripheral nerve was transiently suppressed at the exact moment of the spontaneous EMG suppression (Fig. 9). Thus, there is a strong likelihood that

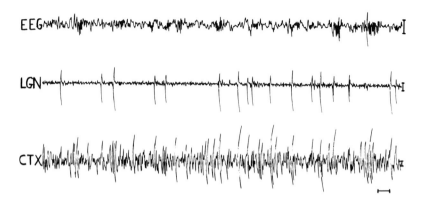

Fig. 5. NREMS in the cat. This figure illustrates PGO spikes during NREM epochs that do not immediately precede REMS. It also documents the principle that the EEG is to some extent a function of the recording technique. In the top tracing (EEG), electrical activity is being recorded from two silver discs cemented to the outer surface of the skull above the frontal sinus. In the bottom tracing (CTX), the electrical activity is being recorded from two screws, the uninsulated points of which rest directly on the cortical surface. It seems likely that the screws are picking up high amplitude waves which are highly localized and whose amplitude totally obscures the more diffuse low amplitude spindling. When the electrodes are at some distance from the brain, local activity is minimized, higher gains are required, and the net effect is probably integration which highlights the more diffuse and coherent spindle activity. Obviously, the top tracing is more analogous to a human stage 2 pattern as is the technique of recording. The LGN (lateral geniculate nucleus) tracing is bipolar and polarity has no particular significance. If a single LGN electrode is referred to a large indifferent reference (monopolar), the spike is seen as a monophasic negative wave. Calibrations: 50 μV, 1 sec.

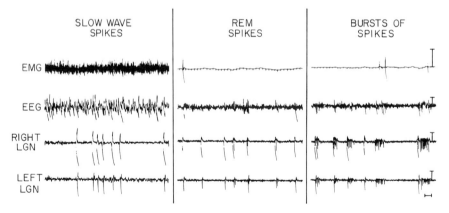

Fig. 6. PGO spikes: the primary phasic response. The large-amplitude, isolated spikes characteristically associated with NREMS are shown on the left, while the low amplitude bursts characteristic of REMS are shown on the right. The middle tracing shows an intermediate example most typical of the final moments of REM periods, or immediately after the REM onset. EMG, electromyogram; EEG, electroencephalogram; LGN, lateral geniculate nucleus. Calibrations: 50 μV, 1 sec. (From Dement *et al.*, 1969a).

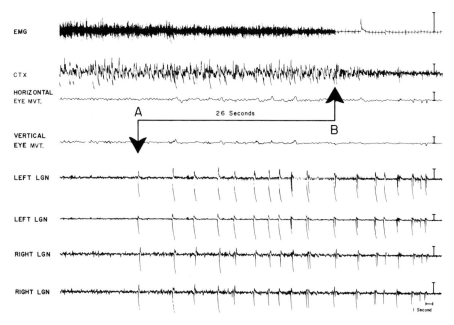

Fig. 7. A typical example from a normal cat of the unvarying sequence of events in going from NREMS to REMS. The arrow B indicates the exact onset of the REM period according to the definition of EEG activation in the presence of PGO spikes and EMG suppression. The arrow at A indicates the first PGO spike in the sequence. This figure may also serve to illustrate the techniques of "spike" deprivation and REM deprivation mentioned somewhat further on in the text. In the latter procedure, the cat would have been aroused at the exact onset of the REM period (B). If the cat had been undergoing spike deprivation, the arousal would have been immediately after the first PGO spike. In this example, such an arousal would have "deprived" the cat of 13 NREM PGO spikes in addition to those that would have occurred in the subsequent REM period. The cat would have also been deprived of 26 sec of NREMS. CTX, cortex; LGN, lateral geniculate nucleus. (From Dement *et al.*, 1969a.)

phasic activity, and perhaps even a discharge analogous to the feline PGO spike, occurs during NREMS in humans. We cannot grant this latter possibility for NREMS without assuming at the same time that PGO spikes also occur in human REM periods.

Additional evidence supporting these possibilities has been independently reported by Rechtschaffen *et al.* (1971) who have described an entirely different kind of phasic event in human sleep.

CNS Arousal:

It is a well-known fact that in many respects the brain in REMS appears to be aroused or awake. Therefore, we postulate some sort of nonspecific arousal process as a third system that operates during REM periods. It is a matter of great puzzlement whether the observed CNS arousal is true wakefulness or a totally different process which merely resembles wakefulness in terms of most of

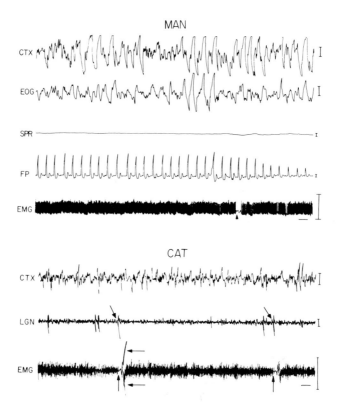

Fig. 8. The occurrence of phasic EMG suppressions in man and cat. In the upper tracings the single vertical arrow indicates the occurrence of a relatively long-sustained phasic EMG suppression during NREM stage 4 sleep in man. CTX, monopolar central (C3/A2) EEG; EOG, bipolar horizontal electrooculogram; SPR, spontaneous skin potential; FP, finger plethysmograph; EMG, bipolar submental electromyogram. In the EMG tracing of the cat two phasic suppressions can be seen (vertical arrows). A biphasic muscle twitch (horizontal arrows) occurs near the end of the first suppression. Note the close temporal correlation between geniculate spiking (arrows, LGN derivation) and phasic EMG suppressions. CTX, visual cortex; LGN, lateral geniculate nucleus; EMG, electromyogram recorded from the posterior cervical muscles. Calibrations: 1 sec, 50 μV. (From Pivik and Dement, 1970.)

the nonspecific measures of CNS activity levels such as brain temperature, EEG activation, cerebral blood flow, and so forth.

While it is perfectly apparent that the animal or human subject in REMS is not perceiving the external world in the way he does when awake, it is not clear that he cannot. In other words, if one is situated in a quiet, dark room, is totally paralyzed, and preoccupied with some kind of intense, internally generated experience (phasic activity, dreaming), it would seem almost inevitable that one would ignore the external world. I would further speculate that if phasic

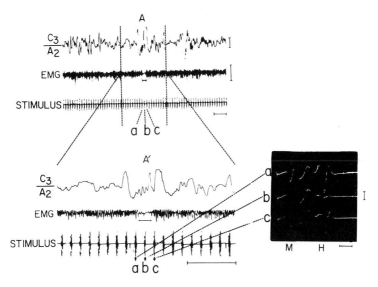

Fig. 9. A phasic EMG suppression (underscored) and associated EEG recorded at standard (A) and enhanced (A′) speeds together with the muscular responses elicited by the three consecutive stimuli (a, b, c) overlapping the suppression. The muscular responses (a, b, c) pictured to the right of A′ correspond, respectively, to the lettered stimuli in A′ directly under the suppression. In the tracings of the muscular responses note the stability of the direct response (M wave) and the inhibition of the H reflex in tracing b, the stimulus for which occurs coincident with the phasic EMG suppression. Calibrations: A and A′: 1 sec, 50 μV; oscilloscope tracings: 10 msec, 500 μV. (From Pivik and Dement, 1970.)

activities were not being generated, a REM period would be essentially identical to a cataplectic attack (Fig. 10). There would be nothing to distract an individual from the external world, and so that attack would be quickly terminated.

The question may be raised again whether the failure to perceive the external environment during REMS is simply a matter of neurological occlusion in which the internally generated phasic activity dominates the perceptual apparatus, or whether this domination is favored simply because there is so little competing external input during the usual time of REMS. Along this line, we might suggest that the portions of REMS between bursts of phasic activity would more closely resemble wakefulness and that response thresholds would be near or at waking levels if tested at these precise moments. There is evidence that external input can be perceived and remembered during REMS at certain times (Berger, 1963; Dement and Wolpert, 1958), and it seems possible that in certain special cases, waking perceptions and REMS associated phasic activity could become extensively intermingled as, for example, in delirium tremens (Gross *et al.*, 1966).

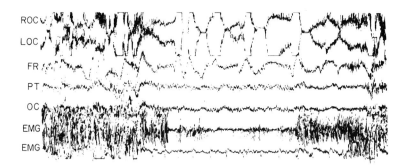

Fig. 10. Polygraphic recording during a cataplectic attack. The patient slumped in her chair for about 10 sec, during which time EMG discharge was dramatically reduced. She was immediately requested to move her eyes from side to side, which she did without difficulty, as may be seen in the two tracings. The EEG patterns during the attack were identical with the patient's normal waking rhythms. ROC, right outer canthus; LOC, left outer canthus; FR, frontal; PT, parietal; OC, occipital; top EMG, submental placement; bottom EMG, supraclavicular. All derivations, except EMG, are monopolar to ears; paper speed: 15 mm/sec. (From Dement and Rechtschaffen, 1968.)

It should be obvious from a consideration of all the foregoing material that a number of possibilities exist for dissociative reactions. Cataplexy, for example, can be regarded as an instance in which the tonic motor inhibitory process, ordinarily occurring in association with phasic activity and CNS arousal, takes place in the waking state. Thus, we may assume that the elimination of one of the three major behavioral states only means that its components do not occur in their typically and therefore recognizably simultaneous fashion. It does not guarantee that these components will not occur in atypical, and therefore not easily recognizable, isolation at other times. We will return to this line of argument in a later section.

THE DYNAMISM OF SLEEP STATES AND TOTAL SLEEP DEPRIVATION

At this point, I would like to take up the question of the dynamics of the establishment and maintenance of states of vigilance. This will lead to a critical examination of total sleep deprivation and whether or not it is really possible to accomplish on either a theoretical or practical basis. For purposes of a manageable discussion, I will limit my consideration to EEG patterns (activation and deactivation) as the primary indicators of NREMS on the one hand, and REMS and wakefulness on the other. Semiphilosophical arguments about whether sleep is the lack of wakefulness, or vice versa, and so forth, will be avoided. In my opinion, the best model of the temporal organization of NREMS and arousal (wakefulness and REMS) is that both conditions are associated with active processes which mediate their occurrence, and whether basically facilitatory or inhibitory, are antagonistic to each other. It seems likely that both processes involve biochemical mechanisms, and at the present time, the only serious candidates for the putative neurotransmitters are catecholamines (CA) mediating arousal (Jouvet, 1969; Jones *et al.*, 1969), and serotonin (5-HT) mediating NREMS (Jouvet, 1969; Koella, 1969).

NREMS and arousal, or more properly, their characteristic EEG correlates, are easily reversible, and such reversals would seem to be able to occur at fairly high rates. Unfortunately, the commonly employed scoring systems utilize epoch lengths that are too large to show rapid alternations in EEG stages. However, the simple fact of the matter is that rats, cats, and even humans, can enter and leave any one of the major behavioral states in a definitive manner during the passage of only a few seconds. Accordingly, it is possible for several clear-cut changes in behavioral state to occur within a single scoring epoch of the usual half or whole minute duration. As long as everyone believes that these brief changes are not important, there is no problem. However, we began to feel otherwise at the Stanford Sleep Laboratory and decided to develop a scoring system for the cat that would be sensitive to brief changes. Accordingly, we began scoring sleep stages to the nearest 3 sec, i.e., we adopted a 3-sec scoring epoch. The actual choice of 3 sec as opposed to 2 or 4 or 5 sec was determined by the grid lines on the EEG paper. This scoring system gives us one order of magnitude greater resolution of the states of vigilance than our previous system which employed a 30-sec epoch. In this system, each successive 3-sec epoch is assigned to one of the states of sleep or wakefulness. This requires the scoring of 28,800 epochs for each 24-hr recording period, and since we often record around the clock for 20 or more consecutive days, the immensity of the task confronting scorers is obvious.

In addition to wakefulness (W), which is defined as EEG activation in the absence of PGO spikes and EMG suppression, our laboratory defines three states in the sleeping cat. *Slow wave sleep* (S) is defined mainly by the EEG pattern recorded from special anterior cortical electrodes which maximize the occurrence of sleep spindles. Any epoch which contains slow waves and/or spindles in the EEG in the absence of PGO spikes above a certain rate and in the absence of waking behavior is scored as S. *REMS* (R) is defined by EEG activation in the presence of PGO spikes. As is obvious, we feel that PGO spikes are an invariable concomitant of REMS in the cat. EMG suppression is helpful, but is not invariably a concomitant of REMS. Accordingly, we do not use it as a defining characteristic any longer. *Slow wave sleep with PGO spikes* (X) is defined by the presence of slow waves and/or spindles and the occurrence of two or more PGO spikes within no more than five successive 3-sec epochs. The total duration of the state interval is from the epoch with the first spike to the epoch with the last spike. S and X may be combined to give total NREMS.

Let me give one example to illustrate that this seemingly ridiculous level of precision can, at times, be helpful. Among other things, the use of the 3-sec epoch permits us to score and tabulate all of the brief interruptions of REM periods that we knew existed but have heretofore ignored. In several cats, we compared the number of interruptions of REM periods during a baseline period with the number of interruptions on the first recovery day following selective REMS deprivation. To our great surprise, there were many more interruptions on the recovery day. Previous work had led us to expect that REMS following deprivation would be more preemptive, more intense, and, as a consequence, less prone to interruptions. Most of the interruptions were quite brief, and the change would not have been apparent if 30-sec scoring epochs had been used.

Even though such changes may be revealed, our willingness to make use of a smaller scoring epoch depends upon our belief that the cat can really enter and leave a particular behavioral state during the passage of a few seconds. Figures 11-13 show examples that support this possibility. Certainly, all polygraphic changes of this sort are not associated with frank behavioral change, but we have definitely seen soundly sleeping cats raise their heads, open their eyes, look around (with activated EEG patterns), and return to sleep (with slow waves) within 3-5 sec.

Now, if we are ready to accept this approach as valid, at least for descriptive purposes, I would like to tell you how dynamic existence really is. Some of these results were reported at the 1969 Federation Meetings by Dr. James Ferguson (Ferguson *et al.,* 1969b). If we pay attention only to the three major states, W, R, and NREM, we find that an average normal adult cat on a 24-hr *ad lib* sleep schedule can have as many as 785 changes of state per day, or one on the average of every 1 min 50 sec. When X and S are scored separately, the total number of state changes is increased to an average of 1400/day or slightly less than one every minute. We have not subdivided wakefulness into fully alert and drowsy states as could easily be done. One can imagine the number of state changes per day if we did.

The distribution by length of all uninterrupted intervals of W for one day in a representative cat are plotted in Fig. 14. Notice that the curve is markedly skewed: 84% of all W intervals are less than 1 min in length and 70% are less than 30 sec. Although extremely numerous, all the intervals that are 1 min or less account for only about one-fifth of the total amount of W in a day.

The distribution of NREMS (S + X) intervals for this day showed a similar pattern: 82% of all intervals are less than 1 min in length and 73% are less than 30 sec (Fig. 15).

If we think about it for a moment, it will become apparent that these distributions support the formulation mentioned earlier, to wit, that all behavioral states are actively induced. The reason that there are so many changes of states and brief intervals is that when the NREMS mechanisms are in control,

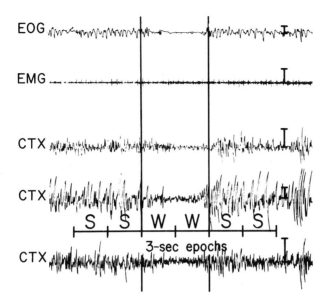

Fig. 11. An example of wakefulness (W) intruding upon NREM sleep (S). EOG, electrooculogram; EMG, electromyogram; CTX, cortex. In this instance, the cat opened his eyes but did not raise his head. No stimulus preceded the change. With larger scoring epochs, such changes are ignored; with the 3-sec epoch, this example qualifies as an unambiguous transition from one behavioral state to another and back within 6 sec. The absence of PGO spikes in lateral geniculate tracings (not shown) confirms the state decision of W as opposed to REM.

W processes remain active and manifest themselves as a series of brief intrusions of W into S or NREM. Conversely, when W is the dominant state, S intervals are continually intruding. Similarly, epochs of S or X intrude in periods of R and R epochs intrude in longer periods of S.

In summary, each of the patterns tells the same story, i.e., the state of vigilance present at any particular moment is determined by a constant interplay of many systems.

As a partial model of this, one can envisage a seesaw mechanism in which two biochemical-neural systems are balanced against each other. When one system has preempted the nervous system and is maximally active, it is exhausting its transmitter, while its antagonist, which is relatively inactive, is conserving its transmitter. At some point, power passes to the system previously held in check, which then becomes active, inhibits its opponent and "takes over." In the absence of other factors, this alteration would be very rapid, since the activity of the systems would simply fluctuate back and forth within a very narrow range around the point of absolute balance.

In order to account for the instances in which any particular state of vigilance

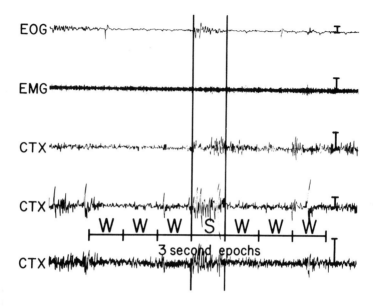

Fig. 12. An example of NREM sleep (S) intruding upon wakefulness (W). EOG, electrooculogram; EMG, electromyogram; CTX, cortex. When slow waves of defined amplitude, frequency, and amount appear in cortical leads and elsewhere, the epoch is scored as NREMS. However, prior to a definitive study, great care is taken to be sure that the EEG change has behavioral significance. In this example, the cat was lying down with his head up, but very relaxed. The 3-sec S epoch was concomitant with a prolonged eye closure.

is maintained for a fairly lengthy interval, we probably must invoke circadian or ultradian changes in enzyme activity which would alter the hypothetical balance of neurotransmitters to favor the dominance of one or other behavioral state during specific periods of time. In addition, sensory stimulation from the environment probably aids in sustaining and consolidating wakefulness, while lack of stimulation effects a similar abetment of sleep. In a free-running cat (to purloin rhythm terminology), by which I mean a cat that is isolated from the environment and continuously recorded without attempting to enforce or reinforce the occurrence of either wakefulness or sleep, the number of state changes per unit time over a 24-hr period is likely to be maximal, and the mean duration of uninterrupted intervals in a particular state is likely to be minimal. When many epochs of W are consolidated into one or several longer periods of wakefulness by means of an enforcing device, such as a treadmill or repetitious nonhabituating stimuli, the number of state changes per unit time is reduced and the mean duration of uninterrupted intervals is increased. Furthermore, greater consolidation of one state favors increased consolidation of its antagonist. It seems obvious that this is beneficial for the organism. In short, the state of

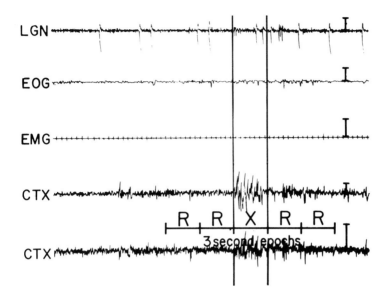

Fig. 13. An example of NREMS (X) intruding upon stage REM (R). LGN, lateral geniculate nucleus; EOG, electrooculogram; EMG, electromyogram; CTX, cortex. Slow waves and/or spindles in the cortical leads determine the shift to NREMS. If the epoch contains PGO spikes, it is scored X as opposed to S. In this instance, there is no clear behavioral concomitant except that muscular twitching is rarely, if ever, present. PGO spikes are usually higher in amplitude and do not occur in bursts.

wakefulness, in order to be effectively utilized, must be sustained, and the same is presumably true for the states of sleep.

Given the adaptive desirability of lengthier uninterrupted periods of wakefulness and sleep, there is nonetheless a point where the continued enforcement of wakefulness is no longer beneficial. After an excessively long period of wakefulness, the state of sleep becomes preemptive. When we enforce wakefulness, we are probably preventing or minimizing activity in the neural systems that subserve sleep induction and maintenance. As the potency of these systems increases during the period of their induced inactivity, they may begin to intrude upon wakefulness in an ever more aggressive manner. A crude analogy for this process would be the damming of a stream. Eventually, the water begins to overflow the banks in many little rivulets.

In terms of all the foregoing, it is very easy to understand that the notion of total sleep deprivation could be somewhat illusory, and could result merely in a redistribution of activity in sleep and arousal systems in which NREMS would occur in the form of hundreds of microsleeps. These episodes could conceivably be so brief that in human subjects they would not be readily detectable even in the scalp EEG. By the same token, it is almost impossible to envisage any

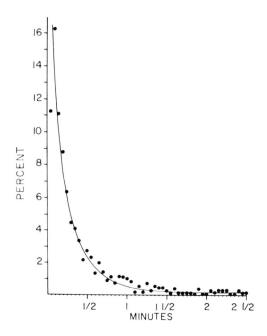

Fig. 14. Distributional plot of all uninterrupted intervals of wakefulness scored to the nearest 3 sec that occurred during a single 24-hr period in a cat. Ordinate, percent of the total of all wake intervals; abscissa, length of intervals in 3-sec increments. Most of the shorter epochs occur as interruptions of NREMS or at definite transition periods when there is a fairly rapid alternation between states. A few intervals of more than 2½ minutes were not included.

situation in which NREMS could be readily prolonged beyond certain limits without a comparable intrusion of "microwakes." The latter process may have something to do with the occasional episodes of disorganization and delirium that occur during the terminal phases of prolonged periods of drug-induced somnolence.

Although we have tended to ignore any notion about daily quotas in our discussion up to this point, it is now appropriate to speculate that the total amounts of arousal and NREMS per day are fixed so that only the degree of consolidation or dispersion can vary. Thus, if we were to add up all the epochs of EEG arousal in the previously mentioned case of the free-running cat, we might find that their sum total would approximate the absolute limit for the longest uninterrupted period of arousal we could achieve by enforced consolidation.

To sum up, the analysis of short recording epochs has led to an appreciation of the extreme frequency of minor shifts in states of vigilance. We have seen that a single "level" of arousal is not maintained for a very long period of time unless its continuance is enforced. However, we can only enforce the prolongation of

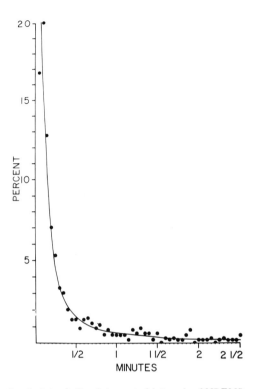

Fig. 15. Distributional plot of all uninterrupted intervals of NREMS scored to the nearest 3 sec that occurred during a single 24-hr period in a cat (the same day and cat as Fig. 14). Ordinate, percent of the total of all NREM intervals; abscissa, length of intervals in 3-sec increments. A very few intervals of more than 2½ minutes in length were not included. Shifts from S to X or from X to S were ignored in constructing this graph.

wakefulness. The ensuing prolongation of sleep occurs passively. There is probably an optimal amount of enforced consolidation and, in view of the fact that microsleeps occur so readily, it is likely that enforcing wakefulness much beyond 24 hr only creates a situation of "modified" arousal in which NREMS continually intrudes. This formulation casts considerable doubt upon our ability to understand the function of sleep by eliminating it for prolonged periods of time.

SELECTIVE DEPRIVATION OF
RAPID EYE MOVEMENT SLEEP

As should be obvious from the many speculations in the previous section, we have made the slightly ambiguous and questionable assumption that the brain is capable of operating in one of *only two* basic modes, and, of course, gradations thereof. These two modes are defined mainly by the EEG and are an activated

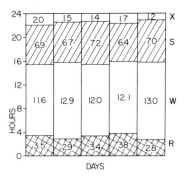

Fig. 16. Total time spent in each of the behavioral states on five consecutive days in a cat. Daily totals of W + R vary less (15.1-15.9 hr) than W alone (11.6-13.0 hr) or even R alone 2.8-3.8 hr). On a percentage basis, the disparity is even more striking: W + R (−3.2 to +1.9%) vs R (−14.9 to +15.9%) or W (−5.9 to +5.5%) or even total sleep time, S + X + R (−5.8 to +6.2%).

mode which can be either wakefulness or REMS, depending upon the function or nonfunction of certain specific systems, and the deactivated mode which is NREMS. If, as was considered earlier, the ability or capacity of the organism to be aroused is limited, and if arousal or activation includes *both* wakefulness and REMS, then the compartmentalization of behavioral states might be better understood by assuming the existence of a sort of reciprocity between these two states. With this in mind, we have examined data from successive 24-hr recordings in adult cats. It is possible to state that there is a distinct tendency for the daily amount of wakefulness and REMS to vary in a reciprocal fashion. This has the effect of allowing total sleep time (TST) (REM + NREM) to undergo a fairly marked fluctuation from day to day while the NREM (deactivated) fraction is relatively constant. As an illustration of this principle, data from a single cat are plotted in Fig. 16

A new way of accounting for the REMS deprivation-compensation phenomenon suggests itself on the basis of the foregoing assumptions. It is possible that the REM deprivation technique fosters a redistribution of NREMS into the wakefulness period of the experimental subject, which, in turn, forces the brain to spend more time in the activated mode (REMS) during the sleep period. In most of our REM deprivation studies in both man and animals, the subjects were on 8-hr sleep schedules which required them to remain awake for 16 consecutive hours (on a slowly moving treadmill in the case of the animals) and to sleep as much as possible during the remaining 8 hr. However, sleep was not continuous during this period since each REMS episode was routinely interrupted at its onset. As the 8-hr sleep portion became progressively more disturbed (with progressively less NREMS), it is likely that more and more NREMS (deactivation) occurred during the 16-hr daily period of "wakefulness." EEG recording from cats on a moving treadmill has verified the possibility that large numbers of NREM "microsleeps" can occur during this type of wakefulness enforcement (Ferguson and Dement, 1967), although accuracy of the recording is greatly reduced by movement artifact. We have begun a reexamination of this paradigm with continuous recording of two channels of telemetered EEG during periods of treadmill-enforced wakefulness in cats. At the moment, it is certain that the total amount of NREMS occurring on the treadmill increases progressively during a period of selective REM deprivation. However, it is too early to say whether or not such increases precisely balance the increased amounts of REMS seen during the recovery period.

If the REMS rebound following selective deprivation is not accounted for in terms of the above formulation, it would suggest that REMS possessed some unique property *not* convertable, on an equal basis, to so many minutes of waking arousal. However, if we wish to retain the notion of reciprocity between the brain activation of REMS and the brain activation of wakefulness for the time being, we must seek elsewhere for unique functions, if any, performed by REMS. In recent years, we have focused on the phasic activities of REMS, and, in particular, the PGO spikes, as events uniquely discharged during REM periods which might account for the effects of selective REMS deprivation more parsimoniously than previously proposed explanations. However, it is important to keep in mind that PGO spikes also occur in NREMS, and that, under certain conditions, they also appear to occur during wakefulness. Once again, we are faced with the difficulties involved in regarding NREMS, wakefulness, and REMS as totally independent and unique states of being, having activities and functions which are not discharged at any other time.

Let us leave these general considerations for the moment and attempt to deal specifically with the known effects of selective REM deprivation in adult mammalian organisms and the issue of whether or not the daily occurrence of a certain amount of REMS is a vital necessity. A major difficulty associated with the various REM deprivation procedures is the possible effect of stress. It is presumed that a certain amount of stress is an inevitable concomitant of whatever technique is used to prevent the occurrence of REM periods, and, in certain experiments, of NREM periods for portions of the day. It is the contention of some that when stress has been virtually eliminated* by painstaking procedural manipulations, the consequences of REM deprivation are not altered.

Our group at Stanford University concluded some years ago that REM periods per se were not necessary for the survival of adult mammalian organisms (Dement *et al.*, 1967). These conclusions were based on experiments in which

---

*In the cat, REM deprivation has been carried out by holding the polygraphically monitored cat and gently stroking it at the onset of REM periods. In such instances, the cat usually wakes up, interrupting REM, and starts purring.

cats were deprived of REMS for long durations up to 70 consecutive days with no serious impairment. In addition, we have concluded that REMS deprivation per se will not necessarily lead to behavioral changes suggestive of psychosis in animals or, as far as we know, in man (Dement *et al.*, 1969a). These conclusions have been supported by the recent report of Wyatt *et al.* (1969) on the effect of prolonged treatment with monoamine oxidase (MAO) inhibitors on sleep in man. These compounds are potent suppressors of REMS in both man and animals. REMS has apparently been eliminated for nearly a year in some narcoleptic and depressive patients with no obvious ill effect. This does not, however, deal with the possibility of dissociation. As has been noted elsewhere, the phasic events of REMS also occur in NREMS. In order to settle the question, we would have to know whether or not this phasic event discharge satisfied a "need" for REMS independent of the occurrence of REM periods.

Regardless of "need," selective deprivation of REMS by the nondrug method of interrupting REM periods just before they begin does produce some consequences. These may be listed under five categories: effects on sleep, effects on behavior, effects on brain excitability, effects on pharmacological responsiveness, and biochemical effects.

Effects on Sleep

Characteristic changes in sleep patterns in man and several other species both during and immediately following selective REMS deprivation have been described by many groups of investigators. These changes include the so-called REM rebound during which the fraction of TST occupied by REMS can reach very high levels, an increase in the "intensity" of REMS measured by size and frequency of muscle twitches and eye movements, and a more frequent occurrence of REM period onsets during the deprivation interval. The postdeprivation increase in REM time is so consistent that its failure to occur is considered by some to be cause for alarm. Such failure has been associated with both psychiatric (Zarcone *et al.*, 1968, 1969) and pharmacologically induced (Dement, 1969; Dement *et al.*, 1969b) abnormalities.

Some recent work in our laboratory has clarified the notion that REMS following selective deprivation is more "intense." In most cats, there does not appear to be an increase in overall rate of PGO spike discharge during REM periods following REM deprivation. There is, however, a dramatic increase in the tendency of PGO spikes to occur in bursts and in the rate and number of spikes in an individual burst. Since more intense bursts of spikes seem to produce, or are at least consistently associated with, more vigorous muscle twitches and more intense bursts of ocular motility, this process could be the major determinant of the "intensity" changes previously reported by Ferguson and Dement (1968).

Behavioral Changes

A few kinds of behavioral changes appear to be well established as a typical consequence of prolonged REM deprivation. They include changes in sexual behavior and eating behavior in cats (Dement *et al.*, 1967), and an augmentation of both aggressive behavior and sexual behavior in rats (Morden *et al.*, 1968a, b). In humans, there have been several inconclusive reports of rather ill-defined motivational changes during periods of REMS deprivation (Clemes and Dement, 1967; Sampson, 1966; Greenberg *et al.*, 1970). The overall concensus is probably that the behavioral change induced by deprivation is trivial when compared to the massive effort required to eliminate REMS for long periods of time.

Brain Excitability

An alteration of brain excitability is perhaps the most predictable consequence of REMS deprivation with the exception of the REM rebound. Experimental findings include decreased electroconvulsive shock (ECS) threshold in rats (Cohen and Dement, 1965), decreased ECS threshold in cats (Cohen *et al.*, 1970), prolongation of the tonic phase of tonic-clonic induced convulsions in mice (Cohen and Dement, 1970), more rapid recovery of auditory EP's in cats (Dewson *et al.*, 1967), and a change in the attention differential of EP's in human adults (Koppel *et al.*, 1971). These changes were all described during wakefulness.

Pharmacological Changes

The REM-deprived animal may undergo some change in his response to certain drugs. In general, the effective dose of REM-suppressive drugs is much higher if animals have been deprived of REMS for fairly lengthy periods. Unpublished results from the Stanford University Sleep Laboratory have shown that this is true for MAO inhibitors (nialamide and pargyline), barbiturates, and amphetamines. REMS deprivation may render a cat immune to the effects of *p*-chlorophenylalanine (PCPA), and there is a definite change in the response to reserpine. A fairly systematic study by Ferguson *et al.* (1969a) showed a differential response to 5-hydroxytryptophan (5-HTP) in the REM-deprived cat. These investigators suggested a change in 5-HT turnover as the basis for their findings. Finally, injections of *d*-amphetamine induce aggressive and sexual behavior in REM-deprived rats while identical injections in controls produce only restlessness and repetitive locomotor activities (Ferguson and Dement, 1969).

Biochemical Changes

Pujol *et al.* (1968a, b) have reported increased turnover of both noradrenaline (NA) and 5-HT in the brain of REM-depirved rats. Their results pertaining to 5-HT have been confirmed by Weiss *et al.* (1968) and pertaining to NA by Mark *et al.* (1969b). In addition to the monoamines, various investigators have reported changes in the metabolism of other brain constituents (Mark *et al.*, 1969a; Bowers *et al.*, 1966; Karadzic and Mrsulja, 1969).

In addition to the items listed above, casual observations in the laboratory led us to consider the possibility that multiple episodes of REMS deprivation in the same animal might produce either permanent change in some waking function or a progressively altered compensatory response after each successive deprivation episode (Dement, 1968). In a specific test of long-lasting change in waking functions, rats were tested for aggressiveness with shock-induced fighting as the measure. Six weeks after the last of four separate episodes of REMS deprivation, the experimental group was significantly more aggressive than a matched control group (Morden *et al.*, 1968a). On the other hand, we found no change in REM rebounds after successive deprivation episodes of equal duration. Two cats were deprived of REMS for 26 consecutive days, and 11 months later they were again deprived of REMS for exactly 26 days. The recovery REM rebounds following the first and second episodes were identical in both cats. Similar results were obtained with 2- and 5-day REM-deprivation episodes in rats. Not only did successive deprivations fail to elicit larger rebounds, but there were no differences in size of rebound compared to the response to a coincident first deprivation in age-matched controls. I have mentioned these findings in some detail because of their developmental implications.

In view of the failure to demonstrate a vital need for REMS or some component thereof in adult mammals by the technique of long-term REM deprivation, and in view of the fact that at least one component of REMS, namely, PGO spiking, also occurs in NREMS, we have considered the possibility that the major function of REMS is to discharge phasic activity. Such consideration can include an additional assumption that a "need" for REMS is satisfied when phasic activity can occur in sufficient quantity in NREMS during a period of REM deprivation, and this assumption might be invoked to explain the fact that there is no further increase in the amount of "extra" REMS after a certain duration of REM deprivation has been exceeded (Dement *et al.*, 1969a).

In order to test the crucial nature of phasic activities, Ferguson and his colleagues (Dement *et al.*, 1969a; Ferguson *et al.*, 1968) carried out experiments referred to as "spike deprivation" (Fig. 7). In these studies, cats were deprived of REM periods and, in addition, extraordinary efforts were made to prevent the occurrence of NREM PGO spikes. The effects of this procedure were compared to "classical" REMS deprivation in the same cats. Finally, a third procedure was instituted in which REM-deprivation arousals were conducted in such a way as to maximize the occurrence of PGO spikes in NREMS.

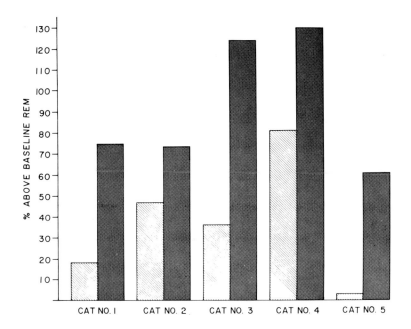

Fig. 17. Spike deprivation vs REM deprivation. The percentage elevation in total REM time on the first recovery day following 2 days of either REM deprivation (light bar) or spike deprivation (dark bar) is shown for all five cats in the series. Spike deprivation elicited a higher rebound in every instance. Large numbers of NREM PGO spikes occurred during the REM deprivation period of cat No. 1 and particularly of cat No. 5 which may have accounted for the relatively small rebounds (see text). (From Dement *et al.,* 1969a).

It was found that 2 days of spike deprivation were followed by larger REM rebounds than identical durations of "classical" REM deprivation, and that the latter was followed by higher rebounds than similar durations of REM deprivation which allowed maximal occurrence of NREM PGO spikes. Some of these results are shown in Fig. 17. Thus, in all three situations, an equal amount of REMS was eliminated and the size of the ensuing rebound appeared to be inversely related to the number of PGO spikes that occurred in NREMS during the deprivation period. However, these differential rebounds were only obtained in cats who were on 8- or 12-hr daily sleep schedules with the remainder of the period spent on a treadmill. When we attempted the same studies on cats who were recorded around the clock and could sleep *ad lib*, spike deprivation did not induce a higher rebound than REM deprivation. At the moment, we are at a loss to explain this result. We have also tested the possibility that there is a daily "quota" of phasic activity by counting the total number of PGO spikes/day in cats on a variety of sleep-wakefulness schedules. Even after lengthy periods of adaptation to each schedule, the postadaptation daily PGO spike totals show markedly different totals depending upon the particular schedule. However, it must be admitted that quantification of PGO spikes probably gives results of questionable accuracy, because of the wide variations in amplitude of individual spikes. Furthermore, the PGO spikes may not occur on a 1:1 basis with bursts of neural discharge in the putative system that generates phasic activity.

DISSOCIATIVE ASPECTS OF SLEEP AND WAKEFULNESS: IMPLICATIONS FOR SELECTIVE AND TOTAL SLEEP DEPRIVATION

We have suggested that the mammalian organism exists in one or other of three basic states. We know which state is present, by definition, when two or more specifically indicated independent neural processes are operating simultaneously. Obviously, total independence of any process or system in one brain is an idealized construct. Nonetheless, at least partial independence is strongly suggested when the activity or process appears to be able to function with relative ease at times other than during the state with which it is ordinarily associated. An example of this principle might be the occurrence of PGO spikes and phasic EMG suppressions in NREMS.

In addition to such instances of overlap that appear to be part of the normal organization of the sleep mechanisms, a number of dissociations have been produced by more drastic pharmacological and surgical manipulations, or are associated with disease. The classical finding in this vein is described in a report by Wikler (1952) on the effects of high doses of atropine in dogs. These animals showed waking behavior simultaneous with clear-cut NREMS patterns in the EEG (slow waves and spindles).

A very striking dissociation in cats can be accomplished by administration of compounds which cause a marked reduction in the level of 5-HT in the brain, notably PCPA and reserpine (Dement *et al.,* 1969b; Delorme *et al.,* 1965). In the former case, adequate treatment is associated with a spectacular occurrence of PGO spikes during what otherwise appears to be a normal waking state. A sample tracing from such an animal is shown in Fig. 18. In the animal given reserpine, PGO spikes, brain activation (low voltage, fast EEG), high levels of EMG activity, and somnolent behavior all occur simultaneously. By surgical ablation of the Nuc. locus coeruleus, Jouvet and Delorme (1965) have apparently produced a cat in whom REM periods are *not* associated with tonic or phasic motor inhibition. The disease of narcolepsy is characterized by multiple dissociative aspects (Dement, 1965a; Rechtschaffen and Dement, 1967); cataplectic attacks represent the dissociative occurrence of tonic motor inhibition, sleep paralysis may be regarded similarly, and finally, hypnagogic hallucinations may represent the dissociative activity of whatever neural system or systems ordinarily produce the dream imagery associated with REM periods.

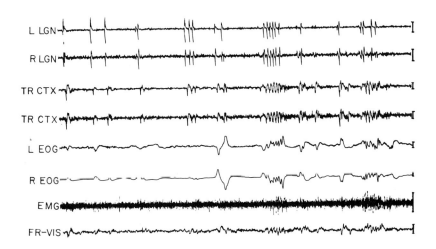

Fig. 18. Polygraphic sample from cat treated with *p*-chlorophenylalanine. LGN, lateral geniculate nucleus. TR CTX, transcortical EEG right and left visual cortex; EOG, electrooculogram; EMG, electromyogram from posterior neck muscles; FR-VIS, standard electrocorticogram from visual area. The animal is quiet, but completely awake. Except for the EMG, the sample could be typical of a REM period. Calibrations: 50 μV. (From Dement *et al.*, 1970. Reprinted with permission of the publisher.)

It seems clear that a frequent consequence of procedures which presumably damage the sleep mechanisms is some sort of dissociative manifestation. More to the point, the major behavioral states consist of several distinct and characteristic processes that occur simultaneously, and it appears possible to achieve a temporal dissection of these processes by experimental intervention. Given the results with surgical ablation and drugs, the next question is, can similar dissociations be produced by manipulations which are somewhat less damaging or drastic and complicated? We are, of course, speaking about the several deprivation approaches. Can total, partial, or selective sleep deprivation initiate or augment dissociative responses in the various sleep processes?

In terms of the latter question, the selective deprivation of REMS may give the clearest answer, because it is the one manipulation which can be accomplished with a high order of precision. The transition point between NREMS and REMS can be specified, in the cat at least, almost to the nearest second.

What are some of the dissociative consequences of REMS deprivation? We have alluded several times to the fact that the phasic activity most characteristic and defining of REM periods (PGO spiking) also occurs to a much lesser degree in NREMS. REMS deprivation appears to augment this tendency in at least two ways. In the "classical" technique of arousing the cat at the onset of each REM period, the frequency of such arousals increases markedly (i.e., the animal attempts to have REMS much more frequently). This means that the overall frequency of events immediately antecedent to the REM period onsets will also, by definition, be markedly increased. Since PGO spikes *always* precede REM periods (Fig. 7), the net result is to shift more phasic activity to NREMS. In addition, the phasic activity (PGO spikes) that takes place in NREMS is more intense. Thus, as Dement *et al.* (Dement *et al.,* 1969a; Dement, 1966) have speculated, this shift may finally result in the same amount of phasic activity occurring in NREMS during REMS deprivation as previously took place mostly within REM periods during the baseline sleep before the deprivation procedure was actually initiated.

A provocative possible consequence of REMS deprivation would be the shift of phasic activity to the waking state. We have recently demonstrated that such a shift can occur in the cat. Dr. Harry Cohen and Mr. George Mitchell REM-deprived two cats by arousing them at the onset of each successive REM period. The arousals took place during a daily 8-hr polygraphically recorded sleep session. During the remaining 16 hr of the day, they placed the cats on a slowly moving treadmill and monitored their PGO spike activity and EEG simultaneously and continuously via telemetry. They found a progressive increase in the occurrence of unequivocal REM-type PGO spike activity during wakefulness and/or drowsiness on the treadmill from one deprivation day to the next.

It is well known that in the sequence of physiological events characterizing the organismic shift from NREMS to REMS, EMG suppression usually precedes EEG activation by a few seconds, occasionally by a minute or more. In one of the early studies of long-term REMS deprivation in humans, Dement (1965b) reported that the gap between EMG suppression and EEG activation (NREM stage 2 to REM stage 1) underwent a steady enlargement. We have made similar observations again and again in feline REM deprivation studies. As far as is known, EMG suppression has never been shifted to the waking state, which is tantamount to saying that experimental cataplexy has never been produced by long-term REMS deprivation (Dement and Rechtschaffen, 1968). Along this line, it would be very informative to see if the frequency of cataplectic attacks during the day were increased by REM-depriving narcoleptic patients at night. Parenthetically, sleep onset REM periods are also a characteristic feature of the narcoleptic illness, and they have been produced by long-term REMS deprivation in both humans and animals (Dement *et al.*, 1967; Dement, 1965b). Of course, with regard to the premature occurrence of EMG suppression during NREMS, it is not clear whether this represents a shift of tonic motor inhibition into NREMS or a persistence of NREM EEG patterns into the REM period. Either way, a disturbance of the state regulating mechanisms is suggested, and the problem of defining whether or not the organism is in a given state is complicated.

It should also be mentioned that the opposite tendency is often seen, that is, a maintenance of tonic EMG activity well past the onset of the REM period unequivocally defined by EEG activation, eye movements, and muscular twitching (plus PGO spikes in the cat) in a recumbent subject. In our laboratory, this dissociation is most commonly observed in "free-running" cats who are being recorded on a 24-hr basis. Were it not for the directly observed occurrence of waking behavior, the totally insomniac PCPA cat would appear to be having essentially normal REM periods marred only by the persistence of tonic EMG potentials (Fig. 18). Finally, the occasional failure of EMG suppression during REM periods has been reported in chronic schizophrenics (Gulevich *et al.*, 1967).

Penile tumescence appears to be a consistent concomitant of REM periods in humans and monkeys (Fisher *et al.*, 1965; Karacan and Snyder, 1966). It has been reported that erections begin to occur in NREM sleep in humans if REM sleep is prevented from occurring (Karacan and Goodenough, 1966). If wild speculation is allowed, we might suggest that the increased sexual manifestations previously described as a behavioral consequence of REMS deprivation actually represented a dissociative shift to the waking state (as opposed to NREMS) of sexual activity ordinarily associated with REMS.

The selective deprivation of NREMS, leaving REMS intact, is not a feasible procedure. However, a short period, perhaps 2 or 3 days, of total sleep deprivation can be regarded as a close approximation to selective NREM deprivation, because the amount of NREMS that is lost is about three times greater than REMS, and a comparable duration (2 or 3 days) of selective REMS deprivation has a relatively small effect on the organism other than eliciting the characteristic recovery rebound. In other words, changes during 1, 2, or 3 days of total sleep loss (prolonged wakefulness) can be ascribed to the loss of NREMS. Partial sleep deprivation may represent the same thing to a lesser degree, since a partial reduction of total nightly sleep time in humans disproportionately effects REMS, because it occurs in larger amounts toward the end of the night. In rats and cats, on the other hand, the higher proportion of REMS is seen in the earlier parts of the sleep period.

At any rate, if we look at the consequences of total sleep deprivation, we see immediately that they can be regarded as dissociative. An extreme example was reported by Armington and Mitnick (1959) who found that sleep deprivation eventually produced subjects who appeared to be behaviorally awake, while their concomitantly recorded brain wave patterns were more or less continuously at the NREM stage 1 level. The most consistent result of modest amounts of total sleep loss in humans is the occurrence of "lapses" or "microsleeps" (Williams *et al.*, 1959). The elegant work of Harold Williams and his colleagues has firmly established the perceptual, behavioral, and EEG correlates of these microsleeps (Williams *et al.*, 1959, 1962; Lubin and Williams, 1959).

If we recall our discussion from an earlier section, the general mechanism of these consequences seems obvious. Additionally, it is no surprise to find that the frequency of microsleeps increases in a progressive fashion throughout any period of sleep loss. Since there is often no apparent interruption of gross waking behavior, we can regard these lapses as the dissociated occurrence of NREMS episodes in the waking state. Presumably, since perceptual shutdown can occur *before* EEG changes are apparent at the onset of sleep under ordinary circumstances (Fig. 1), there may be many more such episodes in sleep deprived subjects than EEG patterns alone would suggest. If we follow this line of evidence to its logical conclusion, we must assume that during an unusually long period of sleep loss, the increasing number of microsleeps would finally add up to a daily total that would, in effect, fulfil the organism's sleep requirement.

We were discussing results from adult human subjects in the foregoing paragraph. It is clear that microsleeps can occur even more readily in cats and rats. In a sense, the NREM systems become preemptive more quickly in these species. The same may also apply to newborn human infants, although prolonged sleep deprivation has not, and hopefully will not be done in such subjects. Thus, we may assume that experimental animals have no unusual difficulty discharging their NREMS requirement on a treadmill or any other sleep deprivation device during a period of sleep deprivation. In our laboratory, we find that when a cat is being "totally" sleep-deprived by confinement on a slowly moving treadmill, he quickly learns to walk to the front and ride back. The brief periods associated with each ride gradually develop into periods of full-blown EEG sleep, even though the animal is standing or sitting up. Eventually, the sleep episodes associated with rides begin to approach the amount of sleep seen in baseline recordings.

Although temporary psychosis does not appear to be a necessary consequence of prolonged sleep loss (Gulevich *et al.,* 1966), psychotic episodes during sleep deprivation have been reported by several groups of investigators (Bliss, 1967; West, 1967). We do not wish to dicuss this controversial area exhaustively, but we may speculate that deprivation-associated hallucinations, mood changes, and delusions represent the dissociated occurrence of REMS equivalents during wakefulness.

CONCLUSIONS

In view of all the things we have considered in this paper, we have arrived at the rather disappointing conclusion that it may be impossible for sleep deprivation studies to give us clear answers about the basic purpose or function of one or other of the major behavioral states, and at the very least, will certainly require heroic precautions to ensure that *all* manifestations of the state in question are completely eliminated for the entirety of the period, however brief.

The experimental and theoretical material that we examined suggests that a behavioral state may only represent an optimal situation for the occurrence of certain activities, and that under "pressure," these activities will readily occur at some other time. Thus, although we may be willing to entertain the hypothesis that any or all components of the two major sleep states are in some way an absolute necessity, we cannot easily design a crucial test. In other words, the consequences of the absence of the state of REMS or of NREMS cannot be fully explored because the "pressure" caused by deprivation techniques "pushes" the activity of the component systems into another state. In short, selective or total sleep deprivation are abstractions which cannot really be accomplished.

It is our tentative opinion, therefore, that we must begin to move away from the tendency to attribute unique and mysterious functions to the states of sleep and wakefulness. It may be better to view these states, rigorously defined to be sure (Anders *et al.*, 1971; Berger *et al.*, 1968), as the net result and outward manifestation of a confluence of several specific processes. This confluence has undoubtedly been encouraged by natural selection and may be partially understood in the light of the adaptive advantages gained therefrom. At this point, we may refer to the evolutionary theory of Snyder and Washburn (1966) which states that sleep has great adaptive advantages for mammals in fostering the conservation of caloric energy. Well and good, but the problem, in view of the short duration of NREM episodes previously mentioned, is to *maintain* sleep for long durations. It is our tentative speculation that REM periods fulfil this function, i.e., by providing a means by which the arousal systems can discharge and the NREM systems can "rest" without interrupting behavioral sleep.

In terms of this formulation, we might expect that REMS time would be enhanced when a large amount of behavioral sleep was advantageous, and would diminish (as would NREMS) if wakefulness was more advantageous, as in the mating season, when pursuing game, etc. In order for such an arrangement to work efficiently, there should be some kind of signal which tells the organism to remain asleep and to enter the REM state, as opposed to interrupting sleep and entering the aroused state. Such a signal should be activated by fatigue or prior periods of prolonged wakefulness, and indeed, many mammals respond to prolonged wakefulness by increasing *both* REMS and NREMS. Thus, from an adaptive point of view, the development of REM in mammals essentially constitutes an additional exploitation of the advantages of remaining asleep.

The large amounts of REMS in the newborn period may be considered as (a) a process which favors a minimum of physical activity and the conservation of caloric energy in the growing and helpless infant, (b) a way of providing internal stimulation to the developing nervous system, and (c) simply a consequence of neocortical immaturity which accordingly precludes the possibility of inhibiting REMS and arousal or some combination of the above.

At the present time, hard facts about the role of the sleep states, if any, in both the adult and developing organisms are in short supply. We may assume only that all of these processes and mechanisms are intimately involved in the overall developmental process.

REFERENCES

Anders, T., Emde, R., and Parmelee, A. (1971). "A Manual of Standardized Terminology, Techniques, and Criteria for Scoring of States of Sleep and Wakefulness in Newborn Infants." UCLA Brain Information Service/BRI Publications Office, Los Angeles, California.

Armington, J., and Mitnick, L. (1959). Electroencephalogram and sleep deprivation. *J. Appl. Physiol.* **14**, 247-250.

Berger, R. (1963). Experimental modification of dream content by meaningful verbal stimuli. *Brit. J. Psychiat.* **109**, 722-740.

Berger, R., Dement, W., Jacobson, A., Johnson, L., Jouvet, M., Monroe, L., Oswald, I., Roffwarg, H., Roth, B., and Walter, R. (1968). *In* "A Manual of Standardized Terminology, Techniques, and Scoring System for Sleep Stages of Human Subjects" (A. Rechtschaffen and A. Kales, eds.), Publ. No 204, US Govt. Printing Office, Washington, D.C.

Bliss, E. (1967). Sleep in schizophrenia and depression—studies of sleep loss in man and animals. *In* "Sleep and Altered States of Consciousness" (S. S. Kety, E. V. Evarts, and H. L. Williams, eds.), pp. 195-210. Williams & Wilkins, Baltimore, Maryland.

Bowers, M., Hartmann, E., and Freedman, D. (1966). Sleep deprivation and brain acetylcholine. *Science* **153**, 1416-1417.

Brooks, D., (1967). Localization of the lateral geniculate nucleus monophasic waves associated with paradoxical sleep in the cat. *Electroencephalogr. Clin. Neurophysiol.* **23**, 123-133.

Brooks, D., and Bizzi, E. (1963). Brain stem electrical activity during deep sleep. *Arch. Ital. Biol.* **101**, 648-665.

Broughton, E. (1968). Sleep disorders: Disorders of arousal? *Science* **159**, 1070-1078.

Clemes, S., and Dement, W. (1967). Effect of REM sleep deprivation on psychological functioning. *J. Nerv. Ment. Dis.* **144**, 485-491.

Cohen, H., and Dement, W. (1965). Sleep: changes in threshold to electroconvulsive shock in rats after deprivation on "paradoxical" phase. *Science* **150**, 1318-1319.

Cohen, H., and Dement, W. (1970). Prolonged tonic convulsions in REM-deprived mice. *Brain Res.* **22**, 421-422.

Cohen, H., Thomas, J., and Dement, W. (1970). Sleep stages, REM deprivation and electroconvulsive threshold in the cat. *Brain Res.* **19**, 317-321.

Delorme, F., Jeannerod, M., and Jouvet, M. 1965). Effets remarquables de la reserpine sur l'activité EEG phasique ponto-geniculo-occipitale. *C. R. Soc. Biol.* **159**, 900-903.

Dement, W. (1965a). An essay on dreams: the role of physiology in understanding their nature. *In* "New Directions in Psychology," Vol. II, pp. 135-257. Holt, New York.

Dement, W. (1965b). Studies on the function of rapid eye movement (paradoxical) sleep in human subjects. *In* "Aspects anatomofonctionnels de la physiologie du sommeil" (M. Jouvet, ed.), pp. 571-611. CNRS, Paris.

Dement, W. (1966). Toward an evolutionary theory of dreaming: discussion. *Amer. J. Psychiat.* **123**, 136-142.

Dement, W. (1968). The psychophysiology of REM sleep, its function and possible clinical relationships. *In* "Mind as a Tissue" (C. Rupp, ed.), pp. 214-236. Harper, New York.

Dement, W. (1969). The biological role of REM sleep (circa 1968). *In* "Sleep: Physiology and Pathology" (A. Kales, ed.), pp. 245-265. Lippincott, Philadelphia, Pennsylvania.

Dement, W. (1970). The nature and function of sleep. *In* "Neuroelectric Research: Electroneuroprosthesis, Electroanesthesia, and Nonconvulsive Electrotherapy" (D. Reynolds and A. Sjoberg, eds.), pp. 171-204. Thomas, Springfield, Illinois.

Dement, W., and Rechtschaffen, A. (1968). Narcolepsy: Polygraphic aspects, experimental and theoretical considerations. *In* "The Abnormalities of Sleep in Man" (H. Gastaut, *et al.*, eds.), pp. 147-164. Aulo Gaggi Editore, Bologna.

Dement, W., and Wolpert, E. (1958). The relation of eye movements, body motility, and external stimuli to dream content. *J. Exp. Psychol.* 55, 543-553.

Dement, W., Henry, P., Cohen, H., and Ferguson, J. (1967). Studies on the effect of REM deprivation in humans and in animals. *In* "Sleep and Altered States of Consciousness" (S. S. Kety, E. V. Evarts, and H. L. Williams, eds.), pp. 456-486. Williams & Wilkins, Baltimore, Maryland.

Dement, W., Ferguson, J., Cohen, H., and Barchas, J. (1969a). Nonchemical methods and data using a biochemical model: the REM quanta. *In* "Psychochemical Research in Man" (A. Mandell and M. P. Mandell, eds.), pp. 175-325. Academic Press, New York.

Dement, W., Zarcone, V., Ferguson, J., Cohen, H., Pivik, T., and Barchas, J. (1969b). Some parallel findings in schizophrenic patients and serotonin-depleted cats. *In* "Schizophrenia: Current Concepts and Research" (S. Sankar, ed.), pp. 775-811. PJD Publications, New York.

Dement, W., Halper, C., Pivik, T., Ferguson, J., Cohen, H., Henriksen, S., McGarr, K., Gonda, W., Hoyt, G., Ryan, L., Mitchell, G., Barchas, J., and Zarcone, V. (1970). Hallucinations and dreaming. *In* "Perception and its Disorders" (D. Hamburg, ed.), pp. 335-359. Williams & Wilkins, Baltimore, Maryland.

Dewson, J., Dement, W., Wagener, T., and Nobel, K. (1967). Rapid eye movement sleep deprivation: a central-neural change during wakefulness. *Science* 156, 403-406.

Ferguson, J., and Dement, W. (1967). The effect of variations in total sleep time on the occurrence of rapid eye movement sleep in cats. *Electroencephalogr. Clin. Neurophysiol.* 22, 2-10.

Ferguson, J., and Dement, W. (1968). Changes in the intensity of REM sleep with deprivation. *Psychophysiology* 4, 380-381.

Ferguson, J., and Dement, W. (1969). The behavioral effects of amphetamine on REM deprived rats. *J. Psychiat. Res.* 7, 111-118

Ferguson, J., Henriksen, S., McGarr, K., Belenky, G., Mitchell, G., Gonda, W., Cohen, H., and Dement, W. (1968). Phasic event deprivation in the cat. *Psychophysiology* 5, 238.

Ferguson, J., Henriksen, S., Cohen, H., and Dement, W. (1969a). The effect of REM sleep deprivation on the response to 5-hydroxytryptophan in cats. *Psychophysiology* 6, 221.

Ferguson, J., Cohen, H., Barchas, J., and Dement, W. (1969b). Sleep and wakefulness: a closer look. *In* Neurohumoral Aspects of Sleep Wakefulness." *Fed. Amer. Soc. Exper. Biol.* 1969.

Fisher, C., Gross, J., and Zuch, J. (1965). Cycle of penile erection synchronous with dreaming (REM) sleep. *Arch. Gen. Psychiat.* 12, 29-45.

Greenberg, R., Pearlman, C., Fingar, R., Kantrowitz, J., Kawliche, S. (1970). The effects of dream deprivation: implications for a theory of the psychological function of dreaming. *Brit. J. Med. Psychol.* 43, 1-11.

Gross, M., Goodenough, D., Tobin, M., Halpert, E., Lepore, D., Perlstein, A., Sirota, M., Dibianco, J., Fuller, R., and Kishner, I. (1966). Sleep disturbances and hallucinations in the acute alcoholic psychoses. *J. Nerv. Ment. Dis.* 142, 493-514.

Gulevich, G., Dement, W., and Johnson, L. (1966). Psychiatric and EEG observations on a case of prolonged (264 hours) wakefulness. *Arch. Gen. Psychiat.* 15, 29-35.

Gulevich, G., Dement, W., and Zarcone, V. (1967). All-night sleep recordings of chronic schizophrenics in remission. *Comp. Psychiat.* 8, 141-149.

Hodes, R., and Dement, W. (1964). Depression of electrically induced reflexes ("H-reflexes") in man during low voltage EEG sleep. *Electroencephalogr. Clin. Neurophysiol.* 17, 617-629.

Jones, B., Bobillier, P., and Jouvet, M. (1969). Effets de la destruction des neurones contenant des catécholamines du meséncephale sur le cycle veille-sommeils du chat. *C. R. Soc. Biol.* **163**, 176-180.

Jones, H., and Oswald, I. (1968). Two cases of healthy insomnia. *Electroencephalogr. Clin. Neurophysiol.* **24**, 378-380.

Jouvet, M. (1969). Biogenic amines and the states of sleep. *Science* **163**, 32-41.

Jouvet, M., and Delorme, F. (1965). Locus Coeruleus et sommeil paradoxal. *C. R. Soc. Biol.* **159**, 895-899.

Jouvet-Mounier, D., Astic, L., and Lacote, D. (1970). Ontogenesis of the states of sleep in rat, cat, and guinea pig during the first postnatal month. *Develop. Psychobiol.* **2**, 216-239.

Kales, A., Jacobson, A., Paulson, M., Kales, J., and Walter, R. (1966). Somnambulism: Psychophysiological correlates. I. All-night EEG studies. *Arch. Gen. Psychiat.* **14**, 586-594.

Karacan, I., and Goodenough, D. (1966). REM deprivation in relation to erection cycle during sleep in adults. *Pap., Ass. Psychophysiol. Study Sleep.*

Karacan, I., and Snyder, F. (1966) Erection cycle during sleep in *Macaca mulatta.* (Preliminary report.) *Pap., Ass. Psychophysiol. Study Sleep.*

Karadzic, V., and Mrsulja, B. (1969). Deprivation of paradoxical sleep and brain glycogen. *J. Neurochem.* **16**, 29-34.

Koella, W. (1969). Neurohumoral aspects of sleep control. *Biol. Psychiat.* **1**, 161-177.

Koppel, B., Zarcone, V., de la Pena, A., and Dement, W. (1971). Changes in selective attention as measured by the visual averaged evoked potential following REM deprivation in man. *Electroencephalogr. Clin. Neurophysiol.* (1972, in press).

Lubin, A., and Williams, H. (1959). Sleep loss, tremor, and the conceptual reticular formation. *Percept. Motor Skills.* **9**, 237-238.

Mark, J., Godin, Y., and Mandel, P. (1969a). Biosynthesis of aspartic, glutamic, gamma-aminobutyric acids and glutamine in brain of rats deprived of total or paradoxical sleep. *J. Neurochem.*, **16**, 1263-1272.

Mark, J., Heiner, L., Mandel, P., and Godin, Y. (1969b). Norepinephrine turnover in brain and stress reactions in rats during paradoxical sleep deprivation. *Life Sci.* **8**, 1085-1093.

Michel, F., Jeannerod, M., Mouret, J., Rechtschaffen, A., and Jouvet, M. (1964). Sur les mécanismes de l'activité de pointes au niveau du système visuel au cours de la phase paradoxale du sommeil. *C. R. Soc. Biol.* **158**, 103-106.

Morden, B., Conner, R., Mitchell, G., Dement, W., and Levine, S. (1968a). Effects of rapid eye movement (REM) sleep deprivation on shock-induced fighting. *Physiol. Behav.* **3**, 425-432.

Morden, B., Mullins, R., Levine, S., Cohen, H., and Dement, W. (1968b). Effect of REMs deprivation on the mating behavior of male rats. *Psychophysiology* **5**, 241-242.

Mouret, J., Jeannerod, M., and Jouvet, M. (1963). L'activité électrique du système visuel au cours de la phase paradoxale du sommeil chez le chat. *J. Physiol. (London)* **55**, 305-306.

Noda, H., and Adey, W. (1970). Firing of neuron pairs in cat association cortex during sleep and wakefulness. *J. Neurophysiol.* **33**, 672-684.

Pivik, T., and Dement, W. (1970). Phasic changes in muscular and reflex activity during non-REM sleep. *Exp. Neurol.* **27**, 115-124.

Pivik, T., Halper, C., and Dement, W. (1969). NREM phasic EMG suppressions in the human. *Psychophysiol.* **6**, 217.

Pompeiano, O. (1969). Sleep mechanisms. *In* "Basic Mechanisms of the Epilepsies" (H. H. Jasper, A. A. Ward, and A. Pope, eds.), pp. 453-473. Little, Brown, Boston, Massachusetts.

Portnoff, G., Baekeland, F., Goodenough, D., Karacan, I., and Shapiro, A. (1966). Retention of verbal materials perceived immediately prior to onset of non-REM sleep. *Percept. Motor Skills* 22, 751-758.

Pujol, J., Hery, F., Durand, M., and Glowinski, J. (1968a). Augmentation de la synthèse de la setotonine dans le tronc cérébral chez le rat après privation selective du sommeil paradoxal. *C. R. Acad. Sci.* 267, 267-372.

Pujol, J., Mouret, J., Jouvet, M., and Glowinski, J. (1968b). Increased turnover of cerebral norepinephrine during rebound of paradoxical sleep in the rat. *Science* 159, 112-114.

Rechtschaffen, A., and Dement, W. (1965). Effect of visual stimuli on dream content. *Percept. Motor Skills* 20, 1149-1160.

Rechtschaffen, A., and Dement, W. (1967). Studies on the relation of narcolepsy, cataplexy, and sleep with low voltage random EEG activity. *In* "Sleep and Altered States of Consciousness" (S. S. Kety, E. V. Evarts, and H. L. Williams, eds.), pp. 488-505. Williams & Wilkins, Baltimore, Maryland.

Rechtschaffen, A., Molinari, S., Watson, R., and Wincor, M. (1971). Extraocular potentials: a possible indicator of PGO activity in the human. *Psychophysiology* (1972, in press)

Sampson, H. (1966). Psychological effects of deprivation of dreaming sleep. *J. Nerv. Ment. Dis.* 143, 305-317.

Snyder, F., and Washburn, S. (1966). Toward an evolutionary theory of dreaming. *Amer. J. Psychiat.* 123, 121-142.

Verdone, P. (1968). Sleep satiation—extended sleep in normal subjects. *Electroencephalogr. Clin. Neurophysiol.* 24, 417-423.

Weiss, E., Bordwell, B., Seeger, M., Lee, J., Dement, W., and Barchas, J. (1968). Changes in brain serotonin (5HT) and 5-hydroxy-indole 3-acetic acid (5HIAA) in REM sleep deprived rats. *Psychophysiology* 5, 209.

West, L. (1967). Psychopathology produced by sleep deprivation. *In* "Sleep and Altered States of Consciousness" (S. S. Kety, E. V. Evarts, and H. L. Williams, eds.), pp. 535-554. Williams & Wilkins, Baltimore, Maryland.

Wikler, A. (1952). Pharmacologic dissociation of behavior and EEG "sleep patterns" in dogs: morphine, N-allylnormorphine, and atropine. *Proc. Soc. Exp. Biol. Med.* 79, 261-265.

Williams, H., Lubin, A., and Goodnow, J. (1959). Impaired performance with acute sleep loss. *Psychol. Mongr.* 73, 1-26.

Williams, H., Granda, A., Jones, R., Lubin, A., and Armington, J. (1962). EEG frequency and finger pulse volume as predictors of reaction time during sleep loss. *Electroencephalogr. Clin. Neurophysiol.* 14, 64-70.

Wyatt, R., Kupfer, D., Scott, J., Robinson, D., and Snyder, F. (1969). Longitudinal studies on the effect of monoamine oxidase inhibitors on sleep in man. *Psychopharmacologia* 15, 236-244.

Zarcone, V., Gulevich, G., Pivik, T., and Dement, W. (1968). Partial REM phase deprivation and schizophrenia. *Arch. Gen. Psychiat.* 18, 194-202.

Zarcone, V., Gulevich, G., Pivik, T., and Dement, W. (1969). REM deprivation and schizophrenia. *Biol. Psychiat.* 1, 179-184.

INVITED DISCUSSION: HOWARD P. ROFFWARG

Dr. Dement has reexamined some of his conceptualizations, and he has attempted to update or "derigidify" our concepts of the REM and NREM "states." Those not in sleep research may wonder why he has taken such great pains to define the periods of REMS and

NREMS as "temporal conglomerations" of particular biochemical and neurophysiological processes rather than "temporally topographical states." It is because the former conception allows for the potential independence of mechanisms of systems that are customarily grouped within each state. The sleep states are not always absolutely distinct in time or in their physiological processes. Phenomena generally peculiar to one state are seen in the other. Surprisingly, however, sleep researchers at first were very taken with the idea that REM and NREM represented two qualitatively differentiated states; that certain systems operated wholly in one state and not in the other. Some revision of these concepts is long overdue and Dr. Dement is not alone in this effort.

Just as the boundary between waking and sleep may be indeterminate, the evidence is of course plain that within sleep we are not dealing with biologically unique states. For example, in the waking state (if we can forget for purposes of discussion that waking has many levels), we may get drowsy and a few lucky ones may even get to nap. Nevertheless, we know that sleep, once in progress, may occasionally be broken by arousals, as wakefulness may be "broken" by intervals of sleep. Hence, one does not consider it alarming that states or individual physiological features of states, may interrupt each other. So, too, certain processes of one sleep state may infrequently cross over to other sleep states. The K complex seen in the midst of REMS is not infrequent and is even legitimated by the latest scoring rules.

However, I should like to suggest that Dr. Dement refrain from blurring too many of the properties of REMS and NREMS. For no sooner will someone like Dr. Dement come along to speak against a too-static conception of sleep states than someone else in our field will claim that REM and NREM are differentiated hardly at all in the sense that "you see only a little more of this in one stage and a bit less of that in another stage, so are the stages really expressions of different states?" Before you know it, the recognition that dissociation and crossover of biological systems between states may be observed will be bastardized to support a unitary notion of sleep.

When it comes to defining sleep as a general state, I do not have a hard and fast notion. The determination of sleep vs waking rests largely on a descriptive behavioral base. Along with many others, I subscribe to the loose but seemingly unimprovable criterion that sleep is the behaviorally reversible situation when the eyes are closed and the individual is out of touch with his environment. In sleep, manifold yet highly specific neurophysiological and neurochemical systems operate and particular functions are executed. They comprise activating and inhibitory functions. But we should not lose sight of the fact that during behavioral sleep (don't call it sleep if you wish), two major groupings of processes cycle in tandem which are likely responsible for two generally different sets of functions.

Now let us take up the notion that so far as we know the PGO spikes are a kind of measurable physiological sine qua non of REMS. There is seeming perplexity over why PGO spikes appear in NREMS. They are first seen when slow waves are very much in evidence, before the commencement of the REM period as scored from the cortical EEG, eye movements, and EMG. According to Dr. Dement's figures, 15% of all PGO spikes occur in NREMS. Is not that fact in contradiction with the concept that PGO spiking is linked to the triggering of phasic phenomena in REMS? But who says that NREMS continues until and REMS begins at the point in time defined by cortical desynchronization and REM? Such scoring depends on criteria established before we knew of the existence of the PGO spike. State transitions in biological systems can never take place without a transition period. I think there is little doubt that a more supportable "beginning" of REMS corresponds to the inception of the PGO activation that leads to the final EEG desynchronization, dropout of muscle tone, and introduction of eye movements. In other words, REMS may very well begin before NREMS ends during a transition period.

In terms of the quandary as to whether the PGO spikes observed in (cortically defined) NREMS, before the beginning of the REMS period per se, are part of NREM or REM, I would like to afford you a military analogy. Let us say that there is a company of soldiers living in a camp. There is also a company command post where a colonel and his staff do their planning. The camp usually has a certain (basal) level of activity when the soldiers are going about camp functions and are not in combat. This level of activity in the camp corresponds to a certain level of activity in the company command post. One can determine that in such periods the colonel and his aides are in the command post a predictable number of hours per day. Messages go in and out of the command post and everything is quite routine.

Now let us say that tomorrow the company is going on maneuvers or into combat. If a Martian, or worse yet, a Viet Cong observer, were monitoring the level of activity in the command post (doing an objective count of how many people were going in and out, how long the lights were on, and the level of activity inside), he would notice an increase in these measures in relation to previous days. However, in spite of the increased activity in the command post, he would observe that the camp itself is still apparently functioning as before. Nevertheless, the observer would see that the following day the level of activity in the camp rises as the soldiers prepare to move out.

Now, if one were to ask if the elevated level of activity in the command post on the day before the soldiers moved out was part of the rest period or the combat period, how would one approach the problem? The orders relayed from the command post resulted in finally getting the troops out. Clearly, then, the heightened activity observed in the command post on the last day that the camp was functioning routinely had more to do with combat than with noncombat operations. One would not seriously claim that because one part of the camp worked for combat while the other part persisted in routine, it would mean that noncombative and combative enterprises could not be functionally differentiated. I hope the parallel to pre-REM PGO spikes is not overdrawn. The point is, that even if they occur in NREMS, they are features of REM activation.

Dr. Dement then goes further. He says that although most of the PGO activity found in NREMS falls into the period just in advance of REMS, one may actually record some PGO spiking all through NREMS. These sorts of dissociations and crossovers are prominent, as he points out, when REMS has been disturbed by deprivation of one sort or another. Nevertheless, Dr. Dement asks whether there are not "more apparent than real qualitative distinctions between the two sleep states." I think the distinctions are real but in a special sense. Let us first ask what is meant by the question, are the sleep states qualitatively different? First of all, it is problematical whether any two states entered into by a biological organism can be wholly different from each other from a qualitative point of view. In the case of an individual who is waking and sleeping, we have the same individual, the same brain, the same fundamental circuitry and neurochemical chains, but the organization of switch mechanisms in these systems and their levels of activity are probably state-related. The state differences are essentially a matter of the type of integration of manifold processes common to both states. These processes may be temporarily dissociable. For example, PGO spike activity may "break into" NREMS. This may indicate the possibility of predominant and subordinate states in simultaneous operation, or alternatively temporary interruptions of one state by a component of another. But this phenomenon does not make PGO activity willy nilly a feature of NREMS. If you will pardon another military example, surely we would agree that if a soldier unwittingly found himself behind enemy lines, he would not perforce have been transformed into a member of the enemy army.

In summary, I would accept Dr. Dement's implication that qualitative differences between states may be more apparent than real (though states can have qualitatively different functions). Differences between states can certainly be explained adequately by quantitative and organizational differences in the operation of systems. After all, ice and steam differ only in degree. But I ask Dr. Dement not to throw out the state baby with the qualitative bath water. For the concept of state differences in sleep need not be discarded simply because we are obligated to note that a state, or "temporal conglomeration" of particular processes, may be transitorily interrupted, mobilized, or incomplete in its operation. The concept of physiological state is probably meaningful only in signifying a predominant grouping of functioning systems which tend generally to remain in operation for a period of time. Specifically, states within sleep are most likely no less subject to temporary variation than are sleep and wakefulness.

This work concerns developmental aspects of sleep and Dr. Dement's paper is based on studies of sleep loss, so I will briefly turn now to a study undertaken by Tom Anders and me in which we sought to investigate sleep loss in infancy. Before summarizing our findings, however, I would like to acknowledge the fact that several investigators at the meeting have referred to the so-called "Roffwarg hypothesis." For the benefit of those present who are not familiar with this proposal, allow me to mention it. I have to implicate Dr. Dement, too, for we published this together in 1966 (Roffwarg *et al.*, 1966). Our idea of a "functional consequence of REMS significant to development" grew out of our joint findings that in the neonatal period there are short REMS-NREMS cycles, and sleep onset REM periods as well as an abundance of REMS which diminishes in amount with maturation. These findings have now been widely confirmed in other studies of developing neonates, and based on them we proposed that the REMS mechanism of the brain stem constitutes a CNS autostimulating system particularly important during uterine development and early postnatal life. These are times when the young organism is relatively cut off from external stimulation. Since there is evidence that growth and maintenance of neural tissue may be enhanced by stimulation, we suggested that the cyclic excitatory activation provided to much of the brain from within the brain during REMS might serve to augment differentiation of neuronal structures and help to lay down the rudiments of neurophysiological discharge patterns in the developing CNS. Accordingly, the consequence of this process would prepare the CNS for the influx of external stimulation as it progressively increases when uterine protection terminates and wakefulness replaces sleep. REMS would thus serve a "link trainer" function for the developing CNS.

Anders and I reasoned that one indirect way of working with this hypothesis, though not a direct test of it, was to investigate REM deprivation in the newborn. Specifically, we wondered whether deprivation of an interfeeding period of REMS would result in large rebounds of REMS. Sharp and exaggerated rebounds of REMS would tend to support a hypothesis that REMS is essential and vital to the functioning of the developing organism. Suffice it to say that we could not even effectively deprive the newborn of REMS. Perhaps this indicates how hard the newborn holds onto it. Furthermore, in a study of total sleep deprivation during interfeeding periods of newborns, REMS was not made up selectively any more than NREMS. As a support for the Roffwarg hypothesis, these results represent a failure. But one thing we learned was how difficult it is to deprive a baby of sleep. Even heroic efforts could not always arouse the infant.

REFERENCE

Roffwarg, H. P., Muzio, J. N., and Dement, W. C. (1966). Ontogenetic development of the human sleep-dream cycle. *Science* **152**, 604-619.

GENERAL DISCUSSION

Dr. Morgane: I am in accord with Dr. Dement's thesis that sleep is the product of a constant interplay of many systems. I do not think this point can be given enough emphasis when we consider the neural substructure underlying the sleep states to be a heterogeneous complex of cholinergic, noradrenergic, and serotonergic systems, among others. Of course, one of the main problems is to determine the nature of this interaction, and the systems serve as checks and balances on each other. A second key point Dr. Dement discusses is that a confluence of systems is "balanced" against one another, and when one has preempted the nervous system, it may actually be exhausting the transmitter. This is an extremely interesting concept, since it has usually been accepted that in a particular sleep state the biochemical mechanism for that state should be concomitantly elevated in the brain. However, if one looks at it the way Dr. Dement suggests, i.e., that the state is actually utilizing the neurochemical as a sort of "fuel" to burn on, then it is clear that at the end of such a state the biochemical substrate would be at a very low level in the brain. Biochemical measurements in these circumstances are just the opposite of what one might normally be tempted to think they should be. This relates to so-called concomitants of a behavioral state and when the animal, during a sleep phase, is actually killed to get the brain for chemical analysis. I think very few workers kill animals with intracardiac perfusion techniques while an animal is in a particular sleep state. I would stress that this is an extremely important point and deserving of much consideration by those who manipulate the brain biochemically after a given state has been dominant for a previous epoch.

Dr. Sterman: In terms of your scoring in the cat, Dr. Dement, we have found that posture is an exceedingly important determinant of EEG patterns in this animal. If the cat happens to be in a sphinx or sitting position instead of lying flat on the floor, spindle bursts are reduced and altered. He may start to go into an REM state, and then the loss of muscle tone awakens him and we find ourselves saying, "Dammit, lie down!" It seems to me, after seeing this sort of thing often, that a lot of what we observe in terms of these polygraphic patterns is rather capricious and dependent upon posture or other aspects of the animal's behavior. I believe that when you exhaust the animal on the treadmill, he lies down and then shows nice spindles.

Dr. Dement: I think posture is absolutely critical. We are really concerned that that is why animals, PCPA animals, stay awake. We call the peculiar position assumed by PCPA-treated cats the "PCPA crouch." We think that if the cat would only lie down flat, he would go to sleep. But we push him down and he gets up and goes into that crouch. Whenever the head drops, it seems to wake him up and we think there is something about that posture that just seems to preclude full-blown sleep. We have not been able to think of a way to eliminate that postural tendency. I think some of the individual differences we see in cats in 24-hr recordings may be a function of posture. One cat is really relaxed; he just drops down. Another cat will sit there in that darn crouch.

Dr. Clemente: If PGO spikes are considered an important correlate of the REM state, can you tell us whether these spikes have been recorded in immature animals? Are they seen in the newborn, for example?

Dr. Dement: The only work I am familiar with is Garma's work in the rabbit (Verley *et al.*, 1969), where PGO spikes appear to be present in the newborn. An interesting finding was that the actual unit activity in the vicinity of cortical PGO spikes was not nearly as great as in the adult. But the PGO spikes are present in the newborn rabbit. Therefore, these electrical changes, and also muscle twitches and so on, indicate something is going on in the brain stem, if not the immature cortex.

Dr. Weitzman: When is an organism awake vs when is an organism conscious? We clinicians who see patients with neurological lesions are familiar with the syndrome resulting from lesions around the third ventricle and upper mesencephalic areas of the brain stem, in which the patient will have a sleep-waking cycle but never become conscious, that is, they are unable to have any perceptual or cognitive interaction. They respond in a minimal and primitive manner to their environment. One cannot verbally communicate with them and yet they will keep their eyes open, will sit, and if food is put in their mouths, they will chew it and swallow it. Some have used the term "coma vigil" to describe this peculiar state. In considering this issue, I have come to the conclusion that one can have a sleep-waking cycle go on, but not necessarily the ability to be conscious—i.e., to be aware of and respond to one's environment. I wonder whether wakefulness and consciousness really should not be separately considered in our understanding of these fundamental biological rhythmic processes?

Dr. Dement's view of the trading off of REM and wakefulness is an interesting concept. When we inverted the sleep-wake cycle in normal subjects, we found that we would awaken during the latter part of the day sleep period and thereby not have REMS. The time when REM should have occurred in those last 2 hr of the day's sleep would be taken by waking instead. This partially REM-deprived the subject and forced REMS to occur earlier in the sleep period. NREM stage 3-4 sleep, however, shifted immediately. These results will support the notion that REM and waking are somehow in a kind of reciprocal relationship.

Dr. McGinty: I can support Dr. Dement's observations on frequent changes in state during sleep and wakefulness. In the rat we see frequent changes in state during sleep, about every 100 sec. These events are very clear in the rat. The rat will wake up briefly, on the average of every 90 or 100 sec. We have quantified this; there seems to be a cyclicity in these brief arousals during sleep. I also wanted to comment on the augmentation of reflexes during active sleep in the kitten. The augmentation of reflexes is not specific to these brain stem reflexes. They have been described in ankle flexor and extensor monosynaptic reflexes. There is some evidence the augmentation is a presynaptic process and the motoneurons themselves are inhibited as they are in the adult. Iwamura (1971) stimulated the motoneuron pool directly and saw that postsynaptic inhibition is present in the neonate.

Dr. Anders: If an infant is kept awake for 210 min and then allowed to sleep undisturbed during the following interfeeding period, his recovery sleep exhibits the expected ratio of REM and NREM percents. We had predicted that there might have been a selective rebound of NREMS during the recovery sleep period.

Dr. Parmelee: We have been analyzing our baby sleep records in small epochs much the same way Dr. Dement has been analyzing his cat sleep records. We use 20-sec epochs which may be comparable to his 3-sec epochs in the cat, which has shorter state cycles than babies. As I tried to show in my presentation yesterday, when one looks at sleep states in small epochs like this, one finds that the 32-week premature has no more REMS than the term infant. This is because only 50% of the 20-sec epochs have eye movements at both ages. On the other hand, if one looks at longer epochs, ignoring short periods without eye movements, then the 32-week premature can be said to have much more active sleep (REMS). I am suggesting that the premature really does not have more REMS than the term infant.

This raises some questions about Dr. Roffwarg's theory of the significance of increased REM states in prematures, since his theory is based on the analysis of large epochs, ignoring the many small epochs within these that have no eye movements.

Dr. Dement: The actual movements of the eyes seem to be fairly vulnerable to alteration as opposed to more primary events. For example, a little barbiturate will wipe out eye movements but will not change REMS time much in the adult. Another thing is that you get large individual variation of what we call the PGO spike-to-eye movement ratio among cats. For some reason, some cats have much more eye movement per spike than other cats. We are assuming that PGO spikes are more primary. At any rate, I do not know how well eye movements reflect more important changes.

Dr. Parmelee: I think you missed my point. While the individual parameters of state change somewhat with maturation, the main difference between the premature and term infant is that the term infant can consolidate many small epochs of REMS into a continuous well-defined cycle of consecutive 20-sec epochs with eye movements.

REFERENCES

Iwamura, Y. (1971). Development of supraspinal modulation of motor activity during sleep and wakefulness. *In* "Brain Development and Behavior" (M. B. Sterman, D. J. McGinty, and A. M. Adinolfi, eds.), pp. 129-143. Academic Press, New York.

Verley, R., Garma, L., and Scherrer, J. (1969). Aspects ontogénètiques des états de veille et de sommeil chez les mammifères. *Bordeaux Med.* 2, 877-893.

16

Development of Sleep Patterns in Autistic Children*

Edward M. Ornitz

In this chapter, I will report a series of investigations of age-related changes during sleep in autistic children. The subjects suffer from a severe developmental disturbance of early childhood. The distinctive features of this syndrome are the inability to relate in the ordinary way to people and situations from the beginning of life, failure to use language for communication, and an anxious desire to maintain sameness in the environment (Eisenberg, 1968; Kanner, 1943). This is childhood autism which is manifestly a disorder of interpersonal and object relations (Kanner, 1949; Rank, 1949; Despert, 1951) and language (Rutter, 1968).

*Supported by a grant from NIMH (MH-13517).

CLINICAL CONSIDERATIONS

While the disturbances of interpersonal and object relationships and language are predominant features of the syndrome of childhood autism, there are other important clusters of symptomatology. There are disturbances of motility (Bender, 1947; Ornitz and Ritvo, 1968b) and the modulation of sensory input (Ornitz and Ritvo, 1968b; Bergman and Escalona, 1949; Goldfarb, 1961, 1963, 1964; Ornitz, 1969). Both the disturbances of motility and perception are characterized by symptoms suggesting behavioral excitation and behavioral inhibition. The motor excitation involves hand-flapping, excited whirling and circling, darting and lunging movements, and toe-walking. In contrast, motor inhibition is manifested by posturing and prolonged immobility. Those perceptual disturbances suggesting excitation involve facilitation of sensory input and are manifested both as overawareness of sensory stimuli and overreactivity to sensory stimuli. As examples of the heightened awareness of sensation, autistic children attend to sounds which they induce by scratching surfaces, banging on their own ears, and grinding their teeth. They regard detail overlooked by the normal child. They rub surfaces, noting subtle differences in texture. Examples of overreactivity to sensory stimuli include fearful reactions to both novel and intense sounds, distaste for foods with rough textures, and agitation induced by the proprioceptive and vestibular input provided by equilibrium play, elevators, and moving vehicles. Inhibition of sensory input is a prominent part of the syndrome. Autistic children disregard speech, may be underreactive to loud or sudden sounds, show complete disregard of their visual surroundings, let objects fall out of hand as if there were no tactile representation of the object, and may fail to react to painful bumps and falls. Thus, motor hyperactivity and hypoactivity are paralleled by disturbances of perception which are characterized by sensory overreactivity and underreactivity.

When the autistic child's environment is held constant, episodes of spontaneous sensory and motor overreactivity alternate randomly with periods of sensory and motor underreactivity (Sorosky *et al.*, 1968). A comprehensive view of the total behavior of these children thus suggests fluctuating states of consciousness characterized by excitation and inhibition. While in the normal child there is a balance and mutual regulation between internally generated facilitory and inhibitory influences and effects, in the autistic child the symptoms reflect an imbalance and failure of this regulation. In the normal child, excessive excitation is automatically and smoothly damped. In the autistic child, it persists or, alternatively, overinhibition occurs.

NEUROPHYSIOLOGICAL CONSIDERATIONS

In attempting to develop a neurophysiological approach to the above considerations, the work in my laboratory has been directed at the study of states of consciousness characterized by facilitation and inhibition of behavior. I have been particularly interested in a state of consciousness in which simultaneous facilitation and inhibition of motor expression and sensory responsivity occurs. Disturbance in such a state might provide a parallel to the behavioral state of the autistic child.

Rapid eye movement sleep (REMS) is characterized by both a state of tonic inhibition and tonic excitation. The tonic inhibitory state is manifested by muscular atonia, increased vestibular and mesencephalic reticular formation threshold for arousal, depression of H reflexes, and a tendency to decreased amplitude of sensory evoked responses (Ornitz and Ritvo, 1968a). Tonic excitation is suggested by an EEG similar to that of the waking state and also by heightened autonomic activity (Snyder *et al.*, 1964). Embedded in this matrix of tonic physiological balance between excitation and inhibition there are more significant phasically recurring episodes of heightened neurophysiological excitation and inhibition which are more extreme than the tonic events and may be mediated by different neurophysiological systems (Pompeiano, 1967a, b). The phasic excitatory events include the bursts of REM, reduced threshold for cortically stimulated movements, phasic dilation of the pupil, myoclonic twitching of the distal extremities, twitching of the middle ear muscles, enhancement of pyramidal discharges, and bursts of rapid-firing unit discharges from the medial and descending vestibular nuclei and other subcortical centers, and a heightened lability of heart rate, respiration, and blood pressure. The phasic inhibitory events include reduced amplitude of sensory-evoked responses, enhanced elevation of vestibular and mesencephalic reticular formation thresholds for arousal, and enhanced depression of H reflexes (Ornitz and Ritvo, 1968a). In general, the phasic excitation tends to involve the motor and autonomic systems, while the phasic inhibition tends to involve the sensory pathways.

In summary, REMS is a special state of consciousness characterized by a balance between strong excitatory and inhibitory influences which involve the regulation of motor expression and sensory receptivity. The most profound excitation and inhibition occur simultaneously during discrete periods of time synchronous with the bursts of REM themselves.

Work with autistic children in my laboratory has been based on the notion that if an imbalance between the excitatory and inhibitory influences of REMS exists, we would have a condition analogous to the behavioral state of childhood autism. For its heuristic value, I have taken this notion one step further and made the assumption that if the unbalanced and therefore unmodulated phasic excitatory and inhibitory events of REMS were to invade the waking state, we would have not only an analogy to the behavior of childhood autism but also a possible cause of it (Ornitz and Ritvo, 1968a). We have therefore studied certain of the neurophysiological events of REMS in young autistic and age-matched normal children. We have particularly looked at the phasic events synchronous with the REM bursts, because it is at such times that the excitatory and inhibitory influences are the strongest.

DEVELOPMENTAL CONSIDERATIONS

An important consideration in most studies of children is the changes with age that occur in the parameters under observation. Many of the symptoms of childhood autism, particularly those of inadequately modulated motor expression and sensory receptivity, seem to represent deviances from earlier developmental levels. For example, the echolalia of autistic children can be observed in normal toddlers around the 18- to 20-month level. The use of the other person as an extension of the self, characteristic of autistic children, may be observed in the 15- to 18-month-old child. The disturbances of motility and perception also suggest a maturational influence. The extensive rocking and head-banging of autistic children are transiently part of normal development (de Lissovoy, 1961). Toddlers may go through a brief period of toe-walking, which, in the autistic child, becomes a permanent part of his behavior (Colbert and Koegler, 1958). The hand-flapping of autistic children may be seen in 1- to 2-year-old children as a brief transient behavior associated with states of excitement. The difference, of course, is that in the normal toddler this behavior rapidly drops out, and when it does occur, it is spontaneously and automatically turned off. In the autistic child, on the other hand, it persists, often over many years, and the flapping episodes may not be transient but rather the flapping may reverberate for many seconds, and may recur frequently throughout the day. Sensory hypersensitivity and awareness of fine detail are also seen in early infancy. The rate and sequence of development is not characterized by either an even retardation or precocity in the achievement of developmental landmarks. Rather, development is characterized by a random sequence of spurts, lags, and plateaus. All of these observations have suggested a dysfunction of the maturational process in autistic children. This was originally suggested by Bender, based on observations of deviations of behavior from developmental norms at every level of development from birth on (Bender and Freedman, 1952).

This being the case, we can anticipate that in autistic children parameters of REMS, reflecting excitation and inhibition, might be similar to those of normal children at a younger age. Furthermore, since spontaneous improvement in the disturbances of motility and perception often occurs as autistic children grow older, we might expect that any abnormal parameters of REMS in younger autistic children would tend toward more normal values with increasing age. With these considerations in mind, we have studied some of the events of REMS in normal individuals of different ages.

SLEEP STUDIES IN NORMAL SUBJECTS

The percent of total sleep time during which REMS occurs and the period of the REMS-NREMS cycle were studied as a measure of the global organization and maturation of sleep patterns. Higher percentages of REMS time tend to be associated with immaturity. This has been demonstrated in comparative studies of the sleep cycle of neonates and older infants (Stern *et al.*, 1969; Roffwarg *et al.*, 1966). The amount of EEG activity in the frequency range of sleep spindles occurring during REMS was quantified as a measure of the differentiation of REMS from NREMS. Decreased differentiation is associated with immaturity. An increased amount of transitional sleep is found in premature babies (Parmelee *et al.*, 1967), and REMS patterns containing spindle frequencies occur in the premature and neonate but disappear in the 3-month-old baby (Parmelee *et al.*, 1968a,b). The number and the duration of the eye movement bursts were studied as an index of the phasic motor excitatory activity of REMS. The relative amplitude of the averaged auditory evoked response (AER) to clicks during the eye movement bursts of REMS was studied as a measure of phasic sensory inhibitory activity during REMS.

After adaptation to the sleep laboratory, a group of six nonpsychotic children, ranging in age from 4½ to 10½ years showed a mean value of 20.2% REMS time

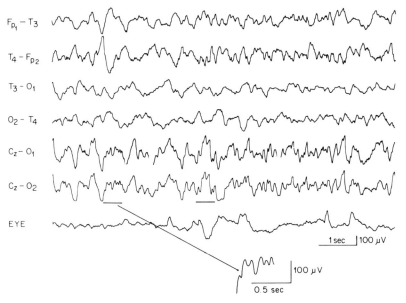

Fig. 1. Underlined segments of EEG were judged as 10.5-15.0 Hz waves. Note proximity of this activity to a burst of rapid eye movements in 8-month-old baby.

(Ornitz *et al.*, 1965). This result is consistent with that of other laboratories.

The number of occurrences of EEG activity in the frequency range of sleep spindles per minute of REMS time was determined in a group of 6- to 8-month-old normal babies and a group of 19- to 45-month-old normal children. The first two REMS periods of the night were compared. The EEG was scored second by second from the first to the last REM burst. Any spindle frequency activity that did not occur within 60 sec of an eye movement burst was considered a transition to stage 2 EEG and was therefore not scored. Each episode must be at least 0.5 sec in duration to be scored. Figure 1 shows the appearance of this activity in a baby. Figure 2 compares the amount of spindle frequency activity during REMS in babies and older normal children. The babies' REMS EEG contained significantly more of this activity (Ornitz *et al.*, 1971). This suggests that the REMS EEG is not fully differentiated until after the first year of life.

The number and duration of REM bursts were measured in the same groups of

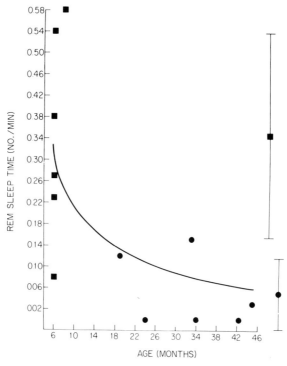

Fig. 2. The amount of spindle frequency activity (10.5-15.0 Hz) during the first two REM sleep periods as a function of age in normal babies and children. (■) 6 babies, 6-8 months; (●) 6 normal children, 19-45 months. A hyperbolic curve was fitted to the data by the least squares method. Means and standard deviations for the groups of babies and children are also shown. There is significantly more of this activity during REM sleep in the babies than in the children ($P = 0.012$).

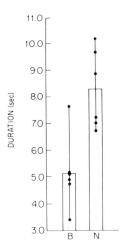

Fig. 3. Group mean and individual values for the duration of rapid eye movement bursts during the first two REM sleep periods in normal babies and children. The babies had significantly shorter bursts than did the children ($P = 0.004$). B = babies, 6-8 months; N = normal children, 19-45 months.

normal babies and children. An eye movement burst was defined as three or more successive eye movements, the interval between any two eye movements not exceeding 3 sec. Horizontal, vertical, and oblique eye movements were monitored on five channels of electrooculogram. The number of eye movement bursts was not significantly different in the babies and the children, but the duration of the eye movement bursts was significantly longer in the children (Ornitz *et al.,* 1971.) (Fig. 3). This finding suggests that the initiation of the epochs of phasic excitation is not decreased with immaturity, but that there is a diminished tendency to sustain the excitation in the first year of life.

The relative amplitude of a long-latency component (wave N-2) of the averaged AER to clicks was measured at the vertex during the REM bursts of REMS in babies, children, and adults (Ornitz *et al.,* 1967, 1969b). Clicks were presented every 2 sec throughout the night at a constant intensity. Recording was bipolar (C_z-O_1 or C_z-O_2) and response amplitudes measured peak to peak were expressed relative to amplitudes obtained from stage 2 sleep of the same night for each subject. Figure 4 shows the relatively large amplitude of wave N-2 during the REM bursts of REMS in a baby. Figure 5 shows the suppression or inhibition of wave N-2 which takes place in an older child during the eye movement bursts of REMS. Relative amplitudes of the averaged AER were expressed as ratios of amplitudes during the eye movement bursts of REMS to amplitudes during stage 2 sleep (Fig. 6). These relative amplitudes are high in infancy and decrease rapidly in early childhood to more mature levels. This finding suggests that phasic inhibition during REMS is not fully developed in the first year of life and that its complete expression may be part of a normal maturational sequence.

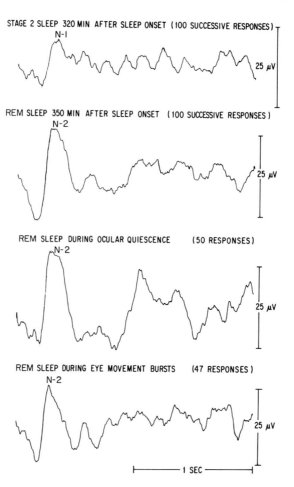

STAGE 2 SLEEP 320 MIN AFTER SLEEP ONSET (100 SUCCESSIVE RESPONSES)

REM SLEEP 350 MIN AFTER SLEEP ONSET (100 SUCCESSIVE RESPONSES)

REM SLEEP DURING OCULAR QUIESCENCE   (50 RESPONSES)

REM SLEEP DURING EYE MOVEMENT BURSTS   (47 RESPONSES)

Fig. 4. Averaged auditory evoked responses during stage 2 and REM sleep in a normal 6-month-old baby boy (vertex-occiput). Summations during ocular quiescent and eye movement burst epochs of REM sleep are not successive responses (From Ornitz *et al.*, 1969b.)

Studies in many laboratories have shown that the newborn spends about 50% of sleep time in the state of REMS (Stern *et al.*, 1969; Roffwarg *et al.*, 1966). This figure drops to about 20% by 3 years of age and the greatest decrement occurs in the first 12-18 months of life. It is during this same period of time that we found a rapidly increasing differentiation of the REMS EEG from NREM EEG patterns as evidenced by decreasing spindle frequencies. Of greater importance, it is during or just after this time that we found evidence for the rapid development of phasic excitatory mechanisms (increased eye movement burst duration) and phasic inhibitory mechanisms (increased inhibition of AERs). Thus the postnatal reduction of REMS time is accompanied by

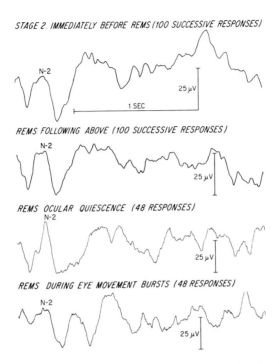

STAGE 2. IMMEDIATELY BEFORE REMS (100 SUCCESSIVE RESPONSES)

N-2

25 µV

1 SEC

REMS FOLLOWING ABOVE (100 SUCCESSIVE RESPONSES)

N-2

25 µV

REMS OCULAR QUIESCENCE (48 RESPONSES)

N-2

25 µV

REMS DURING EYE MOVEMENT BURSTS (48 RESPONSES)

N-2

25 µV

Fig. 5. Averaged auditory evoked responses in a normal child (female, 5 years 7 months old). Note suppression of wave N-2 during eye movement bursts of REM sleep. (Vertex-occiput.)

increasing differentiation and neurophysiological organization of this particular state of consciousness. The evidence suggests that motor excitation and sensory inhibition increase concurrently.

SLEEP STUDIES IN AUTISTIC CHILDREN

When autistic children were compared to normal individuals with respect to age and the parameters of REMS just described, several findings emerged. After suitable adaptation to the sleep laboratory, a group of seven 5- to 12-year-old autistic children showed no difference in the percent of REMS time when compared to age-matched normal children. Nor was the gross pattern of the REMS cycle within a night's sleep remarkable (Ornitz *et al.*, 1965). Figure 7 shows a stage 1 EEG associated with REM occurring in association with diminished chin muscle tone and increased autonomic reactivity in an autistic child. However, detailed examination of the EEG of REMS revealed activity in the frequency range of sleep spindles in the younger autistic children (Fig. 8). This activity diminished as the autistic children became older. When this activity was quantified for the first two REMS periods of each night, the younger autistic children had significantly more of this activity than age-matched normal

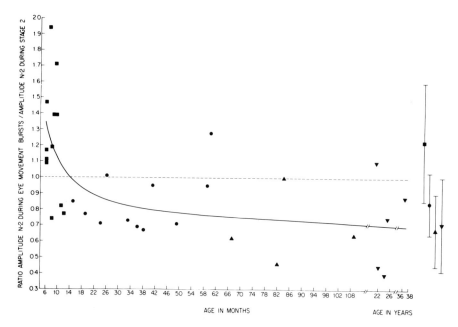

Fig. 6. Ratios of mean amplitudes of wave N-2 during the eye movement burst epochs of REM sleep compared with stage 2 sleep in normal babies, children, and adults. (■) 12 babies, 6-12 months; (●) 10 normal children, 19-60 months; (▲) 4 normal children, 67-109 months; (▼) 5 normal adults, 21-36.6 years. Ratios greater than 1.0 signify relatively larger mean amplitudes during eye movement bursts. Data are derived from Ornitz *et al.* (1967, 1968, 1969b). A hyperbolic curve was fitted to the data by the least squares method. Means and standard deviations for the different age groups are also shown. The babies had significantly higher ratios than those of the younger children (P = 0.006). The 15-month-old normal child was not included in this comparison.

children (Ornitz *et al.*, 1969a) and had values similar to those of normal babies. The data suggest that the decrement in amount of the spindle frequencies occurs at the same rate in respect to age in the autistic and normal children, but that the decrement begins later in life in the autistic children (Fig. 9). It can be concluded that the development of the differentiation of the REMS EEG is delayed in autistic children.

Quantification of the REM activity of the first two REMS periods of the night, using the eye movement burst as the unit of analysis, revealed shorter eye movement bursts in the younger autistic children as compared to the age-matched controls (Ornitz *et al.*, 1969a). The eye movement burst duration of the autistic children was similar to that of the normal babies and tended to increase as the autistic children became older (Fig. 10). In contrast the number of bursts per minute of REMS time was not different in the autistic and normal children. Therefore, it seems that those factors initiating phasic excitation during

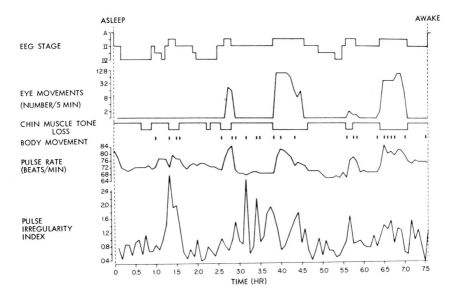

Fig. 7. One night's sleep in a 64-month-old autistic child. (Adapted from Ornitz *et al.*, 1965.)

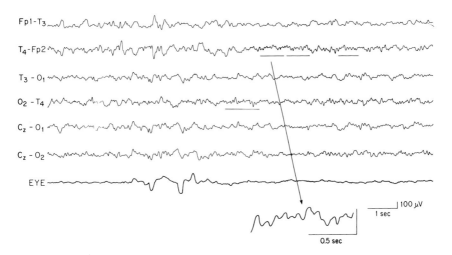

Fig. 8. 10.5-15.0 Hz activity during REM sleep in 31-month-old autistic boy. Underlined segments of EEG were judged as 10.5-15.0 Hz waves. Note proximity of this activity to a burst of rapid eye movements (From Ornitz *et al.*, 1969a).

REMS are not impaired in the autistic children. Rather, the influences sustaining the phasic excitatory events seem to be delayed in their development.

Comparison of the relative amplitude of the AER to clicks during the eye movement bursts of REMS in young age-matched autistic and normal children demonstrated a lack of phasic inhibition of the AER in the autistic children (Ornitz *et al.*, 1968). In fact, the autistic children tended to have relatively enhanced response amplitudes similar to those of normal babies (Ornitz *et al.*, 1969b). As the autistic children became older, there was a tendency toward lower relative amplitudes during the eye movement bursts (Fig. 11). Therefore, the development of phasic inhibition of afferent input is delayed in autistic children.

In summary, there is some evidence from these sleep studies of a maturational delay in the differentiation of sleep EEG patterns and the development of phasic excitatory and inhibitory mechanisms during REMS in autistic children. The delayed development of phasic excitation involves motor activity, while the delay in establishing phasic inhibition involves sensory input.

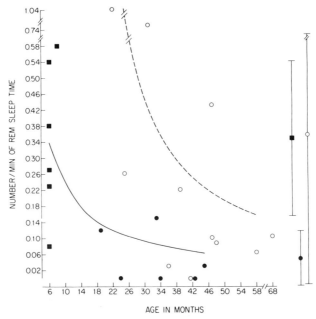

Fig. 9. The amount of spindle frequency activity (10.5-15.0 Hz) during the first two REM sleep periods in normal and autistic children. (■) 6 babies, 6-8 months; (●)6 normal children, 19-45 months; (○) 8 autistic children, 22-47 months. Data are derived in part from Ornitz *et al.* (1969a). Hyperbolic curves were fitted to the data by the least squares method. Means and standard deviations for the different age and diagnostic groups are also shown. The values for the eight autistic children between 22 and 47 months old are similar to those of the normal babies but are significantly greater than those of the six normal children ($P = 0.048$). The three extra values for the autistic children represent additional recordings when three of the autistic children were older.

CENTRAL VESTIBULAR MECHANISMS

To understand the nature of these maturationally related changes in phasic excitation and inhibition during REMS in autistic children, we can turn to experimental data obtained during the awake state. However, it is necessary to consider first the mechanism underlying these phasic events during REMS. It has been demonstrated in the experimental animal that all of the phasic excitatory and inhibitory events involving motility and perception during the ocular activity of REMS are mediated by and depend on the integrity of central vestibular mechanisms. This finding and its implications for a neurophysiology of sensorimotor integration should be credited to the brilliant and exhaustive studies of Dr. Ottavio Pompeiano and his colleagues at the University of Pisa (Pompeiano, 1967a, b). They have shown in the cat that lesions of the medial and descending vestibular nuclei eliminate all phasic inhibition of sensory input and spinal reflexes and all motor output associated with the REM bursts, including the eye movements themselves. They have further demonstrated an intense spontaneous discharge from neurons of these same vestibular nuclei synchronous with the ocular activity. In the human subject, the influence of vestibular mechanisms on the phasic activity of REMS has received partial confirmation. Nystagmus evoked by rotation can be most readily induced during sleep at the time of the REM bursts of REMS (Reding and Fernandez, 1968). In Wernicke-Korsakoff's disease, in which the vestibular nuclei are often damaged,

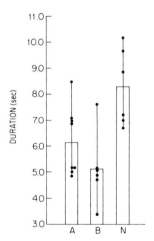

Fig. 10. Group mean and individual values for the duration of rapid eye movement bursts during the first two REM sleep periods in (B) normal babies (6-8 months), (N) normal children (19-45 months), and (A) autistic children (22-47 months). The values for the autistic children are not significantly greater than those of the normal babies but are significantly less than those of the normal children (*P* = 0.022). (Adapted from Ornitz *et al.*, 1971.)

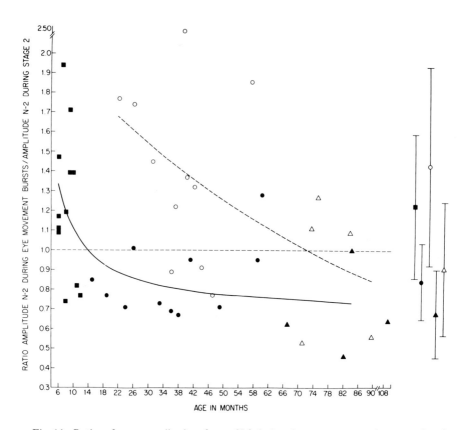

Fig. 11. Ratios of mean amplitudes of wave N-2 during the eye movement burst epochs of REM sleep compared with stage 2 sleep in normal and autistic children. (■) 12 babies, 6-12 months; (●) 10 normal children, 19-60 months; (○) 11 autistic children, 22-57 months; (▲) 4 normal children, 67-109 months; (△) 5 autistic children, 71-89½ months. Ratios greater than 1.0 signify relatively larger mean amplitudes during eye movement bursts. (Data are derived from Ornitz *et al.*, 1968, 1969b.) Hyperbolic curves were fitted to the data by the least squares method. Means and standard deviations for the different age and diagnostic groups are shown. The values for the younger autistic children are not significantly different from those of the normal babies, but are significantly greater than those of the younger normal children ($P = 0.003$). The 15-month-old normal was not included in these comparisons.

the REM are absent during REMS (Appenzeller and Fischer, 1968). An age-related development of phasic inhibition of auditory AER's during the ocular activity of REMS, and an age-related increase in the duration of the REM bursts themselves have been described in normal subjects in this paper. It can be inferred, therefore, that central vestibular influence underlies these phasic events, and that central vestibular control of phasic activity is not fully developed at birth but, rather, follows a maturational schedule.

Some analogous data are available from animal studies. In the adult cat, there is tonic suppression of the digastric reflex during REMS with maximal inhibition during the REM bursts. In the 2-week-old kitten, the digastric reflex is highly variable, and the pattern of inhibition does not develop until 4 weeks of age (Chase, 1970).

The implications of these considerations for a proposed pathoneurophysiology of central vestibular mechanisms in both childhood autism and adult schizophrenia have been developed elsewhere (Ornitz, 1970). In this chapter, I am suggesting that the maturational delay in the development of phasic inhibition and excitation during REMS may be related to a disturbance of central vestibular mechanisms in autistic children. Partial corroboration of this notion may be found in studies of vestibular reflexes in autistic children in the waking state. These studies have involved investigation of vestibularly induced nystagmus in autistic children.

When autistic children were rotated in a Barany chair, 10 revolutions in 20 sec, in a free visual field, the duration of the postrotatory nystagmus was markedly

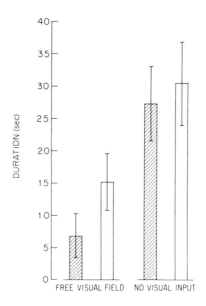

Fig. 12. The duration of postrotatory nystagmus in 22 normal children (☐) and 28 autistic children (▨) in a free visual field and in darkness. The values for the autistic children are similar to those of the normals in darkness but are significantly reduced in the free visual field ($P < 0.0001$). (Adapted from Ritvo *et al.*, 1969.)

reduced compared to age-matched normal children (Ritvo *et al.*, 1969). The nystagmus was measured by a DC electrooculogram, and the results were consistent with previous findings based on visual inspection of both postrotatory and calorically induced nystagmus (Colbert *et al.*, 1959). Thus, autistic children show reduced ocular motility, both in association with the spontaneous vestibular excitation during the eye movement bursts of REMS and in response to induced vestibular excitation in the waking state.

The reduced eye movement burst duration during REMS in autistic children is associated with a failure to manifest the normal phasic inhibition of sensory input, as described above. This suggests that the reduced eye movement burst activity may be related to excessive excitation from the sensory systems. In the waking situation, too, the reduced ocular activity is also related to sensory excitation. The reduced duration of the postrotatory nystagmus in the autistic child only occurs in the presence of visual input and does not occur in the dark (Ritvo *et al.*, 1969) (Fig. 12). Normally, activity of the vestibular nuclei may lead to inhibition of transmission of visual input at the level of the lateral geniculate nucleus (Pompeiano, 1967b; Marchiafava and Pompeiano, 1966). We might speculate, then, that this central vestibular control of sensory transmission may be disordered in autistic children. During REMS, there is the failure of vestibularly mediated inhibition of sensory evoked responses. In the waking state, this speculation is much more inferential; we can, however, imagine that the overinhibition of postrotatory nystagmus may compensate insufficient suppression of visual input at the time of the nystagmoid eye movements. A normal suppression of visual input at the time of voluntary eye movements has been demonstrated (Duffy and Lombroso, 1968).

CONCLUSION

In conclusion, the maturational delay in the organization and control of motor expression and sensory receptivity is paralleled by a delay in the maturation of the REMS EEG and the development of phasic excitation and inhibition during REMS in autistic children. Considerations derived from the experimental neurophysiology of REMS and studies of vestibular nystagmus in autistic children implicate central vestibular mechanisms in the genesis of this disorder. Centrally, the vestibular system may be involved in the modulation and integration of motor output and sensory transmission. This seems to be the case, both in the waking state and during REMS (Pompeiano, 1967b; Cook *et al.*, 1968; Lenzi *et al.*, 1968).

The experiments reviewed in this chapter provide some tentative evidence that this central regulatory function of the vestibular system suffers a maturational disruption in autistic children. It is possible that this postulated vestibular dysfunction disrupts the modulation of motor output and sensory input, both during waking and REMS in the autistic child. An alternative possibility is that the postulated vestibular dysfunction may permit the inadequately modulated phasic motor and sensory events of REMS to break into the waking state.

SUMMARY

Clinical observations of autistic children have suggested that fundamental symptoms of the syndrome of childhood autism involve disturbances of motility and perception. The nature of these disturbances indicates a maturational delay in the development of complex motor patterns and the modulation of sensory input. The behavior of autistic children also suggests an imbalance between excitatory and inhibitory CNS influences. Sleep studies have provided some evidence for a maturational delay in the differentiation of REMS patterns and the development of phasic excitatory and inhibitory mechanisms during REMS in these children. These findings implicate a failure of central vestibular control over sensory transmission and motor output during REMS. The notion that there is a dysfunction of central vestibular mechanisms underlying the delayed organization and differentiation of the REMS state is supported by observations of altered vestibular nystagmus in the waking state in autistic children.

REFERENCES

Appenzeller, O., and Fischer, A. P., Jr. (1968). Disturbances of rapid eye movement during sleep in patients with lesions of the nervous system. *Electroencephalogr. Clin. Neurophysiol.* **25**, 29-35.

Bender, L. (1947). Childhood schizophrenia. Clinical study of one hundred schizophrenic children. *Amer. J. Orthopsychiat.* **17**, 40-56.

Bender, L., and Freedman, A. M. (1952). A study of the first 3 years in the maturation of schizophrenic children. *Quart. J. Child Behav.* **4**, 245-272.

Bergman, P., and Escalona, S. K. (1949). Unusual sensitivities in very young children. *Psychoanal. Stud. Child.* **3-4**, 333-352.

Chase, M. H. (1970). Brain stem polysynaptic reflex activity in the kitten and adult cat during sleep, wakefulness and arousal. *Annu. Meet., Ass. Psychophysiol. Study Sleep, 1970.*

Colbert, E. G., and Koegler, R. (1958). Toe walking in childhood schizophrenia. *J. Pediat.* **53**, 219-220.

Colbert, E. G., Koegler, R., and Markham, C. H. (1959). Vestibular dysfunction in childhood schizophrenia. *Arch. Gen. Psychiat.* **1**, 600-617.

Cook, W. A., Jr., Cangiano, A., and Pompeiano, O. (1968). Vestibular influences on primary afferents in the spinal cord. *Pfluegers Arch. Gesamte Physiol. Menschen Tiere* **299**, 334-338.

de Lissovoy, V. (1961). Head banging in early childhood. A study of incidence. *J. Pediat.* **58**, 803-805.

Despert, J. L. (1951). Some considerations relating to the genesis of autistic behavior in children. *Amer. J. Orthopsychiat.* **21**, 335-347.

Duffy, F. H., and Lombroso, C. T. (1968). Electrophysiological evidence for visual suppression prior to the onset of a voluntary saccadic eye movement. *Nature (London)* **218**, 1074-1075.

Eisenberg, L. (1968). Psychotic disorders in childhood. *In* "The Biologic Basis of Pediatric Practice" (R. Cooke, ed.), pp. 1583-1591. Mc-Graw-Hill (Blakiston), New York.

Goldfarb, W. (1961). "Childhood Schizophrenia." Harvard Univ. Press, Cambridge, Massachusetts.

Goldfarb, W. (1963). Self-awareness in schizophrenic children. *Arch. Gen Psychiat.* **8**, 47-60.

Goldfarb, W. (1964). An investigation of childhood scizophrenia: A retrospective view. *Arch. Gen. Psychiat.* **11**, 620-634.

Kanner, L. (1943). Autistic disturbances of affective contact. *Nerv. Child.* **2**, 217-250.

Kanner, L. (1949). Problems of nosology and psychodynamics of early infantile autism. *Amer. J. Orthopsychiat.* **19**, 416-426.

Lenzi, G. L., Pompeiano, O., and Satoh, T. (1968). Input-output relation of the vestibular system during sleep and wakefulness. *Pfluegers Arch. Gesamte Physiol. Menschen Tiere* **299**, 326-333.

Marchiafava, P. L., and Pompeiano, O. (1966). Enhanced excitability of intrageniculate optic tract endings produced by vestibular volleys. *Arch. Ital. Biol.* **104**, 459-479.

Ornitz, E. M. (1969). Disorders of perception common to early infantile autism and schizophrenia. *Compr. Psychiat.* **10**, 259-274.

Ornitz, E. M. (1970). Vestibular dysfunction in schizophrenia and childhood autism. *Compr. Psychiat.* **11**, 159-173.

Ornitz, E. M., and Ritvo, E. R. (1968a). Neurophysiologic mechanisms underlying perceptual inconstancy in autistic and schizophrenic children. *Arch. Gen. Psychiat.* **19**, 22-27.

Ornitz, E. M., and Ritvo, E. R. (1968b). Perceptual inconstancy in early infantile autism. *Arch. Gen. Psychiat.* **18**, 76-98.

Ornitz, E. M., Ritvo, E. R., and Walter, R.,D. (1965). Dreaming sleep in autistic and schizophrenic children. *Amer. J. Psychiat.* **122**, 419-424.

Ornitz, E. M., Ritvo, E. R., Carr, E. M., Panman, L. M., and Walter, R. D. (1967). The variability of the auditory averaged evoked response during sleep and dreaming in children and adults. *Electroencephalogr. Clin. Neurophysiol.* **22**, 514-524.

Ornitz, E. M., Ritvo, E. R., Panman, L. M., Lee, Y. H., Carr, E. M., and Walter, R. D. (1968). The auditory evoked response in normal and autistic children during sleep. *Electroencephalogr. Clin. Neurophysiol.* **25**, 221-230.

Ornitz, E. M., Ritvo, E. R., Brown, M. B., La Franchi, S., Parmelee, T. M., and Walter, R. D. (1969a). The EEG and rapid eye movements during REM sleep in normal and autistic children. *Electroencephalogr. Clin. Neurophysiol.* **26**, 167-175.

Ornitz, E. M., Ritvo, E. R., Lee, Y. H., Panman, L. M., Walter, R. D., and Mason, A. (1969b). The auditory evoked response in babies during REM sleep. *Electroencephalogr. Clin. Neurophysiol.* **27**, 195-198.

Ornitz, E. M., Wechter, V., Hartman, D., Tanguay, P. E., Lee, J. M. C., Ritvo, E. R., and Walter, R. D. (1971). The EEG and rapid eye movements during REM sleep in babies. *Electroencephalogr. Clin. Neurophysiol.* **30**, 350-353.

Parmelee, A. H., Jr., Wenner, W. H., Akiyama, Y., Schultz, M., and Stern, E. (1967). Sleep states in premature infants. *Devel. Med. Child Neurol.* **9**, 70-77.

Parmelee, A. H., Jr., Akiyama, Y., Schultz, M. A., Wenner, W. H., Schulte, F. J., and Stern, E. (1968a). The electroencephalogram in active and quiet sleep in infants. *In* "Clinical Electroencephalography of Children" (P. Kellaway and I. Peterson, eds.), pp. 77-88. Almqvist & Wiksell, Stockholm.

Parmelee, A. H., Jr., Schulte, F. J., Akiyama, Y., Wenner, W. H., Schultz, M. A., and Stern E. (1968b). Maturation of EEG activity during sleep in premature infants. *Electroencephalogr. Clin. Neurophysiol.* **24**, 319-329.

Pompeiano, O. (1967a). The neurophysiological mechanisms of the postural and motor events during desynchronized sleep. *In* "Sleep and Altered States of Consciousness" (S. S. Kety, E. V. Evarts, and H. L. Williams, eds.), pp. 351-423. Williams & Wilkins, Baltimore, Maryland.

Pompeiano, O. (1967b). Sensory inhibition during motor activity in sleep. *In* "Neurophysiological Basis of Normal and Abnormal Motor Activities" (M. D. Yahr and D. P. Purpura, eds.), pp. 323-372. Raven Press, New York.

Rank, B. (1949). Adaptation of the psychoanalytic technique for the treatment of young children with atypical development. *Amer. J. Orthopsychiat.* 19, 130-139.

Reding, G. R., and Fernandez, C. (1968). Effects of vestibular stimulation during sleep. *Electroencephalogr. Clin. Neurophysiol.* 24, 75-79.

Ritvo, E. R., Ornitz, E. M., Eviatar, A., Markham, C. H., Brown, M. B., and Mason, A. (1969). Decreased postrotatory nystagmus in early infantile autism. *Neurology* 19, 653-658.

Roffwarg, H. P., Muzio, J. N., and Dement, W. C. (1966). Ontogenetic development of the human sleep-dream cycle. *Science* 152, 604-619.

Rutter, M. (1968). Concepts of autism: A review of research. *J. Child Psychol. Psychiat.* 9, 1-25.

Sorosky, A. D., Ornitz, E. M., Brown, M. B., and Ritvo, E. R. (1968). Systematic observations of autistic behavior. *Arch. Gen. Psychiat.* 18, 439-449.

Snyder, F., Hobson, J. A., Morrison, D. F., and Goldfrank, F. (1964). Changes in respiration, heart rate and systolic blood pressure in human sleep. *J. Appl. Physiol.* 19, 417-422.

Stern, E., Parmelee, A. H., Akiyama, Y., Schultz, M. A., and Wenner, W. H. (1969). Sleep cycle characteristics in infants. *Pediatrics* 43, 65-70.

17

Sleep in Mental Retardation

Olga Petre-Quadens

Investigations of the polygraphic aspects of sleep in man have shown that both the amount and type of sleep undergo extensive modifications as a function of physiological or pathological conditions (Petre-Quadens, 1969).

Changes in the patterns of sleep have been described in senescence with declining intellectual function and in elderly patients suffering from chronic brain syndrome (Lairy *et al.*, 1962; Passouant *et al.*, 1965; Feinberg *et al.*, 1965). There are, however, relatively few studies of sleep alterations as a function of mental retardation in young children.

There are many different types of mental retardation. Some of the varieties may be identified by clinical, anatomopathological, or biochemical methods. It was first hypothesized that by comparing the sleep alterations as they occur in identified cases, some of the physiopathological mechanisms of their sleep-waking cycle might be identified, and that electrophysiological variations might be specifically related to different etiological groups of mental retardation.

Reciprocally, it was thought that this approach would provide some interpretation of the sleep characteristics seen in normal children.

It was at first sight a seductive hypothesis: mental retardation means indeed a "retarded maturation," but we shall see that the idea of a simple dissociation between somatic age and the development of the central nervous system (CNS) cannot be accepted without caution. One cannot exclude that a delay in maturation may be superimposed upon an early decline of some brain functions, as we shall see later.

We first tried to determine which alterations in sleep patterns are similar in different groups of oligophrenics. A number of our subjects were examined from birth. It would have been ideal to follow them for a long period of time, but we were able to do so in only a few cases. Most of the subjects were examined only once for a few consecutive nights.

Polygraphic night sleep recordings were made in 150 mentally retarded subjects (Tables XI, XII). They ranged in age from birth to 62 years. The electroencephalogram (EEG), electromyogram (EMG), respiratory rhythm, and electrooculogram (EOG) were recorded simultaneously.

In the analysis of the records, correlations between the features of the different parameters were made every 20 sec. Most of the subjects were recorded twice at a few days' interval. In our analysis, only the first recording was taken into account.

The results obtained in the mentally retarded subjects were compared to those of normal subjects of similar age taken as controls.

Every period of 40 sec during which two or more eye movements occurred was called rapid eye movements sleep (REMS) or paradoxical sleep (PS). The other sleep stages were classified according to Dement and Kleitman (1957). Moreover, a *new abnormality* appeared: more or less long periods of the sleep record were characterized by a low-voltage EEG with "sawtooth waves," without eye movements, and without EMG activity. This "indetermined sleep" (IS) does not belong to any of the classic sleep stages described by Dement and Kleitman (1957). It was not seen in all of the mentally retarded, and it was variable in the same subject from night to night. A small amount of IS was also seen in normal subjects.

QUANTITATIVE VARIATIONS
OF THE SLEEP STAGES

Variability in Type of Sleep during Consecutive Nights

In the normal adult, there is a progressive increase in the percentage of PS on consecutive nights. In the mentally retarded subjects, there was an extreme variability of PS percentage and total sleep time (TST) on consecutive nights.

TABLE I *TST and PS (REM) Percentage of Two Mentally Retarded Subjects Followed for Protracted Periods[a]*

Name	Age	TDS (min)	(%)[b]REMS
P. Fr.	42	346	12.6
	43	496	23.7
	43	420	14.4
	43	525	29.2
	43	489	24.4
T. Cl.	30	420	3.8
	36	315	16.1
	36	237 min 40 sec	6.4
	37	422	16
	37	201 min 40 sec	12.2
	38	412	17.8
	38	500	17.2
	38	520	22.1
	38	498	24.4

[a]From Petre-Quadens (1969).
[b]The last four percentages for each subject are for consecutive nights.

For this reason, in order to have a homogeneous series, we compared the results of the first night only in both groups of subjects (Table I).

Variability as a Function of Age

Since sleep research has proved to be a rich way of exploring the function of CNS, we compared the changes in percentage of the different sleep stages from childhood through adulthood in normal and mentally retarded subjects. The percentages of the various stages were calculated according to the TST. The periods of awakening during the night were not included as part of the TST.

Total Sleep Time (TST)

TST decreases with age in both mentally retarded and normal subjects. No differences in TST may be seen between mentally retarded and control subjects below age 5. Between ages 5 and 20 years, the TST decreases in the mentally retarded as compared to the control subjects (Table II). Between ages 20 and 35 years, the TST is variable in both groups.

Paradoxical Sleep (PS) Percentage

The percentages of the various sleep stages undergo considerable change as a function of age. The percentage of PS decreases after the age of 15 years in the mentally retarded, whereas it remains constant in the normal subjects until 62

TABLE II *Mean TST in Minutes, as a Function of Age, in Normal and Mentally Retarded Subjects[a]*

Age (years)	1-5	5-10	10-15	15-20	20-35	35-46	62
TST (min)[b] Normal subjects	388 (10)	509 (2)		458 (3)	388 (9)	–	277 (1)
Mentally retarded subjects	384 (8)	411 (14)	420 (7)	372 (6)	305 (5)	349 (4)	295 (1)

[a]From Petre-Quadens (1969). Numbers in parentheses: cases corresponding to each series.

TABLE III *Mean PS Percentage as a Function of Age in Normal and Mentally Retarded Subjects[a]*

Age (years)	1-5	5-10	10-15	15-20	20-35	35-45	62
PS (%) Normal subjects	23.8 (10)	17.8 (2)	18.9 (3)	18.9 (3)	21.6 (9)	–	20.8 (1)
Mentally retarded subjects	17.6 (8)	15.2 (14)	17.3 (7)	8.2 (6)	10.2 (5)	9.9 (4)	10.2 (1)

[a]From Petre-Quadens (1969). Numbers in parentheses: cases corresponding to each series.

(Table III). Since PS percent is the ratio of REM time to TST, its decrease could reflect either a decrease in the amount of eye movements or an increase in TST. Table II shows that in our subjects, the TST is similar in normal and mentally retarded adults. It therefore appears that the decrease in PS percent is due to a decrease in REM time (Table III).

States 1, 2, and 3

The percentage of stages 1, 2, and 3 taken together increases regularly with age in both groups. Below the age of 10 years, the mean percentage of these stages is lower in the mentally retarded than in the control subjects. After age 10, the percentage of stages 1, 2, and 3 is almost equal in both groups (Table IV). The data in the subjects over 35 are given *pro memoria* since their number is limited. Simultaneously, with a decrease in percentage of these stages below age 10 in the mentally retarded, a decrease in the amount of sleep spindles may be seen. We shall analyze this fact later on.

Stage 4

The percentage of stage 4 which regularly decreases with age in the normal subjects, is irregularly distributed in the mentally retarded. Below the age of 10,

TABLE IV *Mean Percent of Stages 1, 2, and 3 as a Function of Age* [a]

Age (years)		1-5	5-10	10-15	15-20	20-35	35-45	62
Stages 1, 2, 3 (%)	Normal subjects	54.9 (10)	59 (2)	62.2 (3)	62.2 (3)	69.8 (9)	–	76.5 (1)
	Mentally retarded subjects	45 (8)	49.7 (14)	62.5 (7)	66.8 (6)	71.8 (5)	75.1 (4)	64 (1)

[a]From Petre-Quadens (1969). Numbers in parentheses: cases corresponding to each series.

TABLE V *Mean Percent of Stage 4 as a Function of Age*[a]

Age (years)		1-5	5-10	10-15	15-20	20-35	35-45	62
Stage 4 (%)	Normal subjects	19.2 (10)	18.5 (2)	16.5 (3)	16.5 (3)	7.5 (9)	–	0 (1)
	Mentally retarded subjects	14.1 (8)	14.7 (14)	16.5 (7)	17.8 (6)	11.9 (5)	11.8 (4)	24 (1)

[a]From Petre-Quadens (1969). Numbers in parentheses: cases corresponding to each series.

the mean percentages are, however, lower in the mentally retarded than in the control subjects. The results beyond the age of 35 are given *pro memoria* because of the small number of cases (Table V).

Variability of the Sleep Stage Percentages as a Function of Total Sleep Time (TST)

In the mentally retarded subjects the percentage of PS increases when TST increases. On the other hand, in the normal subjects, the percentage of PS remains constant, whatever the TST may be (Table VI).

When extending this kind of analysis to stages 1, 2, and 3, we see that their percentage decreases from 89.4 to 41.7 as a function of TST in the mentally retarded, whereas it remains constant in the control subjects. Similar analysis of stage 4 percentage shows that it increases from 9.4 to 20.8 in the retarded, whereas it decreases from 15.8 to 10.9 in the control group (Table VI).

Discussion

Sleep alterations in mentally retarded subjects are rather complex. Percentages of the various sleep stages in the retarded approximate those of normal subjects between 10 and 15 years of age. On the one hand, we observe a significant decrease of PS percentage in the mentally retarded subjects. On the other hand, the increase of PS percentage in some subjects below the age of 15 exceeds the

TABLE VI　*Mean Percentages of Different Sleep Stages as a Function of Total Sleep Time (TST)*

	TST (min)	0-100	100-200	200-300	300-400	400-500	500-600	600
PS (%)	Normal subjects		20.7 (1)	21 (5)	19.2 (4)	22.6 (13)	23.8 (2)	
	Mentally retarded subjects	0.6 (2)	0 (2)	11.3 (8)	10 (14)	17.5 (9)	21.5 (7)	32.9 (9)
Stages 1, 2, 3 (%)	Normal subjects		58.5 (1)	62.4 (5)	65.9 (4)	61.7 (13)	62 (2)	
	Mentally retarded subjects	89.4 (2)	76 (2)	52.9 (8)	62.4 (14)	56.2 (9)	56.1 (7)	41.7 (9)
Stage 4 (%)	Normal subjects		15.8 (1)	15.5 (5)	12.1 (4)	11.8 (13)	10.9 (2)	
	Mentally retarded subjects	9.4 (2)	7.7 (2)	13.9 (8)	15.7 (14)	18.4 (9)	20.7 (7)	20.8 (9)

[a] From Petre-Quadens (1969). Numbers in parentheses: cases corresponding to each series.

normal values of REM and reaches 40%, i.e., that of normal and mature newborns (Fig. 1).

The maximal percentage of PS per sleep cycle (40%) seems never to be exceeded. One may wonder why in the human being, except after REM deprivation, this proportion of REMS constitutes a limit. Also, one may wonder why in certain young mentally retarded subjects, the percentage of REMS is similar to that of the normal newborn, while the lowest values for REM are found, without exception, in adult retarded subjects. The significance of this decrease of REMS with age and its increase in some young retarded subjects is still unknown.

The decrease in percentage of PS is correlated with a decrease in eye movement density. Similar observations have been made by Feinberg *et al.* (1965) in older subjects with chronic brain syndrome. He termed REM every 20-sec epoch showing eye movement activity. He found a significant correlation between the degree of mental retardation, measured by the Wechsler test of intelligence, and the amount of REM.

The decrease of REM in mentally retarded subjects has been confirmed by Schmidt *et al.* (1968). They report observations similar to ours as regards the increase in the amount of sleep spindles toward puberty.

The decrease of TST in our subjects is related to the number of awakenings during the night. The mentally retarded are unable to sustain sleep for protracted periods. This relative insomnia does not seem to be due to anxiety as

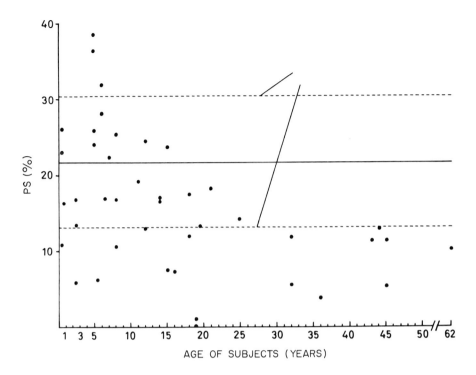

Fig. 1. PS percent as a function of age in 43 oligophrenics. Solid line, mean PS percent in control subjects; dotted lines, limits of PS percent in a normal population (= 2 s.d. from the mean value). (From Petre-Quadens, 1969.)

shown by the variability of sleep during consecutive nights (Table I). However, there is some evidence for a "first night effect." The awakenings appear often at the onset of a PS epoch but may also occur during any other stage, as shown by Feinberg (Feinberg *et al.*, 1965).

We do not find many changes in percentage of stage 4. The same observations have been made in adult retarded subjects (Lairy *et al.*, 1965; Gibbs and Gibbs, 1950).

Conclusions

In the oligophrenics, the following has been demonstrated: (1) The decrease in REM is correlated with a decrease in eye movement activity. (2) The decrease in percentage of stages 1, 2, and 3, below age 10, is accompanied by a decrease in sleep spindles. Spindles occur in shorter bursts and their frequency is slightly lower than in normal subjects. (3) No significant changes in percentage of stage 4 are seen. It has also been demonstrated that the sleep stage percentages vary as a function of TST.

TABLE VII *Mean Percentages of Different Sleep Stages as Compared to Four Normal Children of Same Age (5-15 years)*[a]

Subjects	No.	Stages 1, 2, 3 (%)	Stage 4(%)	PS (%)	IS (%)	TST (min)
Normal	4	60.6	17.5	18.3	2.3	415
Mongolians	10	54.98	20.08	20.39	3.2	501
Typus amstellodamensis	8	55.27	19.94	21.63	3.5	470

[a] From Petre-Quadens (1969).

RELATIONSHIP OF ETIOLOGY TO SLEEP VARIABLES IN THE MENTALLY RETARDED

Mongolism

Ten subjects with mongolism, who ranged in age from 5 to 15 years, had a normal percentage of PS, of stage 4, and of IS. An increase in TST and a decrease in the percentage of stages 1, 2, and 3 combined could be seen (Table VII).

The children with mongolism were clinically typical Down's syndrome but had not undergone chromosomal examination. This is emphasized because it is known that there are oligophrenics with the signs of Down's syndrome without chromosomal abnormalities.

Since mongolism is considered in its typical form to be related to a chromosomal error, it was of interest to analyze the sleep of children with other diseases of the same group.

Typus amstellodamensis

Eight children with *Typus amstellodamensis,* the Cornelia De Lange syndrome, have been studied (Table VII). Analysis of their sleep records showed changes similar to those found in mongolism. They had a normal percentage of PS, stage 4, and IS. TST was less increased, and the percentage of stages 1, 2, and 3 was less decreased than in the subjects with mongolism. One of our cases of *Typus amstellodamensis* has been confirmed by karyographic examination.

Metabolic Diseases

Among the congenital metabolic diseases, data were obtained from patients with phenylketonuria (PKU), homocystinuria, and glycinuria.

Cystinuria. Among the mentally retarded subjects examined, four were cystinuric siblings with hypotonia (Table VIII). They ranged in age from 9 months to 6 years. If the results of their night records are compared with those of normal children of the same age, a significant decrease in the percentages of

TABLE VIII   *Mean Percentages of Different Sleep Stages in Cystinuric Children as Compared to Normal Children of Same Age (1-5 years)[a]*

Subjects	Stages 1, 2, 3 (%)	Stage 4 (%)	PS (%)	IS (%)	TST (min)
Normal children, 1-5 years (10 cases)	54.9	19.2	23.8	9	388
Cystinurics (4 cases)	50.7	11.7	14.32	22.3	316

[a]From Petre-Quadens (1969).

TABLE IX   *Mean Percentages of Different Sleep Stages in PKU Children as Compared to Normal Children of Same Age (1-5 years)[a]*

Subjects	Stages 1, 2, 3 (%)	Stage 4 (%)	PS (%)	IS (%)	TST (min)
Normal children, 1-5 years (10 cases)	54.9	19.2	23.8	9	388
Phenylketonurics, 2½-7 years (6 cases)	52.2	12.8	15.7	19.3	349

[a] From Petre-Quadens (1969).

PS and stage 4 and a small decrease in the percentage of stages 1, 2, and 3 are seen. On the other hand, an important increase of IS and a decrease of TST is observed. In 1942, Van Creveld and Grünbaum had already described sleep disorders in cystinuric patients.

Phenylketonuria. Nine PKU subjects, including two pairs of twins, were recorded several times and the data compared with that obtained from normal subjects of the same age range. Both Tables IX and X show that the PKU subjects differ from normal subjects in their PS and IS percentages. There were no differences in the sleep stage percentages between the children with cystinuria and those with PKU.

Other Etiologies. A group of subjects with retardation of undetermined origin (Prader's disease and others) showed changes in their sleep stage percentages similar to those seen in other metabolic diseases. We also studied thesaurismosis, gargoylism, and Tay-Sachs diseases. In spite of the extent of the lesions, either neuronal, myeloaxonal, or mixed, these diseases do not lend themselves to anatomophysiological correlations. We mention them for reference only because the extreme variability of the results does not allow valid conclusions (Tables XI and XII).

TABLE X   *Mean Percentages of Different Sleep Stages in PKU Adults as Compared to Normal Adults (20-35) years)[a]*

Subjects	Stages 1, 2, 3 (%)	Stage 4 (%)	PS (%)	IS (%)	TST (min)
Normal adults, 20-35 years (9 cases)	69.8	7.5	21.6	1.8	388
Phenylketonurics, 19½ and 28 years (3 cases)	73.7	9.9	8.6	7.8	324

[a] From Petre-Quadens (1969).

TABLE XI *Mean Percentages of Different Sleep Stages in Various Types of Mental Retardation*

Diagnosis	No. of cases	Age (years)	Stages 1, 2, 3 (%)	Stage 4 (%)	PS (%)	IS (%)	TST (min)
Ataxia-telengiectasia	3	3½-8	38.6	1.4	15.1	44.9	348
Prader's disease	2	4 and 8	67.5	2.4	15.2	14.9	241
Tay-Sachs disease	2	1½ and 3½	30.1	3.4	22.4	44.1	400
Niemann-Pick disease	1	5	33.1	24	24.7	18.2	369
Bourneville's tuberous sclerosis	1	5½	52	3.1	5.5	39.4	107
Crouzon's disease	1	6	54.4	7.4	26.8	11.4	383
Lowe's disease	1	9	41.7	11	18	29.3	464
Francescetti's disease	1	9	59.2	12.8	22.1	5.9	348

Discussion

By further exploring the biochemical disorders in retarded subjects, correlations with the biochemical mechanisms of sleep may arise. Recent studies have shown that the metabolism of catecholamines (CA) and 5-HT is closely related to sleep mechanisms (Jouvet *et al.*, 1967).

In mongolism, the decrease in brain 5-HT is perhaps responsible for some of the pathological features of sleep (Schwartz-Tiene and Caredou, 1962). PKU, characterized by impaired conversion of phenylalanine (PA) into tyrosine,

TABLE XII   *Clinical Symptoms in Various Types of Mental Retardation*

Diagnosis	No. of cases	Age of our patients (years)	Clinical signs
Ataxia-telangiectasia	2	3½-8	Conjunctival telangiectasia, ataxia, mental retardation, recurrent bronchitis
Cranial dysostosis (Crouzon)	1	6	Cranial malformations, exophthalmia, optic neuritis, facial malformations, mental retardation
Glycinuria	1	5½	Nephrolithiasis, osteomalacia, glycosuria
Homocystinuria (Field *et al.*)	4	0.75-6	Mental retardation, osteoporosis, hyperlaxity, ocular impairment
Phenylketonuria (Fölling)	9	(6 cases) 2½-7 (3 cases) 19½-28	Blond hair, light blue eyes, special odor, convulsions, motor disorders, mental retardation
Tay-Sachs disease	2	1½ and 3½	Amaurosis, cherry-red macula, hypotonia or hypertonia, severe mental regardation
Mongolism (Down)	10	5-15	Particular aspect of the eyelids, tongue, feet, and hands
Niemann-Pick's disease	1	5	Hepatosplenomegaly, mental retardation, yellowish pigmentation of the skin, cherry-red macula, generalized hypertonia
Tuberous sclerosis (Bourneville)	1	5½	Mental retardation, epilepsy, adenoma sebaceum, shagreen skin
Lowe's disease	1	9	Male, glaucoma or cataract, mental retardation, hypotonia, tubular renal insufficiency
Franceschetti's disease	1	9	Mandibulo-facial dysostosis, mental retardation
Prader's disease	2	4 and 8	Absence or reduction of fetal movements, hypoglycemia, hypothyroidism, muscular hypotonia, mental retardation
Typus amstellodamensis (Cornelia de Lange)	8	5-15	Congenital muscular hypertrophy, extrapyramidal disorders, hirsutism, microcephalic, mental retardation

involves a disturbance of hydroxylation processes. In cystinuria, the enzyme deficiency involves the deaminating processes (Fanconi, 1945). It has to be kept in mind that cystinuria and PKU, characterized by disorders of the deamination and hydroxylation processes, respectively, show similar features in their sleep record.

Should we conclude that in all cases of mental deficiency, whatever their etiology, metabolic disorders of the monoamines occur? Or is the sleep disturbance a nonspecific phenomenon expressing a disorder of brain function? Whatever the case, the constancy of PS percentage which characterizes sleep in the normal human being, is considerably disturbed in the mentally retarded subjects. Similar findings in mentally ill patients (Lairy *et al.*, 1965) seem to indicate that the homeostasis of PS is closely linked to normal mental function. The "normalization" of the sleep stages of the mentally retarded subjects towards puberty, however, calls attention to a possible relationship to humoral and hormonal factors.

QUALITATIVE VARIATIONS

Besides the modifications in the amount and type of sleep, characteristic changes occurred within the sleep patterns of the mentally retarded. (1) Abolition of muscle tone at the level of the chin muscles exceeded considerably the REM epochs and could be seen with any EEG or EOG pattern. (2) Sleep spindles were rare. Their frequency was slightly decreased, and the bursts were shorter as compared to normal subjects. (3) During PS, the quantity of eye movements was decreased.

Muscle Tone

The disappearance of EMG activity has been considered to be one of the parameters defining PS (Jacobson *et al.*, 1964; Berger, 1961). In the retarded, the abolition was almost constant during PS but could occur in any other stage. The epochs of muscular activity and inactivity had a more "normal" distribution during sleep in the subjects with mongolism and the subjects with *Typus amstellodamensis* than in the others. With sleep stage percentages, positive correlations were found with age rather than with etiology. The epochs of abolition of muscle tone during stages 1, 2, 3, and 4 were, in the normal subject, longer when the child was younger. In the mentally retarded subjects (including subjects with mongolism and *Typus amstellodamensis*) hypotonia reached a minimum from age 10 to 15 years (Tables XIII and XIV).

Our data bear exclusively on the variations in tone of the chin muscles. In the normal subject, Berger (1961) noticed that the tonus was diminished in the

TABLE XIII *EMG Activity (Percent) during Sleep[a]*

Subjects	Stages 1, 2, 3		Stage 4		IS	
	EMG +	EMG −	EMG +	EMG −	EMG +	EMG −
Normal	94.4	4.6	99	1	−	−
Mongolians	79.7	21.3	67	33	−	100
Typus amstellodamensis	87.7	12.3	99.4	0.35	−	100
Cystinurics	3.4	96.6	−	100	4.8	95.2
Phenylketonurics	39.9	60.1	28.6	71.4	−	100
Unknown etiologies	82.6	17.3	66.3	33.7	−	100
Prader's disease	23.2	76 6	−	100	12.2	87.7
Gargoylism	−	100	−	100	−	100
Albinism	7.3	92.7	−	100	7.6	92.3

[a]From Petre-Quadens (1969).

TABLE XIV *Abolition of the EMG Activity (Percent) during Sleep (Stages 1, 2, 3, 4)[a]*

Age (years)	Normal subjects[b]	Mentally retarded subjects[b]
¼-5	14.7 (10)	55 (8)
5-10	9 (2)	55.7 (14)
10-15	9 (2)	12.8 (7)
15-20	2.4 (4)	30.4 (5)
20-25	2.4 (4)	30 (6)
25-30		30 (6)
35-40		37.5 (4)
62	0.9 (1)	56.1 (1)

[a]From Petre-Quadens (1969).
[b]Parentheses: number of cases.

external laryngeal muscles during PS. Hodes and Dement (1964) have shown that the reflex response evoked by stimulation of the posterior tibial nerve in man disappears during the epochs of eye movements. Jacobson *et al.* (1964) emphasize the fact that the submental EMG is abolished in only a small proportion outside PS. As regards the mentally retarded subjects, the abolition of the EMG is not a criterion of PS. There is thus a dissociation between the EMG and the other parameters (EEG and EOG) of PS. The "normalization" of the EMG in the retarded during stages 1, 2, 3, and 4 toward puberty (Table XIV) suggests, as do the changes in the sleep stage percentages, a possible endocrine or humoral influence.

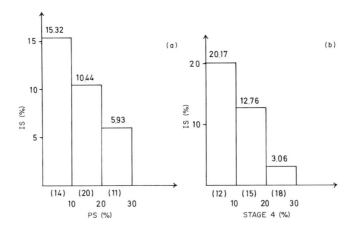

Fig. 2. (a) Percent of IS as function of PS percent. Number of cases in parentheses. (From Petre-Quadens, 1969.) (b) Percent of IS as function of stage 4 per cent. Number of cases in parentheses. (From Petre-Quadens, 1969.)

Spindles and Indetermined Sleep (IS)

We have seen that the epochs of IS in retarded subjects were longer below the age of 10 and that they decreased with age. They also decreased when the TST increased. It is difficult not to compare this relationship of the longest IS epochs to the shortest TST's with Table II showing that lower PS percentages correspond to shorter TST's. One might be tempted to assimilate the IS epochs with REMS without eye movements or during which the eye movements could have been so discrete that they had escaped both the recording and the observer. In order to verify this hypothesis, the distribution of IS as a function of PS and of stage 4 was studied (Fig. 2a, b). It appeared that IS developed simultaneously as a function of each one of these two sleep stages. As a result, one might question the relationship of IS to the spindle sleep stages.

Therefore, the sleep tracings of 29 mentally retarded subjects, ranging in age from 1 to 10 years, were selected and compared to those of 12 normal subjects of similar age taken as controls. Their mental deficiency was due to various causes. We compared these two groups, aged more than 1 year, cognizant of the fact that in each one of these groups, the subjects differed to some extent in brain maturation.

When analyzing the tracings, the percentages of the sleep stages were first calculated. Then the sequential association of PS with the other stages was determined, without reference to their respective duration. While spindles are considered to belong to stage 2, they may occur during stage 3. For simplification, all the 20-sec epochs of spindle sleep were called "stage 2." The following results were obtained.

TABLE XV *Mean Percentages of Stage 2, Indetermined Sleep, and Sum in Normal and Mentally Retarded Subjects[a,b]*

Age: 1-10 years	N	Stage 2 (%) [c]	IS (%) [d]	Stage 2 + IS (%)
Normal	12	48 S.D. = 5.44	7.3 S.D. = 5.33	55.3
Mentally retarded	29	32.6 S.D. = 16.91	24.3 S.D. = 15.44	56.9

[a]From Petre-Quadens (1969).
[b]Standard deviation is of mean values; individual values have a gaussian distribution.
[c]$p < 0.005$.
[d]$p < 0.001$.

1. Percentage of stage 2 was lower in the mentally retarded than in the normal subjects. On the other hand, IS percentage was higher in the retarded than in the normal children. The sum of the stage 2 and IS percentages was similar in both groups of subjects (Table XV).

2. The sequential association of PS with the other sleep stages was determined. In the normal subjects, PS most often preceded and followed stage 2 (Table XVI). In the retarded, PS was preferentially preceded and followed by IS (Table XVI). The sum of stage 2 and IS epochs (in percent) preceding PS is similar in mentally retarded and normal subjects. The same holds true for stages 2 and IS epochs following PS.

Table XVI shows that there is an inverse relationship between the amount of sleep stages with spindles and the amount of IS epochs without spindles. This inverse relationship is found by adding up the total amount of stage 2 and IS epochs during the night (Table XV), as well as by determining their frequential association with PS (Table XVI). The results suggest that IS in the mentally retarded subjects is the equivalent of stage 2. In parallel with the vanishing of stage 2, the retarded show a decrease of PS. Since we have assimilated with stage 2 all the epochs with spindles, the question of the relationship of sleep spindles to PS was raised. In the normal subject, Brebbia and Altschuler (1968) studying the metabolism of O_2 and CO_2 during sleep, showed that there is a significant parallelism between metabolic exchanges and sleep stages. These exchanges are maximal during PS, minimal during stages 3 and 4, and intermediate during stage 2.

In the newborn we noted that spindles occurred immediately before and at the beginning of PS, and we suggested that spindles might be related to one of the mechanisms responsible for the releasing of PS (Petre-Quadens, 1965, 1966). The vanishing of stage 2 in the retarded raises the question of whether the decrease of spindles is linked to the decrease of PS.

Metcalf and Jordan (1971) showed that the amount of spindles increases

TABLE XVI *Frequential Association of the Different Sleep Stages with Reference to REM[a]*

Subjects	Stage 1 → REM (%)	Stage 2 → REM (%)	Stage (3-4) → REM (%)	IS → REM (%)	Awake → REM (%)
Normal[b]	17.4	64.2	6.4	10.9	2
	(7)	(29)	(3)	(5)	(1)
Mentally retarded[c]	14.4	20.4	4	51.8	9.2
	(36)	(51)	(10)	(129)	(23)

	REM → Stage 1 (%)	REM → Stage 2 (%)	REM → Stage 3-4 (%)	REM → IS (%)	REM → Awake (%)
Normal[d]	18.2	56.1	0	11.3	13.6
	(8)	(26)	(0)	(5)	(6)
Mentally retarded[e]	12.4	21.6	0.8	50.2	14.8
	(31)	(54)	(2)	(125)	(37)

[a] From Petre-Quadens (1969).
[b] Number of REM in parentheses (total: 45). Stage 2 + IS → REM = 75.1%.
[c] Number of REM in parentheses (total: 249). Stage 2 + IS → REM = 67.4%.
[d] Total REM: 45. REM → Stage 2 + IS = 72.2%.
[e] Total REM: 249. REM → Stage 2 + IS = 71.8%.

rapidly in the normal child below 2 years of age. This increase slows down toward the age of 2 to 3 years, and the morphology of the spindles becomes steady. Later on, from ages 4 to 9 years, the stability of the spindles breaks down again.

The structures responsible for spindles have been located in the intralaminar thalamic nuclei. In cats, the orbital region of the frontal cortex seems also to be involved in their appearance (Velasco and Lindsley, 1965). The orbital cortex seems to be essential in the function of the thalamocortical synchronization mechanisms and to be part of a nonspecific system responsible for internal inhibition and sleep.

> The fact that in the mentally retarded subjects, behavior is particularly impaired in the areas of symbolic thought, language, and manual ability, fits in with the relative vulnerability of the supralimbic lobes of the brain during the prenatal and postnatal periods. The neuromorphological correlates of this behavioral impairment in mentally retarded subjects are to be found in the architectonic deviations of the supralimbic lobes, i.e., the reduction in the configuration of the supralimbic sulcus in the brain of the mentally retarded subjects (Yakovlev, 1959).

There are more spindles observed in normal children than in adults. We may reasonably assume that the thalamic structures are mature very early. The increase of spindles with maturation might therefore be attributed to the development of cortical function during the first years of life (Metcalf and Jordan, 1971).

However, in some mentally retarded subjects, hyperspindling has been described (Gibbs and Gibbs, 1962). Bixler and Rhodes (1968) recently reviewed this problem and found these "extreme spindles" in mildly retarded subjects. The retarded subjects in our study were suffering from severe mental deficiency. Spindles were missing and learning was extremely impaired. Although "extreme spindles" were found in five of our patients, they were associated with bruxism. Since bruxism has been reported to be related to the occurrence of "extreme spindles" (Reding *et al.*, 1968), we did not include these in our series.

In patients with mental illness, Lairy (1968) and Snyder (1965) described separately a sleep stage similar to the IS in retarded subjects. Greenberg (1966) showed that in lesions of the parietal lobe, spindles disappeared in the injured hemisphere, and PS decreased.

GENETIC ASPECTS OF SLEEP

Studies were made on the genetic aspects of some sleep abnormalities, such as narcolepsy (Sours, 1963), and its occurrence in identical twins (Imlah, 1961). Two pairs of identical twins were selected by strict criteria from our PKU patients.

Tables XVII and XVIII represent the mean percentages of the various sleep stages recorded for two consecutive nights in identical twins suffering from PKU with severe oligophrenia. The twins Len (Table XVIII) were recorded twice, at the age of 6 and again at age 7 years. It is remarkable that PS percentages remained constant in each of them over a 1-year interval. Since it was impossible to estimate the differences in stage percentages observed in these twins, the sleep patterns of the twins Ro and Wi (Table XVII) were compared with those of their sibling (Hu) suffering from the same disease. The only important difference resides in the low percentage of PS in Hu. His age is most likely the determining factor in this difference. As far as the other sleep stage percentages are concerned, they are not closer in twins than in siblings (Tables XVII-XIX).

An attempt to analyze phenotypes was made by a comparative study of sleep in siblings. Table XIX represents four siblings suffering from cystinuria and mental retardation. Table XX gives the data of the sleep records in two mildly retarded siblings suffering from an ill-defined metabolic abnormality (Sfaello and Hariga, 1967). Detailed clinical and biochemical data of the cases to which the six following figures refer, appeared in previous publications (Clara and Lowenthal, 1965). The data indicated that the sleep stage percentages in twins (Tables XVII and XVIII) did not differ from those found in siblings (Tables XIX-XXI). This fact indicates that the sleep stage alterations were dependent on some nonspecific factor perhaps related to learning capacities. Therefore, sleep

TABLE XVII *Sleep Stage Percentages in Three Mentally Retarded Siblings with Phenyl-ketonuria[a]*

Siblings[b]	Age (years)	PS	Stage 1	Spindles	Stage 4	IS
Ro	19	9.2	71.2	10.3	8.6	6.1
Wi	19	14.6	48	15.4	6.9	9.4
Hu	28	1.2	70.2	15.3	9.4	3.5

[a] From Petre-Quadens (1969).
[b] Ro and Wi are identical twins.

TABLE XVIII *Sleep Stage Percentages in Mentally Retarded Identical Twins with Phenylketonuria. Showing One-Year Differences[a]*

Twins	Age (years)	PS	Stage 1	Spindles	Stage 4	IS
Da	6	17.1	17.9	33.5	12.3	20.4
Gui	6	15.5	13.4	25.9	15.1	30.6
Gui	7	15.2	11.6	45.4	26.5	0.8
Da	7	18.8	9.2	50.6	21.9	0

[a] From Petre-Quadens (1969).

TABLE XIX *Sleep Stage Percentages in Four Mentally Retarded Siblings with Cystinuria[a]*

Siblings	Age (years)	PS	Stage 1	Spindles	Stage 4	IS
Ed	2	15.7	10.6	49.5	5.3	37.4
Na	5	8	27.3	24.5	14.1	31.1
Be	6	15.7	4.8	42.7	14.6	18.5
Pa	0.75	16.2	22.1	26.2	0.4	33.6

[a] From Petre-Quadens (1969).

patterns were investigated in mentally retarded patients and in their healthy siblings as well.

Table XXII gives the sleep stage percentages of five siblings. Four of them (Cl, Ja, Ch, and Li) were suffering from glycinuria, but only one (Cl) was severely retarded. Ja was a mildly retarded child. Two other siblings, Ch and Li, were glycinuric but mentally normal. Only in the two mentally retarded children was a decrease in PS percentage found. The PS percentage of their two siblings, also glycinuric but mentally normal, did not differ from that of their sibling Chris, only child of the family who was biochemically undamaged. The sleep tracing of their mother showed a normal PS percentage. She was glycinuric but mentally normal.

In conclusion, the percentages of the various sleep stages, compared in identical twins and in siblings, all mentally defective and with metabolic diseases,

TABLE XX *Sleep Stage Percentages in Three Mentally Retarded Siblings with Ataxia-Telangiectasia[a]*

Siblings	Age (years)	PS	Stages 1, 2, 3	Stage 4	IS
Lu	8	13.7	44.5	0	68.1
Lic	6	17.5	38.6	5.6	34.6
Ka[b]	1	15.6	51.4	3.7	29.1
Ka[b]	3	13.1	40.5	1.5	40.2

[a] From Petre-Quadens (1969).
[b] Ka was recorded twice at a 2-year interval.

TABLE XXI *Sleep Stage Percentages in Undifferentiated Mildly Retarded Siblings[a]*

Siblings	Age (years)	PS	Stage 1	Stage 2	Stage 3	Stage 4	IS
De	6	21.5	4.5	22.1	48.9	23	8
Pa	7	16.4	12.2	22.4	18	23.2	6.2

[a] From Petre-Quadens (1969).

were not different. Data in another family showed that the PS percentages were similar in siblings with metabolic disease, but mentally undamaged, and in a completely healthy sibling (Table XXII). The data are insufficient to draw a firm conclusion but support a relationship between sleep and cognition. Our results are similar to those obtained recently by Schmidt *et al.* (1968).

THE EYE MOVEMENTS OF SLEEP

The EOG recording is based upon the corneoretinal potential described by Dubois-Reymond (1848). From this discovery, we know that the eye is a polarized system, the retinal part of which is negatively charged as compared to the cornea. The difference in potential, independent of the lighting, is 5-6 μV.

Electrodes placed at the external epicanthi and the upper and lower orbits induce deflections on the EOG when eye movements occur. Changes in the corneoretinal dipole entail variations in the electric field between the electrodes. Moreover, the amplitude and the direction of the deflection vary according to the amplitude and the direction of the eye movements.

The EOG is calibrated at 6 mm for 50 μV, and the time constant is 0.3 sec.

This method has the advantage of demonstrating the eye movements when observation is difficult, but it is somewhat inaccurate. Indeed, brain waves or other artifacts may be recorded, and mislead the investigator. Within the framework of this study, it was, however, a minor problem because the same

TABLE XXII *Sleep Stage Percentages in Five Siblings and Their Mother*[a]

Subjects	Age (years)	PS	Stages 1, 2, 3	Stage 4	IS
Cl [b]	12	0	0	0	100
Li[c]	2	24.1	54.6	14.6	3.5
Ch[c]	4	31.3	47	14.8	5.1
Chris[d]	5	25.3	60.4	6.4	15.3
Ja[e]	10	10.9	66	25	0
Mother	33	18.5	77	14.8	5.1

[a] From Petre-Quadens (1969).
[b] Glycinuric and severely retarded.
[c] Glycinuric but mentally normal.
[d] Normal metabolically and mentally.
[e] Glycinuric and mildly retarded.

recording techniques were used for all subjects, and the same criteria were used for recognition of the eye movements.

The time intervals separating consecutive eye movements were measured in 22 subjects—15 mentally retarded and 7 normals. The mentally retarded subjects were selected by assessments of intellectual function by administration of the Wechsler scale of intelligence: I.Q. below 30 for 11 mental retardates; I.Q. close to 60 for 4 mental retardates. We included PKU and cystinuric patients as well as patients with metachromatic leucodystrophy and Prader's disease. As normal subjects, only children and adults without major physical, psychological, or cultural impairment were selected. The recordings, made at the clinic or at home, covered about 10 hr of physiological sleep for two consecutive nights. Of those two tracings, we considered only the second one, the record of the first night being frequently affected by experimental conditions.

PS was selected according to the following criteria: fast low-voltage tracing and the presence of REM. Measurements were made within the REM epochs, arbitrarily defined. In the analysis of the EOG, all clear-cut deflections of the baseline *not accompanied by a simultaneous deflection in the EEG* were considered as being eye movements. We were perhaps overscrupulous and therefore neglected genuine eye movements because they coincided with slow waves occurring in the EEG. However, owing to the present controversy regarding the recognition of eye movements, we hoped to escape some criticism from a technical point of view. A total of 41.843 eye movements were counted.

For each of our subjects, the distribution of the vertical and horizontal eye movements was studied separately. Rather than resort to an arbitrary method of classification, the interval histogram method was used. Attention was paid to the time intervals, in seconds, separating the consecutive eye movements. Absolute frequencies were obtained first, noting the occurrence of each interval, for the various PS stages. These absolute frequencies were converted into relative frequencies with respect to 100 sec PS in order to control the time variable (i.e., the real duration of PS).

The sequence of the intervals during the night was investigated and their distributions were compared between groups of subjects, between subjects, and within the same subject. This was justified because the distribution of the eye movements is not rigorously homogeneous during PS (DeLee and Petre-Quadens, 1968).

For the statistical analysis, we referred to the absolute frequencies.

Quantitative Data

Comparison of Time Intervals between Eye Movements (I) in Mentally Retarded and Normal Subjects

The histograms of the relative frequencies showed that, in the normal subjects, the modal value of the results is represented by intervals shorter than 1 sec, whereas in the mentally retarded subjects, it might concern the intervals longer than 1 and shorter than 2 sec. Nevertheless, the histograms show, for all PS stages, the same negative exponential distribution. The histograms of the vertical and horizontal eye movements in mentally retarded and normal subjects are given in Fig. 3.

For the absolute frequencies, we compared the mean values of both groups for the following intervals: (1) shorter than 1 sec; (2) equal or longer than 1 sec and shorter than 2 sec; (3) equal or longer than 2 sec. The results are given in Table XXIII. The t of Student shows for the three types of I and for both vertical and horizontal eye movements highly significant differences ($p < 0.001$) between the mentally retarded and the normal subjects.

Vertical vs Horizontal Eye Movements

No significant difference in the mean frequencies between vertical and horizontal eye movements are seen in retarded or normal subjects for any of the three types of I. Therefore, our results are in disagreement with those of

TABLE XXIII *Mean Frequencies of the Different Types of I*[a]

	Mentally retarded subjects		Normal subjects	
	VEM	HEM	VEM	HEM
1 sec < I	20.89	15.92	164.99	124.53
1 sec ≤ I < 2 sec	14.39	10.46	56.14	46.69
2 sec ≤ I	37.12	31.55	80.48	71.55

[a]From Petre-Quadens (1969). VEM = vertical eye movements; HEM = horizontal eye movements.

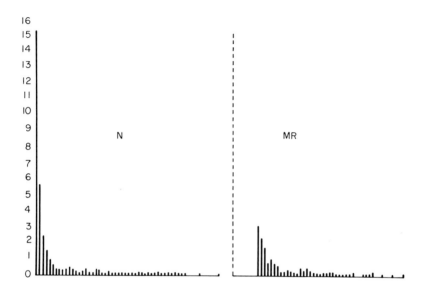

Fig. 3. Histogram of the time intervals separating the eye movements in the 1- to 6-year age group. I < 1 sec: α = 0.001; 1 sec ≤ I < 2 sec: α = 0.001. N = normal subjects (2); MR = mentally retarded subjects (4). Ordinate: Percent I for 100 sec PS. Abscissa: Different types of I. E.g.: The first vertical line represents the I < 1 sec; the second, the intervals: 1 sec ≤ I < 2 sec; the third, the intervals: 2 sec ≤ I < 3 sec; etc. (From Petre-Quadens, 1969.)

Roffwarg *et al.* (1968) who observed a slight dominance of the horizontal eye movements, but our results are in agreement with those of Prechtl and Lenard (1967). We may thus consider the horizontal and vertical eye movements together. The mean frequencies obtained this way for the intervals shorter that 1 sec and for the whole of the intervals equal or longer than 1 sec are given in Table XXIV.

It should be noted that in the normal subjects, the difference between the percentage of intervals shorter than 1 sec and of the intervals equal or longer than 1 sec was not significant, though the frequency of the I < 1 sec was higher than that of the I ≥ 1 sec (Table XXV). These results confirm the "constancy of the oculomotor distribution" considered by Mouret (1964) as being characteristic of the eye movement distribution in PS. Mouret has shown that the amount of eye movements in the discharges and the amount of isolated eye movements are similar. The same holds true in our study for the intervals shorter than 1 sec and the intervals equal or longer than 1 sec. The high frequency of the shortest intervals might be due to the fact that our criteria are less rigorous than Mouret's. This similarity was, however, not seen in the mentally retarded subjects since the differences between the two kinds of intervals were statistically significant (α = 0.01).

TABLE XXIV *Mean Frequencies of the I < 1 sec and I ⩾ 1 sec[a]*

	Mentally retarded subjects	Normal subjects
I < 1 sec	18.88	177.37
I ⩾ 1 sec	47.77	130.56

[a]From Petre-Quadens (1969).

TABLE XXV *Correlation between the Mean of PS Time and the Mean Frequency of I[a]*

	Mentally retarded subjects	Normal subjects
ΣI	0.74	0.86
I < 1 sec	0.42	0.72

[a]From Petre-Quadens (1969).

Correlations between PS Percentage and the Density in Eye Movements

The mean duration of PS was 7 min for the mentally retarded and 11 min for the normal subjects. This difference was significant at $\alpha = 0.05$.

Spearman's correlation coefficient allowed us to determine the relationship between PS time and the occurrence of eye movements. Considering the sum of the I, their correlation with the mean PS time is significant in the mentally retarded as well as in the normal subjects. Considering only the intervals shorter than 1 sec, this correlation remains significant for the normal subjects, whereas it no longer holds true for the mentally retarded subjects. Table XXIII already showed a dramatic decrease in the amount of short intervals in the mentally retarded subjects.

Evolution of the Small Intervals during Consecutive PS Stages

Reverting to the relative frequencies of I, we may now observe the evolution of the shortest intervals during the various PS stages. In the normals, their density was alternatively high and low as if their appearance depended on some excitatory phenomenon occurring irregularly during consecutive PS stages. One might also consider the low density REM as epochs of increased inhibition. However, in the mentally retarded subjects, the intervals shorter than 1 sec did not seem to be under the influence of those alternatively excitatory and inhibitory functions.

Figure 5 shows that there is a large variability in the short intervals from one PS stage to the next. This variability stands out against a general tendency toward an increase of the short intervals during the night. This characteristic was more pronounced for the intervals shorter than 1 sec and, in the normal subjects, it was more marked for the vertical eye movements than for the horizontal ones. The mentally retarded subjects showed less variability in the eye movement

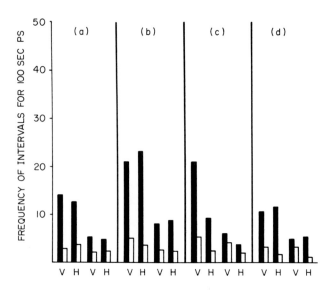

Fig. 4. Frequencies of the short intervals (I < 1 sec (left) and 1 sec < I < 2 sec (right) during PS in normal subjects (black columns) and in mentally retarded subjects (white columns). V = intervals between vertical eye movements; H = intervals between horizontal eye movements; (a) 1-6 years: 4 mentally retarded and 2 normal subjects; (b) 6-8 years: 4 mentally retarded and 1 normal subject; (c) 8-12 years: 2 mentally retarded and 2 normal subjects; (d) 20-25 years: 3 mentally retarded and 2 normal subjects. (From Petre-Quadens, 1969).

density, as if they were not under the influence of these excitatory or conversely inhibitory factors.

Correlations with Age of the Subjects

Correlations with age are given in Fig. 4 for the I shorter than 1 sec and the I equal to or longer than 1 sec and shorter than 2 sec. The corresponding frequencies, for the three types of intervals determined above, are found in Table XXVI.

For the statistical analysis of the results, we could not use the t of Student because of the fractioning of our population. Therefore, we used the Mann-Whitney U test.

1. We noticed that the mentally retarded children differed from the normals for the I < 1 sec at $\alpha = 0.002$, for the 1 sec $\leq$ I < 2 sec at $\alpha = 0.05$ and for the I $\geq$ 2 sec at $\alpha = 0.02$. The mean duration of the PS stages was 8 min in the mentally retarded and 14 min in the normal children. This difference was

TABLE XXVI *Mean Value of I for Normal and Mentally Retarded Children and Adults[a]*

	Mentally retarded subjects		Normal subjects	
	Children	Adults	Children	Adults
1 sec > I	18.25	7	168.12	106
1 sec ≤ I < 2 sec	13.88	6.70	69.75	48.15
2 sec ≤ I	33.33	15.20	76.56	72.01

[a]From Petre-Quadens (1969).

TABLE XXVII *Correlation between the Mean Duration of the PS Stages and the Eye Movement Density[a]*

	Mentally retarded children	Normal children
ΣI	0.53	0.95
I < 1 sec	0.20	0.90

[a]From Petre-Quadens (1969).

significant at $\alpha = 0.02$. Correlations between the mean duration of the PS stages and the amount of eye movements in the children are given in Table XXVII.

This correlation was high in normal children but was not significant in the mentally retarded children. In the retarded, the degree of correlation for the intervals shorter than 1 sec was low. This fact indicates a more specific disturbance of the bursts of REM in the mentally retarded.

As far as the adults were concerned, this kind of correlation could not be made because of the small number of subjects in both groups. The data indicated, however, that the results would have been similar to those in children (Fig. 5).

2. Data of children and adults have been correlated. We limited ourselves, for the same reason, to the observation of the graphic representation (Fig. 4). Age difference did not entail perceptible changes in the I of mentally retarded subjects. In the normal subjects, a correlation with age was found for the I shorter than 1 sec only. This was, however, significant. Figure 4 confirmed that in the mentally retarded subjects, the frequency of eye movements did not vary much with age, whereas the normal subjects, aged 6-10 years, showed higher eye movement density within the bursts of REM. The same high density REM seemed to be maintained from ages 10 to 14, with a preference for the vertical eye movements. Furthermore, greater individual variations were found in the vertical eye movements than in the horizontal ones in both the normal and mentally retarded subjects.

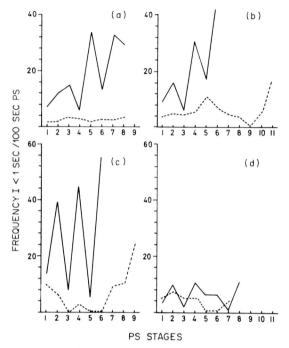

Fig. 5. Frequency of the I < 1 sec between vertical eye-movements during consecutive PS stages. (—) Normal subjects; (. . .) mentally retarded subjects. (a) 1-6 years; (b) 6-8 years; (c) 8-10 years; (d) 20-25 years. (From Petre-Quadens, 1969).

Correlations with I.Q. as Determined by the Wechsler Scale

Correlation of REM density to I.Q. gave surprising results. Percentage of I shorter than 1 sec in three children with I.Q. = 60 was shown to be higher than in three severely retarded subjects with I.Q. below 30; but it was lower than in two brilliant children with I.Q. above 125 (Table XXVIII). The eight children of this group were in the same age range, 6-8 years.

Discussion

We know that learning capacities are maximal in the child and that they considerably diminish in adulthood. We are also aware of severe learning deficiencies in the mentally retarded. The finding of a correlation between intellectual function and REMS would further support the sleep cognition hypothesis. But the correlation, if the hypothesis is correct, is not a simple one. Indeed, the I < 1 sec increase considerably during pregnancy when important humoral and hormonal changes occur (Petre-Quadens *et al.*, 1967).

TABLE XXVIII *Percentage of I < 1 sec in Eight Children*[a]

	I.Q. < 30 (3)	I.Q. ± 60 (3)	I.Q. > 125 (2)
I < 1 sec	1.65	8.68	24.33

[a]From Petre-Quadens (1969). Number of subjects in parentheses.

Qualitative Observations

It appears impossible to describe a pattern of eye movements, because of the great intraindividual and interindividual variations. As far as their amplitude and distribution are concerned, it appears that some characteristics are common to the different groups of subjects. In the mentally retarded, the EOG waves were small and the bursts rare. When bursts appeared in some subjects they did so during the last PS stages only, as if the releasing mechanisms required a more or less long running-period. In any case, REM density is smaller in retarded than in normal subjects, and this phenomenon was even more characteristic in retarded adults. The REM of the normal subjects were well-differentiated and longer. They were grouped in bursts from the first PS stages. Later during the night, the bursts lasted until 80 sec in the children. They were shorter in the adults. Moreover, the distribution of the eye movements was not homogeneous. Eye movements were rare at the onset of a PS stage. Their frequency increased rapidly when PS progressed, and decreased again toward the end of the stage.

EEG activity fluctuated during REM even when the EMG was abolished. Bursts of 6 Hz waves appeared on a flat tracing, sometimes related to bursts of eye movements.

Direct observation data were rather poor in retarded subjects during REM. In the normal subjects, the behavior changed, the respiratory rhythm became irregular, small incoordinated jerks animated fingers, legs, and arms. The eyelids were half-open and some of our children were smiling, crying, and murmuring.

Discussion

The eye movements during sleep have been analyzed only recently (Aserinsky, 1967; Mouret, 1964), and the interval histogram method has been applied even more recently (Prechtl and Lenard, 1967; Feinberg, 1968). In a study on eye movement patterns in newborns, Prechtl and Lenard (1967) found a negative exponential distribution similar to ours. In the newborn, also, the distribution of the amount of eye movements showed a fast increase when PS stage started, and toward the end a progressive decrease. In older children, the distribution of eye movements does not seem to vary much during maturation (Gabersek and

Scherrer, 1966). According to the same authors, the REM are preceded by slow eye movements in PS.

We have also noticed slow or isolated eye movements in the newborn. They appeared in the right part of the interval histogram and thus corresponded with the long intervals. As pointed out by Prechtl and Lenard (1967) and Mouret (1964), it seems that the short intervals or bursts of eye movements belong to a population different from the long intervals or slow eye movements.

Dement (1964) showed that in the adult, REM are highly organized and precise. This holds true in normal children but not in the mentally retarded. For Mouret (1964) and Jeannerod (1968; Jeannerod *et al.*, 1965), the eye movements of PS differ from those of wakefulness in their speed and distribution.

A number of studies have shown that PS is not a steady state. Phasic variations appear within the various physiological parameters of PS. They are synchronous with bursts of eye movements. REM have been correlated in cats with an increase of heart rate (Gassel *et al.*, 1964a), a phasic dilation of the pupil (Berlucchi *et al.*, 1964; Hodes and Dement, 1964), and with small movements of the limbs (Gassel *et al.*, 1964b). The monosynaptic reflexes, depressed during PS, are even more depressed during the bursts of eye movements (Baldissera *et al.*, 1966; Gassel *et al.*, 1964c). Presynaptic inhibition during PS has been found in the trigeminal nerve (Baldissera *et al.*, 1966) and in the visual (Bizzi, 1966) and auditory afferents (Berlucchi *et al.*, 1966). Similar correlations of bursts of REM with other phasic phenomena have been described in man (Snyder *et al.*, 1964; Dement, 1964; Wolpert, 1960; Prechtl and Lenard, 1967). Prechtl and Lenard (1967) explain the absence of organized patterns in the EEG during PS by the absence of sensory input in the CNS due to presynaptic and postsynaptic sensory inhibition. Aserinsky (1967) has shown that the amount of eye movements vary in the consecutive PS stages, and even within the same PS stage.

Our results in mentally retarded subjects support the sleep cognition hypothesis. But the increase of eye movement density during pregnancy and, as we shall see later, in the mature newborn, indicates that the relationship of REM to learning is indirect, and may be linked to some neuroendocrine feedback mechanisms. The study of Reiss (1963) and of Hamburg (1966) strongly support the concept that hormonal factors influence learning capacities. It has also been shown (Michael, 1965) that labeled estrogens are fixed in the hypothalamus, the limbic, septal, and preoptic areas. Those areas are part of the limbic midbrain circuit, described by Nauta and Kuypers (1960), spreading from the limbic system down to the midbrain, in which sleep mechanisms have been identified.

An increase in eye movement density has been found in newborns (Petre-Quadens *et al.*, 1971). Correlative studies on the sleep patterns in normal newborns and in newborns with mongolism have shown that toward term, there is a decrease in REMS in those with mongolism (Petre-Quadens, 1966, 1969)

(Fig. 6). This decrease is correlated with a decrease in the amount of I < 1 sec as compared to normal newborns. Correlation of the distribution of the I < 1 sec during consecutive REM in newborns with mongolism to that seen in normal newborns and prematures is shown in Fig. 7.

We considered the intervals between the vertical eye movements only. Data, however, indicated that similar results would have been obtained with horizontal eye movements. In the newborns with mongolism, the variability in the distribution of the short intervals between successive REM stages is small and looked similar to that in premature babies. In the full-term newborns, there is a large variability in those intervals from one REM stage to the next one. This variability stands out against a general tendency toward a gradual increase of the short intervals during consecutive REM stages of the same sleep cycle. This phenomenon was even more pronounced in children of older age groups. This points to the development of an inhibitory process exerting its influence upon the eye movements. The variability of the eye movement density would reflect the variability of this process. Indeed, the I < 1 sec are alternatively dense and far apart, as if their appearance depended on some excitatory process occurring irregularly during consecutive REM stages. One might also consider the low densities as periods of increased inhibition. It seems that in newborns with mongolism, as in the prematures, the intervals shorter than 1 sec are not subjected to these alternatively excitatory and inhibitory processes.

Investigations on the biochemical aspects of sleep, as well as the extensive studies of Bazelon *et al.* (1967) and Lee *et al.* (1969), on the effects of 5-HT on psychomotor functions in children with mongolism, have led us to correlate the effects of 5-HTP administration with the sleep patterns of infants with mongolism and with their psychomotor development. Only preliminary data can be given here.

In one child, 5-HTP, a precursor of 5-HT, was given at a dosage of 0.5 mg/kg body weight. Total night sleep was recorded before and after increase of the dosage. REM intervals were analyzed according to the same method. Histograms of the I < 1 sec are given in Fig. 8(a). A shows the data of the control record of the baby aged 10 months, before drug administration. Beginning at that age, this baby received daily 5-HTP at a dosage of 0.30 mg/kg body weight. New records were taken at age 12 months (b, solid lines). At that age, the dosage of 5-HTP was increased to 0.50 mg/kg (b, broken lines). REM density increased, whereas total sleeping time decreased. An increase in sleep spindles was observed. Two months later, at age 14 months, a new sleep record showed a decrease in REM density as if habituation had occurred (c, solid lines). A new increase of the dosage to 0.75 mg/kg body weight was followed by a new increase in REM density (c, broken lines). At age 18 months, the baby was still at the same dosage of 5-HTP. But since the record showed only a slight decrease in REM density and the baby seemed to develop well, treatment remained unchanged. At

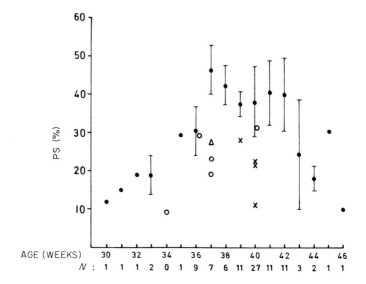

Fig. 6. PS percent as function of gestational age in normal and abnormal newborns. (●) Normal; (○) dysmatures; (X) mongols; (△) microcephalics. Vertical lines around black symbol give the standard deviations of the mean PS percent in the normal babies. *N* = number of babies in each age group. (From Petre-Quadens, 1969).

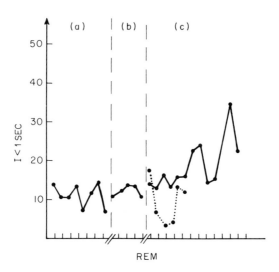

Fig. 7. Frequency of I < 1 sec for 40 sec PS time during consecutive REM. (——) Prematures and normal newborns: (a) 6 babies, 33-36 weeks; (b) 5 babies, 37-39 weeks; (c) 13 babies, 40-41 weeks. (· · ·) Newborns with mongolism: (c) 3 babies, 40-41 weeks.

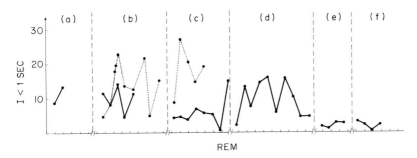

Fig. 8. Frequency of the I < 1 sec for 40 sec epochs during consecutive REM in one patient with mongolism. (a) Age 10 months, control before 5-HTP administration; (b) age 12 months: continuous line, receives 5-HTP daily for 2 months; broken line, 2 weeks after dosage had been increased; (c) age 14 months: continuous line, same dosage as in broken line in (b); broken line, 2 weeks after dosage had been increased further; (d) age 18 months, same dosage 5–HTP as in broken line in C; (e) age 23 months, without 5-HTP; (f) age 24 months, without 5-HTP.

age 22 months, 5-HTP was stopped. Total night sleep records taken at ages 23 and 24 months showed a dramatic decrease in REM density (e and f). These are, of course, only preliminary data, but they show a trend to an increase in REM density with 5-HTP. Clinically, an increase in muscle tone was observed with an improvement of motor behavior, as shown by Bazelon *et al.* (1967). However, the question of the biological significance of the decrease in PS in the oligophrenics entails teleological speculations. The association of PS with dreaming is well known, though dreaming may occur in all sleep stages. The decrease of REM in oligophrenics can be understood if we assume (Hernández-Peón, 1965) that dreaming could be "an effect or an epiphenomenon associated with the recovery process of mnemic inhibitory neurons essential for normal waking behavior and logical thought." This concept, of course, does not explain the given facts, but could be a hypothesis for future investigations.

SUMMARY

Investigations on mentally retarded subjects of all ages and all etiologies have shown changes in the proportions not only of PS but also of all other sleep stages. In this study, the greatest problem was in the quantification of these changes. The time intervals separating 42.320 eye movements have been measured in mentally retarded and normal subjects. This method also provided an estimation of the density of eye movements. When converting time intervals into percentage with respect to a conventional duration of 100 sec PS, we made them independent from the duration of each PS epoch, and consequently comparable. In our analysis, we separated the vertical and horizontal eye movements, but there were no statistically significant differences between them.

In normal subjects, the frequency of the intervals shorter than 1 sec was four to six times higher than in retarded subjects, and the frequency of those between 1 and 2 sec were two to three times higher in normal subjects. It seems thus that very short intervals are lacking in retarded subjects.

From the whole investigation, the notion of the nonspecificity of the sleep cycle alterations became apparent. Therefore, it is not possible to establish a differentiation between various types of mental retardation on the basis of sleep characteristics, at least quantitatively. On the other hand, it appears clear that the sleep cycle alterations seem to be related to the maturation of cerebral function, i.e., with the age of the studied subjects.

The trend to normalization of the sleep stage percentages in the retarded subjects at the time of puberty has raised the question of a possible influence of the endocrine system in the regulation of the sleep mechanisms.

REFERENCES

Aserinsky, E. (1967). Physiological activity associated with segments of rapid eye movement periods. *In* "Sleep and Altered States of Consciousness" (S. S. Kety, E. V. Evarts, and H. L. Williams, eds.), pp. 338-350. Williams & Wilkins, Baltimore, Maryland.

Baldissera, F., Broggi, G., and Mancia, M. (1966). Monosynaptic and polysynaptic spinal reflexes during physiological sleep and wakefulness. *Arch. Ital. Biol.* 104, 112-133.

Bazelon, M., Paine, R. S., Cowie, V. A., Hump, P., Houck, J. C., and Mahanand, D. (1967). Reversal of hypotonia in infants with Down's syndrome by administration of 5-hydroxytryptophan. *Lancet* 1, 1130-1133.

Berger, R. (1961). Tonus of extrinsic laryngeal muscles during sleep and dreaming. *Science* 134, 840.

Berlucchi, G., Moruzzi, G., Salvi, G., and Strata, B. (1964). Pupil behavior and ocular movements during synchronized and desynchronized sleep. *Arch. Ital. Biol.* 102, 230-244.

Berlucchi, G., Munson, J. B., and Rizzolatti, G. (1966). Auditory evoked responses in cats with tenotomized middle ear muscles during sleep. *Pfluegers Arch. Gesamte Physiol. Menschen Tiere* 292, 80-82.

Bixler, E. O., and Rhodes, J. M. (1968). Spindle activity during sleep in cultural familial mild retardates. *Psychophysiology* 5, 212 (abstr.).

Bizzi, E. (1966). Changes in the orthodromic and antidromic response of optic tract during the eye movements of sleep. *J. Neurophysiol.* 29, 861-870.

Brebbia, D. R., and Altschuler, K. Z. (1968). Stage related patterns and nightly trends of energy exchange during sleep. *Proc. World Congr. Psychiat., 4th, 1968,* pp. 319-335.

Clara, R., and Lowenthal, A. (1965). Aminoacidurie tubulaire congénitale et familiale avec nanisme grave et hypotonie musculaire à évolution favorable chez quatre enfants d'une même fratrie. *Acta Neurol. Psychiat. Belg.* 65, 911-936.

DeLee, C., and Petre-Quadens, O. (1968). Les mouvements oculaires de sommeil. *Acta Neurol. Psychiat. Belg.* 68, 327-331.

Dement, W. C. (1964). Eye movement during sleep. *In* "The Oculomotor System" (M. B. Bender, ed.), pp. 366-416. Harper, New York.

Dement, W. C., and Kleitman, N. (1957). Cyclic variations in EEG during sleep and their relation to eye movements, body motility and dreaming. *Electroencephalogr. Clin. Neurophysiol.* 9, 673-690.

Dubois-Reymond, E. (1848). "Untersuchungen uber Theirische Electricität," 2 tomes in 3 vols. Reimer, Berlin.

Fanconi, G. (1945). Kasuistischer Beitrag zur den Kalkstoffwechselstörunger rezidivierde Tetanie mit Verkalkungsstörungen am Skelett. *Helv. Paediat. Acta.* 1, 85-91.

Feinberg, I. (1968). Eye movement activity during sleep and intellectual function in mental retardation. *Science* 159, 1256.

Feinberg, I., Koresko, R., Gottlieb, F., and Wender, P. (1965). Sleep electroencephalographic and eye movement patterns in patients with chronic brain syndrome. *J. Res.* 3, 11-26.

Gabersek, V., and Scherrer, J. (1966). Etude électroencephalographique de sommeil de l'enfant. *Rev. Neuropsychiat. Infant.* 14, 121-138.

Gassel, M. M., Marchiafava, P. L., and Pompeiano, O. (1964a). Phasic changes in muscular activity during desynchronized sleep in unrestrained cats. *Arch. Ital. Biol.* 102, 449-470.

Gassel, M. M., Marchiafava, P. L., and Pompeiano, O. (1964b). Tonic and phasic inhibition of spinal reflexes during sleep in unrestrained cats. *Arch. Ital. Biol.* 102, 471-479.

Gassel, M. M., Berlucchi, G., Marchiafava, P. L., and Pompeiano, O. (1964c). Phasic changes in blood pressure and heart rate during rapid eye movement episodes of desynchronized sleep in unrestrained cats. *Arch. Ital. Biol.* 102, 530-544.

Gibbs, E. L., and Gibbs, F. A. (1950). Electroencephalographic changes with age during sleep. *Electroencephalogr. Clin. Neurophysiol.* 2, 351-363

Gibbs, E. L., and Gibbs, F. A. (1962). Extreme spindles: Correlation of electroencephalographic sleep pattern with mental retardation. *Science* 138, 1106-1107.

Greenberg, R. (1966). Cerebral cortex lesions: the dream process and sleep spindles. *Cortex* 2, 357-366.

Hamburg, D. A. (1966). Effects of progesterone on behaviour. *In* "Endocrines and Central Nervous System" (R. Levine, ed.), pp. 251-265. Williams & Wilkins, Baltimore, Maryland.

Hernández-Peón, R. (1965). A neurophysiologic model of dream and hallucinations. *J. Nerv. Ment. Dis.* 141, 623-650.

Hodes, R., and Dement, W. C. (1964). Depression of electrically induced reflexes ("H-reflexes") in man during low-voltage EEG sleep. *Electroencephalogr. Clin. Neurophysiol.* 17, 617-629.

Imlah, N. W. (1961). Narcolepsy in identical twins. *J. Neurol., Neurosurg. Psychiat.* 24, 158-160.

Jacobson, A., Kales, A., Lehman, D., and Hoedemarker, F. S. (1964). Muscle tonus in human subjects during sleep and dreaming. *Exp. Neurol.* 10, 418-424.

Jeannerod, M. (1968). Principes et méthodes de l'enregistrement des mouvements oculaires chez l'homme. *Progr. Ophthalmol.* 19, 52-99.

Jeannerod, M., Mouret, J., and Jouvet, M. (1965). Etude de la motricité oculaire au cours de la phase paradoxale du sommeil chez le chat. *Electroencephalogr. Clin. Neurophysiol.* 18, 554-566.

Jouvet, M., Bobillier, P., Pujol, J. F., and Renault, J. (1967). Suppression du sommeil et diminution de la serotonine cérébrale par lésion du système du raphé chez le chat. *C. R. Acad. Sci.* 264, 360-362.

Lairy, G. C. (1968). Le rêve chez les malades mentaux. *In* "Rêve et Conscience" (P. Wertheimer, ed.) 4th trim., pp. 199-224. P. U. F., Paris.

Lairy, G. C., Cor-Mordret, M., Faure, R., and Ridjanovic, S. (1962). Etude EEG du sommeil du vieillard normal et pathologique. *Rev. Neurol.* **107**, 188-202.

Lairy, G. C., Barte, H., Goldsteinas, J., and Ridjanovic, S. (1965). Sommeil de nuit des malades mentaux. *In* "Le sommeil de nuit normal et pathologique" (G. Masson, ed.), pp. 353-379. Masson, Paris.

Lee, J. C. M., Ornitz, E. M., Tanguay, P. E., and Ritoo, E. R. (1969). Sleep EEG patterns in a case of Down's syndrome before and after 5-HTP. *Electroenceph. Clin. Neurophysiol.* **27**, 686.

Metcalf, D. R., and Jordan, K. (1971). EEG ontogenesis in normal children. *In* "Drugs, Development and Cerebral Function" (W. L. Smith, ed.). Thomas, Springfield, Illinois (in press).

Michael, R. P. (1965). Oestrogens in the central nervous system. *Brit. Med. Bull.* **21**, 87-90.

Mouret, J. (1964). Les mouvements oculaires au cours du sommeil paradoxal. Thesis, Imprimerie des Beaux-Arts, Lyon.

Nauta, W. J., and Kuypers, H. B. (1960). Some ascending pathways in the brain stem reticular formation of the brain. *In* "Reticular Formation of the Brain" (H. H. Jasper, ed.), pp. 3-30. Little, Brown, Boston.

Passouant, P., Cadilhac, J., Delange, M., Gallamand, M., and El Kossabgui, M. (1965). Age et sommeil de nuit, variations électrocliniques du sommeil, de la naissance à l'extrême vieillesse. *In* "Le sommeil de nuit normal et pathologique" (G. Masson, ed.), pp. 87-113. Masson, Paris.

Petre-Quadens, O. (1965). Etude du sommeil chez le nouveau-né normal. *In* "Le sommeil de nuit normal et pathologique" (G. Masson, ed.), pp. 149-155. Masson, Paris.

Petre-Quadens, O. (1966). On the different phases of the sleep of the newborn with special reference to the activated phase or phase *d*. *J. Neurol. Sci.* **3**, 151-161.

Petre-Quadens, O. (1969). Contribution a l'étude de la phase dite paradoxale du sommeil. Thesis. *Acta Neurol. Psychiat. Belg.* **69**, 769-898.

Petre-Quadens, O., de Barsey, A. M., and Sfaello, Z. (1967). Sleep in pregnancy: Evidence of foetal-sleep characteristics. *J. Neurol. Sci.* **4**, 600-605.

Petre-Quadens, O., De Lee, C., and Remy, M. (1971). Eye movement density during sleep and brain maturation. *Brain Res.* **26**, 49-56.

Prechtl, H. F. R., and Lenard, H. G. (1967). A study of eye movements in sleeping newborn infants. *Brain Res.* **5**, 477-493.

Reding, G. R., Zepelin, H., Robinson, J. R., Jr., Smith, V. H., and Zimmerman, S. O. (1968). Sleep pattern of bruxism: A revision. *Psychophysiology* **4**, 396 (abstr.).

Reiss, M. (1963). Endocrine research in psychiatry. *Proc. World Congr. Psychiat., 3rd, 1961,* Vol: 1, pp. 121-127.

Roffwarg, H. P., Frankel, B., and Persah, M. (1968). The nocturnal sleep pattern in pregnancy. *Psychophysiology* **5**, 227.

Schmidt, H. S., Kaelbling, R., and Alexander, J. (1968). Sleep patterns in mental retardates: Mongoloids and monozygotic twins. *Psychophysiology* **5**, 212.

Schwartz-Tiene, E., and Caredou, P. (1962). Alterzioni del metabolismo del triptofanonella fenilchetonuria nell'ipsaritmia nel mongolismo e in alcune cerebropatic infantil. *Minerva Pediat.* **14**, 1471-1481.

Sfaello, Z., and Hariga, J. (1967). Monilethrix associé à la débilité mentale. Etude d'une famille. *Arch. Belg. Dermatol. Syphiligr.* **23**, 363-371.

Snyder, F. (1965). Progress in the new biology of dreaming. *Amer. J. Psychiat.* **122**, 377-391.

Snyder, F., Hobson, J. A., Morrison, D.,F., and Goldfrank, F. (1964). Changes in respiration, heart rate, and systolic blood pressure in human sleep. *J. Appl. Physiol.* **19**, 417-422.

Sours, J. A. (1963). Narcolepsy and other disturbances in the sleep-waking rhythm. A study of 115 cases with review of the literature. *J. Nerv. Ment. Dis.* **137**, 525-542.

Van Creveld, S., and Grünbaum, A. (1942). Renal rickets and cystinuria. *Acta Paediat. Scand.* **29**, 183-210.

Velasco, M., and Lindsley, D. B. (1965). Role of orbital cortex in regulation of thalamo-cortical electrical activity. *Science* **149**, 1375-1377.

Wolpert, E. A. (1960). Studies in psychophysiology of dreams. II. An electromyographic study of dreaming. *Arch. Gen. Psychiat.* **2**, 231-241.

Yakovlev, P. I. (1959). Anatomy of the human brain and the problem of mental retardation. *In* "Mental Retardation" (P. W. Bowman and H. V. Mautner, eds.), pp. 1-43. Grune & Stratton, New York.

18

Maternal Toxemia, Fetal Malnutrition, and Bioelectric Brain Activity of the Newborn*

F. J. Schulte, Gabriele Hinze, and Gerlind Schrempf

Neurological studies of motor behavior (Saint-Anne Dargassies, 1955, 1966; Amiel-Tison, 1968; Brett, 1965; Robinson, 1966; Graziani *et al.*, 1968). the electroencephalogram (Dreyfus-Brisac, 1964; Parmelee *et al.*, 1968; Nolte *et al.*, 1969), cortical evoked responses (Engel and Benson, 1968; Graziani *et al.*, 1968; Akiyama *et al.*, 1969), and nerve conduction velocity (Schulte *et al.*, 1968; Ruppert and Johnson, 1968; Dubowitz *et al.*, 1968) have led to the concept that fetal brain development is dependent on conceptional age rather than on body weight. Basically, this concept is correct and well supported by anatomical studies (Larroche, 1962). However, more sophistication in methodology, on one hand, and subdivision of small-for-gestational-age infants, on the other, enabled us to detect rather consistent deficits. It is the purpose of this paper to

*Supported by grants from the Deutsche Forschungsgeneinschaft (SFT 33). Computing assistance was obtained from the Health Sciences Computing Facility, UCLA, sponsored by a grant from NIH (FR-3).

document deviations with regard to bioelectric brain maturation in small-for-gestational-age newborn infants of toxemic mothers.

SUBJECTS

Twenty-two small-for-gestational-age newborn infants of toxemic mothers were matched for both age from conception and from birth with 22 normal newborn infants. The gestational age was calculated from the first day of the mother's last menstrual period until birth. Conceptional age means gestational age plus age from birth until the examination was carried out. Infants were included in this study only when their mothers were certain about their last menses.

The Abnormal Group

From mothers with toxemia, only small-for-gestational-age newborn infants were included, that is, all the abnormal infants had a birth-weight below the 10th percentile of the Hosemann (1948) intrauterine growth curves. Conceptional ages ranged from 36 to 45 weeks, birthweights from 1460 to 2610 g. Maternal toxemia was defined as consistently elevated systolic blood pressure above 140 mmHg with either proteinuria or edema. Five infants had postnatal asphyxia of slight degree (oxygen therapy) and three required artificial ventilation for not more than 15 min. Three infants were delivered by caesarean section, 19 had a normal vaginal delivery. Eight infants received i.v. infusions of 5-10% glucose since they were originally suspected as having "symptomatic hypoglycemia," i.e., they had both neurological symptoms and a blood glucose level below 30 mg/100 ml. All infants of the abnormal group were referred to the Universitäts-Kinderklinik from other hospitals, since the obstetricians found the infants either abnormal or "at risk." Thus, the group is selected toward severe pathology.

In this study, the main interest was to investigate the effects of intrauterine malnutrition on bioelectric activity. However, many other factors, notably perinatal hypoxia and postnatal hypoglycemia, may well mask the influence of intrauterine malnutrition on the infant's brain. Therefore, we will have to classify our results as being obtained from infants who are from toxemic mothers as well as being small-for-gestational-age. On the other hand, in studying the nervous maturity of malnourished fetuses, it is not justifiable to exclude infants with adverse intrauterine factors. Otherwise, only "normal" small-for-gestational-age infants who may not have suffered from any restriction whatsoever are left in the study. It is not surprising that their neurophysiology is comparable to normal weight infants. Thus, in studying the effects of placental insufficiency and intrauterine malnutrition on the human fetal brain, our results are either bound to be contaminated with a variety of adverse effects, mainly hypoxia, or they are only representative of infants who apparently did not suffer at all from placental dysfunction. The EEG's of seven infants were subjected to numerical spectrum analysis. Four of these EEG's were recorded from small-for-gestational-age newborn infants of toxemic mothers and three from normal control infants matched for age. The four abnormal infants were selected because their case histories were representative for this study. Their prenatal intranatal, and postnatal histories are given in detail.

(a)(P. J.) Pregnancy was complicated by severe toxemia with elevated blood pressure of constantly 170/105-220/140 mmHg, generalized edema and proteinuria, oliguria, and disturbance of vision. At 38 weeks of gestation, a dysmature 2500-g infant was delivered by caesarean section. No asphyxia or any other postnatal problems were observed; pH, base reserve and pCO_2 were normal. The infant was slightly hyperexcitable with spontaneous myoclonic motor activity. She received 80,000 units of penicillin daily for 6 days. Blood glucose concentrations were 41, 31, 48 mg/100 ml, and, at the time of EEG recording 83 mg/100 ml; Hct 60%; serum calcium 10.1 and 10.5 mg/100 ml. Polygraphic recording was done on the 5th day in an incubator.

Visual analysis of EEG without knowledge of the case history: underestimation of age by 1 week; some low amplitude spikes particularly during active sleep; conclusion: abnormal EEG. Spectrum analysis of the EEG: no 4-5 Hz power peak. Large amount of high frequency activity with unusually strong coherence during active sleep.

(b)(H. D) Pregnancy was complicated by a moderate degree of toxemia with elevated blood pressure of constantly 160/110-180/130 mmHg, proteinuria, and slight edema. The placenta was small and had numerous calcified infarctions. Delivery of a 1460-g dysmature infant occurred spontaneously after 35 weeks of gestation. Postnatal asphyxia was briefly present with subsequent mild acidosis: base deficit 11.3 mEq/liter, pCO_2 22.5 mmHg, pH 7.335. The remainder of the postnatal course was uneventful except for skeletal muscle hypertonia. Blood glucose concentrations were 26, 46, 27, and 52 mg/100 ml. On the first day of life, a shortlasting infusion of fructose and bicarbonate was given. The polygraphic recording was done 5 weeks after birth (41 weeks conceptional age) in a crib.

Visual analysis of EEG without knowledge of the case history: overestimation of age by 1 week; high amplitude slow waves and sleep spindles even during active sleep; conclusion: abnormal EEG. Spectrum analysis of the EEG: poorly developed 4-5 Hz peak. Large amount of high frequency activity.

(c)(J. F.) Pregnancy was complicated by mild toxemia with elevated blood pressure of 135/110 mmHg, occasional albuminuria, and edema. After 39 weeks of gestation a dysmature 2300-g infant was spontaneously delivered. No asphyxia or any other postnatal illness was noted. Motor behavior was normal.

Blood glucose concentrations were 29 and 49 mg/100 ml, and, at the time of EEG recording 60 mg/100 ml. Hct 64%, serum calcium 10.6 and 10.2 mg/100 ml. Polygraphic recording was done on the 3rd day in a crib. Visual analysis of EEG without knowledge of the case history: overestimation of age by 2 weeks; otherwise normal EEG. Spectrum analysis of the EEG: poorly developed 4-5 Hz power peak.

(d)(D. E.) Pregnancy was complicated by severe toxemia with convulsions (no medical care during pregnancy). Blood pressure 170/140 mmHg. Proteinuria. After 40 weeks of gestation a 2580-g infant was delivered by caesarean section. No asphyxia or any other postnatal illness was noted. Skeletal muscle tone was slightly increased. Blood glucose concentrations were 55, 40, and 77 mg/100 ml, and, at time of EEG recording 89 mg/100 ml. Serum calcium 9.3, 8.9, and 9.2 mg/100 ml. Hct 62%. Polygraphic recording was done on the 6th day in a crib. Visual analysis of EEG without knowledge of the case history: underestimation of age by 2 weeks: no 4-5 Hz power peak. Moderately increased amount of high frequency activity.

The Control Group

The 22 infants of this group had an uneventful prenatal course and normal vaginal delivery, although, for comparison with the study group, an equal number of these infants were preterm. The postnatal courses were without complications and the pediatric examinations were normal. All infants of this group were born in the Universitäts-Frauenklinik Göttingen and had a birthweight between the 25th and the 75th percentile of the Hosemann (1948) intrauterine growth curves.

METHODS

Blood Glucose Determinations

Enzymic, colorimetric blood glucose determinations with uranyl acetate deproteinization were done immediately after admittance and repeated usually once a day until normal values were obtained. Three infants with severe hypoglycemia each had three estimations within 24 hr. With the enzymic colorimetric blood glucose determination (glucose oxidase method) after uranyl acetate deproteinization we are not measuring pure glucose alone. Particularly on the first 2 days of life blood glutathione content contributes to falsely low blood glucose values (Relander and Räihä, 1963; Ek and Daae, 1967). However, a strong correlation of $r = 0.68$ on the first and second day and of $r = 0.99$ on the fifth day exists between the glucose oxidase and the hexokinase method (Wolf, unpublished data). The values obtained with the hexokinase method, in which true glucose is determined, are always a little higher (Bachmann, 1969) than with the glucose oxidase method after uranyl acetate deproteinization. Therefore, the glutathione contamination does not influence the conclusions drawn from our data: none of our study infants, in fact, had symptomatic hypoglycemia. The true glucose levels were even a little higher than indicated in this article.

In order to evaluate the degree, duration, and resistance of hypoglycemia to therapy, not only the minimum blood glucose level but also an additional scoring system was used for the correlation with neurological findings. In this scoring system for each blood glucose estimation below 30 mg/100 ml one point was added to one, below 20 mg/100 ml two points, and below 10 mg/100 ml three points. Long-lasting resistant hypoglycemia is heavily weighted by these scores. Such a scoring system seemed to be advantageous for correlation with neurological findings, since infants with resistant hypoglycemia are probably at higher risk than those with only short-lasting low glucose levels (Gentz *et al.*, 1969).

Polygraphic Recording

Polygraphic sleep recording of 2-3 hr duration between afternoon feedings were obtained from each infant between 3 and 11 days after birth. Only two infants, 1 normal and 1 abnormal, were recorded 5 weeks after birth. Special care was taken to guarantee nearly identical conditions during the sleep recording. All normal and 19 abnormal infants were recorded in the same room in a crib. Only three infants were recorded in an incubator.

Polygraphic recordings were done on an eight-channel Offner Dynograph Type T and comprised: (1) Observed eye movements, registered by a push button; (2) respiration, registered by a thermistor attached to the infant's nose; (3) electromyogram of chin muscle activity; (4) facial and body activity, continuously observed during the recording and indicated by a code on the paper writeout; (5) EEG recorded with silver/silver chloride stick-on electrodes in 6 bipolar leads from frontocentral, centrotemporal, and centrooccipital regions. The electrode resistance was reduced to 5 kΩ or less. Pen deflection was 9 mm/50 μV, the time constant was 0.3 sec, and the paper speed was 1.5 cm/sec.

The following criteria were used for the differentiation of sleep states. Active sleep: rapid eye movements (REM), irregular respiration, continuous EEG activity, and presence of various patterns of phasic facial muscle and body activity. Quiet sleep: Absence of rapid eye movements (NREM), regular respiration, discontinuous EEG activity consisting of high-amplitude bursts of slow waves (*Schlafgruppen* of Schroeder and Heckel, 1952) alternating with intervals of attenuated activity, i.e., *tracé alternant* (Dreyfus-Brisac, 1964) and absence of phasic facial muscle and body activity.

All sleep states which could not be classified as either active or quiet sleep by rigidly applying our criteria were regarded as "transitional" or "ill-defined" sleep and were not considered in this study.

The maturational changes in EEG patterns during sleep in preterm and fullterm infants have been described by Dreyfus-Brisac (1962, 1964). On the basis of her observations, Parmelee *et al.* (1968) and Schulte *et al.* (1969a) established an EEG pattern coding system. Expanding this coding system we were able to recognize 11 different EEG patterns between 36 and 44 weeks of conceptional age indicated by certain code numbers (Fig. 1). In the polygraphic recordings from all infants the EEG was coded page by page (20-sec epochs) during REM and NREM sleep. Subsequently, the examiner estimated the infants conceptional age on the basis of the EEG patterns. While coding the EEG and estimating the menstrual age, the examiner did not know the infant's age, gestational history, or neonatal condition.

From earlier studies (Schulte *et al.*, 1969b) it seemed promising to examine the sleep cycle behavior at least in one small-for-gestational-age infant of a toxemic mother in more detail. The respiration rate was determined. The regularity of respiration was indicated by the ratio between the shortest and the longest breath-to-breath interval in each 20-sec epoch (Monod and Pajot, 1965), this ratio being almost one for very regular respiration and close to zero for highly irregular respiration.

Computer Analysis

Seven EEG's which were visually analyzed have also been examined by means of numerical spectrum analysis. We wish to emphasize that the computer part of this study is still preliminary. Its results were not yet treated by any statistical procedure. They can, therefore, only be regarded as single examples which are, however, able to improve our visual interpretation of neonatal EEG records, both normal and abnormal.

During both active and quiet sleep, artifact-free samples of 3 min duration each were subjected to the computer analysis. Mathematical functions useful in this study are the autospectrogram, or power spectrum, and the coherence spectrum. The mathematical definition of these quantities and their applicability to EEG analysis have been discussed in detail by Walter (1963).

The autospectrogram resolves an EEG recording into frequency components assigning higher intensity values to those frequencies at which the bioelectric activity is most pronounced and most regular. The more subtle variations in the activity at higher frequencies are best seen by plotting the logarithm of intensity against frequency.

The coherence function provides a quantitative measure of the interdependence of the bioelectric activity in different areas of the brain, as exhibited by different channels of EEG tracings. The magnitude of the coherence lies

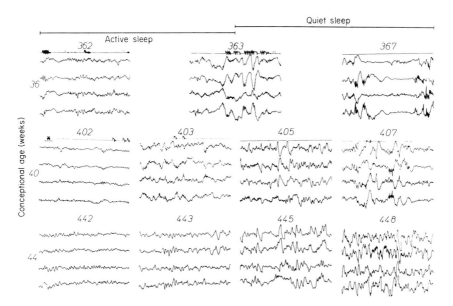

Fig. 1. Between 36 and 44 weeks of conceptional age, 11 EEG patterns can be identified as being typical for a certain conceptional age and for a particular behavioral state. For a detailed description of these patterns, see Parmelee *et al.* (1968) and Schulte *et al.* (1969b). The code number for each pattern consists of three digits: the first two indicate the conceptional age in weeks and the third digit indicates the EEG patterns usually seen in specific behavioral states: 1 occurs during awake (not depicted in this figure), 2 and 3 during active sleep, 7 and 8 during quiet sleep. From 1 to 8 the amplitude and the amount of slow wave activity in the EEG increases. Code no. 7 is always a discontinuous pattern (*tracé alternant*), no. 8 is a slow wave pattern with spindles.

between 0 and 1, indicating the relative linearity of the relation between two tracings. This quantity is the analog of the correlation coefficient of elementary statistics.

The EEG data were digitized and the power and coherence spectra computed using a general program for "Time Series Spectrum Estimation" (program no. BMDX 92, Dixon, 1969).

RESULTS

Compared with the control infants, the small-for-gestational-age infants of toxemic mothers had significantly more immature EEG patterns (Fig. 2), both in active and quiet sleep. Thus, conceptional age was frequently underestimated in the growth-retarded infants, whereas the estimation was rather correct in normal babies (Table I) as it was in our earlier studies (Parmelee *et al.*, 1968; Schulte *et*

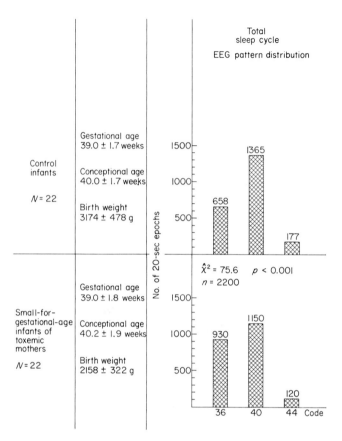

Fig. 2. EEG pattern distribution indicated by the first two digits of our codes along the *x* axis in normal and in small-for-gestational age newborn infants of toxemic mothers. 100 artifact-free EEG epochs of 20-sec duration each were coded for every single infant during both active and quiet sleep. In the abnormal infants significantly more immature EEG patterns (36) and in the normal infants significantly more mature EEG patterns (40 and 44) are found. The EEG interpreter did not know the infants' conceptional ages or fetal histories.

al., 1969a). It was difficult to estimate the age from some EEG's, since their patterns were not characteristic for any age. Such an EEG is depicted in Fig. 3. The discontinuous, "spikey" *tracé alternant* during quiet sleep is usually present in normal 36-week-old infants. In contrast, however, the high frequency activity during active sleep is not compatible with 36 weeks conceptional age. Such discordant or abnormal EEG's were found much more often among the small-for-gestational-age newborn infants of toxemic mothers than among the control babies (Table II).

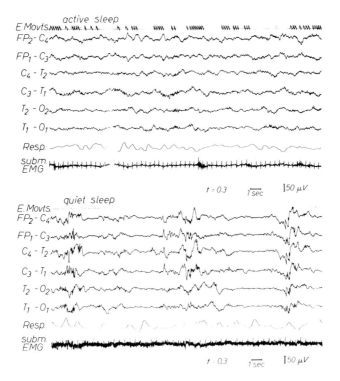

Fig. 3. Infant of toxemic mother; 39 weeks conceptional age; 2500 g. The EEG of this infant is dominated by rather high frequency bioelectric activity during active sleep (see Fig. 4a) and by a very marked *tracé alternant* pattern with some spikes during quiet sleep. If at all normal, the active sleep pattern is consistent with 40 weeks conceptional age, but the quiet sleep pattern is more typical for immature infants of 36-38 weeks. t = time constant (sec); E.Movts. = eye movements; Resp = respiration; subm. EMG = submental electromyogram with EKG artifacts.

In Fig. 4, autospectra of the EEG's during active sleep of four pairs of infants are depicted, one of each pair being a control and the other one a small-for-gestational-age newborn infant of a toxemic mother. The pairs were matched for conceptional age. Figure 4 contains the autospectra of the EEG during active sleep depicted in Fig. 3. Two abnormal infants showed more power in the high frequencies. Moreover, the power peak at about 4-5 Hz, indicating an emerging basic frequency during active sleep, is absent or small in all the abnormal but only in one control infant. No consistent differences could be detected between the control and the abnormal infants of this study in the power spectra during quiet sleep.

The bioelectric coherence between the two hemispheres was rather similar in the abnormal and in the control infants during both active and quiet sleep (Fig.

TABLE I *Maturation of EEG Patterns*[a]

	Gestational age (weeks)	Conceptional age (weeks)	Birth weight (g)	Conceptional age estimate amount of error in weeks						
				−5	−4	−3	−2	0 ± 1	+2	+3
Control infants N = 22	39.0 ± 1.7	40.0 ± 1.7	3174 ± 478	0	0	1	2	16	2	1
Small-for-gestational-age infants of toxemic mothers N = 22	39.0 ± 1.8	40.2 ±1.9	2158 ± 322	1	1	4	4	10	2	0

[a]Based on the codes given to each 20-sec epoch of EEG the conceptional age estimate is rather accurate in the normal but frequently underrated in the abnormal infants.

TABLE II *Evaluation of EEG*[a]

	N	Normal	> 2 weeks retarded	Abnormal	Abnormal + > 2 weeks retarded
Control infants	22	21	0	0	1
Small-for-gestational-age infants of toxemic mothers	22	7	5	9	1

[a]EEG's containing patterns which could not be classified as being typical for a certain conceptional age or containing patterns of different developmental maturity are called abnormal. With one exception, such EEG's are found only in the abnormal infants. This evaluation was done without knowledge of the infants' conceptional ages or fetal histories.

5). The coherence was always stronger in the lower (below 8 Hz) than in the higher (over 7.5 Hz) frequencies. For 0.5-7.5 Hz activity the coherence was consistently higher in the frontocentral than in the centrotemporal leads. These two findings were significant at a 0.05 probability level. The EEG, depicted in Fig. 3 which was visually classified as abnormal and whose unusual power spectra are given in Fig. 4, was unique in showing a rather high coherence of the 7.5-24 Hz activity during active sleep (Fig. 6).

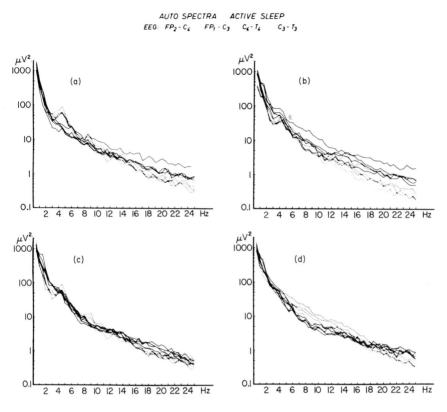

AUTO SPECTRA   ACTIVE SLEEP
EEG: FP₂-C₄   FP₁-C₃   C₄-T₄   C₃-T₃

Fig. 4. The EEG power spectra are very consistent, provided that the infants compared are of identical conceptional ages and in the same behavioral states. (a) (1/m) P. J.: 39/0 weeks, 2500 g; (...) G. B.: 38/4 weeks, 3000 g. (b) (1/m) H. D.: 40/4 weeks. 1460 g; (...) D. Z.: 41/2 weeks, 2150 g. (c) (1/m) J. F.: 39/1 weeks, 2300 g; (...) G. B.: 38/4 weeks, 3000 g. (d) (1/m) D. E.: 40/5 weeks, 2400 g; (...) A. Sch.: 41/0 weeks, 3400 g. In all abnormal infants (dotted lines), but only in one normal infant (solid lines), the 4-5 Hz power peak is missing. In the abnormal infants (a), (b), and less marked in (c), the amount of high-frequency activity is increased.

Some small-for-gestational-age newborn infants of toxemic mothers showed a disturbed sleeping behavior with poorly coordinated quiet sleep. As shown in Fig. 7, quiet sleep states were often short and respiration was not as regular as in the corresponding control infant. The regularity of respiration during quiet sleep was more than two standard deviations from the normal mean (Schulte *et al.*, 1969b). We did not study these phenomena statistically in all the infants of toxemic mothers, since it has been reported from various centers to be a rather consistent finding in many abnormal newborn infants with quite different diseases (for references, see discussion).

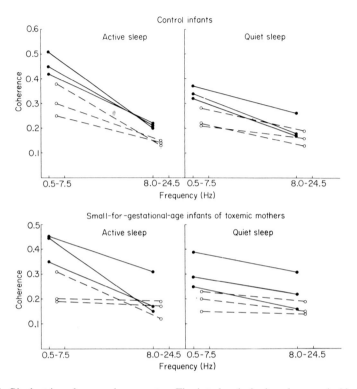

Fig. 5. Bioelectric coherence in neonates. The interhemispheric coherence in bioelectric activity indicated by the linear correlation coefficient is always higher for the low frequencies and over the frontocentral area of the brain. There are no significant differences detectable so far between active and quiet sleep. The coherence is less consistent in the abnormal infants and one of them shows a rather high level of coherence particularly for the high frequencies (see also Fig. 6). (●) Frontocentral; (○) centrotemporal.

Some small-for-gestational-age newborn infants of toxemic mothers had low blood glucose values. However, the EEG abnormalities occurred almost as frequently in those infants who had never been hypoglycemic, but a little more frequently in those who had low blood glucose values for a prolonged period (Fig. 8). However, at the time of recording, in all 10 hypoglycemic infants (below 30%) blood glucose levels had stabilized above 40 mg/100 ml.

DISCUSSION

In 1968, Dreyfus-Brisac and Minkowski reported on abnormalities and developmental retardation in EEG's of small-for-dates infants, without quantitatively comparing the results with a control group. Three abnormal neonatal

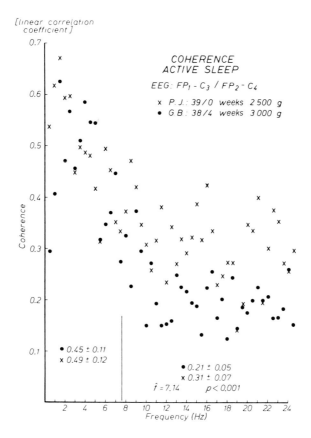

Fig. 6. Compared with all other control infants, baby P. J., whose EEG is depicted in Fig. 3, with its power spectra in Fig. 4a, has a significantly high interhemispheric coherence for the high-frequency activity of the frontocentral cortical area. (*t = t* test.)

EEG phenomena, i.e., developmental retardation, bioelectric patterns of different maturity in the same EEG, and unusual patterns which normally do not occur, have since been worked out by Dr. Dreyfus-Brisac. In this study, a significant number of EEG's of small-for-gestational-age newborn infants of toxemic mothers was not appropriate for the infant's conceptional age. For this statement, it is important to know that both groups of infants, normal and abnormal, were comparable in conceptional ages. The inclusion of more preterm infants in the growth-retarded group, as compared with the control group, would have led to the same result. Therefore, the identity in conceptional ages of both groups of infants was not only ascertained by carefully evaluating the mothers' dates but also by measurement of nerve conduction velocity in each infant. The means and first standard deviations for ulnar nerve conduction velocity were

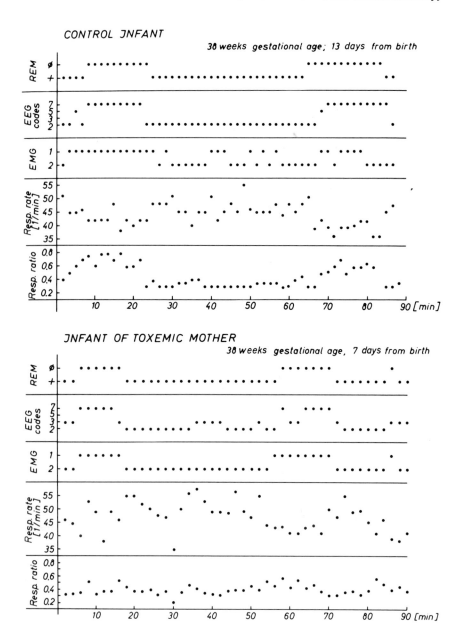

Fig. 7. Compiled polygram of one normal and one small-for-gestational-age newborn infant. In the abnormal infant the durations of the two quiet sleep periods are shorter. Moreover, in the abnormal infant the EEG patterns are inconsistent and the respiration remains irregular during quiet sleep. REM: ϕ = absent; + = present. EEG codes: (Fig. 1). EMG: 1 = tonic submental muscle activity; 2 = phasic or absent submental muscle activity. Respiration ratio: shortest/longest breath-to-breath interval within 20-sec epoch.

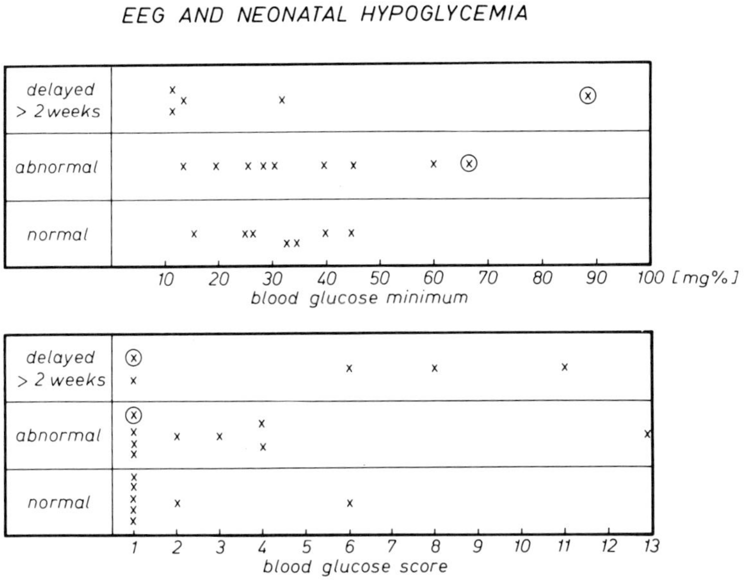

EEG AND NEONATAL HYPOGLYCEMIA

delayed > 2 weeks	x x x ⊗
abnormal	x x x x x x x x ⊗
normal	x xx x x x x

```
          10   20   30   40   50   60   70   80   90   100 [mg%]
                     blood glucose minimum
```

delayed > 2 weeks	⊗ x x x x
abnormal	⊗ x x x x x x x
normal	x x x x x x x

```
          1    2    3    4    5    6    7    8    9    10   11   12   13
                     blood glucose score
```

Fig. 8. EEG and neonatal hypoglycemia. Abnormal and retarded EEG patterns are found a little more frequently in small-for-gestational-age newborn infants with low postnatal blood glucose values, particularly in those with long-lasting hypoglycemia. However, at the time of recording, all blood glucose values were normalized. X = These infants had been given glucose before the first blood glucose estimations had been done.

very similar for both groups (Schulte *et al.*, 1971) indicating that the conceptional ages were the same (Schulte *et al.*, 1968; Blom and Finnström, 1968; Ruppert and Johnson, 1968; Dubowitz *et al.*, 1968).

Computer analysis showed patterns which we are tempted to regard as abnormal for various reasons in at least two small-for-gestational-age infants. (Fig. 4a, b). The spectrum analysis of the EEG during active sleep showed a tendency toward an increase in high frequency activity with low interhemispheric coherence. This activity may therefore be speculatively regarded as cortical noise, i.e., a highly asynchronous random activity in the cortical neurones. In the same abnormal infants, there was a lack in the development of dominating rhythms at about 4-5 Hz. Further investigations are necessary to determine whether this 4-5 Hz activity peak can be regarded as bioelectric maturational milestone, which is not yet attained in small-for-gestational-age newborn infants of toxemic mothers.

The area of any computer analysis of neonatal EEG's is still such new territory that all findings can only be interpreted with caution since we do not yet know the developmental sequence. This is particularly true for coherence studies which determine degrees of coordination of bioelectric activity between corresponding locations on the two hemispheres. Since this coordination is dependent upon the developing thalamocortical synaptic connections, its evaluation seems to be particularly promising for developmental studies. We would like to leave the interpretation of our normal coherence values in full-term infants until a later time, when similar studies in both older and younger infants have been done. However, it is interesting to note that one small-for-gestational-age newborn infant of a toxemic mother had a significant increase in interhemispheric coherence of high-frequency activity in the frontocentral part of the brain. This most likely indicates that a common centrencephalic pacemaker was abnormally active during active sleep. We do not think that the large amount of coherent high-frequency activity is due to aliasing, because frequencies only a little higher than indicated are automatically filtered out in BMDX 92.

It is important to mention that some small-for-gestational-age newborn infants of toxemic mothers had an EEG nearly normal for their conceptional age. However, all the abnormal EEG's showed a similar type of abnormality.

In normal sleep of infants, specific patterns of physiological variables and motor behavior recur periodically and are stable over a length of time before changing to another pattern. These cycle fluctuations imply that coordinative and homeostatic mechanisms must be active in the newborn, and we visualize the interrelationships as schematically illustrated in Fig. 9. The mechanisms for the maintenance of quiet sleep over a certain period of time seems to be one of the most vulnerable in the newborn brain. It is only in the last few weeks before term that the infants are able to sustain quiet sleep with all its characteristics (regular respiration and heart rate, no body or eye movements, tonic submental muscle activity, high voltage *tracé alternant* EEG (Parmelee *et al.*, 1967). With various kinds of prenatal or perinatal pathology, the neonatal brain loses this recently acquired ability to coordinate all these parameters and/or to maintain the still very labile state of quiet sleep for a normal period of about 10-15 min (Monod *et al.*, 1967; Prechtl, 1968; Schulte *et al.*, 1969b). This vulnerability of the quiet sleep state was also shown in one small-for-gestational-age infant of a toxemic mother, whose sleep behavior was similar to that of a preterm infant.

In small-for-gestational-age newborn infants, hypoglycemia has been discussed very extensively as being one of the etiological factors of central nervous system (CNS) dysfunction (Cornblath *et al.*, 1959, 1964; Neligan *et al.*, 1963; Creery, 1965; Haworth, 1965; Reisner *et al.*, 1965; Pilders *et al.*, 1967). In the infants of this study, the abnormal bioelectric phenomena cannot be regarded as symptomatic hypoglycemia, since (1) the bioelectric abnormalities were identical in infants with and without hypoglycemia, and (2) at the time of recording the blood glucose levels had stabilized at values above 40 mg/100 ml. Moreover, it seems unlikely that a significant number of study infants suffered from posthypoglycemic brain dysfunction, since no significant relation between postnatal blood glucose and abnormal EEG could be detected. In order to avoid

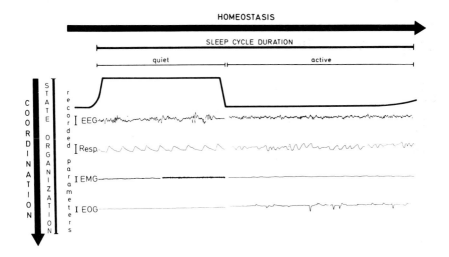

Fig. 9. The maintenance of certain sleep states over a period of time is called homeostasis. The state-appropriate function of all systems, is called coordination (Lenard, 1970). Active sleep with irregular respiration and rapid eye movements (REM). Quiet sleep with regular respiration and tonic muscle activity in the electromyogram of the submental muscles. Each state (active or quiet sleep) is characterized by certain parameters, only a few of which are depicted in this schematic diagram. Many biochemical and endocrine functions are also changing with sleep states.

any misunderstandings, we wish to emphasize that we certainly do not doubt the existence of neonatal symptomatic hypoglycemia and the importance of its prevention by early feeding and glucose infusions (Cornblath and Reisner, 1965; Gentz *et al.*, 1969). In fact, in some of our study infants we may have prevented further brain damage by these precautions. However, for some neonates with brain dysfunction and hypoglycemia we are tempted to propose another hypothesis. The low blood glucose values of the infants in this study may have been just another manifestation of the poor homeostatic brain mechanisms as documented by the impaired maintenance of quiet sleep. We know that some endocrinological and metabolic parameters are as closely related to the sleeping states as the neurophysiological ones monitored in this study (Mandell and Mandell, 1969). It is possible that the same adverse effects which impaired the CNS feedback mechanisms controlling behavioral states, affected brain stem metabolic control systems as well. In the infants of this study, it is also likely from the results on their motor behavior (Schulte *et al.*, 1971) that poor blood glucose control was a symptom rather than the cause of brain dysfunction (Etheridge and Millichap, 1964).

It is obvious from our data that the bioelectric abnormalities were, in general, not caused by intranatal or postnatal hypoxia, which occurred only in 3 of the 16 infants with visible EEG abnormalities or retarded EEG's and only in one of the infants with deviant EEG computer data. Furthermore, the rather consistent abnormal bioelectric phenomena occurred in the absence of any other overt postnatal illness. Recent investigations into the biochemical results of severe malnutrition during intrauterine development disclosed defective myelinization (Dobbing, 1965-1966; Widdowson *et al.*, 1960) as well as neurocellular growth retardation (Zamenhof *et al.*, 1968; Winick and Rosso, 1969; Winick, 1970).

That the bioelectric abnormalities are the functional correlates of brain cell reduction and myelinization deficits is an unproven though intriguing hypothesis. We do not think that our findings are specific for small-for-gestational-age newborn infants of toxemic mothers. In large-for-gestational-age infants of diabetic mothers, for instance, we were able to demonstrate similar abnormalities (Schulte *et al.*, 1969a, b). The number of neurophysiological reactions to adverse effects is limited and different pathological circumstances may result in quite similar patterns of abnormal brain function. Whatever the interpretation and the cause of our findings may be, the broad statement that nervous system maturation progresses independently of the nutritional status of the fetus is no longer feasible and the above-mentioned biochemical and anatomical results of Dobbing (1965-1966), Widdowson *et al.* (1960), Zamenhof *et al.* (1968), and Winick (1970; Winick and Rosso, 1969) may well have a functional correlate. We do not think that the abnormalities of bioelectric brain maturation in infants of toxemic mothers represent only developmental retardation. Indeed, what looked like immature EEG patterns could in reality be abnormal. Certain findings in individual infants, like the occurrence of EEG patterns of different maturity and, certainly, the abnormally high coherence, are indicative of developmental pathology rather than developmental retardation.

SUMMARY

The bioelectric brain development of 22 small-for-gestational-age newborn infants of toxemic mothers were compared with an equal number of normal neonates matched for both age from conception and age from birth.

1. The development of age-related EEG sleep patterns was significantly retarded. Thus, from their EEG's, the conceptional age of newborn infants of toxemic mothers was frequently underestimated.

2. Many small-for-gestational-age newborn infants of toxemic mothers showed abnormal EEG patterns which could not be classified as characteristic of any age.

3. EEG numerical spectrum analysis during active sleep showed certain peculiarities in the high frequency and/or in the 4-5 Hz range.

4. With one exception, interhemispheric coherence was normal, being higher over the frontocentral than over the centrotemporal area of the cortex. Low frequency waves were more coherent than 7.5-24 Hz activity.

5. The abnormal EEG phenomena occurred in the absence of any other overt postnatal illness and without hypoxia and hypoglycemia. CNS maturation does not proceed independently of the nutritional status of the fetus.

REFERENCES

Akiyama, Y., Schulte, F. J., Schultz, M. A., and Parmelee, A. H. (1969). Acoustically evoked responses in premature and full-term newborn infants. *Electroencephalogr. Clin. Neurophysiol.* **26**, 371-380.

Amiel-Tison, D. (1968). Neurological evaluation of the maturity of newborn infants. *Arch. Dis. Childhood* **43**, 89-93.

Bachmann, K. D. (1969). Die Hypoglykämien des Neugeborenen. *Monatsschr. Kinderheilk.* **117**, 230-234.

Blom, S., and Finnström, O. (1968). Motor conduction velocities in newborn infants of various gestational ages. *Acta Paediat. Scand.* **57**, 377.

Brett, E. M. (1965). The estimation of foetal maturity by the neurological examination of the neonate. *In* "Gestational Age, Size and Maturity" (M. Dawkins and W. G. MacGregor, eds.), pp. 105-115. Heinemann, London.

Cornblath, M., and Reisner, S. H. (1965). Blood glucose in the neonate and its clinical significance. *New Engl. J. Med.* **273**, 378-381.

Cornblath, M., Odell, G. B., and Levin, E. Y. (1959). Symptomatic neonatal hypoglycemia associated with toxemia of pregnancy. *J. Pediat.* **55**, 545-562.

Cornblath, M., Wybregt, S. H., Baens, G. S., and Klein, R. J. (1964). Symptomatic neonatal hypoglycemia. *Pediatrics* **33**, 388-402.

Creery, R. D. G. (1965). Hypoglycemia in the newborn. *Can. Med Ass. J.* **92**, 861-863.

Dixon, W. J. (1969). BMDX92–time series spectrum estimation. *In* "Biomedical Computer Programs," X-Ser. Suppl., pp. 198-224. Univ. of California Press, Berkeley. (Univ. of Calif. publication in automatic computation, No. 3.)

Dobbing, J. (1965-1966). The effect of undernutrition on myelination in the central nervous system. *Biol. Neonatorum* **9**, 132-147.

Dreyfus-Brisac, C. (1962). The electroencephalogram of the premature infant. *World Neurol.* **3**, 5-15.

Dreyfus-Brisac, C. (1964). The electroencephalogram of the premature infant and the full-term newborn: normal and abnormal development of waking and sleeping patterns. *In* "Neurological and Electroencephalographic Correlative Studies in Infancy" (P. Kellaway and I. Petersen, eds.), pp. 186-207. Grune and Stratton, New York.

Dreyfus-Brisac, C., and Minkowski, A. (1968). EEG maturation and low birth weight. *In* "Clinical Electroencephalography of Children" (P. Kellaway and I. Petersen, eds.), pp. 49-60. Almqvist & Wiksell, Stockholm.

Dubowitz, V., Whittaker, G. F., Brown, B. H., and Robinson, R. (1968). Nerve conduction velocity. An index of neurological maturity of the newborn infant. *Develop. Med. Child Neurol.* **10**, 741-749.

Ek, J., and Daae, L. N. W. (1967). Whole blood glucose determination in newborn infants, comparison and evaluation of five different methods. *Acta Paediat. Scand.* **56**, 461-466.

Engel, R., and Benson, R. C. (1968). Estimate of conceptional age by evoked response activity. _Biol. Neonatorum_ **12**, 201-213.

Etheridge, J. E., and Millichap, J. G. (1964). Hypoglycemia and seizures in childhood. The etiologic significance of primary cerebral lesions. _Neurology_ **14**, 397-404.

Gentz, J. C. H., Perrson, B. E., and Zetterström, R. (1969). On the diagnosis of symptomatic neonatal hypoglycemia. _Acta Paediat. Scand._ **58**, 449-459.

Graziani, L. J., Weitzman, E. D., and Velasco, M. S. (1968). Neurologic maturation and auditory evoked responses in low birth weight infants. _Pediatrics_ **41**, 483-494.

Haworth, J. C. (1965). The neurological and developmental effects of neonatal hypoglycemia: A follow-up of 22 cases. _Can. Med. Ass. J._ **92**, 861-863.

Hosemann, H. (1948). Schwangerschaftsdauer und Neugeborenengewicht. _Arch. Gynaekol._ **176**, 109-123.

Larroche, J. C. (1962). Quelques aspects anatomiques du development cérébral. _Biol. Neonatorum_ **4**, 126-153.

Lenard, H. G. (1970). "Polygraphische Schlafuntersuchungen bei Gesunden und Kranken Säuglingen und Kleinkindern." Habilitationschrift der Universität, Göttingen.

Mandell, A. J., and Mandell, M. P. (1969). Peripheral hormonal and metabolic correlates of rapid eye movement sleep. _Exp. Med. Surg._ **27**, 224-236.

Monod, N., and Pajot, N. (1965). Le sommeil du nouveau-né et du prématuré. _Biol. Neonatorum_ **8**, 281-307.

Monod, N., Eliet-Flescher, J., and Dreyfus-Brisac, C. (1967). Le sommeil du nouveau-né et du prématuré. III. Les troubles de l'organisation du sommeil chez le nouveau-né pathologique: Analyse des études polygraphiques. _Biol Neonatorum_ **11**, 216-247.

Neligan, G. A., Robson, E., and Watson, J. (1963). Hypoglycemia in the newborn. Sequel of intrauterine malnutriton. _Lancet_ **1**, 1282-1284.

Nolte, R., Schulte, F. J., Michaelis, R., Weisse, R., and Gruson, R. (1969). Bioelectric brain maturation in small-for-dates infants. _Develop. Med. Child Neurol._ **11**, 83-93.

Parmelee, A. H., Wenner, W. H., Akiyama, Y., Schultz, M., and Stern, E. (1967). Sleep states in premature infants. _Develop. Med. Child Neurol._ **9**, 70-77.

Parmelee, A. H., Schulte, F. J., Akiyama, Y., Wenner, W. H., Schultz, M. A., and Stern, E. (1968). Maturation of EEG activity during sleep in premature infants. _Electroencephalogr. Clin. Neurophysiol._ **24**, 319-329.

Pilders, R., Forbesa, E., O'Connor, S. M., and Cornblath, M. (1967). The incidence of neonatal hypoglycemia: A completed survey. _J. Pediat._ **70**, 76-80.

Prechtl, H. F. R. (1968). Polygraphic studies of the full-term newborn. II. Computer analysis of recorded data. _In_ "Studies in Infancy" (M. S. Bax and R. C. MacKeith, eds.), pp. 22-40. Heinemann, London.

Reisner, S. H., Forbes, A. E., and Cornblath, M. (1965). The smaller of twins and hypoglycemia. _Lancet_ **1**, 524-526.

Relander, A., and Räihä, C. E. (1963). Differences between the enzymatic and O-toluidine methods of blood glucose determination. _Scand. J. Clin. Lab. Invest._ **15**, 221-224.

Robinson, R. J., (1966). Assessment of gestational age by neurological examination. _Arch. Dis. Childhood_ **41**, 437-447.

Ruppert, E. S., and Johnson, E. W. (1968). Motor nerve conduction velocities in low birth weight infants. _Pediatrics_ **42**, 255-260.

Saint-Anne Dargassies, S. (1955). La maturation neurologique du prématuré. _Etudes Neo-natales_ **4**, 71-83.

Saint-Anne Dargassies, S. (1966). Neurological maturation of the premature infant of 28-41 weeks gestational age. _In_ "Human Development" (F. Faulkner, ed.), pp. 306-325. Saunders, Philadelphia, Pennsylvania.

Schroeder, C., and Heckel, H. (1952). Zur Frage der Hirntätigkeit beim Neugeborenen. *Geburtsh. Frauenheilk.* **12**, 992-999.

Schulte, F. J., Michaelis, R., Linke, I., and Nolte, R. (1968). Motor nerve conduction velocity in term, preterm and small-for-dates infants. *Pediatrics* **42**, 17-26.

Schulte, F. J., Lasson, U., Parl, U., Nolte, R., and Jürgens, U. (1969a). Brain and behavioural maturation in newborn infants of diabetic mothers. Part II. Sleep cycles. *Neuropaediatrie* **1**, 36-43.

Schulte, F. J., Michaelis, R., Nolte, R., Albert, G., Parl, U., and Lasson, U. (1969b). Brain and behavioural maturation in newborn infants of diabetic mothers. Part I. Nerve conduction and EEG patterns. *Neuropaediatrie* **1**, 24-35.

Schulte, F. J., Schrempf, G., and Hinze, G. (1971). In preparation.

Walter, D. O. (1963). Spectral analysis for electroencephalograms: Mathematical determination of neurophysiological relationships from records of limited duration. *Exp. Neurol.* **8**, 155-181.

Widdowson, E. M., Dickerson, J. W., and McCance, R. A. (1960). Severe undernutrition in growing and adult animals. IV. The impact of severe undernutrition on the chemical composition of the soft tissues of the pig. *Brit. J. Nutr.* **14**, 457-471.

Winick, M. (1970). Cellular growth in intrauterine malnutrition. *Pediat. Clin. N. Amer.* **17**, 69-78.

Winick, M., and Rosso, P. (1969). The effect of severe early malnutrition on cellular growth of human brain. *Pediat. Res.* **3**, 181-184.

Zamenhof, S. E., van Marthens, E., and Margolis, F. L. (1968). DNA (cell number) and protein in neonatal brain: Alteration by maternal dietary protein restriction. *Science* **160**, 322-323.

GENERAL DISCUSSION

Dr. Roberts: The last data presented are quite in keeping with the failure of normal development of inhibitory neurological mechanisms in abnormal children, or a delay in the development of these mechanisms which are responsible for very finely tuned neural regulation. They may also be involved in metabolic regulation by the hypothalamus, which is in control of homeostatic regulation.

Dr. Anders: There appears to be a discrepancy between the two sets of data presented by Dr. Schulte and Dr. Petre-Quadens. Dr. Schulte reports that his infants have a reduction or inability to maintain quiet sleep; and Dr. Petre-Quadens has shown a disturbance in PS in her group. I wonder whether this discrepancy reflects a difference in scoring sleep stages or whether there are real differences between the subject groups resulting, perhaps, from their different ages and diagnoses.

Dr. Petre-Quadens: I do not think there is a real discrepancy. Dr. Schulte's test was quiet sleep and he showed that in abnormal babies there is an inability to sustain quiet sleep. We took, as a test, REMS and showed the children's inability to sustain REMS. There is, in the abnormal infants, an inability to *organize* sleep. This points to their lack of behavioral inhibition needed for the maintenance of both quiet and REMS.

Dr. Schulte: The data of Dr. Petre-Quadens cannot be compared with ours, since I think we have to specify and to subdivide mental retardation. Different etiology may account for different results. Hypothyroid infants, for example, have a very specific type of disorganization of sleep: during active sleep, they have few eye movements; during quiet sleep, they have few spindles, both almost quantitatively increasing with therapy (Schultz *et al.,* 1968; Schulte *et al.,* 1971). The lack of spindles in hypothyroidism is quite in contrast to the high amount of sleep spindles in PKU. If we were looking at the retarded in general, we would have missed this point.

Dr. Metcalf: I have two questions. Maybe you can answer them both. In the area of the difficulty of controlling and maintaining quiet sleep, is there one of the variables, as you add them up, for quiet sleep that is particularly prone to poor control and disturbance? What do you think this might mean if this is the case?

Dr. Schulte: In the newborn, poor coordination and homeostasis of quiet sleep is a consistent finding in many abnormal neonates with different pathology. The regularity of respiration seems to be extremely vulnerable. However, I am not yet saying that this is the most vulnerable parameter. A more sophisticated analysis of REMS patterns, power spectra of EEG, or even biochemical parameters may or may not disclose equal vulnerability and sensitivty to abnormal influences during pregnancy and birth.

Dr. Gordon: I wish to put in a specification about the definition of the term "newborn." A lot depends on the number of postnatal hours. A lot depends on whether you are in the delivery room. It is important to know whether toxemic mothers have been treated with magnesium, or whatever, before you use the infants for observation. I think we tend sometimes to lump all newborns together without knowing exactly what circumstances existed before we began to observe them or their mothers.

Dr. Schulte: I should say that in all these babies the data you mentioned are very complete, e.g., pregnancy, birth, and postnatal data. I left them out only to keep the paper short. We had both neurological and biochemical studies done on these infants and on their mothers. The correlation mathematics will keep us busy probably during the next year. However, one point I can make already now: the results are not due to maternal anesthesia with magnesium or any other drug.

Dr. Anders: We, and others (Schulman, 1969), have studied the sleep patterns of newborns delivered to drug-addicted mothers. These babies show atypical and reduced amounts of NREMS.

Dr. Weitzman: I have two questions, the first for Dr. Petre-Quadens and the second for Dr. Ornitz. Since most of your subjects were studied for only one night, and of those studied for more than one night you only used the first night of recording, how would the subject variability influence those results? For example, in one subject, you had a sleep time which ranged from 3½-8½ hr/night, with a range of PS between 3.3 and 24%. It would seem to me it would be very important to establish the stability of these patients, or at least define the degree of instability before one could interpret the results of such a heterogeneous population of patients.

The question I have for Dr. Ornitz regards the issue of using the first two REMS periods of the night as a time to define his measured parameters. Is it possible that daytime activity contaminated or influenced, in the early part of the night, those first two REM periods? Is it not possible, therefore, that your results showing differences could be explained not so much on differences in REMS phenomena, but differences of NREMS phenomena which intruded into and became associated with the REMS period? Thus, the interpretation of this relationship to your phasic excitatory-inhibition theory might be a very different one?

Dr. Petre-Quadens: I wish to answer the question directed to me by referring to Fig. 10. We compiled PS as a function of total sleeping time in mentally retarded subjects and normal subjects. We see in this figure that in the mentally retarded the percent of REMS or PS increases linearly as a function of the TST, whereas in the normal subjects the percent of PS remains approximately the same regardless of the length of TST. Since the variability of TST is greater in normal subjects, the eye movement intervals have been measured in records of subjects with similar TST.

Dr. Ornitz: Dr. Weitzman's point is a very good one. We are going to try to correct this in

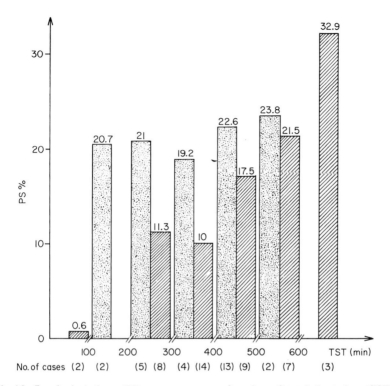

Fig. 10. Paradoxical sleep (PS) percentage as a function of total sleep time (TST) in mentally retarded (▨) and normal (▨) subjects.

future studies. But the nature of children's sleep patterns does not always let us have the same number of REMS periods available on each child.

We have, in fact, data on five REMS periods available on the babies. These data show that the eye movement burst duration is what one might expect, that is, it increases in almost a linear manner across the five successive REMS periods. But for many of the autistic children and the normal children, we were not able to get that many REMS periods per night, so that we could not make the comparison we wanted to make. We did have at least two REMS periods on all of the children and babies studied, and that is why we made the comparison based on the first two REMS periods.

Dr. Weitzman: This point is very important. The whole issue of 24-hr cyclicity, the duration of the night sleep, the preceding daytime activity of these very abnormal children vs a normal group makes it very difficult to compare results in terms of a specific measurement during a specific period of sleep.

REFERENCES

Schulman, C. (1969). Alterations of the sleep cycle in heroin addicted and "suspect" newborns. *Neuropaediatrie* **1**, 89-100.

Schulte, F. J., Lenard, H. G., and Bell, E. (1972). In preparation.
Schultz, M. A., Schulte, F. J., Akiyama, Y., and Parmelee, A. H. (1968). Development of encephalographic sleep phenomena in hypothyroid infants. *Electroencephalogr. Clin. Neurophysiol.* **25**, 351-358.

19

Summary and Concluding Remarks

Donald B. Lindsley

There have been excellent presentations and discussions of a wide variety of topics by experts representing several disciplines. It would be presumptuous, indeed, for me to assume that I could do justice in a brief summary to the great variety of materials and challenging ideas presented. I should like to make some general remarks about the history of this subject, define its terms, and discuss some of the foregoing chapters. I will also make some remarks about the rapid development of science and technology during the past few decades, as well as the constraints this seems to have placed upon us generally, and in the field of this particular work.

HISTORICAL BACKGROUND

As we all know, the past four decades have witnessed a tremendous increase in interest in the study of the brain and nervous system. So far as the brain is concerned it has been an era dominated by neurophysiology, and more specifically by electrophysiology (both electrical stimulation and recording), which over the years before 1920 had been slow to take shape, largely due to the lack of suitable instrumentation. Sherrington, Forbes, Lucas, Adrian, and others had been concerned with studies of reflexes, using electrical stimulation and electrical recording with the string galvanometer and electrometer prior to 1920. Following the development of radio for use in World War I, Forbes and Thacher (1920) first adapted vacuum tube amplification for use in electrophysiology, thereby making it possible to use less sensitive recording devices but with higher frequency-response characteristics, and Erlanger and Gasser first employed the Braun tube (cathode ray oscilloscope) in about 1923. Thereafter, the recording of electrical activity in peripheral nerves, receptors, and muscles began in earnest. In 1928 Adrian published *The Basis of Sensation,* to be followed later in 1932 by *The Mechanism of Nervous Action,* both landmarks in the study of neural mechanisms.

By the end of the 1920's, Berger (1929) had described the human electroencephalogram (EEG) and by 1932 had noted the effect of sleep on the EEG. He had also observed developmental changes in the EEG with age (Berger, 1932). Berger's discovery that the brain has a rhythmic electrical beat of its own was a powerful stimulus to further explore the brain electrically, either directly in animals or through the scalp and skull of intact human subjects. Loomis *et al.* (1935, 1937) were the first to utilize the EEG in the study of all-night sleep and outlined the major stages of sleep as reflected in the EEG. Blake and Gerard (1937) and Blake, Gerard, and Kleitman (1939) were also early contributors to our understanding of sleep in terms of the EEG. Lindsley (1936, 1938, 1939) and Smith (1937, 1938a, b, c, 1939) were the first to make systematic cross-sectional and longitudinal studies of the developmental changes in the EEG of infants and children as a function of age. Smith (1938c) also studied changes in the pattern sequence during sleep in infants.

During the 1920's Hess began electrical stimulation studies of the diencephalon of cats and reported changes in emotional behavior. Hess (1929a, b, 1954) also discovered that it was possible by low-frequency, slowly rising pulses to induce sleep by stimulating in the region of the posterior hypothalamus and along the walls of the third ventricle and in the midline nuclei of the thalamus. During the late 1920's and 1930's Ranson and colleagues (see Ranson, 1939; Ranson and Magoun, 1939) explored the brain stem and hypothalamus by electrical stimulation, revealing many autonomic and brain stem reflex mechanisms, including descending and ascending influences. Kleitman began his studies of the physiology of sleep during the 1920's and in 1939 published the first extensive survey of sleep in a book entitled *Sleep and Wakefulness* (Kleitman, 1939). This book has since been revised and expanded (Kleitman, 1963). Bremer (1935) was the first to show by electrocortical recording and behavioral methods that a midbrain transection of the neuraxis (*cerveau isolé* preparation) causes somnolence. This was later shown by Lindsley *et al.* (1949, 1950) to be due to interruption of the ascending reticular activating system rather than deafferentation as proposed by Bremer.

The decade of the 1930's also became one of increased awareness of the importance of neuropharmacology and neurochemistry. The work of Sir Henry Dale (Dale 1935; Dale *et al.*, 1936) and Otto Loewi (Loewi and Navratil, 1926; Loewi, 1936) and their collaborators, which won for them a Nobel award, was well under way on the liberation of acetylcholine at synaptic and neuromuscular junctions. Cannon and Rosenblueth (1937; see also Rosenblueth, 1950) studying the autonomic nervous system, postulated neurohumoral substances in the form of sympathin E and I, terms later to become abandoned in favor of noradrenaline, adrenaline, and others with inhibitory properties.

During the 1940's, dc potentials were first recorded by Libet and Gerard (1941), and microelectrodes were first used by Ling and Gerard (1949); however, both accomplishments were to find their greatest usefulness and fruition during the 1950's and 1960's after further technical advances had come about.

Several electrophysiological studies bearing on thalamocortical relationships were initiated in the early 1940's by Morison and Dempsey (1942a, b) and Dempsey and Morison (1942a, b), but because of the imminence of World War II, their importance was largely overlooked until later. Toward the end of the first half of the 20th century, Magoun and collaborators carried out very important work on the descending and ascending roles of the brain stem reticular formation. In particular, the monumental discovery and clearly formulated theory of the role of the ascending reticular formation in sleep and wakefulness by Moruzzi and Magoun (1949) should be noted.

The study of the brain in learning and conditioned reflexes was ushered in by a realization that behavior could be studied objectively and quantitatively in animals. From the beginning of the 20th century, Pavlov, Thorndike, Franz, Lashley, and others began to point the way. The behaviorists Watson, Holt, Weiss, and others during the 1920's gave psychology a distinctly behavioral bent, and that tradition was to continue strongly up to the present. The understanding of behavior and its underlying mechanisms is, of course, one of the major goals of most of us, and the combining of behavioral, electrophysiological, neuro-pharmacological, neuroanatomical, and other methodologies has been one of the strong features of the past few decades.

The earliest contributions of neuroanatomy and neuropathology date back more than 100 years, but about 100 years ago the development of microscopes with greater resolving power and the development of suitable staining and sectioning methods led to great advances in the study of the fine structure of the nervous system. The German school of architectonics attempted a very elaborate differentiation of cortical areas in terms of their cellular structure, and

Brodmann's numerical labeling is still the principal way of denoting cortical topography. Golgi, Marchi, Ramón y Cajal, and others developed special methods of studying nerve cells and their processes. In the 1880's and 1890's Flechsig, with his myelogenetic approach, was the first to devote special attention to the development of the human brain and cortex in terms of neurohistology (Flechsig, 1920). Nearly 50 years later, Conel (1939-1959) published a monumental series of monographs on the developing human brain, beginning with newborns and carrying the analyses forward to 6 years of age and more. In the past decade, the development of specially refined Golgi silver staining procedures and the application of the electron microscope and microelectrode recording has led to finer and finer approaches to an understanding of the development of the cerebral cortex, structurally and functionally, by such investigators as the Scheibels, Nauta, Collonier, de Robertis, Valverde, Anokhin, Purpura, Scherrer, and others. It is especially important for this conference that some of this work has been directed toward the immature and developing brain about which we are rapidly gaining new and exciting concepts.

I have deliberately added this sketchy historical review to my remarks, because I believe it provides a useful background for the kinds of studies found in this volume. One can see that great progress has been made in methods of study of the brain and behavior; some of this progress has come about through new technical developments, but much of it, as in all science, has come about through the dedicated efforts of many people struggling with the accumulated record of progress in the past and attempting to move things forward a few notches. However slow and disappointing this progress may be at times, I believe all of us must admit that our curiosity, once aroused, is indeed a strong and persistent motivating factor. Also, I believe that all of us can take pride in the fact that we now know enough to talk about the brain and its mechanisms. Even though there remain many lifetimes of effort in unraveling its secrets, we are in a better position to understand how the brain functions in health and disease, how it learns and remembers, how it adapts and adjusts, how it performs in sleep and wakefulness, and how it matures and grows structurally and functionally. In all of these areas there remains much to be learned; progress will undoubtedly be slow, but the importance of the goal will hopefully always keep interest and the level of motivation high.

These last points are the subject of this work. Much knowledge has accumulated about brain structure and function within the past few decades, and many currently advanced techniques are being employed to chart new paths. Also, within the past few decades new findings and interpretations have appeared with regard to sleep behavior. Finally, the developmental approach to behavior and to the study of the brain appears to be one of the most powerful and versatile.

SOME ATTEMPTED DEFINITIONS

Maturation

Maturation, as a process, includes the complex of changes in growth, development, and adaptation of an organism, or its parts, as a function of age. Maturation, as a state, involves the degree to which form and function have attained completeness and unity. In either case, maturation is dependent upon the unfolding of a hereditary pattern or plan which begins with conception. The hereditary limits are set by genic conformation and the potentialities and liabilities within these limits are subject to the interactions of the organism with its environment, both internal and external. The interactions of organisms (or parts of organisms) with their environment, individually and collectively, constitute *behavior*. In this sense behavior may be covert as well as overt, and may be comprised of whole or part reactions.

Brain Mechanisms

Brain mechanisms are the neural, structurofunctional patterns by means of which an organism is enabled to interact with its environment. Some patterns, relatively fixed and vital to life processes, represent the maturational unfolding and development of hereditary patterns. These, sometimes referred to as "built-in" or "soldered-in" connections, result in so-called "instinctive" or unlearned behaviors. Other, more dynamically oriented, structurofunctional patterns permit a wider and more variable range of interactions with the environment and depend upon a plastic or modifiable record of the interactions and their consequences. The memory storage and utilization, over shorter or longer intervals, of such a dynamic record constitutes *learning*. The potential for its adaptive use may be called *intelligence* and the proficiency in learning to adapt, *achievement*.

Sleep and Sleep Behavior

Sleep is a variable function of a circadian life cycle typically alternating periodically with the waking state. It is believed to serve a restorative, recuperative function because it is necessary for the preservation of life and because it markedly reduces interactions with the environment. It is generally characterized by reduced sensory sensitivity, relative relaxation and quiescence, slowed respiration and heart rate, lowered oxygen consumption, and loss of consciousness, except during brief interspersed periods of dreaming of which one is aware. In addition to overt manifestations, the electrical activity of the skin, muscles, and brain may be used to study and assess sleep behavior. Skin resistance typically increases as sleep ensues and deepens. The electromyogram (EMG) characteristically recedes to a near zero baseline level, as relaxation becomes more complete. The EEG characteristically goes through a series of stages from waking to sleeping in which there is a progressive slowing and enlargement of the predominant waves, except for two phasic changes of relatively short duration.

The first of these phasic, transient states is marked in the EEG by the appearance of bursts of ~12-14/sec rhythmic waves which recur periodically at intervals of ~8-10 sec in young infants and more frequently and irregularly in adults. The appearance of these so-called spindle bursts is believed to mark the onset of sleep and is accompanied by loss of consciousness. Drowsiness and partial awareness, with mixed α and low-amplitude slow waves, precedes the spindle burst and slow wave stage denoting onset of sleep, and more profound sleep with mainly slow waves follows it. Although seen more widely, the origin or predominant locus of the spindle bursts appears to be in the midcentral region over the sensorimotor cortex in the neighborhood of the Rolandic fissure. This is especially evident in young infants.

The second phasic change in the EEG occurs typically several times per night of sleep and may range in duration from a few minutes to a half hour or more. Usually there are. periodic interruptions of the large, slow and somewhat irregular waves characteristic of deep sleep, during which the prevailing activity in the EEG suddenly shifts to a low amplitude, faster desynchronized, waking-type pattern associated with rapid eye movements (REM), profound relaxation and quiescence and a tendency on the part of the subject to report awareness and memory for dreams if awakened. This periodically recurring phasic stage of apparently deep sleep (according to some criteria) is called REM sleep (REMS) or sometimes paradoxical sleep (PS) because the EEG pattern is more characteristic of aroused or activated wakefulness than of deep sleep.

SOME COMMENTS ON WORKS IN THIS VOLUME

For a decade or more, Dr. Purpura (Chapter 1) has been concerned with the morphology of developing cortical neurons (Purpura, 1961; Noback and Purpura, 1961) as well as with their correlated structural-functional properties (Purpura *et al.*, 1964, 1965). He and his colleagues have shown that synaptic properties of the immature kitten cortex differ in several ways from those of a more mature animal, as he has explained so elegantly. Especially striking to me were the results reported by Purpura *et al.* (1965), using intracellular recording in sensory cortex of the kitten during stimulation of somatosensory thalamic relay nuclei, in which the long latency of EPSP's and the large magnitude, long-latency and duration of IPSP's, together with a failure of ability to respond to repetitive stimulation, was brought out so clearly.

These results seemed to help clarify at the unit level certain findings for somatosensory, visual, and auditory stimulation with gross recording at the cortical level, especially the changes in the magnitude and latency of the components of the evoked response reported by several groups of investigators (Scherrer and Oeconomos, 1954; Marty *et al.*, 1959; Ellingson and Wilcott, 1960; Rose and Lindsley, 1965, 1968). Furthermore, there were at least fairly good correlations temporally with respect to the onset and development of some of the characteristics of the evoked potential. For example, the predominant visually evoked cortical potential after the first several days was a growing and developing long-latency negative wave, which, after 10-15 days of age in the kitten, was preceded by an emerging positive-negative complex; each of these had long latencies compared to the adult cat or a 1-month-old kitten and the duration of the components was at first long and then shortened as was the latency (Rose and Lindsley, 1968). Also, in the immature brain, whether rabbit, kitten, monkey, or man, repetitive stimulation more rapidly than 1/sec usually gave only a single response at onset and offset of a train of light flashes. Thus it is evident, from what Dr. Purpura has said here and previously, that among other things the properties of immature cortical neurons reflect some of the same properties seen in large aggregates of neurons. In each instance, response components are characterized by slowness, both in latency and duration. In addition, he reports now that inhibitory postsynaptic potentials seem to overshadow excitatory ones in the immature cortex of kittens. Such observations as he and his colleagues have made morphologically and electrophysiologically suggest that the earliest synaptic events occur in the superficial layers of the cortex which he believes receive primary projections quite early in the life of the kitten. Synapses seem to form and become functional there before the axodendritic connections are made farther down along the shaft of the apical dendrite on the developing spines and finally upon basal dendrites and eventually axon connections with the soma or cell body of pyramidal cells.

In keeping with this conclusion are the results of Ata-Muradova (1967) and Ata-Muradova and Chernyshevskaya (1966) in which they found that in the rabbit the early appearing, long-latency surface-negative oscillation could be identified as arising in the most superficial layer of the cortex. These and other studies from Anokhin's laboratory (1961, 1964) have suggested that there are two morphologically separate pathways which develop independently and at different times in the immature brain, one accounting for the negative and one for the positive component of the early developing evoked potentials. A similar view was taken by Rose and Lindsley (1968) in proposing that the long-latency negative component of the visually evoked response, first seen at 4 or 5 days in the kitten, can be identified with a nonspecific system, whereas the later developing (10-15 days) shorter latency positive-negative complex seems to be identified with the specific visual pathways of geniculostriate system. Farber (1968), on the contrary, believes that both the positive and negative components are parts of the same specific sensory system which develop at differential rates due to formation of synapses at different points along a pyramidal cell at different times.

Purpura's results also have opened the possibility of differential and selective development of transmitter mechanisms at these early formed synapses in superficial cortex. This question has also been raised by the work of Marley and Key (1963) who have found differential rates of development of behavioral and electrocortical activity in the kitten subjected to intravenous and intraventricular infusions of sympathomimetic and parasympathomimetic drugs. Also Ata-Muradova and Chernyshevskaya (1966) reported that the different origin of the negative and positive components determines their different physiological properties, such as increased sensitivity of the negative component to heat, urethane, and γ-aminobutyric acid (GABA), and reduced lability as compared to the positive component.

As in the case of all attempted correlations of brain, maturation, and development with behavioral, electrophysiological, and neurochemical changes, the principal difficulty is one of temporal coordination. The problem is how to isolate specific-response components which have particular significance, either from the viewpoint of previously established functional relationships (e.g., synaptic properties), or morphological changes identified at specific points in time, or chemical or neurohumoral properties identified somewhat precisely in time, any of which may be correlated with the others. Purpura, and also Hoffer (Chapter 2) have both resorted to the cerebellum as a model system from which to infer properties about cortical mechanisms.

The Scheibels (Chapter 3) have utilized a very elegant spinal cord model from which to derive properties of developing dendrites and neuronal subsystems. How dendrites form and develop in clusters or bundles seems to be identified better than in more complex structures, such as the cortex. At 12 days of age in the kitten, with this bundling, come the association of diverse cell groups and certain reflex and behavioral developments as a consequence. Thus it is demonstrated that neural morphogenesis and differentiation of function and behavior can be sought in model systems, from which eventual extrapolations can hopefully be made. But the Scheibels have long before this sought and found significant correlations between the state of developing spines on apical dendrites through their advanced Golgi technique, and the onset of certain behaviors, as well as the onset of evoked responses and spontaneous EEG manifestations (A. B. Scheibel, 1962; M. E. Scheibel and Scheibel, 1964a, b). This should remind us that we seek not only correlations between electrophysiologically evoked responses and morphophysiological and neurochemical development, but also correlations for the development of the spontaneous background EEG activity with behavior, neural structure, and neurochemistry. It was long ago shown by Lindsley (1936, 1938, 1939) that the occipital α rhythm first appears as a persistent rhythm at about 3 months of age at 3-4 waves/sec and increases in frequency until an adult average frequency of 10 waves/sec is attained at 10-12 years of age. A similar onset of rhythmic activity occurs in the monkey, and when adjustments are made for a shorter life span, it is found that the onset of the occipital α rhythm in the monkey at 15-20 days of age is roughly equivalent to its occurrence in the human infant at 3 months of age (Caveness *et al.*, 1960; Caveness, 1962). M. E. Scheibel and Scheibel (1964b) have found that the spontaneous rhythms first occur in the kitten at about 10 days of age, as have Marley and Key (1963).

Whereas suggestions have come from the foregoing studies indicating that certain components of developing evoked potentials in immature brains may be related to the presence or absence of transmitter substances, or to their differential rates of maturing, Dr. Roberts (Chapter 4) has shown us some interesting data relative to the presence of GABA or its precursor enzyme γ-aminodecarboxylase (GAD) at the stellate cell level of the cortex in the mouse and in the rabbit from birth to about 30 days. In both instances, GAD was found to increase much more sharply than GABA, especially after the first several days of life. It is evident that we have much to learn about these basic neurochemical capabilities of developing cortex and their temporal relationships to changing behavior and electrophysiology, as well as structure of the cortical matrix.

In the absence of Dr. Jouvet, Dr. Resnick (Chapter 6) commented upon some of Jouvet's conclusions that serotonin (5-HT) is associated with slow wave sleep (SWS) and norepinephrine (NE) with REM or PS. Since SWS is absent at birth in some species, it is interesting to note that 5-HT in the CNS has been found to be minimal or absent; in the goat, which manifests SWS at or shortly after birth, 5-HT is present in the CNS. This is only one of many types of neurochemical correlation which can and should be made, although admittedly with considerable difficulty. Dr. Williamina Himwich (Chapter 7) notwithstanding such difficulties, has sought for differences in GABA, dopamine, and acetylcholine (ACh), during SWS and activated sleep as well as wakefulness, but without very clear-cut differences. She has gone on to chlorpromazine, imipramine, propericiazine, haloperidol, and others, but again without striking results.

Dr. Morgane (Chapter 8) has assembled data from a number of sources relative to amounts of time spent in waking and sleeping, and in SWS and REMS. He has reached out to other laboratories for systematic comparisons of neurochemical data with sleep stage. Such systematic data gathering can be very fruitful in developing leads in connection with unsolved problems. Indeed, Morgane seems to have arrived at a conceptual schema by this method, as well as by his own experimental efforts, to visualize a midbrain-limbic-forebrain system, one pathway of which is via the medial forebrain bundle and NE in type, the other, a more laterally placed system, involves 5-HT. In fact, we need much more of this type of effort and systematization.

It is well known that data have been accumulating at a fantastic rate during the past 20 years or so, and it is also known, though less widely discussed, that many of us have been so busy collecting data and designing new experiments to produce more data that we have scarcely had time to mull over the data already available and awaiting synthesis, comparison, and good honest and serious thought. It seems to have become part of our technological age and scientific culture that we must hurry and get on with the next experiment, and in so doing often make use of our hands rather than our heads!

Dr. Ellingson's work (Chapter 9) is distinctly of this systematization-analytical type in that he surveyed the state of knowledge phylogenetically with respect to the development of sleep EEG patterns and drew up a series of generalizations that could serve as both a summary of the state of affairs in this area, or a challenging point of takeoff for an argument. It is a way of putting down what one thinks one knows and then mulling it all over in search of shortcomings and new ideas. I disagree with his generalization 4 that "sleep spindles appear relatively late, after most of the other elements of the sleep pattern are established," at least so far as the development of the EEG in human infants in concerned. In 25 infants studied during the first 10 days of life, several showed quite distinctly incipient spindles in the sensorimotor region which appeared to be the anlage of sleep spindles, because they increased progressively in amplitude during the second 10 days of life and became full-blown by the third or fourth 10-day periods. In fact, the spindle burst-slow wave pattern of sleep appeared to be as complete at about 1 month of age as it ever became subsequently and it was evident that this phase of the sleep EEG had matured more rapidly than the autonomous sensory α activity which did not become a persistent rhythm over occipital, temporal, or parietal regions until at least a month or so later (usually about 3 months). I am surprised that he has apparently forgotten these observations, because I introduced him to the human EEG when he was a Ph.D. student of mine at Northwestern University and he, in fact, spent many hours with me in 1949 perusing and evaluating these records!

Ellingson's generalization 5, in my opinion, also needs a bit of correction. Amplitude of waking α increases from 3 months of age to about a year and then progressively decreases as a function of age along a curve more or less the reciprocal of that for the increase in frequency of the α rhythm to the age of 10-12 years (Lindsley, 1939). Sometimes the α frequency exceeds the adult level for a year or so around the age of the onset of puberty, especially in females. All other frequency components of the waking EEG I have studied (Lindsley, 1938) show a parallel frequency growth function with age. This includes some slower rhythms not generally seen with contemporary EEG's whose bandwidths and time constants are greatly restricted as compared to those we used in the late 1930's, with also greatly enlarged optically recorded tracings instead of the relatively small inkwriter oscillations characteristic of EEG's today.

Dr. Sterman's report (Chapter 10) opens up an important new consideration, namely, whether rest-activity cycles as a basic biological phenomenon underlie or are superimposed upon sleep-wakefulness cycles. In any event, it is important to understand how these are related and possibly more important how they are related to a variety of circadian rhythms as well as many physiological and behavioral rhythms of much shorter and much longer duration. The late, distinguished mathematician and cyberneticist, Norbert Wiener (1948; 1958) was convinced that the brain harbors a controlling clock mechanism. He based this on considerations of autocorrelations of brain rhythms. Among the many people concerned with the endogenous or exogenous nature of biological clocks and rhythms in plants and animals, may be mentioned a few of the principals, such as Frank Brown (1962) of Northwestern University, a strong advocate of exogenous controlling influences believed to be of geomagnetic or other geophysical nature, Bünning (1967) of Germany, who believes in an endogenous biological "metabolic" clock mechanism which he could demonstrate is influenced by exogenous factors such as temperatures, etc.

Colin Pittendrigh, of Stanford University, J. Woodland Hastings of Harvard University, and Franz Halberg of the University of Minnesota, to mention only a few, are strong advocates of an endogenous regulating mechanism, generally believed to be capable of functioning autonomously but capable of being entrained to internal or external rhythmic variants, such as a day-night cycle. In fact, apparently all concerned now believe that there exists an endogenous clocklike cellular mechanism responsible for biochemical and physiological oscillations (Brown *et al.*, 1970). The main argument hinges upon whether this clock mechanism is relatively autonomous, i.e., a *Zeitgeber* in its own right, or one subject to exogenous influences of local or remote nature. Whatever its nature, the clock's rhythms appear to be capable of entrainment (but only within limits) to imposed rhythms in the environment.

Halberg supplied the term *circadian*, about a day, because of various rhythms corresponding to a 24-hr light-dark cycle, due to the earth's rotation in the presence of light and heat generated by the sun. However, even when these factors are controlled, the rhythm persists, as if "conditioned," or even "genetically conditioned" and therefore "built in" through eons of exposure.

Herein also might lie the importance of Sterman's observations (Chapter 10) that sensorimotor rhythm in the cat can apparently be "conditioned." The rhythm itself presumably remains unchanged, but its periodic occurrence and duration, like circadian rhythms (whether sleep-wakefulness, rest-activity cycles, etc.), may be changed, but again only within limits. The question seems to be broadened with each consideration and each experiment seeking to answer a specific question. Is it not possible that life itself, dependent upon biochemical processes, endows a cell, any cell, with rhythm and even the fluids which bathe it and the membranes which enclose it? These are the processes of metabolism and there is a metabolic cycle for the cell, or for the organism composed of millions of diverse cells. Hastings and his colleagues have been pursuing the biochemical nature of the biological clock, and looking into the matter of specific chemical inhibitors of one or another process involving time periodicity. Interestingly enough, in view of the sleep-wakefulness cycles, rest-activity cycles, REM cycles, etc. which have received intensive treatment and discussion at this conference, Bünning and Tazawa (1957) found in the bean plant seedling a sleep-movement rhythm of almost exactly 24 hr, which could be entrained or modified up and down from 24 hr, and could be phase-shifted on a 24-hr cycle when subjected to appropriate conditions of light and temperature. However, when constant darkness was introduced, under controlled temperature conditions, the original cycle was restored.

Thus we see that this is a vast and complex problem, just as is the problem of rest-activity, sleep-wakefulness, and other rhythmic cycles and one not likely to find simple resolution at the level at which we are approaching it. This does not mean that we should not study such fetal, postnatal, and developmental activities. However, I believe it requires that we do so "with our eyes open" and with full realization that we are studying complicated and interactive processes, ranging from the basic physicochemical properties of protoplasm, membranes, and single cells, to aggregates of cells, tissues, organs, organ systems, and total organisms.

The chasm between the basic and microlevel of approach of Purpura and the Scheibels, dealing with detailed fine and microstructure of neural cells and elements and the nature of postsynaptic potentials (PSP's) recorded intracellularly in single pyramidal cells of the cerebral cortex, and that of Ellingson (Chapter 9), Desmedt (Chapter 12), and others dealing with the scalp-recorded spontaneous and averaged evoked potentials from newborn and developing young infants does indeed seem large and almost insurmountable. But the truth is that bridges are gradually being built. Chemistry underlies these background processes and may help to provide a bridging link. The physicochemical properties of neural cells, individually and in collective aggregates, or functioning in nerve networks connected by synaptic junctions, constitute some of the basic data. Other studies must be concerned with interactive properties of excitation and inhibition, with positive and negative feedback loops operating neurally and humorally, with physiological solutions which bathe and make possible the metabolism of these cells and, indeed, that of the entire organism.

We could, hopefully, learn to understand how our home television set functions, by destroying or disconnecting parts and wires, as we attempt to do by ablation and lesion in the nervous system. We could even attempt to build one by putting parts together according to prescribed or hypothesized wiring diagrams, just as we attempt to follow nature's processes in the unfolding of a genetic plan and the development of behavior and brain rhythms in the newborn infant and maturing child. Our pharmacological and neurochemical colleagues can assist, or lead the way, by showing us how to block or activate particular pathways or systems, by telling us how and when certain chemical changes occur which correlate with or underlie the electrophysiological and behavioral events we observe as a function of age, and maturational development. But we must always realize that the whole is more than the sum of its parts. Even the simplest behavior calls for the integration of numerous neural circuits, and the more complex behaviors, whether socially adapted or maladapted, are dependent not only upon many parts and functions within the organism and the internal environment (*milieu interieur* of Claude Bernard), but also upon the external environment involving interactions between and among organisms.

Thus, important as it is to fractionate and reduce the complexity of the brain and nervous system by attempting to understand what goes on in a single brain cell or even at a single synapse, it is also important to investigate and attempt to understand how large aggregates of brain cells function relative to behavior, and to be constantly aware that the endpoint, or goal, is to understand behavior which involves whole organisms. Electrical phenomena of the brain, as revealed by the EEG, have been studied through the scalp and skull of newborns, young infants, and children, and even *in utero*, as was first described by Lindsley (1942). In some respects, the electrical activity recorded from the brain becomes a substitute for behavior or perhaps, better, an intermediary step between the fractionated activity and behavior. Due to recent technical developments, it is now possible to record three kinds of brain electrical activity from the scalp: (1) spontaneous or autonomous background activity, (2) averaged sensory evoked potentials, and (3) slow negative potential shifts or the contingent negative variation (CNV).

We have heard much about the first type of activity, the classical, ongoing, spontaneous, background activity revealed in the EEG. Its variations have been described for the different states of sleep and wakefulness, or it has been used to identify particular states, such as periods of REMS or NREMS, SWS, and so forth, in order to study reflex and other behavioral manifestations at those times (e.g. reports or discussions by Ellingson (Chapter 9), Parmelee (Chapter 11), Sterman (Chapter 10), Chase (Chapter 13), McGinty (Chapter 13), Dement (Chapter 15), Roffwarg (Chapter 15), Metcalf (Chapter 11), Prechtl (Chapter 14), Ornitz (Chapter 16), Petre-Quadens (Chapter 17), Weitzman (Chapter 14), Schulte (Chapter 14), and others.

The second type of scalp-recorded brain electrical activity, the averaged sensory evoked potentials, has only recently become feasible by algebraically summing responses to repeated stimuli by means of special purpose computers. Dr. Desmedt (Chapter 12) has demonstrated that this can be a valuable tool for investigating the development of sensory fields in the newborn and young infant brain, and Dr. Rosen (Chapter 12) has told us about such studies of the fetal brain at time of birth.

The third type of brain electrical activity, the CNV or negative slow potential, has not been dealt with in this volume. The CNV was first described in human subjects by Walter *et al.* (1964) and was called the contingent negative variation because it appeared to be contingent upon a warning signal followed at varying intervals of time by a stimulus to which the subject was to respond and which was referred to as the imperative or command signal. It has been variously associated with anticipation or expectancy, attention, motivation, conation, etc. Since these processes, reputed to be associated with the CNV, are, or tend to be, related to so-called cognitive functions, the usefulness of the CNV in infants and young children may be somewhat limited. On the other hand, some slow potential shifts have been identified with initiation of activity in the motor cortex, the so-called *Bereitschaftspotential* first described by Kornhuber and Deecke (1965) and further studied by Vaughan *et al.* (1968). (For a recent symposium review of average evoked potentials and related information, including CNV, see Donchin and Lindsley, 1969.)

SOME GENERAL COMMENTS

Finally, I want to say something about technology and its relation to our research activities today. Sometimes I think that the multiplicity of techniques and methodologies of today have gotten in our way, especially in the United States where we have seen so much technical advancement in the past 30 years or so. In general, it has been my impression, that investigators in Europe and Great Britain approach problems more philosophically and logically than we do in the United States. It seems characteristic of them to do an experiment in their minds before they do it in the laboratory; to anticipate alternative outcomes and what they might say about the results if they came out this way or that way. In any event, they appear to be less dominated or intimidated by the requirements of modern technology and the constraints that it imposes upon one, at least so far as problem determination is concerned. I am thinking about the fact that, given a new computer or some other advanced instrumentation, we tend to search around for something we can do with it, instead of formulating problems and critical questions we want to answer, and then searching for appropriate tools, procedures, and methods with which to cope with the problem.

All science has proceeded so rapidly at a technological level and along interdisciplinary lines that no longer can a person be trained broadly enough or monitor the literature adequately to be cognizant of all the programs relevant to his own lines of endeavor. I think we are all aware of that as we face the massive and new literature of today. Thirty or forty years ago it was quite easy to keep abreast of the relatively few journals in which works of this type were published. The rush to get more and more highly specific and often short papers published and not look to more comprehensive and thoroughly studied problems has led us to a point where very few people are conceptualists or theorists. Furthermore, the high degree of concentration in the past 30 years on design of experiments and statistical and quantitative methodology, as admirable as that is and as much as we need it, has led many to rely on the outcome of rather mechanically tabulated data rather than a conceptual or model analysis approach to problems. To some extent, I see this reflected in a conference such as this. None of us, I presume, are to be excluded from this criticism. I think there is need to caution ourselves about pushing descriptive categorizing, and probably extensive quantification, too far, too fast. We need time to philosophize about what we have done and what others have done in order to develop a proper problem-set within a proper perspective. We need more broadly based conceptualizations and logical selection of problems—what one might call a problem-oriented approach. Also we need among us some broadly trained synthesizers who can see the woods as well as the trees, and who are capable of weaving the warp and woof into a fabric of understanding, not only to serve each of us as individual investigators but also to serve the public which supports our enterprises and rightly hopes for health, education, and social welfare benefits.

REFERENCES

Adrian, E. D. (1928). "The Basis of Sensation." Christophers, London.

Adrian, E. D. (1932). "The Mechanism of Nervous Action." Univ. Of Pennsylvania Press, Philadelphia.

Anokhin, P. K. (1961). The multiple ascending influences of the subcortical centers on the cerebral cortex. *In* "Brain and Behavior" (M. A. B. Brazier, ed.), Vol. 1, pp. 139-170. Amer. Inst. Biol. Sci., Washington, D.C.

Anokhin, P. K. (1964). Systemogenesis as a general regulator of brain development. *Progr. Brain Res.* 9, 54-86.

Ata-Muradova, F. (1967). Ontogenetic study on development of secondary components of the evoked response in rabbit. *In* "Developmental Neurophysiology and Neurochemistry" (E. M. Krelsa, ed.), pp. 89-98. Acad. Sci., Leningrad.

Ata-Muradova, F., and Chernyshevskaya, I. (1966). Morphophysiological correlates of evoked potentials in rabbit sensorimotor cortex during postnatal ontogenesis. *Fiziol. Zh. SSSR i I. M. Sechenoya* 52, 1410-1420 [translation in *Neurosci. Transl.,* No. 2, pp. 143-152 (1967-1968)].

Berger, H. (1929). Über das Elektrenkephalogramm des Menschen. I. *Arch. Psychiat. Nervenkr.* 87, 527-570.

Berger, H. (1932). Über das Elektrenkephalogramm des Menschen. V. *Arch. Psychiat. Nervenkr.* 98, 231-257.

Blake, H., and Gerard, R. W. (1937). Brain potentials during sleep. *Amer. J. Physiol.* 119, 692-703.

Blake, H., Gerard, R. W., and Kleitman, N. (1939). Factors influencing brain potentials during sleep. *J. Neurophysiol.* 2, 48-60.

Bremer, F. (1935). Cerveau isolé et physiologie du sommeil. *C. R. Soc. Biol.* 118, 1235-1242.

Brown, F. A. (1962). "Biological Clocks." Heath, Englewood, New Jersey.

Brown, F. A., Hastings, J. W., and Palmer, J. D. (1970). "The Biological Clock: Two Views." Academic Press, New York.

Bünning, E. (1967). "The Physiological Clock." Springer-Verlag, Berlin and New York.

Bünning, E., and Tazawa, M. (1957). Über den Temperatureinfluss auf die endogene Tagesrhythmik bei Phaseolus. *Planta* 50, 107-127.

Cannon, W. B., and Rosenblueth, A. (1937). "Autonomic Neuro-Effector Systems." Macmillan, New York.

Caveness, W. F. (1962). "Atlas of Electroencephalography in the Developing Monkey: Macaca mulatta." Addison-Wesley, Reading, Massachusetts.

Caveness, W. F., van Wagenen, G., and Lindsley, D. B. (1960). Comparison of monkey and human EEG development from birth to puberty (scientific exhibit). *Trans. Amer. Neurol Ass.* 85, 246.

Conel, J. L. (1939-1959). "The Postnatal Development of the Human Cerebral Cortex," Vols. I-VI. Harvard Univ. Press, Cambridge, Massachusetts.

Dale, H. H. (1935). Pharmacology and nerve endings. *Proc. Roy. Soc. Med.* 28, 319-332.

Dale, H. H., Feldberg, W., and Vogt, M. (1936). Release of acetylcholine at voluntary motor nerve endings. *J. Physiol. (London)* 82, 121-128.

Dempsey, E. W., and Morison, R. S. (1942a). The production of rhythmically recurrent potentials after localized thalamic stimulation. *Amer. J. Physiol.* 135, 293-300.

Dempsey, E. W., and Morison, R. S. (1942b). The interaction of certain spontaneous and induced potentials. *Amer. J. Physiol.* 135, 301-308.

Donchin, E., and Lindsley, D. B., eds. (1969). "Average Evoked Potentials: Methods, Results and Evaluations." NASA (Nat. Aeronaut. & Space Admin.), Washington, D.C.

Ellingson, R. J., and Wilcott, R. C. (1960). Development of evoked responses in visual and auditory cortices of kittens. *J. Neurophysiol.* 23, 363-375.

Farber, D. A. (1968). Evolution of specific evoked responses in visual cortex, during ontogenesis. *Fiziol. Zh. i I. M. Sechenova* 54, 778-786 [translation in *Neurosci. Transl.* No. 6, pp. 651-658 (1968-1969)].

Flechsig, P. (1920). "Anatomia des menschlichen Gehirns and Rüchenmarks." Thieme, Stuttgart.

Forbes, A., and Thacher, C. (1920). Amplication of action currents with the electron tube in recording with the string galvanometer. *Amer. J. Physiol.* 52, 409-471.

Hess, W. R. (1929a). Hirnreizversuche über den Mechanismus des Schlafes. *Arch. Psychiat. Nervenkr.* 86, 287-292.

Hess, W. R. (1929b). Loakallisatorische Ergebnisse der Hirnreizversuche mit Schlafeffekt. *Arch. Psychiat. Nervenkr.* 88, 813-816.

Hess,W. R. (1954). The diencephalic sleep centre. *In* "Brain Mechanisms and Consciousness" (J. F. Delafresnaye, ed.), pp. 117-136. Thomas, Springfield, Illinois.

Kleitman, N. (1939). "Sleep and Wakefulness." Univ. of Chicago Press, Chicago.

Kleitman, N. (1963). "Sleep and Wakefulness," (rev. ed.). Univ. of Chicago Press, Chicago.

Kornhuber, H. H., and Deecke, L. (1965). Hirnpotentialänderungen bei Willkürbewegungen und Passiven Bewegungen des Menschen: Bereitschaftspotential und Reafferente Potentiale, *Pfluegers Arch. Gesamte Physiol. Menschen Tiere* 284, 1-17.

Libet, B., and Gerard, R. W. (1941). Steady potential fields and neurone activity. *J. Neurophysiol.* 4, 438-455.

Lindsley, D. B. (1936). Brain potentials in children and adults. *Science* 84, 354.

Lindsley, D. B. (1938). Electrical potentials of the brain in children and adults. *J. Gen. Psychol.* 19, 285-306.

Lindsley, D. B. (1939). A longitudinal study of the occipital alpha rhythm in normal children: Frequency and amplitude standards. *J. Genet. Psychol.* 55, 197-213.

Lindsley, D. B. (1942). Heart and brain potentials of human fetuses *in utero*. *Amer. J. Psychol.* 55, 412-416.

Lindsley, D. B., Bowden, J., and Magoun, H. W. (1949). Effect upon EEG of acute injury to the brain stem activating system. *Electroencephalogr. Clin. Neurophysiol.* 1, 475-486.

Lindsley, D. B., Schreiner, L. H., Knowles, W. B., and Magoun, H. W. (1950). Behavioral and EEG changes following chronic brain stem lesions in the cat. *Electroencephalogr. Clin. Neurophysiol.* 2, 483-498.

Ling, G., and Gerard, R. W. (1949). The normal membrane potential of frog sartorius fibers. *J. Cell. Physiol.* 34, 383-396.

Loewi, O. (1936). Quantitative and qualitative Untersuchungen über den Sympathicusstoff. *Pfleugers Arch. Gesamte Physiol. Menschen Tiere* 237, 504-514.

Loewi, O., and Navratil, E. (1926). Über humorale Ubertragbarkeit Herznervenwirkung. X. Über das Schicksal des Vagus-stoffes. *Pfluegers Arch. Gesamte Physiol. Menschen Tiere* 214, 678-688.

Loomis, A. L., Harvey, E. N., and Hobart, G. (1935). Potential rhythms of the cerebral cortex during sleep. *Science* 81, 597-598.

Loomis, A. L., Harvey, E. N., and Hobart, G. (1937). Cerebral states during sleep, as studied by human brain potentials. *J. Exp. Psychol.* 21, 127-144.

Marley, E., and Key, B. J. (1963). Maturation of the electrocorticogram and behavior in the kitten and guinea-pig and the effect of some sympathomimetic amines. *Electroencephalogr. Clin. Neurophysiol.* 15, 620-636.

Marty, R., Contamin, F., and Scherrer, J. (1959). La double-réponse électrocorticale à la stimulation lumineuse chez le chat nouveau-né. *C. R. Soc. Biol.* 153, 198-201.

Morison, R. S., and Dempsey, E. W. (1942a). A study of thalamocortical relations. *Amer. J. Physiol.* 135, 281-292.

Morison, R. S., and Dempsey, E. W. (1942b). Mechanisms of thalamocortical augmentation and repetition. *Amer. J. Physiol.* 138, 297-308.

Moruzzi, G., and Magoun, H. W. (1949). Brain stem reticular formation and activation of the EEG. *Electroencephalogr. Clin. Neurophysiol.* 1, 455-473.

Noback, C. R., and Purpura, D. P. (1961). Postnatal ontogenesis of neurons in cat neocortex. *J. Comp. Neurol.* 117, 291-307.

Purpura, D. P. (1961). Analysis of axodendritic synaptic organization in immature cerebral cortex. *Ann. N.Y. Acad. Sci.* 94, 604-654.

Purpura, D. P., Shofer, R. J., Housepian, E. M., and Noback, C. R. (1964). Comparative ontogenesis of structure-function relations in cerebral and cerebellar cortex. *Progr. Brain Res.* 4, 187-221.

Purpura, D. P., Shofer, R. J., and Scarff, T. (1965). Properties of synaptic activities and spike potentials of neurons in immature neocortex. *J. Neurophysiol.* 28, 925-942.

Ranson, S. W. (1939). Somnolence caused by hypothalamic lesions in the monkey. *Arch. Neurol. (Chicago)* 41, 1-23.

Ranson, S. W., and Magoun, H. W. (1939). The hypothalamus. *Ergebn. Biol. Chem. Exp. Pharmakol. Physiol.* 41, 56-163.

Rose, G. H., and Lindsley, D. B. (1965). Visually evoked electrocortical responses in kittens: development of specific and nonspecific systems, *Science* 148, 1244-1246.

Rose, G. H., and Lindsley, D. B. (1968). Development of visually evoked potentials in kittens: specific and nonspecific responses. *J. Neurophysiol.* 31, 607-623.

Rosenblueth, A. (1950). "The Transmission of Nerve Impulses at Neuroeffector Junctions and Peripheral Synapses." Wiley, New York.

Scheibel, A. B. (1962). Neural correlates of psychophysiological development in the young organism. *Recent Advan. Biol. Psychiat.* 4, 313-328.

Scheibel, M. E., and Scheibel, A. B. (1964a). Some neural substrates of postnatal development. *Ann. Rev. Child Develop.* 1, 481-519.

Scheibel, M. E., and Scheibel, A. B. (1964b). Some structural and functional substrates of development in young cats. *Progr. Brain Res.* 9, 6-25.

Scherrer, J., and Oeconomos, D. (1954). Réponses corticales somesthésiques du mammifère nouveau-né, comparées à celles de l'animal adulte. *Etud. Neo-Natales* 3, 199-216.

Smith, J. R. (1937). The electroencephalogram during infancy and childhood. *Proc. Soc. Exp. Biol. Med.* 36, 384-386.

Smith, J. R. (1938a). The electroencephalogram during normal infancy and childhood. I. Rhythmic activities present in the neonate and their subsequent development. *J. Genet. Psychol.* 53, 431-453.

Smith, J. R. (1938b). The electroencephalogram during normal infancy and childhood. II. The nature of the growth of the alpha waves. *J. Genet. Psychol.* 53, 455-469.

Smith, J. R. (1938c). The electroencephalogram during normal infancy and childhood. III. Preliminary observations on the pattern sequence during sleep. *J. Genet. Psychol.* 53, 471-482.

Smith, J. R. (1939). The "occipital" and "pre-central" alpha rhythms during the first two years. *J. Psychol.* 7, 223-226.

Vaughan, H. G., Jr., Costa, L. D., and Ritter, W. (1968). Topography of the human motor potential. *Electroencephalogr. Clin. Neurophysiol.* 25, 1-10.

Walter, W. G., Cooper, R., Aldridge, V. J., McCallum, W. C., and Winter, A. L. (1964). Contingent negative variation: An electrical sign of sensorimotor association and expectancy in the human brain. *Nature (London)* 203, 380-384.

Wiener, N. (1948). "Cybernetics." Wiley, New York.

Wiener, N. (1958). Time and the science of organization. *Scientia (Milan) [6]* 52, 1-12.

Subject Index

A

Acetylcholine, 46, 79
Acetylcholine system, effects of isolation
  housing on, 101
Activation response, 46
Active sleep, 166
  physiological criteria for, 264
σ Activity, 168
Adenosine triphosphate (ATP), 86
Alpha rhythm attenuation, 322
Amino acids in development, 131
γ-Aminobutyric acid (GABA), 38, 45
  antagonism, 86
  binding Na$^+$ requirement and, 85

release from brain slices, cortex and
  Purkinje cells, 85
"shunt," 97
  pathway of, 82
system, 79-98
  in cortex, hippocampus, retina, and
    spinal cord, 94
γ-Aminobutyric acid glycine, 79
Aminotransferase, 82
Amphetamine(s), 104
  in neonates, 134
  sleep-waking rhythm and, 191
Antabuse, 114
Area 17, measurements of dendrites of, 65
Arousal of isolated animals, 276
Artifacts, in fetal recordings, 249

461

LBJ Country

Houston *Chronicle* photographs
by Sam Pierson and Richard Pipes

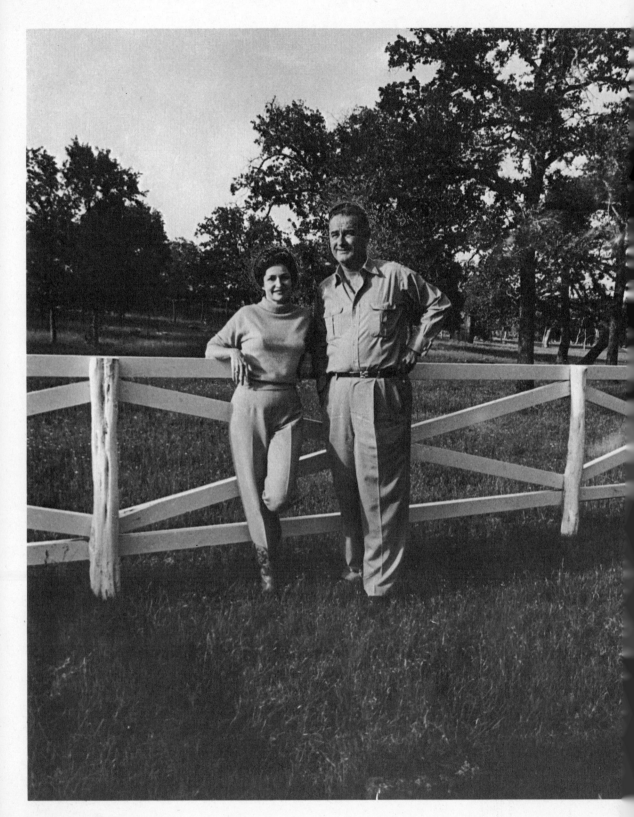

Lady Bird and Lyndon Johnson at home.

BILL PORTERFIELD

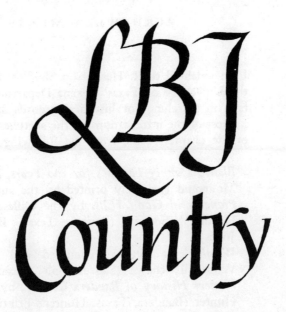

1965
DOUBLEDAY & COMPANY, INC.
GARDEN CITY, NEW YORK

ACKNOWLEDGMENTS

I am indebted to R. Henderson Shuffler, Director of the University of Texas' Texana Department, for his help in searching for historical records and sources.

Most of the information for the sketches at the end of the chapters came from the following books:

Blanco County Families for 100 Years, by John S. Moursund (privately printed by the author)
Pioneers in God's Hills, by the Gillespie County Historical Society (Austin, Texas: Boeckmann-Jones)
Wimberley's Legacy, compiled and edited by Williedell Schawe (San Antonio, Texas: Naylor)
Pioneer History of Bandera County, by J. Marvin Hunter (Bandera, Texas: Hunter's Printing House)

Permission is gratefully acknowledged to use the lore about Creed Taylor, which is taken from *It Occurred in Kimble*, by O. C. Fisher. Copyright 1937 by O. C. Fisher, published by the Anson Jones Press, Salado, Texas.

BILL PORTERFIELD

To William P. Steven
begetter of it all
And for Jo

FOREWORD

A president's hardest task is not to do what is right, but to know what is right.

Yet the presidency brings no special gift or prophecy or foresight. You take an oath, step into an office, and must then help guide a great democracy.

The answer was waiting for me in the land where I was born.

It was once barren land. The angular hills were covered with scrub cedar and a few live oaks. Little would grow in the harsh caliche soil. And each spring the Pedernales River would flood the valley.

But men came and worked and *endured* and built.

Today that country is abundant with fruit, cattle, goats, and sheep. There are pleasant homes and lakes, and the floods are gone.

Why did men come to that once forbidding land?

Well, they were restless, of course, and had to be moving on. But there was more than that. There was a dream—a dream of a place where a free man could build for himself, and raise his children to a better life—a dream of a continent to be conquered, a world to be won, a nation to be made.

Remembering this, I knew the answer.

A president does not shape a new and personal vision of America.

He collects it from the scattered hopes of the American past.

It existed when the first settlers saw the coast of a new world, and when the first pioneers moved westward.

It has guided us every step of the way.

It sustains every president. But it is also your inheritance and it belongs equally to the people we serve.

It must be interpreted anew by each generation for its own needs, as I have tried, in part, to do today.

President Lyndon Baines Johnson
State of the Union Message, 1965

LBJ Country

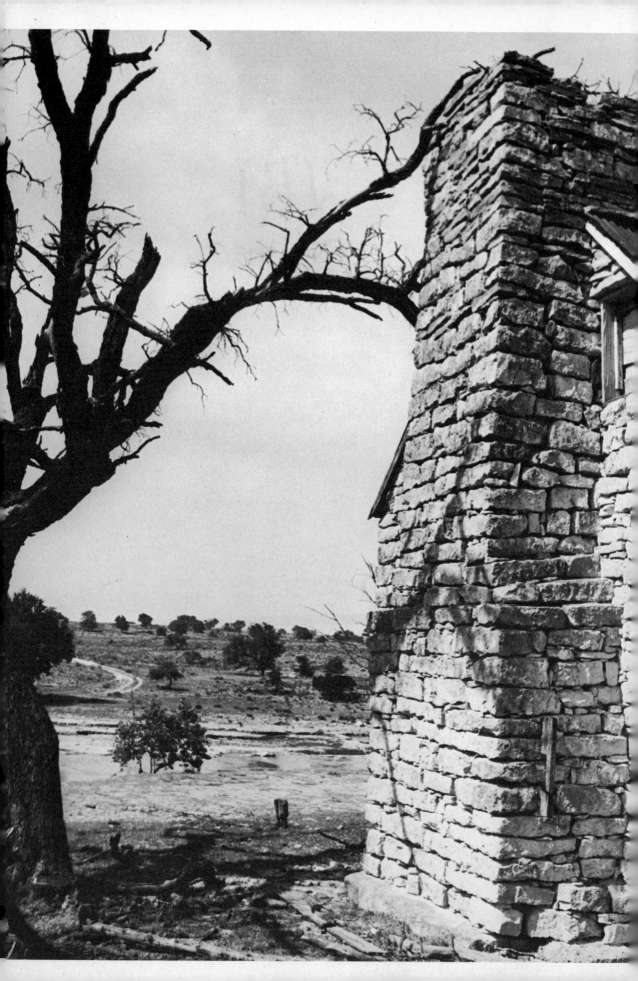

CHAPTER ONE

U.S. 290

climbs a range of small mountains forty-three miles west of Austin, glides through a gap, and drops into a little valley —into a land that will be the stuff of legend as long as Americans dream.

In these hills a president of the United States of America was born and here he grew to manhood.

Because his origin was common and obscure, and because his root and rhythm and destiny took seed and shape here, people will come to these hills when he is gone, when you and I and our children are gone, to look and ponder and dream.

It is a place for dreams, a country of pink granite mountains and purple hills, of golden meadows and green valleys, of blue lakes and clear springs.

There are more deer here than men; more fish and wild turkey and beaver.

But it is not paradise.

When you look closely, it is harsh country.

All life below man seems stunted, compromised. The deer are small, the turkeys scrawny. The hills never quite become mountains. Trees twist out of the rock and reach warped fingers toward the burning sun. The grass on the limestone ranges is dry and barely boot-high. The earth hardens and cracks in the heat. After a long drouth, the rivers run low and lazy; the creeks go down to bedrock; and fish go down to fossils.

A turn in the weather can change all this in a matter of hours, for here is a country of extremes. Torrents of rain— "stump movers" and "gulley washers" they call them—come out of nowhere to flood the canyons and wash away houses and whole herds of cattle. Ranchers who feared their grass was going to burn watch helplessly as tons of topsoil run down the draws.

A cool spring rain will give freshly sheared goats pneumonia.

Opposite page
Though it is abandoned to the elements, neither time nor weather erodes the native stone of this pioneer home near Johnson City.

One August a few years back, Pierce Hoggett of Junction lost five hundred goats because of a shower. The next winter was worse—he lost nine hundred head in a "blue norther" that whistled down from the Panhandle.

The German nesters in these hills used to top their houses with heavy iron to keep the roofs from buckling under the hailstorms.

Yet all things live in this crucible of compromise, where an idealistic tree can somehow take root and grow through a crack in the hardest rock. "Lookit that tree hanging up there where it has no business being," says an old-timer. Bluebonnets bloom in cactus patches. Rattlesnakes rest in rabbit holes and frisky lambs frolic under the patient arc of a gliding buzzard.

This ranch country is hell on a farmer; yet you can find patches of level land where the rock and the plow have come to an understanding, and out of the shallow soil pop pecans, peaches, grains, and arrowheads.

The land and the limitless sky dwarf a man—but make him feel larger than life. This country can coax and coddle and please you with its beauty and resource; and drive you to drink with its willful meanness and dismal poverty. It is a living thing—this country—omnipotent and omniparent, always with you, under your feet, over your head, in your mind and heart.

The heart of Lyndon Baines Johnson is in these highlands; this is where he learned as a boy the lesson of the rock and the tree, and this is where he comes to rest and find the source of his strength.

He sees the cattle rancher live beside the goat rancher, the sheep rancher, and the dude rancher. He knows men who are all of these without contradiction.

He heard his granddaddy talk of the time the Indian, the Negro, the Anglo-American, the German, and the Mormon lived together in these hills.

They did not always live in peace.

The Indian left in anger. The Mormon wandered off in search of God. The Anglo hung the German to a tree because the German refused to enslave the Negro. Most of the Negroes left. The Germans stayed. The Anglos stayed. And they learned to live together with their differences.

This is the country that shaped a president.

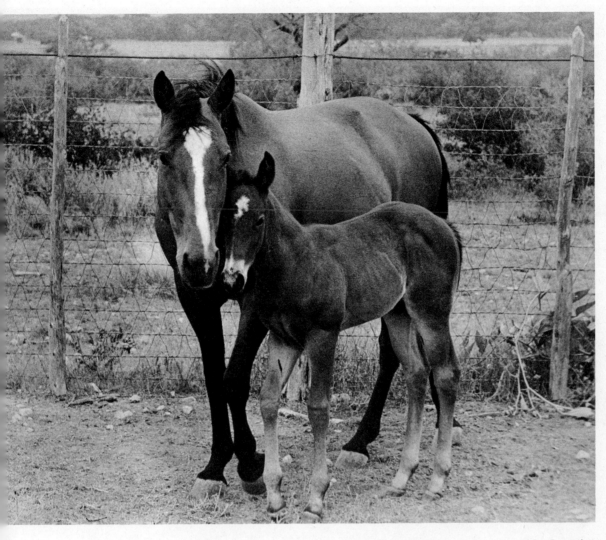

Pastoral poetry embodied in mare and foal on the Jack Hoggett Ranch outside Junction.

3

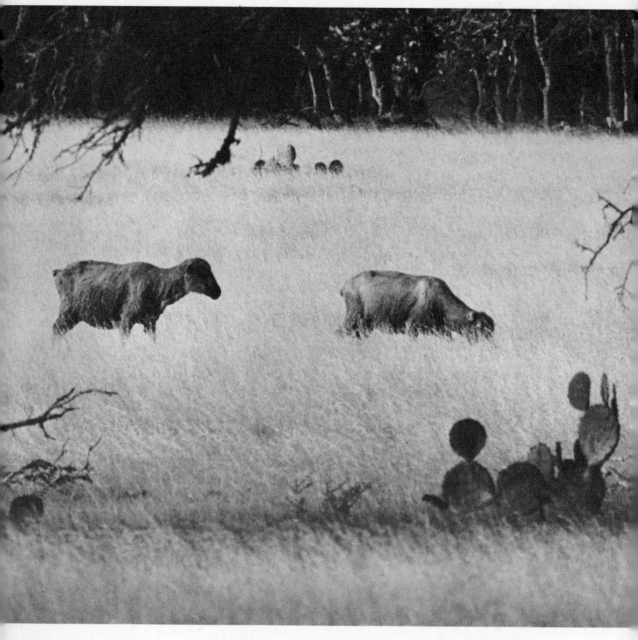

It's a lazy summer day in the hill country and the shorn sheep are in the meadow.

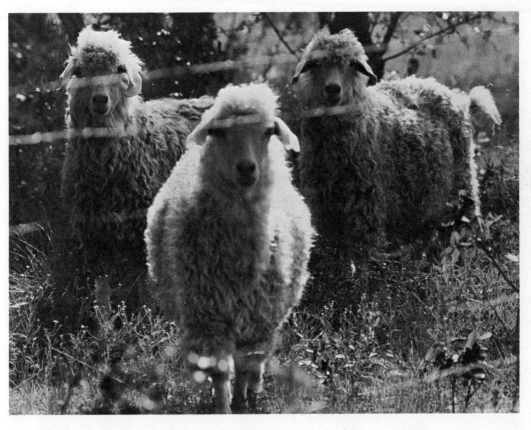

Barbed-wire fences separate the sheep from the goats.

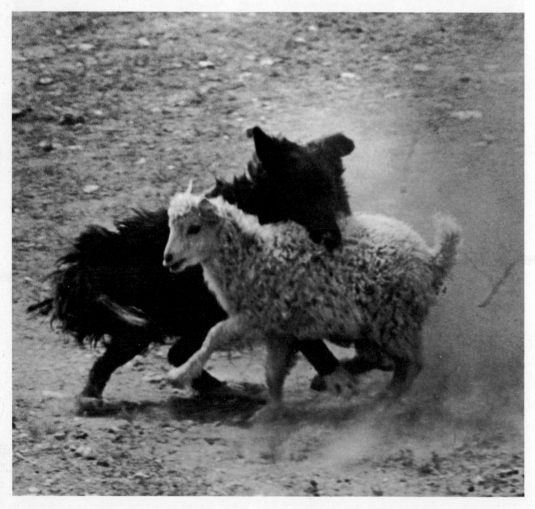

A border collie attends to business with a runaway sheep over in Kimble County.

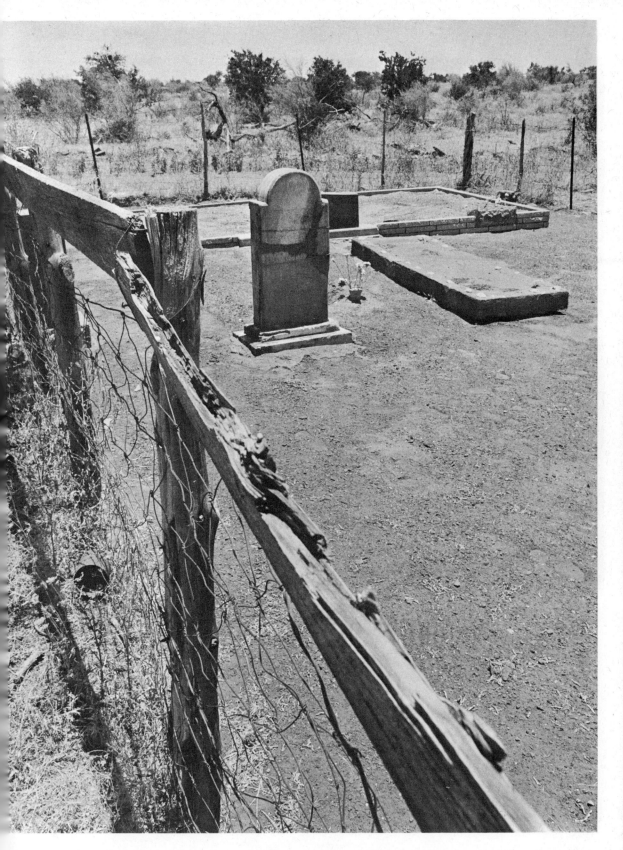

Dust thou art, to dust returneth. In Mason County it hasn't rained in a long time.

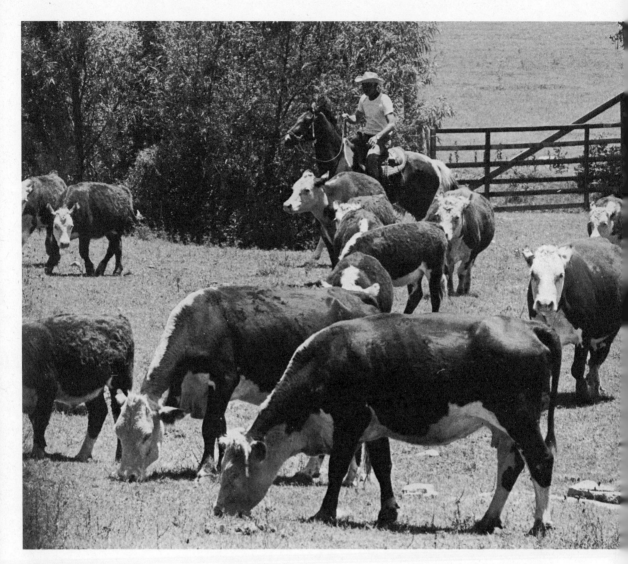

On his Gillespie County homestead, Hondo Crouch rides herd on his white-faced cattle.

THE BALCONES FAULT

Man came late to the Texas hill country. Nature had her way with it for a longer time than man can count. Eons ago, a great sea covered this part of Texas. Through the ages, the bones and shells of sea creatures settled on the ocean floor, building a vast plateau of limestone. At last, Edwards Plateau hove out of the sea. As it rose, it cracked on one end and a crevice ran up the center of the land. Springs gushed from the fault line, forming rivers and streams which coursed through the sloping country, cutting out canyons and gorges and basins. Today, this great crack, called the Balcones Fault, splits the state in half. East of the fault lies the flat farm country. The hilly ranch country rolls west.

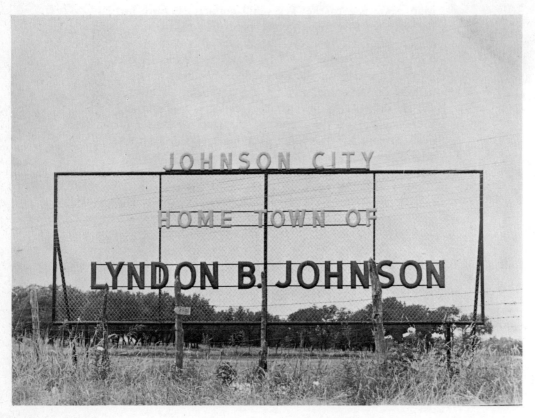

Civic pride rears a monument at the entrance to Johnson City.

CHAPTER TWO

It was almost noon.

Miz Minnie Cox, the secretary of the Johnson City Chamber of Commerce, sat in the chamber's new office on Main Street. Well, the office is really an old gas station. But it has been repainted, the pumps removed and petunias planted in their place. It seems nice and new to Minnie, who used to have to run the chamber's business from her home.

"Hidy."

Minnie nodded. She was a tall, angular woman with a businesslike expression on her face and a hair bun at the nape of her neck.

She sold a pamphlet called *LBJ . . . His Home and Heritage*, handed over a free map of the town, and commanded, "Don't forget to sign our guest register. You're our fourth visitor today."

Three ladies from Michigan had stopped that morning to scribble their names in the book and look around town. They were Mrs. J. Greskiwiak of Detroit, Miss Reta Hines of Ann Arbor, and Mrs. Carmel Scheich of St. Clair Shores.

"If you want to see LBJ's boyhood home, it's one block over on Ninth Street," Minnie said.

"I thought he lived in a shack on the Pedernales River when he was a boy . . . ?"

"Oh, he was born on the Perd 'n' Alice all right," Minnie said. "But after several years, they moved into town here and Lyndon lived over there on Ninth Street until he got out of high school and left home.

"Look, you can see the house from here—the white one with the fence around it. Nobody lives there any more. The family just keeps it looking nice. When they lived here, a wistaria vine used to bloom every summer beside the front porch. It was a pretty purple. When they moved away it died. Now it's trying to come back. Probably'll bloom again next spring."

Miz Minnie locked up and went to lunch. The Johnson place is an old house with a windmill out back. But there isn't much character in the place now. It has that unlived-in but well-kept-by-hired-hands look.

Sparrows chattered in the pecan trees on the courthouse square.

The stucco-and-tin office of the *Record-Courier* was locked, and an old-timer said the editor, Stella Gliddon, was over at the post office. She's postmistress too. She was at lunch. A sign hung in the P.O. window. It said the sophomore class was having a bake sale at Groft's Humble Service Station the next day from 8:30 A.M. until noon.

The lead in the *Record-Courier* was about the ladies of the Blanco County Home Demonstration Council picking Pleasant Hill as the site for the 4-H show. There was a letter on page one from Ensign Alton Felps, a local boy aboard the U.S.S. *Lake Champlain*, somewhere off the Virginia coast. He wrote that his ship collided with a destroyer, and allowed that "it must have been a pure miracle" nobody was killed. The rest of the front page was taken up with a story about a Ladies for Lyndon club, a rundown on the honor graduates of the Lyndon B. Johnson High School, and an item about the coming visit of Miz Mollie Goodpasture, Worthy Grand Matron of the Texas Order of the Eastern Star.

Edna Ferber's notion of Texas, *Giant*, was advertised at the Jaycee Theater. But it wasn't on. The show was closed for the summer. But there was a drive-in movie down back of town which was open on weekends. The man who runs it is a practical sort. The back of his house is the silver screen.

It was dark and cool inside the stone courthouse. The sheriff was out to lunch. A dated proclamation hung on the bulletin board in the hall. It announced the time of the Republican primary, and was signed in a bold hand by Robert Singleton, the G.O.P. county chairman. The county went Democratic anyway.

A couple of cowboys were drinking beer in Red's Place behind the courthouse. Red stuck a sign in his fly-specked window. It said the Alamo Boys would play for the Saturday night dance at the Mustang Tavern on Round Mountain. Red didn't mind posting the notice. He didn't have a dance floor—yet.

The enchiladas were good and oniony at Minnie Pilgrim's Cafe. The jukebox blared. Buck Owens sang through his nose about how his love for some gal was high as a mountain and deep as the sea.

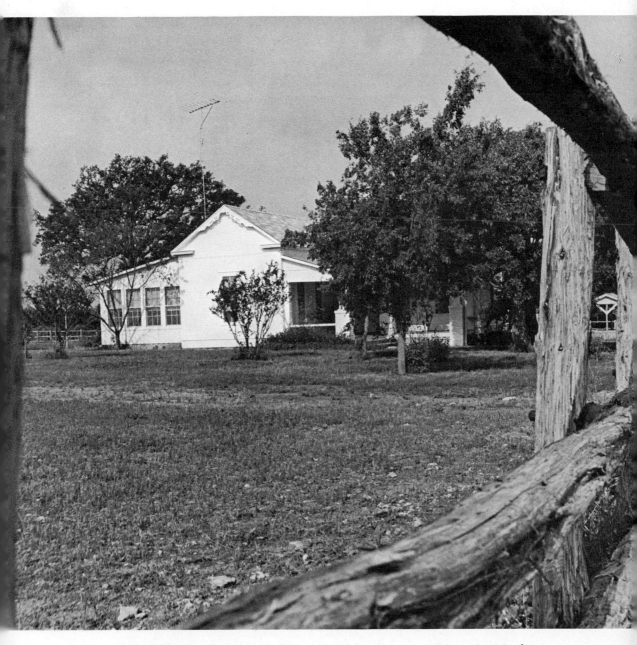

In this little white house with wooden lace on the gable and a big front porch, Lyndon Johnson spent his boyhood.

The highest thing in town, except for a cowpoke at Red's Place, was the water tower. The deepest thing was the frown on Zeke Felps's face. He'd just lost a domino game to James Ealy Johnson, the President's cousin. They sat at a table under the mulberry tree beside Casparis' Cafe. "Shuffle 'em agin," Zeke told Ealy. "Annie won't have dinner ready nohow."

THE FIRST HILL COUNTRY PEOPLE

The first hill country people were not ranchers but hunters. Llano Man stalked the cedar brakes twelve thousand years ago hunting elephants now extinct. The Tonkawa Indians were in the hills when Domingo Teran de los Rios, a Spanish explorer, rode into Central Texas in 1691. Teran was just passing through, but he blazed a bending trail from Mexico to Louisiana which became El Camino Real—The King's Highway—the greatest thoroughfare across Texas for a century and a half. Forty years after Teran, another Spaniard, Domingo Ramon, established three missions along the Colorado River near the present site of Austin. The Comanches and Kiowa Apaches forced Ramon to move his missions down on the San Antonio River. The Comanches and Kiowas were not hill country Indians. They lived in the plains. But they were bold warriors who roamed far from home. The first white man to establish a town in the Texas hills was Don Felipe Roque de la Portilla, who in 1807 laid out the Villa de San Marcos de Neve, on a site in the present town of San Marcos. Roque could get no help against the Comanches and after four years he took his colony to Mexico. Twenty years later, the first Anglo settlers from Stephen F. Austin's colony came up the Colorado and found the offspring of Don Felipe's cattle running wild with the buffalo. The Tonkawas were a small people, fleet of foot, meek of heart. They never fought the white intruders, often became the settler's ally for protection against marauding Comanches and Kiowas. It did no good. The Tonkawas were soon extinguished. Today, not more than fifty Tonkawas are to be found on earth. The last survivors live on a reservation in Oklahoma.

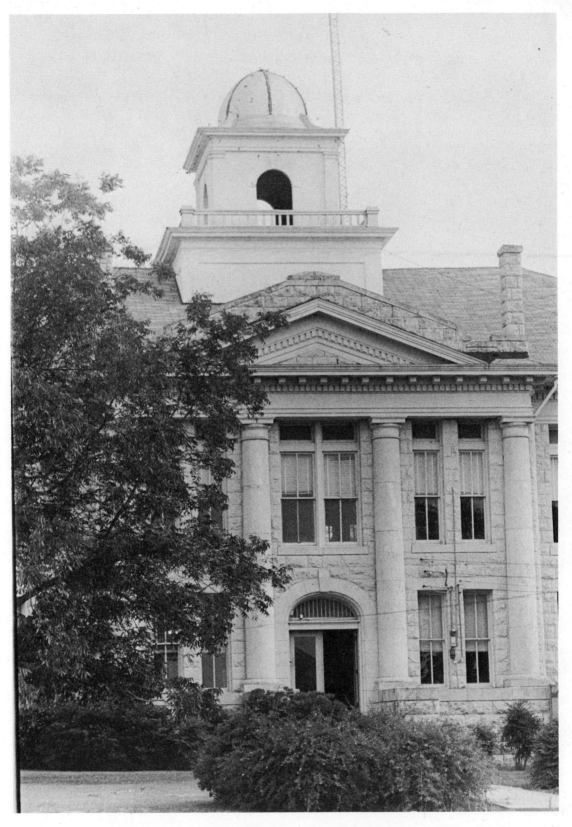

The Johnson County Courthouse has a Palladian pediment and local rock, and is the seat of law and order in Johnson City.

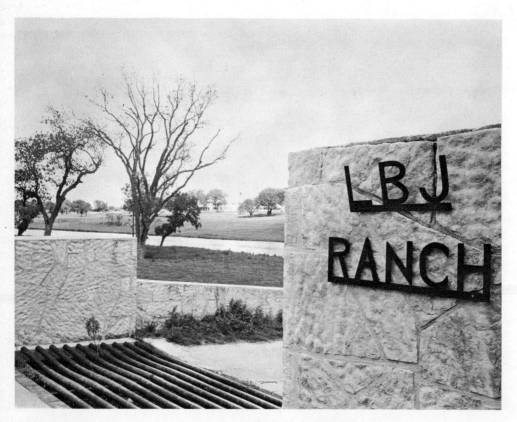

A cattle guard makes the imposing entrance to the LBJ Ranch seem more homelike.

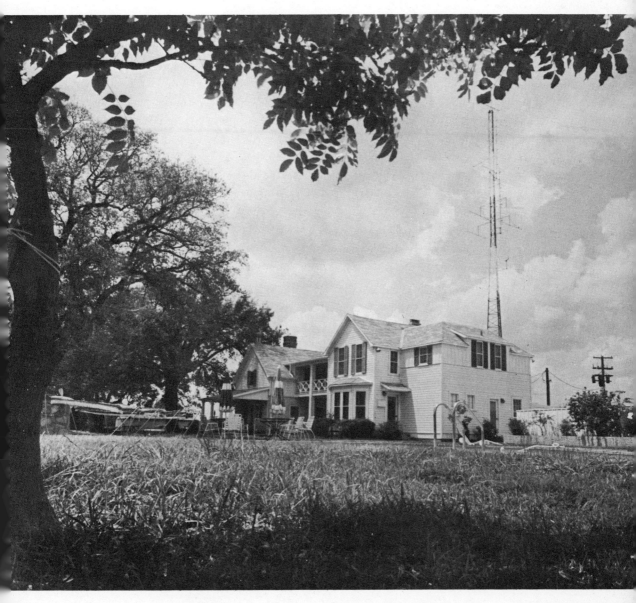

The LBJ Ranch house drowses under the cumulus clouds of the Texas sky.

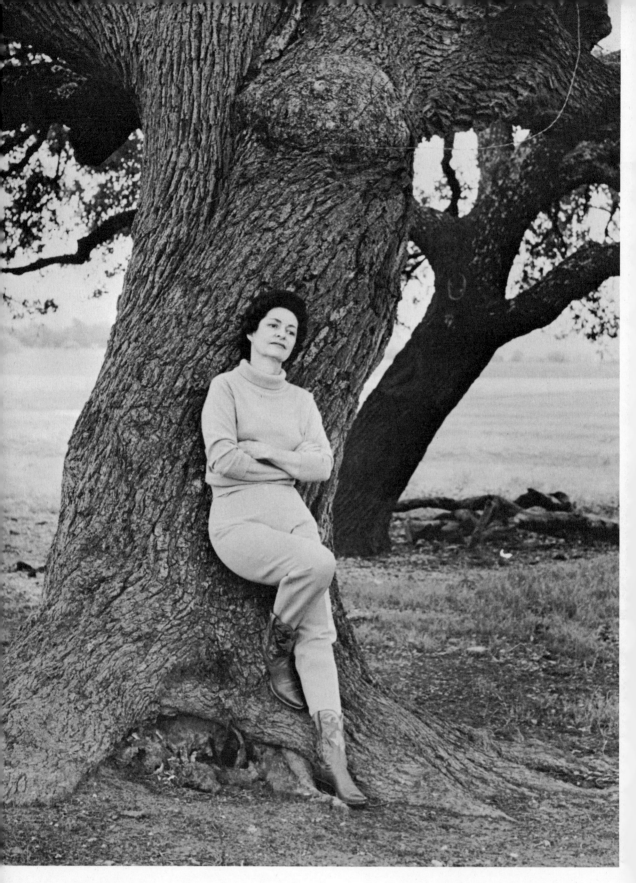

A pause in the day's occupations—Lady Bird Johnson relaxes against a gnarled old live oak.

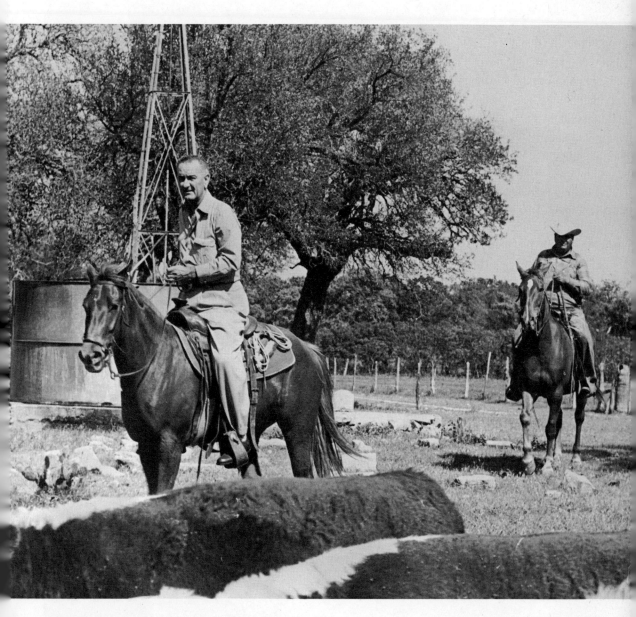

Land and cattle get in a man's blood. Lyndon Johnson takes time out to inspect his herd.

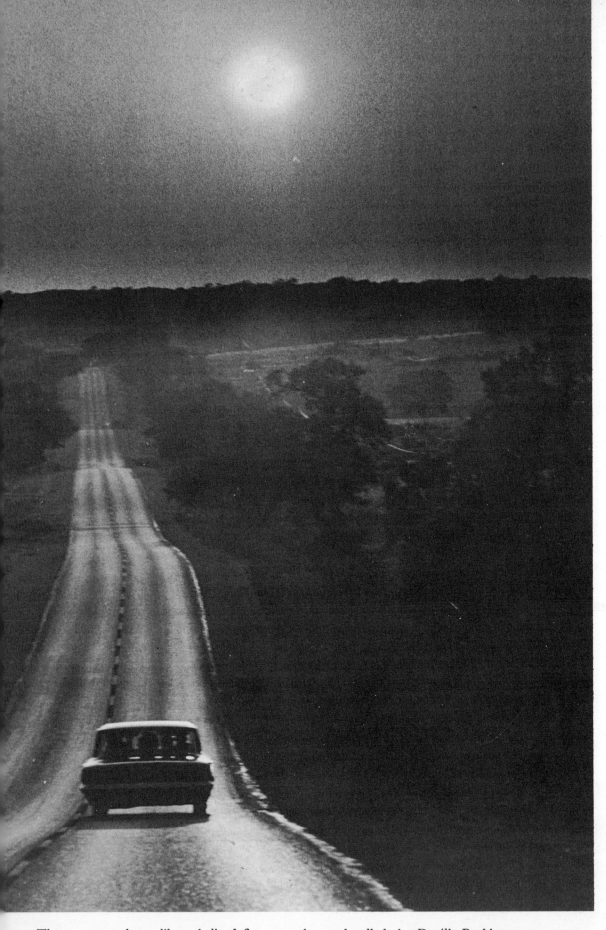

The sun goes down like a ball of fire over the road called the Devil's Backbone.

CHAPTER THREE

It is eight o'clock at night in Johnson City and the fireflies are burning brightly and the sparrows are turning quietly in the pecan trees about the courthouse.

A cat lies in the second story window of the Adams Hotel, silhouetted by the faint glare of a bare bulb burning in the bathroom beyond. She lifts her tail with a violent jerk, then lets it float softly down again. On the porch below, three old men talk in low voices as they rock in creaking chairs. Two wear broad-brimmed hats and one wears no hat at all.

A boy and a girl eat hamburgers and French fried potatoes in Minnie Pilgrim's Cafe. The girl has pimples on her face but she's pretty.

Some baby's daddy sits in the doorway of the automatic laundry waiting for a tub of diapers to spin dry.

Next door at Red's Place, two nesters play dominoes and slowly sip their beer. They wear broad-brimmed hats and Red wears no hat at all.

Miz Waters is out in the yard of her boardinghouse sniffing the larkspur.

Three friendly fellows talk in the Friendly Bar. Two wear broad-brimmed hats and one wears a baseball cap.

The old men on the porch of the Adams Hotel stand stiffly, stretch their skinny arms, and swallow toothless yawns. They go inside and the screen door slaps behind them.

A car rolls up to the hotel. It is Russell Strege, the crippled singer of sad songs, at the wheel. He backs the old car up an alley and parks it on a slope. He knows the car battery will be dead by morning and he wants a downhill start to wherever he is going.

Strege limps to a porch chair, pushes back his (yes) broad-brimmed hat, and strokes a cheap guitar. The sheriff's car moves slowly past, its long antennae swaying like the cat tail in the second story window. Strege swallows a yodel and limps into the darkness where old men and loners sleep.

And that's the way it is around the square in Johnson City,

Texas, U.S.A., at eight o'clock on a summer's night in the year of the ascension of LBJ.

Down back of town, in the Maverick Tavern on old 281, Andrew is talking with Oscar. Andrew is the proprietor. Oscar the customer.

"Tha other day," Andrew says to Oscar, "a tourist came in here and ast me wher tha Prezadent's place was, and I said, 'Which?'

"And he said, 'Which? Don't you know you got a prezadent from here?'

"And I said, 'Course I know we got a prezadent from *here*. He's drunk beer in tha very spot you're standin' on. I meant which place of hiz? He's got a dozen places 'round this country.'

"And you know what that tourist said? He said, 'Hell, I don't see how this place ever made a prezadent.'

"And I said, 'Looky here, boy. This place ain't never *made* nobody. He made hizself. And that's a fact.'"

Oscar shook his head and said, "All them bodyguards. Ever'where he goes. I'd ruther be me. Gimme 'nother beer, Andrew."

BIGFOOT WALLACE

1817–1899

A Goliath backwoodsman who tracked down
runaway slaves when he ran out of Indians to kill,
Bigfoot once ate twenty-seven eggs before walking to
town for a full meal. When a citizen asked for an
Indian boy he was dragging through the streets of
Castroville, Bigfoot replied, "This is my Injun. If you
want an Injun, go and ketch one. Thar be plenty
more whar this 'un cum from."

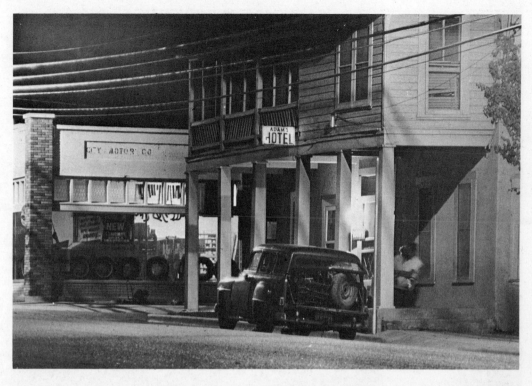

There's not a lot of night life in Johnson City but the Adams Hotel is always open.

You don't really need a reservation.

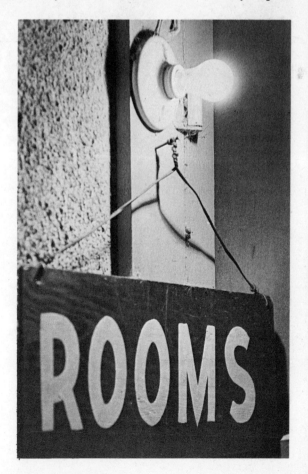

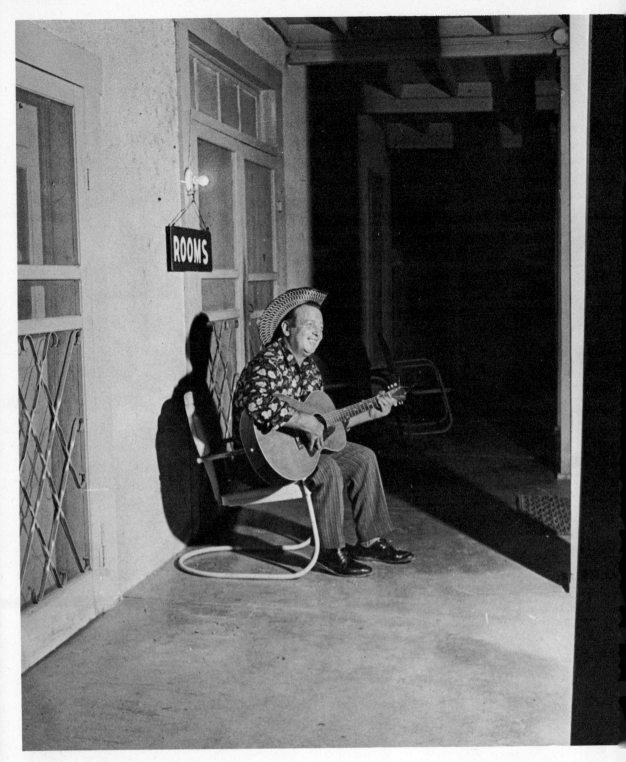

Russell Strege makes his lonesome music on the front gallery of the Adams Hotel.

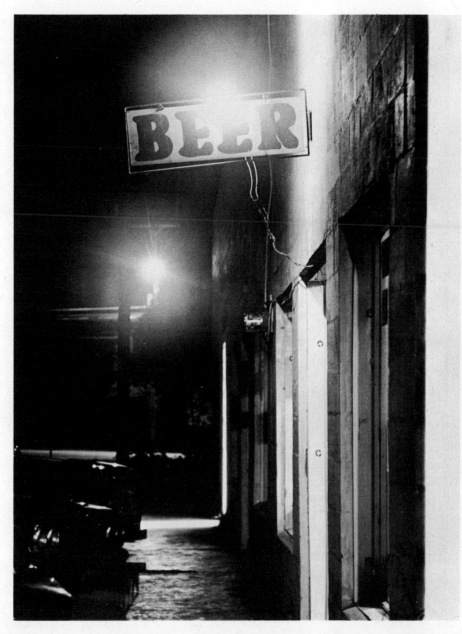

You can always go to Red's Place.

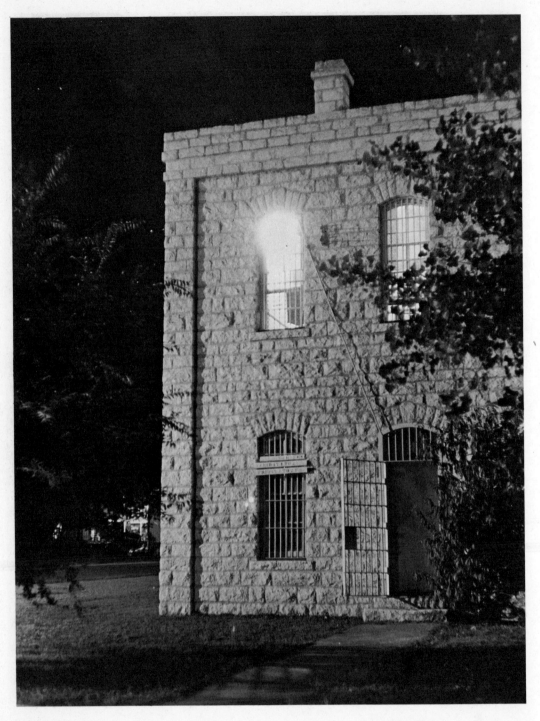

Somebody's singing "Good Night, Irene" down there at the jailhouse.

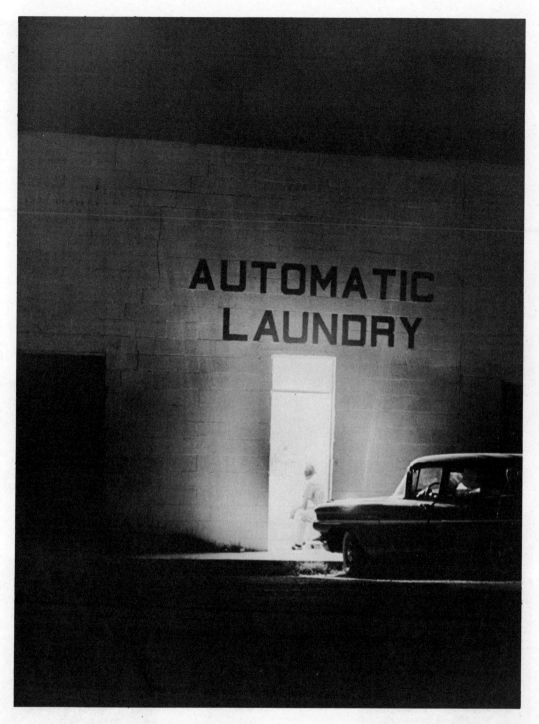

The laundry in Johnson City keeps late hours to accommodate the fathers of families.

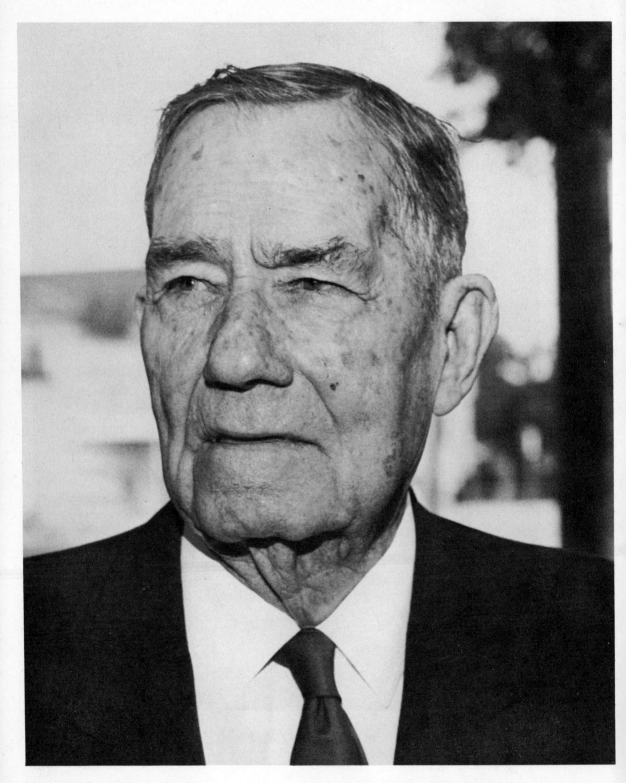

Percy Brigham, Blanco banker, says Lyndon Johnson was a bright, hard workin' boy.

CHAPTER FOUR

Go see Percy Brigham," people used to tell flatlanders who came to Blanco County on business.

Now they say, "Go see A. W. Moursund."

Moursund, the Johnson City lawyer-rancher who takes care of the LBJ family's private interests, is the county's power boss now.

Brigham, the Blanco banker who loaned Lyndon Johnson money to start college on, is the old boss.

Moursund is understandably a busy man. He said he didn't want to hurt anybody's feelings, but he figured that giving out stories on the President's country was a damn waste of time. You couldn't trust what you read. It looked like to him that all the stuff about Blanco County in the national magazines had been conceived by Republicans to embarrass the President.

Brigham, eighty-six, is understandably not so busy. He recently retired after fifty-seven years with the Blanco National Bank. A telephone call from Johnson City found him at home. Sure. He'd talk—face to face.

How long would it take to get there?

"Well," Brigham replied in a soft drawl, "if you're walkin', might take a day or two. But if you're drivin' you'll probably be here before I finish lunch, and I just sat down at the table."

A slow drive through the hills makes the motorist wish his car was air conditioned. He counts more buzzards than houses and wonders if the next road sign will have as many bullet holes as the ones he passed. How could anyone drown in this country? But they say somebody dies every year in the flash floods that roar through the draws.

The town of Blanco lies fourteen miles to the south of Johnson City. Johnson City is the county seat, but Blanco is bigger by about two hundred folks. Both places look much alike—one traffic light and a few stores built around a native stone courthouse.

The courthouse in Blanco stands dark and empty, a symbol of Blanco's defeat in a long-ago rivalry that still hangs in the air like a black curtain separating the towns. Blanco was the county seat until 1890, when Johnson City took it away in a special election. The difference was sixty-five votes.

Welcome signs on the outskirts of both towns hint a new rivalry. Johnson City's sign announces you are entering the "Home Town of Lyndon B. Johnson." Blanco has to settle for the "Homeland" of LBJ.

Blanco was founded in 1853 as Pittsburgh. Johnson City wasn't founded until 1878. It was named after James Johnson, a cousin of the President's grandfather.

Jimmy Finch operates a Texaco service station across the street from Percy Brigham's home in Blanco. A couple drove up in a car with California license plates. "Where's the LBJ Ranch?" the driver asked. Jimmy told him how to get there, and added, "Can't get in, though."

"Why not?"

"Cause that's the summer White House," Jimmy said. "Got guards all over the place."

"So that's Texas hospitality," the tourist snapped, and drove away.

Jimmy shook his gray head. "If they let every peckerwood in that ranch, they'd cart off all the fence posts for souvenirs."

Percy Brigham was finished with lunch. "Let's talk in my office at the bank," he said. "My wife's not feelin' too well today."

He walked slowly to the bank, greeting those he met by their first names. He is a tall man, straight as a stem of prairie hay. He has a rugged face, a strong jaw. But his manner is gentle and there is humor in his eyes.

He said he was born on the Blanco River, son of a rancher. He has been a lawyer, a schoolteacher, an insurance man, a banker and you damn right, a Democrat.

Above his desk is a portrait of Lyndon Johnson taken when Johnson was a senator. It is signed with a fond inscription.

The story goes that when young Johnson decided to go to college, he applied for a loan at the Johnson City bank and got turned down. He went to Brigham, who gave him the money without a question.

Opposite page
A storm uprooted this old dead tree on the highway between Johnson City and Blanco.

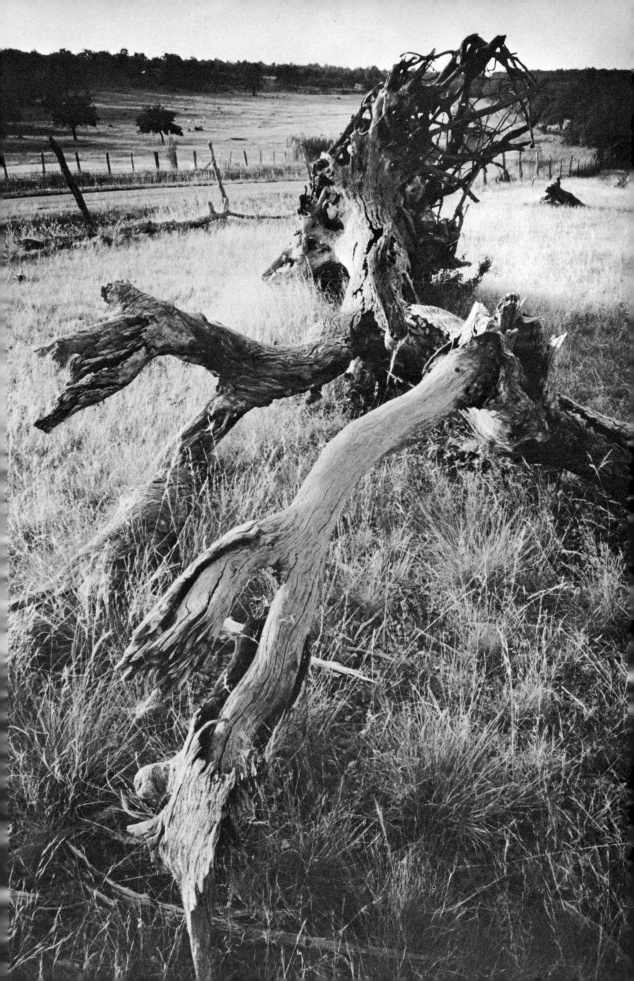

Did Brigham have any idea that the young man before him with a hand out would ever amount to anything?

"Oh, Lyndon was a bright, hard-workin' boy," Brigham said. "But let's don't talk about that loan. That's Lyndon's business and not mine. I can tell you he paid it back promptly."

The old banker said his contact with the Johnson family goes back to the early 1900s, when he worked in the Blanco law office of Judge Joseph W. Baines, the President's maternal grandfather.

"Judge Baines was one of the great men of Texas," Brigham said. "I learned more law under him than I ever did at the University of Texas."

He emphasized that Baines's daughter, Rebekah, the President's mother, was raised in Blanco.

"She was one of the smartest women I've ever known," Brigham said. "That's where Lyndon got his brains. His old daddy, Sam, was straight as a shingle."

The Baineses came from Blanco and the Johnsons from Johnson City! Looked like both places would claim the President. He laughed. Lyndon was a big man. The whole hill country could call him its own. Even Gillespie County, traditionally an island of Republicanism, would go for the native son next election. Yes sir, native son. Lyndon was born in Gillespie County. Folks over there were going to see the light and do him right for a change.* Hadn't he done right by everybody? He had helped bring in electric co-operatives, dams, and soil-saving measures.

Still, Brigham said, not even LBJ has been able to stop the death of the old way of life.

"The ranch folk are selling out," he said. "Selling out to the rich devils from Houston, Austin, and Dallas."

"These playboys are willing to pay high prices for the land," he said. "Prices so high that the little rancher has little choice but to sell. Their kids don't want to stay here in these rocky hills and fight drouth to make a livin', so the old folks put their places on the market and retire on the take. The goin' price for the poorest land here in Blanco County is $105 an acre. You

* Brigham's prediction came true. Lyndon Johnson carried Gillespie County by 421 votes in the 1964 presidential election. The vote was 1879 for Johnson, 1458 for Barry Goldwater.

can't buy an acre of river front property for less than $250—
if you can buy any at all."

How long will this go on?

"A long time," he replied, rather sadly. "It'll be getting worse. They'll put more dams down here. More resort property buyers will come in and there'll come a time when there won't be a legitimate rancher left."

He sat deep in thought.

Was it worth it spending a lifetime here?

"Hell," he said, breaking into a grin, "I feel good. I'm a pioneer. Wouldn't take back a minute of it."

CAPT. JAMES H. CALLAHAN
1814–1856

This Indian fighter and hero of the Texas Revolution established the first settlement in Blanco County in 1853. Callahan was shot and killed in a feud with a neighbor, Woodson Blassengame. Callahan went after Blassengame to avenge Mrs. Callahan's honor, which he thought Blassengame had soiled. A mob of Callahan's friends took Blassengame and his son from guards and murdered them. The grand jury ruled that the Blassengames were murdered "by a company of men unknown to the jury."

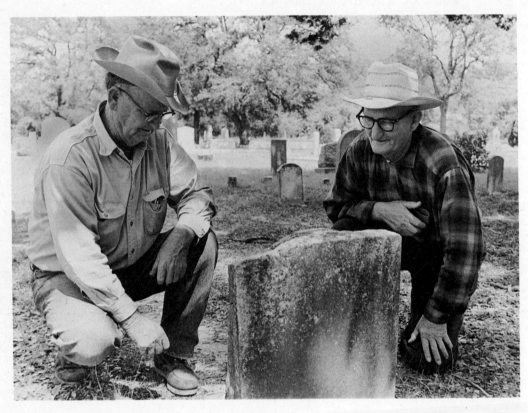

Zeke Felps and friend, Otho Summy, at the grave of Zeke's ancestors in the Miller Creek Cemetery.

CHAPTER FIVE

Zeke Felps sits in a chair up against the cool side of the house teasing Annie about her poppies. He accuses her of growing morphine. She lies belly down on the front room bed. Her head is in the window sill and she laughs through the screen.

Zeke came home happy after an afternoon of victory at the battlefield under the mulberry tree beside Casparis' Cafe. Annie's beans burble on the stove, rattling the lid. The scent seeps out and finds his nose in the yard. It will be a while yet.

The sun hangs over the Pedernales, reluctant to go down. But the turkeys know. They feel in their feathers the death of day. They will be safe on their roosts at the first fall of darkness.

But there is time enough for talk on the cool side of a rock house in a tiny Texas town in the seventy-eighth year of our Zeke. Old men talk at twilight, knowing they may not wake at morning.

"You know," he said, "I'm the oldest Felps man left in the county. There was fifteen kids in my brood. Now two are left. Me and my sister Minnie. Minnie's eighty-two. Lives on the road to Austin."

Blanco County used to be full of his kin. Now there are more Felpses out in Miller Creek Cemetery than there are Felpses walking around.

"Pshaw," he said. "Back when I was a boy, if you met a man south of the Johnson City divide, you could bet he was a Crider. If you met a man north of the divide, you wouldn't go wrong by sayin' 'Hidy, Mr. Felps.' Sure different now."

Annie in the window said Zeke had never been out of the county but one time, when he went down to Del Rio, on the Mexican border, two hundred and fifty miles away.

"Don't make no difference," he said. "I'm known all over the country anyhow."

"I'll swan, just listen to him."

"It's true," he said with mock seriousness. "And I'll tell you

35

why. One of them big magazines carried my picture. They took it when me and the boys were playin' dominoes under the mulberry tree. What was the name of that magazine, Annie?"

"*Life*," she said.

"My daughter out in California saw it," Zeke said with a grin. "She was sittin' under a hair dryer in a beauty shop, thumbin' through the magazine, when she saw her old daddy."

Zeke was born on McCall Creek, ten miles outside Johnson City. His daddy was a rancher, so that's what he took up. He'd still be ranching if some strangers from the city hadn't forced him to sell. He had 602 acres and they offered him $125 an acre. He had bought it in 1919 for less than $9 an acre. What was a man to do? He and Annie moved into town.

He used to hire out for extra money. One time he was working on a road gang with a young fella by the name of Lyndon Johnson. Lyndon's daddy was the foreman. Lyndon drove a pickup truck on the job. The other drivers would back up their trucks to a dirt pile, then get out and help shovel the dirt into the truck bed. Lyndon would back up his truck to the dirt pile, then settle in the seat for a nap while the others shoveled.

"Go on, Zeke Felps!" Annie scolded. "That doesn't sound like the President. Why, he runs everybody else ragged up there in Washington!"

"Lyndon was no fool," he said. "He knew what he was about. He was savin' his energy to run this country."

The cemetery was full of Felpses, and Zeke walked upon his dead kin, stopping here and there to read an epitaph. Uncle Wid was under the spreading branches of a cedar tree. Uncle Brit was beside an oak.

Otho Summy pointed at two headstones and said, "Zeke, there's your granddaddy and grandmama."

Zeke nodded. "I know it, Otho, and you're standing on my daddy and mama." Otho looked down and stepped off them.

Zeke said he and Annie would be buried here when their time came. How did it make him feel to look at his final resting place? Oh, he said, it was a pleasant place for the living and he didn't hear the dead complaining.

It is a nice place in May. The old trees keep the sun out and the graveyard is dark and cool and wildflower-fragrant. You can sit among the tombs and hear the water gurgling down Miller Creek or watch squirrels scamper for acorns. A sweet

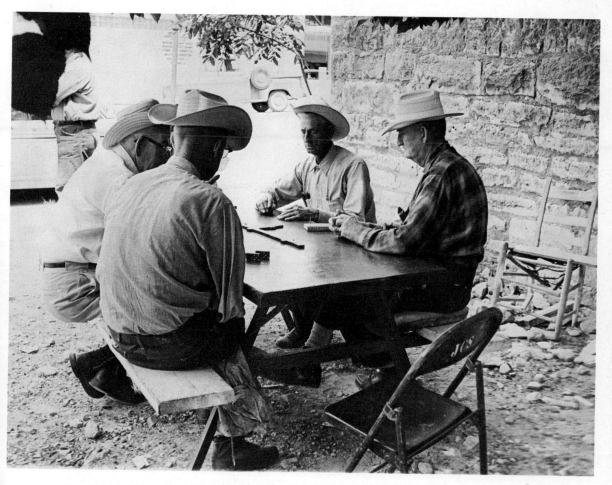

Zeke Felps and cronies in a game of skill and chance under a Texas mulberry tree.

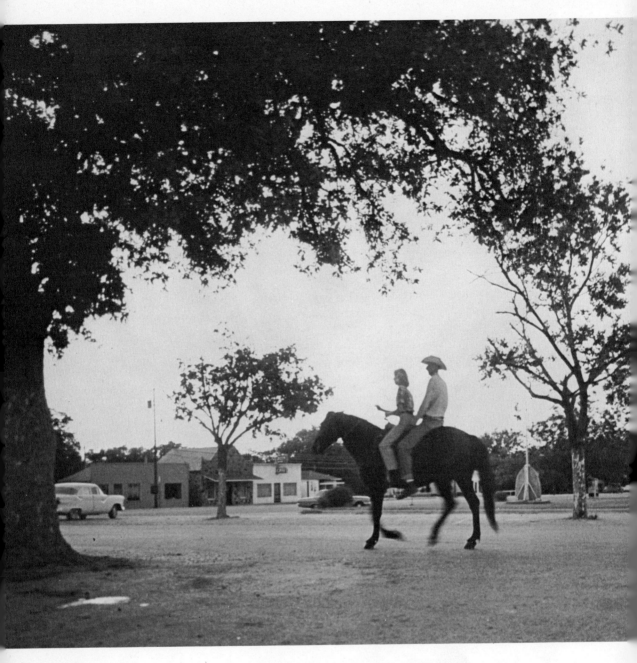

A young couple making the drag around the Courthouse Square in Johnson City.

nostalgia—not a sour sadness or mawkish remembrance—pervades. It is not a Disneyland of the Dead with alabaster angels and chalk Christs and Muzak. It is a country cemetery with a quiet, simple dignity.

Zeke found the grave of Tom and Eliza Felps, who were killed by Comanches and buried together in the same hole. Eliza was the last woman scalped by Indians in Blanco County. They didn't scalp Tom, Zeke said, because Tom had red hair. Tom was Zeke's uncle and a third cousin to Otho Summy.

It happened in 1869, which seems a long time ago. But Miz Jennie Shipp of Johnson City, who'll be one hundred years old in November, remembers the grownups talking about the tragedy. Eliza Felps was nineteen. They say she was a pretty little thing.

Eliza and Tom lived with their children, Callie and Tom, Jr., in a log cabin on Miller Creek. Eliza's daddy was county judge, and whenever Judge White had to sit at court, she and Tom would take the kids and stay with her mother at the White ranch, east of Round Mountain.

That's where the Felpses were on July 21, 1869. Miz White kept the kids while Tom and Eliza went down to Cypress Creek to catch some fish for dinner.

They were sitting on the bank, in the shade of the sumac and Spanish oak, when a Negro boy on a pony rode up and said Indians were coming. Tom and Eliza ran for the house. They never made it. The Comanches took the Negro boy's pony, but they let the boy go. He ran to Miz White with the news.

A posse led by Judge White and Tom's daddy, Jacob, found the bodies the next day. Tom had been shot and stabbed and stripped of his clothes.

Eliza Felps lay naked, an arrow puncturing her breast. She had been scalped alive, but managed to crawl some distance before dying.

The posse rode off in search of the Comanches. One of the deputies was Sam Ealy Johnson, Sr., who left his wife and infant daughter alone in their stone cabin.

Sam's wife was named Eliza too. She was drawing water from a spring near her cabin when she saw Comanches coming through the woods on horses. There wasn't a man in the settlement. She ran to the cabin, grabbed her baby and crawled down into a cellar beneath the cabin floor. She closed the trap door, stuck a stick through the crack, and pulled a braided rug over the door. Then she tied an extra diaper over the baby's mouth to keep it from crying out loud.

The Indians stomped into the cabin and tore up the place. But they didn't find Eliza Johnson and her baby. She heard them go to the barn, get fresh horses, and ride away. She didn't come out of the cellar until Sam got home after dark. He told her they didn't catch the Indians. She pointed to a trunk. The Comanches had destroyed wedding gifts the Johnsons had brought by wagon from Lockhart.

Judge White never got over his daughter's murder. The next year, he and his wife left Blanco County and settled in Austin.

The daughter, Callie, went to live in Austin with the Whites. She never married and died a young woman.

Her brother, Tom, Jr., was raised by his uncle, Wid Felps. When Tom, Jr., was sixteen, he went to California. He came back home only once, in 1910, to appear briefly in a court suit over his granddaddy's estate. After the trial, he stopped by the Miller Creek Cemetery for a few minutes and then went back to California. No one in Blanco County saw him again.

Sam and Eliza Johnson did right well with their lives. Sam and his brother Tom became the biggest trail drivers in seven counties—until Texas drouths and Kansas blizzards killed their cattle and left them broke. But Eliza Johnson bore Sam eight more children, and the fifth child, Samuel Ealy Johnson, Jr., made the family proud. He married a genteel beauty, Rebekah Baines, became a farmer, served in the state legislature for twelve years, and sired a president.

DONATA PELLAR

1858–1959

On her hundredth birthday, this Round Mountain
widow told a friend: "My wedding dress was white
organdy with little white bows. I wore flowers in my
hair, but I can't remember what kind. I believe it was
a wreath of rosebuds. I can still remember everyone
telling me how radiant I looked and how pretty
were the flowers in my hair."

CHAPTER SIX

Every day, Fannie and Austin Casparis get up and let the morning sun come into their little cafe on the square in Johnson City.

Fannie parts the curtains and Austin turns on the floor fan and opens the door. Then they sit in rocking chairs and wait.

Austin waits for the sun to hit half past high noon. Then he'll go out under the mulberry tree for an afternoon of dominoes with James Ealy Johnson, Zeke Felps, Clegg Smith, John Martin, and Lee Green. Sometimes Otho Summy sits in on the game.

Fannie just sits and rocks until time to close. She waits for customers. She knows they will never come.

When people in Johnson City eat out now, they go to Minnie Pilgrim's or Danz's Barbecue or to the two cafes out on the highway.

Customers used to come to Fannie's cafe.

When Lyndon Johnson was a tall, lanky boy he would walk in at noon and Fannie would slide a bowl of chili in front of him. She never had to ask what he wanted. If Lyndon didn't ask for a second helping, Fannie would put her hands on her hips and shake her head in mock disappointment. Lyndon was a schoolmate of Fannie's oldest daughter, Louise.

There's nothing wrong with Fannie's cooking now. Austin still eats it and he's a strong eighty-two. It is just that Fannie had to quit cooking for the public.

Ten years ago, she was peeling potatoes when she fell and broke a hip. Austin locked up and drove her to the hospital. Fannie was sixty-eight at the time, and her bones didn't set the way the doctors wanted. But she got up and about, even opened the cafe again.

But the strain of cooking for crowds and waiting on tables was too much. The kids made her close for good.

Well, Fannie couldn't bring herself to do just that. She compromised. Every morning she went down to the cafe, opened the doors, and placed a "closed" sign in the window. Then she

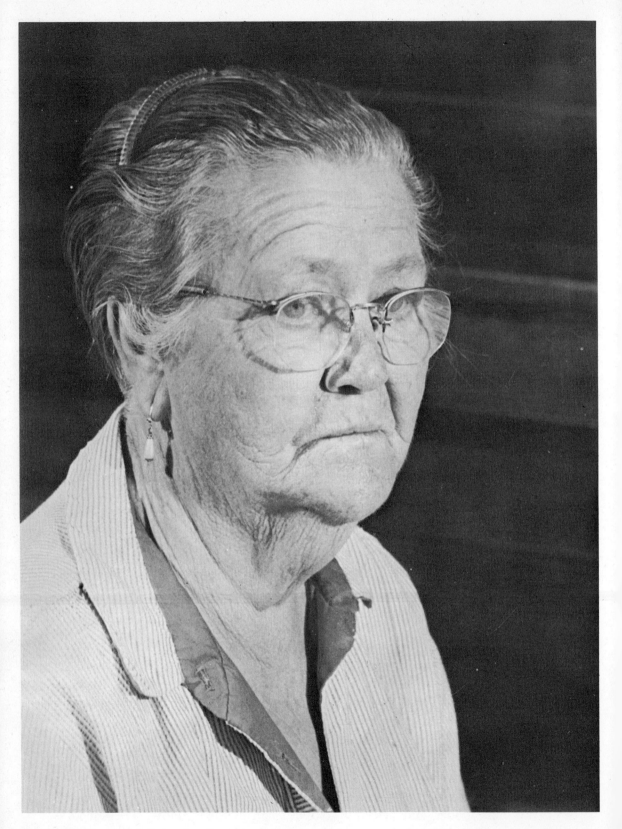

Fannie Casparis helped develop Lyndon Johnson's gourmet taste for chili, before she broke her hip.

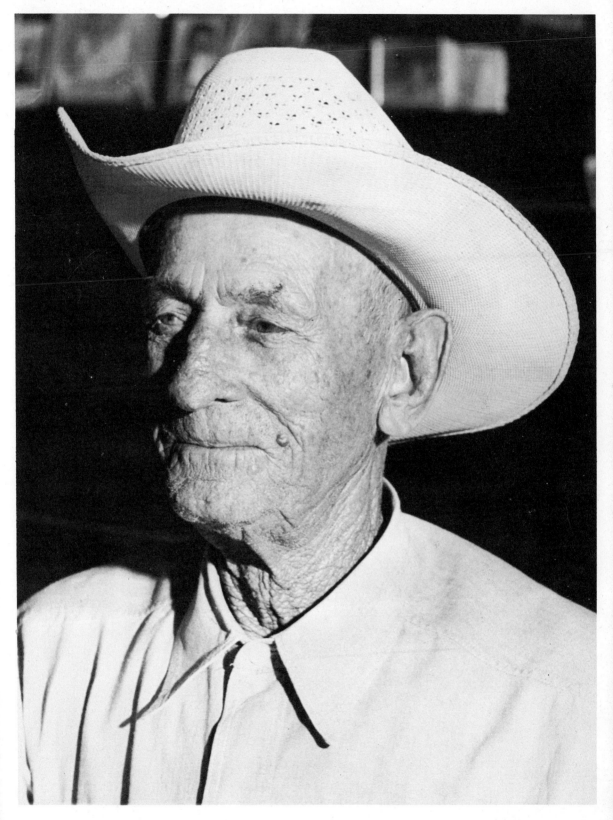

Austin Casparis is luckier than most folks: Fannie still makes chili for him.

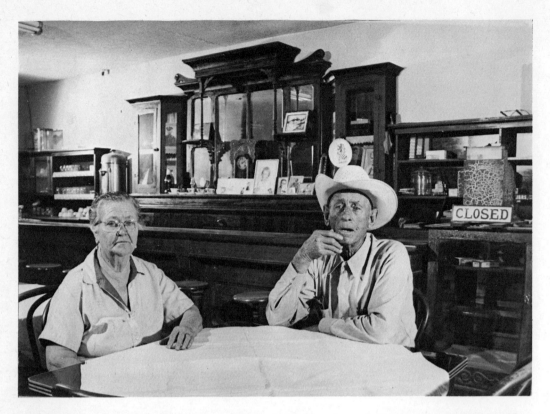

You could write a ballad about Fannie and Austin Casparis' sad cafe.

sat there in her rocking chair, waiting for customers she knew would never come.

Austin joined her. They began having their meals in the cafe. Every night after supper, Fannie would mix up a batch of sour dough just as she did in the old days. She would sit it on the table and they would lock up and walk the half block home. Fannie would be in the cafe early the next morning, and everybody around the square could smell her bread baking. Austin got his fill of bread. One day they moved beds into the back of the cafe. They seldom go home any more.

Twice a week now, Fannie washes and irons the cafe's tablecloths and mops the floor. She keeps fresh salt and pepper and sugar on each table.

The place looks open for business. The "closed" sign is small. A stranger missed it the other day. He walked in and ordered a hamburger. Fannie's eyes lighted up for an instant, then she shook her head sadly and turned him away.

A couple of days ago, Red, one of her six sons, asked if he could use her tables and tablecloths for the dance hall he was opening beside his beer joint.

Fannie agreed.

But when Red came by the next day, she told him, "Son, I couldn't sleep for worryin' about those tables and tablecloths. . . ."

"Okay, Mama," Red said. "I'll leave them alone."

JOHN SPEER

1831–1906

In his diary, Speer, an early Blanco merchant, wrote
of his fellow frontiersmen: "We were not a rough,
uncouth, 'hoosierish' set, not a bit of it; for even in
that day the ladies were well read up on 'Gody' and
'Madame Demorest.' This writer saw ladies dressed in
that most bewitching of all dresses, the full bloomer.
The men, as a general thing, did not put on much
style—hickory shirts with woolen skin leggings, a
six-shooter and a butcher knife, hung by a broad belt
around the waist and with large, jingling spurs. The
Sunday dress was about the same, with the exception
of a calico shirt instead of a hickory one. Very few
had overcoats but used their camp blankets instead.
All carried six-shooters, from the cowboy to the
minister, and, strange to say, there were few personal
difficulties and no quarrels, for a quarrel between
men well-armed meant blood."

CHAPTER SEVEN

Red Casparis says he was an oil tool salesman until the day the big boss from Houston caught him drinking on the job. So he came back to Johnson City and opened a beer joint.

Red could have gone somewhere else and made more money. That's not because people around here don't like beer. Red says where you find domino players you find beer drinkers. Trouble is, there's not a lot of people left around here to buy it. The population of Johnson City is down to 611. In fact, the whole county's population has dropped over the last three census counts.

So it's quiet around here, not exactly a businessman's bonanza. Red came back because he felt like somebody had to look after his mother and daddy, who are up in years. The nine other Casparis children have moved away.

Red's trying to make the best of it. For a year now, he's been mulling over the idea of opening a dance hall next door. The other night he tried it.

He got a band out of Austin to agree to play for 70 per cent of the gate. The band leader, a Negro hipster by the name of Roper, wanted a guarantee. Red wouldn't give it to him. He wasn't sure ten people would come.

By dance time, twenty-one men and two women had showed up, but no band. Everybody waited around for an hour. Red kept looking at the Pearl Beer clock on the wall and mumbling. He'd advertised the dance all over the county, went to a lot of trouble getting tables and chairs and a license. The customers, weary of waiting for a band that apparently wasn't coming, began leaving. As they filed out, Red refunded the seventy-five cents he had charged each of them at the door.

Wes Waugh, eighty-two, couldn't hide his disappointment. He mentioned the dance to everybody he met all week and had even gotten a haircut. The barber, Pancho Althaus, had come with him. Now Wes said he wanted to go home. Naw, said Pancho, stick around, I'll dance with you. They joined Red's cousins at the domino table.

47

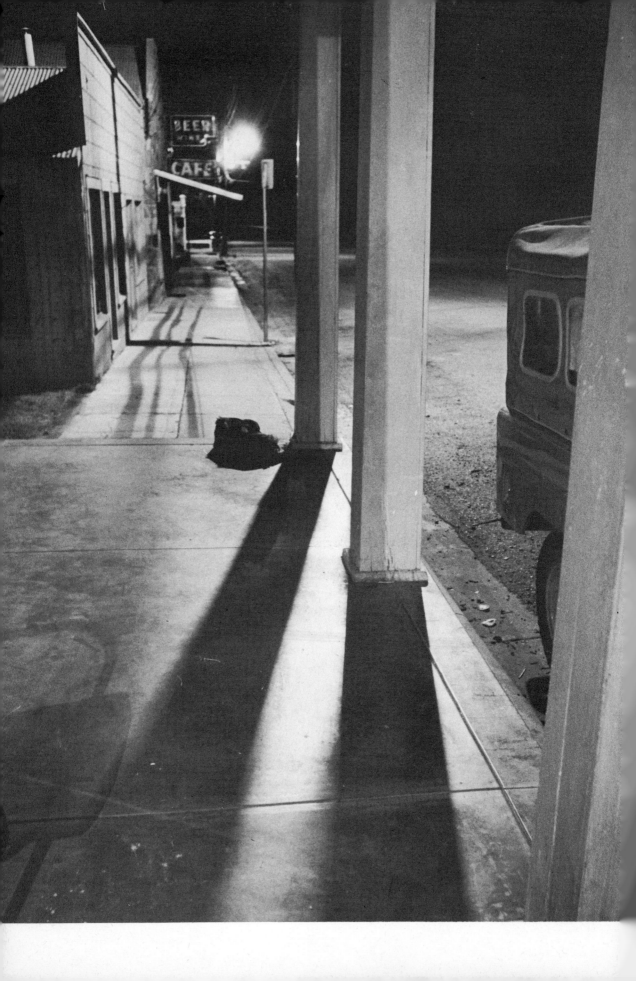

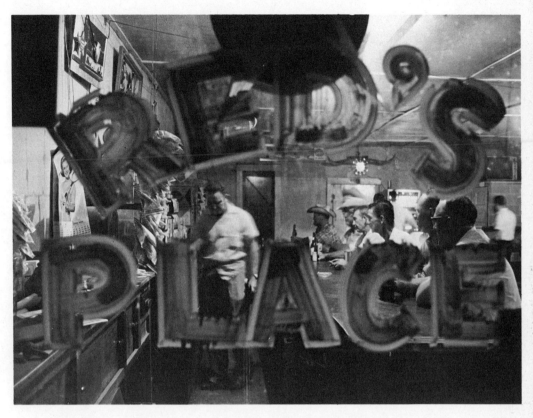

When the evening sun goes down the action is at Red's Place.

Opposite page
Quiet descends on the main street of Johnson City after supper is over.

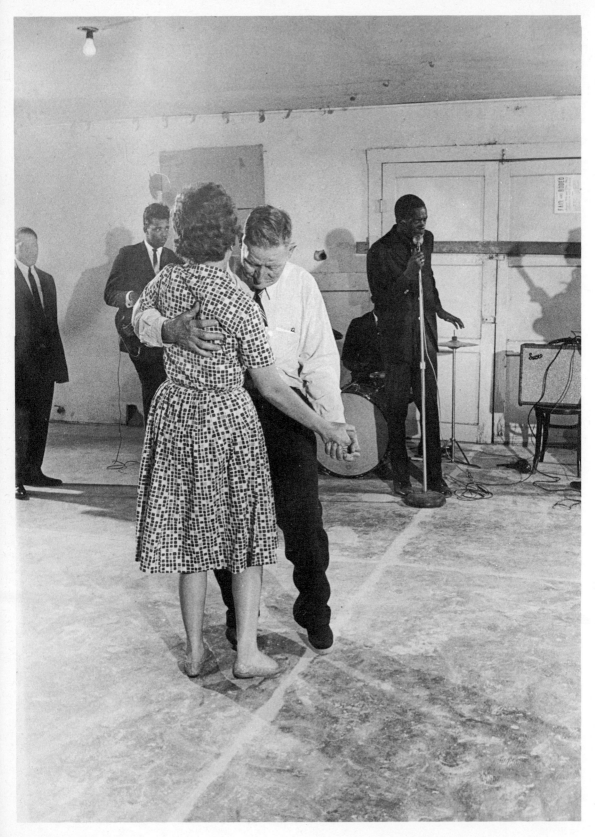

Red hasn't got around to the fad for the discothèque. He still features live music.

They were shuffling the dominoes when the band arrived.

Roper said he was sorry. He had to scramble to get a drummer. Red grumbled a little, but told Roper and his boys to go ahead and start playing. Maybe the noise would wake up the town to the fact that there was going to be a dance after all.

It sure did. And it turned out to be a fairly profitable night for Red. The crowd drifted back, and by the time the dance really got under way there were five women—counting Red's girl—and about thirty men.

Most of the men didn't dance. There weren't enough women to go around and the band was grooved in the rock 'n' roll style. Rock 'n' roll doesn't make much sense to Johnson City polka dancers. As Wes Waugh said, "Why ask a woman to dance if you're not goin' to hold onto her?" But Wes and the barber didn't waste time when the band played an occasional slow piece. Wes danced with Betty, Red's girl, and then Pancho gave her a swing while Wes pulled a fresh-faced blonde around the floor. He'd been itching to dance with the blonde after he watched her twist with her boy friend, a callow youth nobody knew. Wes said she wiggled "ever little ole thang." Somebody said she looked like the Harvey girl. No. The Harvey girl was a little lighter in the ankle. Besides, the Harvey girl *sure* wouldn't make a public exhibition of herself. This gal was from across the county line.

Red sold a lot of beer—more than he would have sold on a routine night—and he got almost eight dollars of the gate. He says he'll try it again—with a different band—if he can find a group who'll play without a guarantee. Roper and his boys wouldn't come back if Red wanted them, which he doesn't. Their take of the gate—and their take for the night—was eighteen dollars. Split that five ways and a man wonders if they even made expenses. They drove from Austin in a fire-engine red automobile so heavy with hardware it must have eaten up ten dollars' worth of gasoline just coming.

J. C. DODGEN

1858–1935

Brother Dodgen was a farmer who felt he had to preach. In fact, he spent more time preaching than he did farming and made little money at either. But he had ten children, and nearly all of them went to college.

CHAPTER EIGHT

Ella Mae is out in the smokehouse melting beer bottles to make into ash trays. Jesse, her husband, is over at Henly, east of the ranch, talking with his brother Jody about opening a barbecue stand on the highway into Johnson City. D, the bachelor brother and oldest of the Smithermans, is across the ranch road watering fig trees he planted last season. The trees are runty. D says nothing grows good on the land. Too much caliche, not enough vitamins. The strip he and Jesse own is some of the sorriest land in the county. Why'd they buy? Somebody had to tackle it. Besides, it's home. They'd been leasing the place since '27.

He and Jesse and Jody came to Blanco County from Kimble County on July 20, 1927. Moved about two thousand head of cattle with them and leased 1280 acres on Flat Creek. Looking back on it all, maybe they shouldn't have left Kimble County. Now that's real ranch country! Up there you can feed cattle cottonseed meal—to prick their appetite—and they'll fill up on old rotten grass and get fat as butterballs. Here it's different. One cow won't get fat on twenty acres. You have to feed them out year round. He and Jesse mix maize with corn and shorts and mineral syrup, which is an expensive proposition. Now, the bottom's dropped out of the beef market. Calves that a year ago would bring $120 now bring about $75.

Jody got out of the partnership and bought him a place over at Henly. Jody married Hazel Herbest and Jesse married Hazel's sister Ella Mae. D never married. He looked after Mother and she lived to be eighty. Now he's seventy. Jody's sixty-five and Jessie's fifty-nine.

D turned off the water and started toward the house. Ella Mae met him at the gate. She said she was going into Johnson City to sell some of her LBJ ash trays.

It was almost noon. D said he'd whip up some dinner. He got out some ground pork sausage, patted it into patties, and dropped them into a frying pan. He cooked them black and crispy, and fried eggs in the leftover grease.

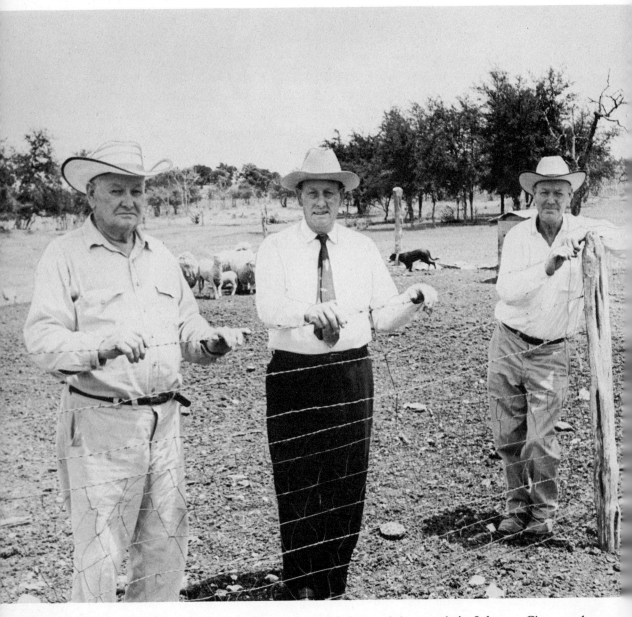

The Smitherman brothers—D, left; Jodie, center; and Jesse, right—on their Johnson City ranch.

Yeah, he thought they had done a pretty good job on the house. He and Jesse built it themselves in 1959 with stone they hauled out of the fields. Jody and some of Ella Mae's brothers helped. The other house was getting so old it was falling down.

He and Jesse now had about 1600 acres. They leased all but 347 acres, which they bought to put the new house on. No. They don't run anywhere near 2000 head of cattle any more. Might have 50 cows. But they ran 350 sheep and that many goats. No. Just had one horse. Tippy, their border collie, took care of the roundups. He's handled cows so much, though, that he's a little rough for sheep.

Jesse came in. He said a barbecue stand down on 290 was bound to be a money-maker. It looked like LBJ was going to be President for eight more years and already the hill country was full of tourists. A man who grew his own beef could run a barbecue stand with a good margin for profit. Might even put in a motel. Ella Mae could sell her ceramics. It was sure something to think about.

D said he had to go down to the barn and turn on the self-feeder. Now that was some contraption. He and Jesse had built it themselves out of scrap. You could push a button and start the whole thing. The milo maize went from a bin to a measuring box and into a hammer mill where it was ground. The mill spat the maize into a mixer, where it picked up corn and shorts and minerals and then was dumped into the feeder trough. They even had the hayloft rigged so that one man could dump the bales into the cow lot without working up a sweat.

Jesse told D they ought to think about getting some Holstein cows. He knew good and well that people were going to keep on drinking milk.

Ella Mae's pickup bounced down the road from Johnson City, its wheels spinning a storm of dust along the road. The dust was so dry it hung in the air like smoke. Jesse wished for rain.

It was cooler. The sun was low and lavender and seemed so close it looked like it was going to fall into Flat Creek. D said it was time for supper.

UNCLE BILLY BARTON

1782–1840

When his nearest neighbor was within ten miles of
his cabin at La Grange, the Daniel Boone of Texas
complained that the country was getting too crowded
and moved into the hills. He settled at the spring
which bears his name in Austin and named two
other springs after his daughters, Eliza and Parthenia.
When the Republic of Texas stationed soldiers near
his cabin to protect the settlers against Indians, Uncle
Billy wrote the President: "Come git your blasted
soldiers. It's a sight more trouble to keep them away
from my daughters than it is to fight Indians."

Opposite page
The sun was low and lavender and seemed so close it looked like it was
going to fall into Flat Creek.

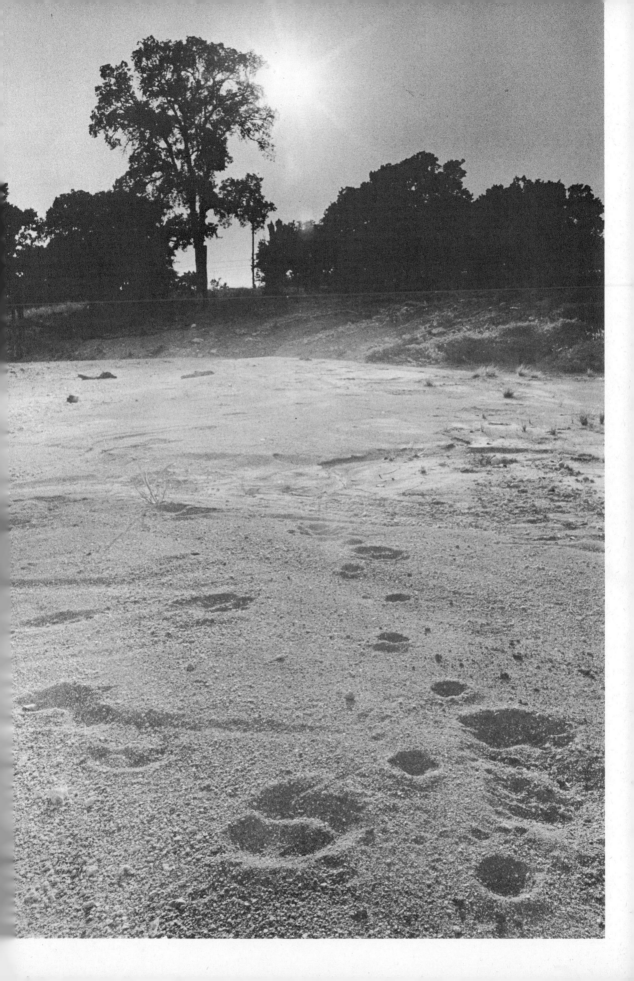

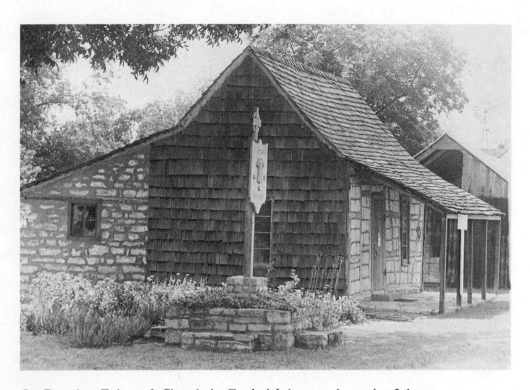

St. Barnabas Episcopal Church in Fredericksburg, where the Johnson family worship.

CHAPTER NINE

Ace Reid, the cowboy cartoonist at Kerrville, remarked the other day that folks at Fredericksburg are beginning to act like Democrats.

Ace was only half teasing. A customer can buy LBJ souvenirs in almost any shop in Fredericksburg, and there's a cafe on Main Street that displays a picture of the President alongside those of Admiral Chester Nimitz, a native son, and Konrad Adenauer, a cousin from the old country.

Fredericksburg is the county seat of Gillespie County, which in 1960 gave Richard Nixon 76.7 per cent of its votes. Lyndon Johnson, who, of course, was the Democratic candidate for vice-president, was born in Gillespie County.

The Republican win in Gillespie County—and in Kerr, Kimble, Mason, and Comal counties—was no personal reflection against Johnson.* He carried the rest of the hill counties and the whole state for John F. Kennedy.

It just points up what everybody in Texas has known for years—that hill country people of German descent are independent-minded and always have been. The reason is rooted in history.

The Napoleonic Wars crippled Germany's economy and sent a wave of unrest through the country. University students, inspired by the French Revolution, began rioting against the Crown. The masses joined them in an open revolt, which the petty German princes mercilessly suppressed. The country became a police state, and Germans of intellect and energy began looking to America.

In the next twenty years, thousands of Germans came to Texas and the hill country. They were intellectuals, artists, musicians, teachers, doctors, and lawyers; skilled craftsmen, farmers, and mechanics. They put down roots in the hills, worked hard, and minded their own business.

* Lyndon Johnson carried twelve of the thirteen hill country counties in the 1964 presidential election. He trailed Barry Goldwater in Kendall County by a vote of 970 to 1173.

Fredericksburg was founded by German immigrants in 1846. The first colonists arrived in twenty ox-drawn wagons. Their first supper was a bear shot by a scout, John Schmidt.

Many died of cholera that first year. A two-wheeled cart was drawn through the streets to pick up the dead. The survivors, too ill to build coffins, wrapped the dead in sailcloth.

The Indians, hostile to the Anglo-American settlers, tended to trust the Germans. The Comanches brought honey, meat, and bear fat to the sick immigrants.

The country seemed to attract nonconformists. In 1847, Lyman Wight set up a Morman colony five miles east of Fredericksburg and called it Zodiac. The Mormons supplied the Germans with meal and lumber and taught them to cultivate the land.

Wight was a strange zealot, known as "The Wild Ram of the Mountains." After Joseph Smith's death at the hands of a mob in 1844, Wight fought Brigham Young for control of the Mormon Church. Young, who attracted the most followers, excommunicated Wight. The Wild Ram and his one hundred and fifty followers came down the Mississippi River into Texas.

One of those flash floods on the Pedernales washed away Wight's mills in 1851 and that was the end of Zodiac. The Wild Ram gathered his flock and wandered about Texas in search of "God's Country." They never found it. When the Civil War rumbled at Fort Sumter, Wight tried to lead his people out of Texas. He fell dead near San Antonio and his people lost hope and scattered like dry leaves in the winds of war.

Texas joined the Confederacy, but most of the hill country counties voted against secession. The Germans opposed slavery and refused to repudiate their loyalty to the United States.

In Gillespie County, where in fifty-three years a president of the *United* States would be born, the vote was 398 to 16 for the Union.

In neighboring Blanco County, where the President would grow up, the vote was two to one against the Union.

Sam Ealy Johnson, Sr., the President's grandfather, left his cattle herds on the Pedernales and fought for the South.

Bands of German men left their families in the hill country and fled to Mexico to join Lincoln's cause. Many were killed before they reached the border. Vigilante gangs murdered Germans in their homes. In 1865, the Blanco County Grand Jury

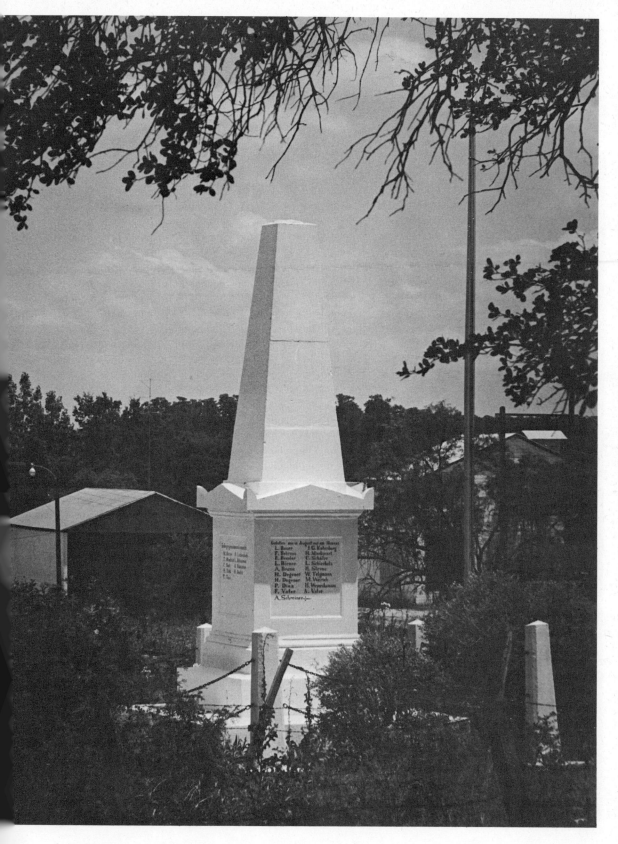

A monument to the Yankee loyalists slain by Confederates, in the town of Comfort, Texas.

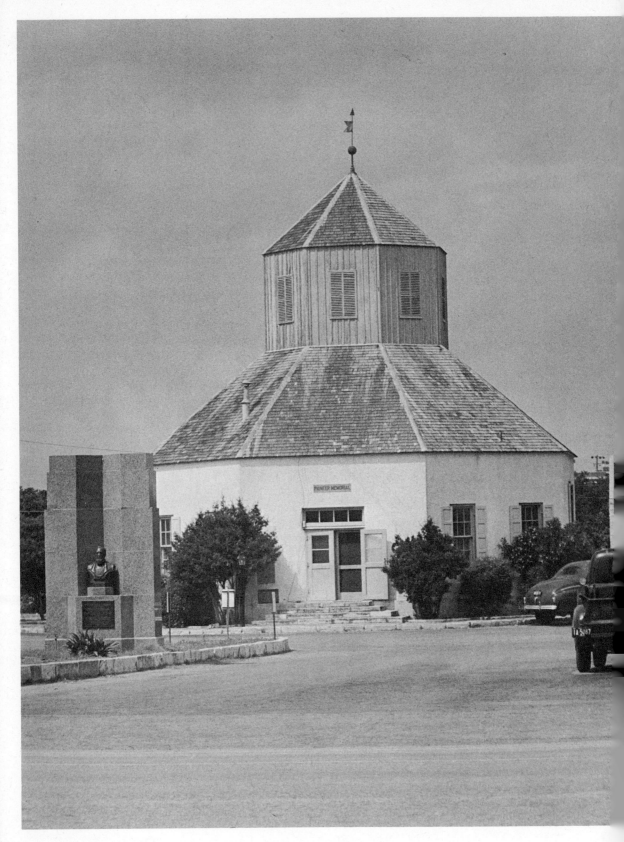

The Fredericksburg Pioneer Memorial in downtown Fredericksburg.

returned seventy-three murder indictments. Few of those charged were ever tried.

It was a long time before the Anglo-Americans in the hills could look at their "Dutchman" neighbors without resentment.

Maury Maverick, Jr., of San Antonio remembers the hate whispers that circulated when his great-uncle, Congressman James Slayden, appointed a "German" boy to the U. S. Naval Academy. But Chester Nimitz made a pretty good sailor anyhow.

It is different now. Disagreements are settled in ballot boxes and not in blood.

GOTTLIEB BURCHARD DANGERS

1811–1869

Pastor Dangers came from Germany to Fredericksburg in 1845 with a new wife, a flute, a zither, and a grand piano. He baptized 1061 persons, married 187 couples, and buried 256 neighbors. His first four children died of diphtheria.

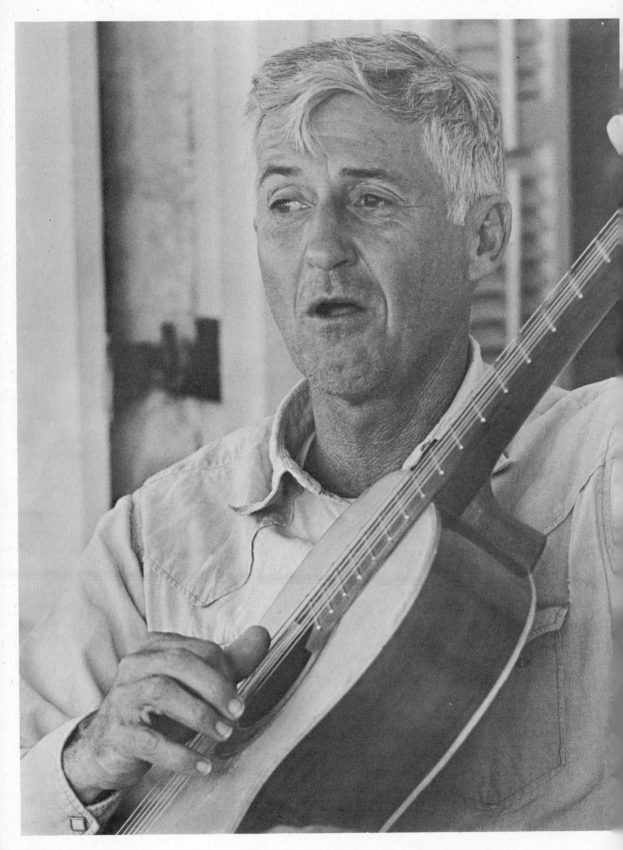

Hondo Crouch, a man of parts, singing a Mexican song in the town of Hye.

CHAPTER TEN

Hondo Crouch sat on the steps of the post office at Hye, a place in the road between Johnson City and Fredericksburg.

He wore a straw hat and blue denim white at the knees. When Hondo saw the car with the out-of-state license roll up, he stuck a stem of hay between his teeth.

"Hello," the driver called.

"Hidy," Hondo said, scratching at his belly.

"How can I get to the LBJ Ranch?"

"Tha what?" Hondo asked, cupping a hand to his ear.

"The Johnson ranch."

"Oh . . ." said Hondo. "The Johnson place. Seems to me I've heard of it. Lemme see . . . Well . . . Nope. Don't know. Sorry . . . I don't live here. Live down the road a mile. . . ."

The tourist shook his head and sped away.

Hondo went limp with laughter.

He had lied on all accounts but one, and his arithmetic was wrong on the honest answer. He lives twenty-five miles down the road from Hye.

But that's Hondo. He never lets facts get in the way of the truth of parody.

Who is Hondo? Well, he's many things; and just about the time you think you have him all collected and pinned under glass with an identification tag, he flutters away.

A newspaper columnist once described him as a country beatnik. But that's not all of Hondo, as we shall see. In some ways he's exactly the opposite.

To readers of the Comfort *News*, Hondo is Peter Cedarstacker, the irreverent bard of Cedar Creek. Cedar Creek is a mythical hill country community populated with people who bear an uncomfortable resemblance to Hondo's own neighbors. Let's look at a typical Cedarstacker report on the doings at Cedar Creek:

"Late Tuesday of this week the Joneses visited the Smiths.

"For those of you who are interested, the coronation gown

of the Gutowsky girl is on exhibit at the Cedar Creek Post O, beer joint and ice house. (Its a 3 piece ensemble). She was chosen Miss Burr Clover in Bear Creek last week and we're proud.

"The Wurstbottoms have remodeled their town house here in Cedar Creek since all their children have left home. Seems kinda sad that the children grew up in a shack on the ranch and now that they'r gone mama and daddy built a nice house with rugs tacked on the floor, beds with no steads, electricity and hidden stoves. It happens every time. Now no one'll enjoy it but the old folks and they wont enjoy it much. They keep the shades down so's the sun wont sad the colors of the rug in the livin room where no bodys been. Then too, they'r gone lots. He goes fishin and she goes to the garden club, beauty parlor, and belongs to the 'Bugs United Together Stand' Club, 'Bird Lovers of Our Precinct' Club, 'Old Home Makers', etc. They dont see much of each other anymore.

"The house is purtier than the shack at the head of the canyon and is cool in the summer and warm in the winter. And instead of a room with a path, they now have two bath rooms and both of 'em are inside. One for her and one for him. They dont see much of each other anymore."

To vaqueros who sip a cool one in the cantinas around Comfort, Hondo Crouch is a compadre with the face of a gringo and the soul of a Mexican. He can sit for hours with his brown brothers, strumming a guitar and wailing ranchero songs in beautiful Spanish.

To goat buyers, Hondo is one of the biggest ranchers in the hills. His daddy-in-law may be the biggest. Hondo lives in a big rock house, off the highway between Fredericksburg and Comfort, with his wife, Shotzie, and their children—Becky, nineteen, Juan, seventeen, Kerry, fifteen, and Cris (a girl), twelve. Hondo says that Becky, a dark-eyed beauty who is an honor student at the University of Texas, is Miss Mohair of the Universe and Cedar Creek.

To the Comfort Chamber of Commerce, Hondo is the owner of the Comfort Wool and Mohair Co., which brings a lot of business to town.

To Democrats, he is an irksome Republican with a barbed-wire tongue. To the University of Texas athletic department, he is a pleasant memory—an All-American on the Longhorn

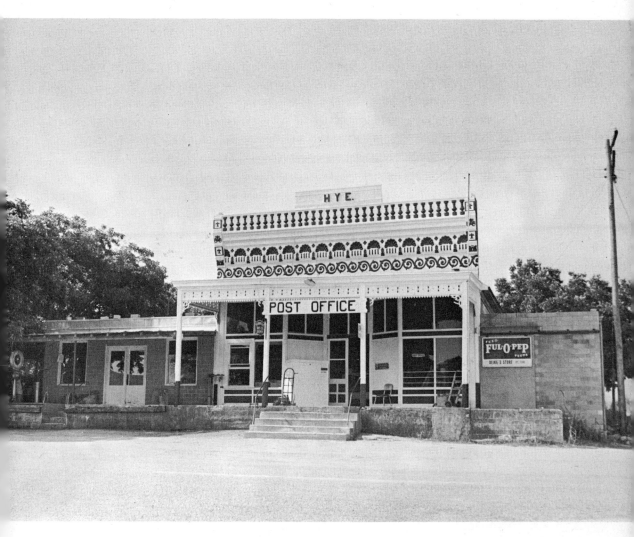

At Hye's decorative post office, Hondo pleasures himself teasing the tourists.

swimming team. And to prying strangers with pad and pencil, Hondo is just plain frustrating.

He sat munching a soft tortilla, telling as straight as he could the story of his life.

"Well, let's see," he said. "I was born in Hondo, Texas. My daddy was a railroad man. I went off to the university and made the swimming team. That was kind of hard for the home folks to understand because there wasn't any water in Hondo. But they forgot that it rained one year and I learned to swim in a cow track.

"A married lady helped me through college—my mother.

"I got out of the university in 1941 and went to Houston, where I taught boys with silk stockings on to swim at a River Oaks boys' club. Then I joined a bigger boys' club—the Air Force.

"After the war, my wife's daddy talked me into buying a goat ranch."

All of a sudden, he gulped down the tortilla and became Peter Cedarstacker. "You know," he said, "sneaking a beer by Jesus is like trying to sneak daylight by a rooster.

"In the newspaper business, which is what I am in as much as anything else, lazy reporters say that no news is good news. That's all wrong, the grammar I mean. News are plural. I heard a German farmer talking about his 'bi-focus glasses' the other day. Now that's a new. Isn't it?

"Did I tell you that my friend Jesus—that's pronounced Hey-soos—McNeel returned this week from a visit to Mexico? Well, he did. And he was telling me that his uncle from Zia-huatanejo on the Chilpacingogo had a little misunderstanding at the bridge last month. The uncle had been hauling barnyard fertilizer across the bridge to Mexico in wheelbarrows. He'd been doing this for ten years. Every load was dug into and sifted by customs inspectors because they knew he was smuggling something worth more than thirty-seven cents but they didn't know what.

"Several times they took the wheel off and searched the bearings and blew through the hollow handles that were full of fertilizer. Well, last week he got caught, not by the customs men but like all big criminals by the internal revenue people. He had not reported his wife as a partner in his wheelbarrow sales. For ten years he'd been smuggling wheelbarrows."

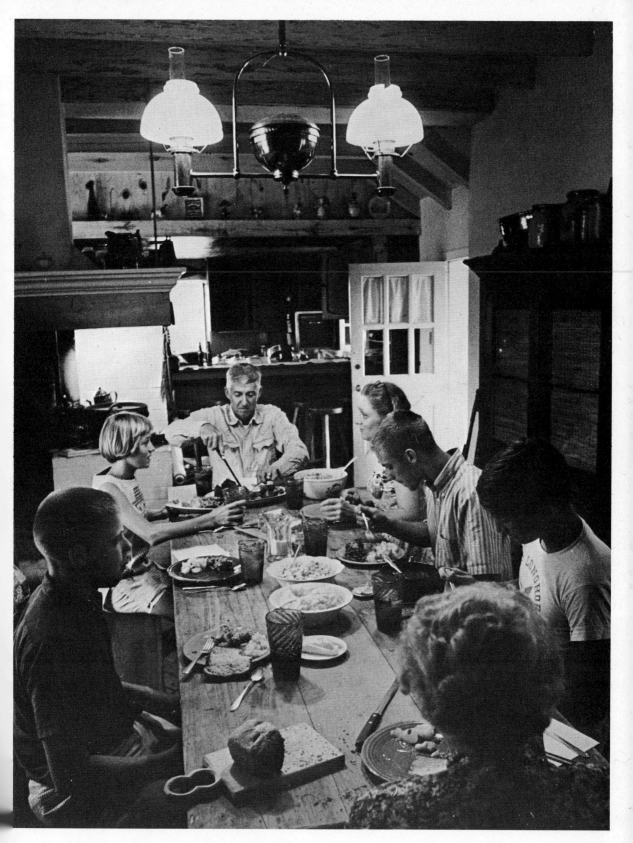

Hondo Crouch carves the roast lamb at dinner with his handsome family.

FRANK (YANKEE) DAVIS

1839–1914

Davis came to Johnson City to gin cotton after the Civil War. They didn't like him up in Shiloh, N.J., because he hired a substitute to fight for him in the Union army. The substitute was killed. They liked him fine in Johnson City.

CHAPTER ELEVEN

Grandpa Holmes and his wife Charlotte are hosts of the Cypress Inn at Comfort. Charlotte cooks and Grandpa waits on customers. Charlotte's meals are tasty, but what really attracts customers like Capt. Eddie Rickenbacker and Lynda Bird Johnson is Grandpa's art work, which he displays on the walls of the cafe.

Grandpa Holmes calls himself the "Grandpa Moses of Texas," but he is much more modern than this indicates. He works mostly in the collage medium, in which the artist stands back and pastes anything he can get his hands on to the canvas. Grandpa's "Springtime in the Rockies" is a good example, perhaps his best. He painted a background of mountains on the canvas, then hung little wire springs from a bunk bed all over it. He sold the work for fifty—cents. It is the only painting he has sold. He's certainly not commercial.

"Abstract art," says Grandpa, "is a product of the untalented sold by the unprincipled to the utterly bewildered."

Avant-garde as he is as a painter, Grandpa Holmes is rather old-fashioned in his appreciation of poets. He has a picture gallery of poets he admires hanging on the wall. They all have bushy beards or long sideburns. Their names are Whittier, Emerson, Longfellow, Lowell, Holmes (no kin to Grandpa), and Bryant. Under their pictures Grandpa has written a bitter legend: "Poets today's school kids never hear about."

A lover of modern poets suggested that Grandpa was showing his age. It didn't faze him. "Would you believe it if I told you I was eighty-four?" he asked the heckler. "No," the man said with surprise. "Good," retorted Grandpa. "I'm only seventy-nine."

Charlotte says Grandpa is a man of zany impulse. She prays that the customers who come in off the long hot highway are in good humor. One time a couple of Grandpa's friends came in with a stranger—editor of some kind of ranching magazine. They ordered steaks and Grandpa asked the stranger if he wanted gravy. "Sure," the man said, "lots of it." Whereupon

Grandpa stuck his bare hand in the gravy bowl, cupped the goo as best he could, and slopped it all over the man's plate. There was a brief silence. The stranger watched Grandpa wiping the gravy from his fingers. Then he looked up at Grandpa and roared with laughter. Grandpa laughed so much he had to sit down.

Grandpa Holmes has his serious side.

He likes to show Comfort visitors the only Civil War monument in the South erected to the memory of Union sympathizers. The bones of nineteen men lie beneath the marker.

In 1862, sixty-eight men, all German immigrants and all loyal to the Union, gathered at nearby Turtle Creek and began a march toward the Mexican border.

They marched and sang songs about "refugeeing to Mexico," unaware that a Confederate force of 120 men was on their trail. The Rebels attacked them on the banks of the Nueces River in Kinney County, killing and wounding nineteen. The wounded were shot and the dead left unburied. Eight others were killed trying to cross the Rio Grande River.

After the war, a group of men from Comfort traveled to the battle scene on the Nueces, picked up the bones of the dead, and returned them home.

Grandpa Holmes knows so much history of Kendall County you are surprised to learn he has lived here but twelve years. He's a Connecticut Yankee!

"I used to travel for a New England manufacturer," he said, "and the first time I came through the Texas hill country I fell in love with it. The landscape and climate are nice and the people . . . well . . . they're like nobody else in the world. They're not in a hurry. They don't just 'take time' to talk with their neighbors. They *like* to get to know one another. Know what I mean?

"So I brought Charlotte down and bought this place. We're here to stay."

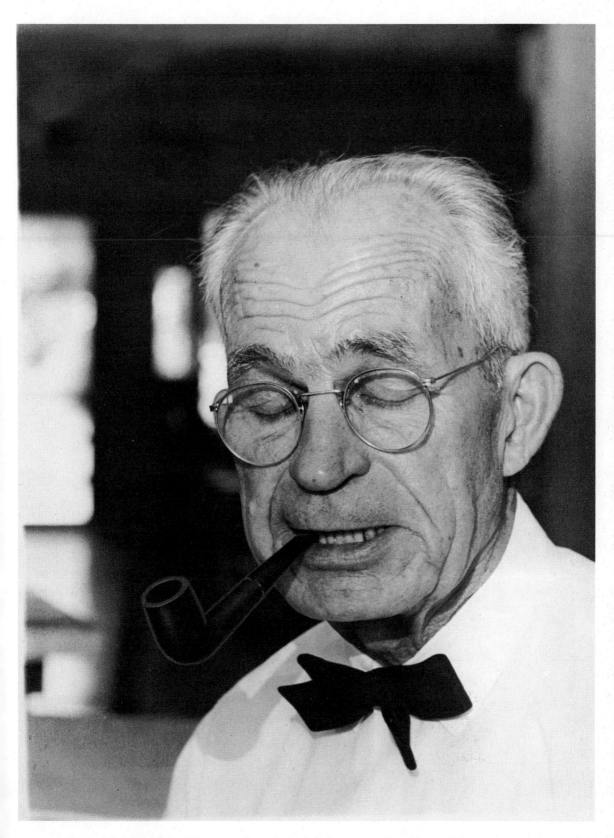

Grandpa Holmes refers to himself as the Grandpa Moses of Texas. He paints.

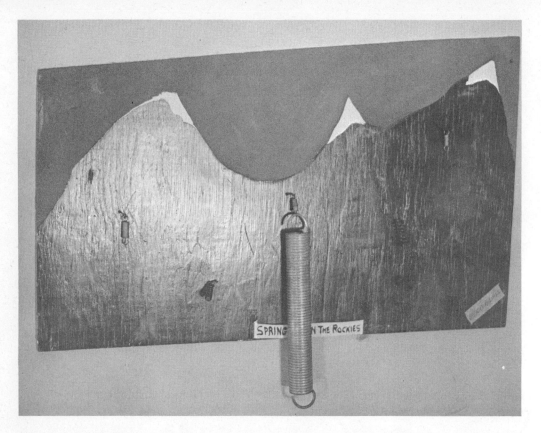

Grandpa Holmes's favorite medium is collage, where you paste what's handy on the canvas.

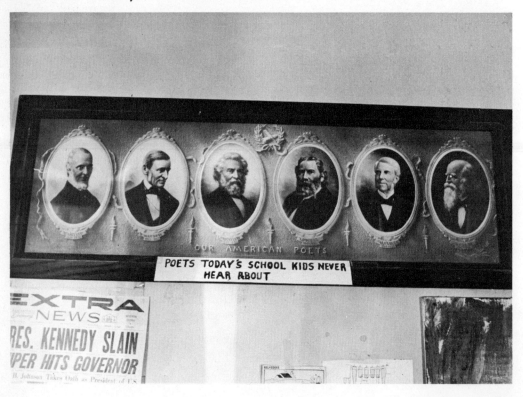

Grandpa Holmes likes modern art but he sticks to old-fashioned poets.

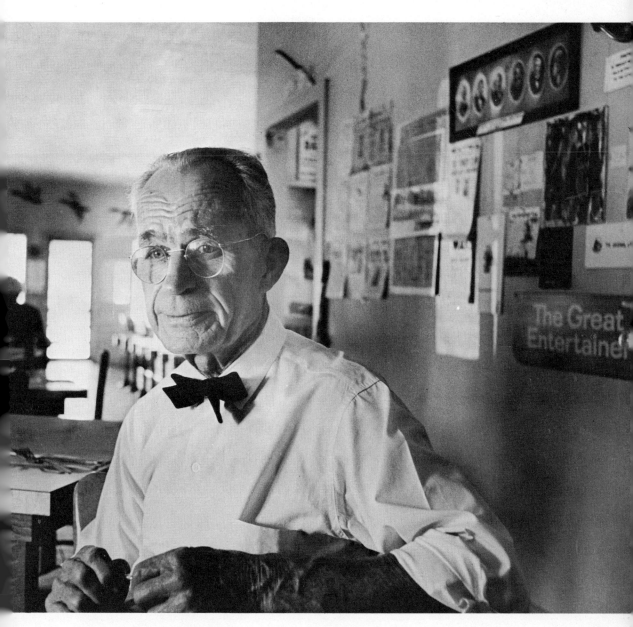

Grandpa at the Cypress Inn in Comfort, which he runs in his spare time.

PETER BERG

1837–1907

Berg came to Fredericksburg, Texas, from Germany
in 1857, worked as a stone mason so he could pay
his fiancée's passage to America. She landed at
Indianola, Texas, married another, and Berg never
saw her again. He withdrew from society, built a
hermitage in a ravine in the woods. He built a stone
tower, in which he studied the stars and made
weather forecasts. He built a pipe organ of brass,
board, and paper and played it particularly well after
several nips of home brew, which he sold for thirty
cents a gallon. He devised a burglar alarm, talked
with the wild animals who drank at his spring, and
shot himself to death at the age of seventy. They
called him the Hermit of the Hills.

CHAPTER TWELVE

Ace Reid was on the telephone talking with Windy Ryon, the Fort Worth saddlemaker. Windy had a problem. Ace and the boys with the Texas Livestock Auction Association had paid him twenty-five thousand dollars to make a fancy saddle, which they were going to give to the President. Would it be all right if he put the presidential seal on the saddle?

"Why shore," Ace said. "Tha'd be real nice. Good idea, Windy."

But was it legal? That was what was bothering Windy.

"Hell, I don't know," Ace said. "You better call Barefoot Sanders. He'd be able to tell you."

Windy said he would call Barefoot. Barefoot is the United States Attorney at Dallas.*

Ace hung up the telephone. "Let's go out on the patio," he said. "I want you to try some good ole home brew beer. Feller over at Comfort makes it. He's the game warden."

Was that legal?

He laughed. "Let's don't ast Barefoot the answer to that one. Naw, it's all right long as you don't sell it. It was give to me. Uumm. Ain't it nice and yeasty?"

A landscaping crew out of Kerrville was sodding Ace's yard. Ace and his family had just moved into the new house. It was low and swank. The studio where Ace draws his cowboy cartoons for a newspaper syndicate was built over a little creek. The place sits back in the hills of his Draggin' S ranch, seven miles north of Kerrville.

"Come on," Ace said. "Let's run over to Chuck Richey's place. Chuck's my model for 'Jake,' the main character in the cartoons. You'll see the resemblance. Chuck's the only man I know who judges people like he sizes up horses. Just wait and see."

Ace pointed out the sights on his ranch as he drove. He said he only had four hundred acres, but that if it was flattened out it would run to four thousand.

* Barefoot has since gone to Washington as assistant deputy attorney general.

Chuck was just like any cowpoke—lean and leathery and bowlegged. He was down in the corral.

"You don't look so good, boy!" Ace said.

"Don't feel so good."

"Whatsamatter?"

"Awww . . . Joe Ramos and his bandito beer joint is gonna make a drunk outa me. Ever'time I get to sleep at night, the music from the jukebox wakes me up. The joint's right down behind the house. So ever'night I have to get up and go down there and tell Joe to turn the dang thang down. Well you know how it is. While you're down there you might as well have a beer. I been gettin' to bed awful late."

Chuck said he and Ace first cowboyed together up in North Texas. "I met Ace on the Triangle Ranch," he said. "We were flankin' calves. Ace was a good hand and we worked together around the country. One day we were breakin' Tennessee Walkers and one kicked ole Ace in the shin. Oh, it hurt. He looked at me and said, 'Richey, there's gotta be a better way to make a livin'.' So he started drawin' pitchers."

Ace said Chuck used the same veterinarian as the President. He was leading up to something.

"I shore do," Chuck said, "and Doc Thomas is a good 'un."

"Is Lyndon Johnson gonna be a good 'un?" Ace asked.

"Huh?"

"Is LBJ gonna be a good prezedent?"

"You durn right he is," Chuck said, "the best tha New Nited States ever had. He's got beeeeg long ears, like a gooooood horse. Ever'thang's beeeeg about his face. A feller with leeeetle bitty eyes and short ears don't thank, and Mr. Johnson is jeeeest the opposite."

Chuck said he had an eighteen-day career in the Navy.

"They let me out because I was crazy," he said. "I told them I didn't know anythang about waters. I guess I was batty. I got that way tryin' to roll up my clothes into a leeeetle bag no bigger'n Armita Matilda's stockin's."

"Armita Matilda was his wife," Ace explained.

"Oh, she was a looker," Chuck said. "Yeller hair and greeeen eyes. But she was so wild I had to chain and feed her after

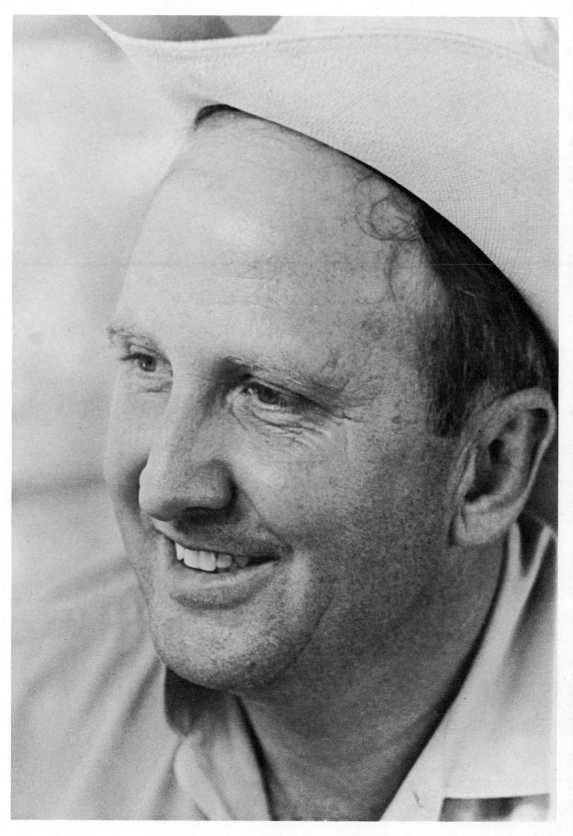

Ace Reid is a cartoonist when not working out at his Draggin' S Ranch near Kerrville.

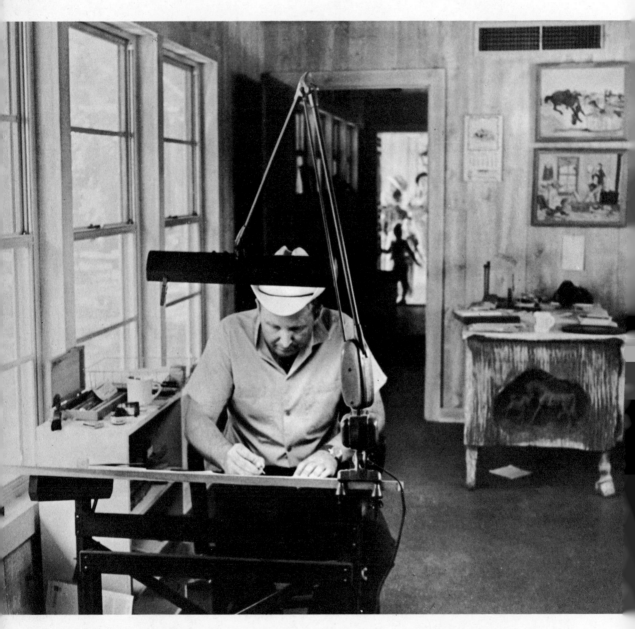

Here's Ace, inventing adventures for "Jake," his cowpuncher cartoon character, now syndicated.

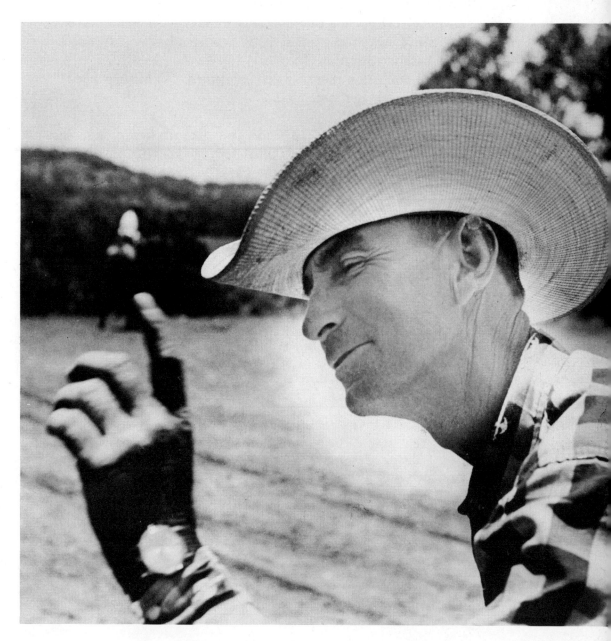

Chuck Richey, a local cowboy, was the inspiration for Ace Reid's "Jake."

dark. She started steppin' out on me when I went off weekends to the rodeos. So I took to lockin' her in the cellar. One weekend I went to the Vernon rodeo and left her in the ground. It come up a haaaard rain, and by the time I got back the cellar was flooded. I opened the door. All I could see was the leeeetle pink tip of her nose. You see, she was standin' on her tiptoes just'a barely a-breathin'."

"Well don't stop there," Ace complained. "What happened?"

"Oh, I drug her out!"

"Whad she say?"

"She said, 'This is the end, you lizzard head,' and she jumped in her roadster and killed ten chickens before she hit the main highway. Never came back."

CAPT. JOSEPH A. TIVY

1818–1892

Captain Tivy, of the white beard and bushy brows, came from Canada to Kerrville in 1870 with two sisters. Tivy promised his sisters he would never marry, spent most of his time surveying Kerr County with Bigfoot Wallace. One day Tivy up and married the Widow Losey. His sisters, hurt to the bone, went back to Canada. Shortly after their marriage, Mrs. Tivy came down with a fatal illness. She asked to be buried on Tivy Mountain, a rock fortress that overlooked the town. They had to build a road up the mountain side and use dynamite to dig a vault in the rock. The blasting could be heard for miles. The casket was drawn up in a hack pulled by mules. The sisters in Canada heard the good news and one of them returned to live out her days with Captain Tivy. Today, the captain, his sister, and his wife lie side by side on the mountaintop. Once a year, members of the Tivy High School senior class make a pilgrimage to the graves.

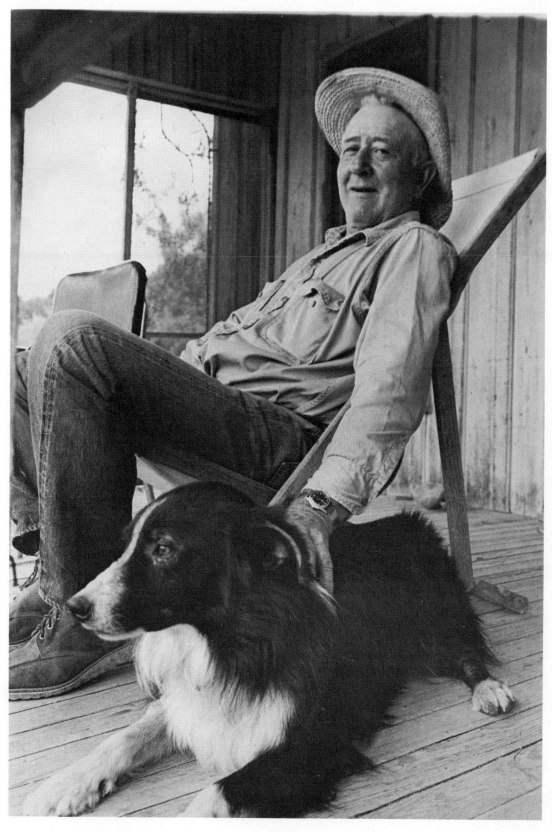

Charlie Bishop relaxes on the front gallery of his Bois d'Arc ranch with his dog.

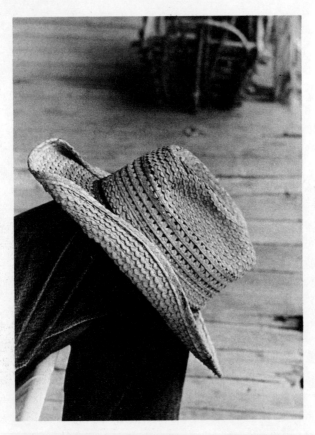

Charlie took off his hat and put it on his knee when he told about the cockfight.

CHAPTER THIRTEEN

Five weeks had passed since Texas Rangers had raided the biggest chicken fight in Kimble County history, and Charlie Bishop down at Bois d'Arc was still talking about it. There were things about it that tickled him, and there were things about it that made him mad.

What tickled him the most was that Providence had kept him away from the fight and therefore out of jail. He was on the promoter's secret mailing list, and an invite had been sent out in his name. But it didn't get to him. It had been mailed by mistake to a Charlie Bishop out near Abilene. The Abilene Charlie had been kicked out of the local cockfights the year before, and it looked like that when he got word of the new tournament the sorehead spilled the beans. This is the thing that made Bois d'Arc Charlie mad. He didn't like poor sports. "I'd been in favor of whuppin' him if it wasn't so far to Abilene," he said.

In a way, Charlie almost wished he had known about it in time to go, because from the way the boys talked it had been something to see.

The Junction boys had won three fights and it looked like they were going to win the pot when the law arrived. The Rangers found thirty dead roosters around the pit and about two hundred spectators. The local boys left their women and children behind and blazed a hundred trails through the cedar brakes. The pit was on Hal Holland's ranch, and they said one of the promoters ran all the way to Arnold Grosenbacher's place—a good five miles away—with a chicken under his arm. Another old boy, carrying a cock under each arm, stepped off eight miles before he discovered that the car at his heels wasn't the law, but just another scared chicken fighter.

The Rangers graciously allowed the women and children to go home, but they chained the abandoned cars to trees. It was a smart move. A lot of the men who tore off through the cedar brakes had second thoughts and came back for their cars. As one of them said, "There was nothing to do but go back and give myself up. My car was worth more than the fine."

Justice of the Peace John Ball said he collected more than a thousand dollars in fines, mostly from fellows from out of the county. They came from as far away as Austin and Abilene. Charlie said they got caught because they didn't know where to run. Hal Holland said he had leased the place where the fights were held to another man and didn't know anything about any cockfights.

Charlie missed all the fun all right, but he came out ahead. He and Steve and Tadpole and Bill played dominoes all that day and into the next morning and Charlie won a hundred dollars.

JIM STOUT

1848–1884

Stout, a handsome gambler, wandered into Junction one day in 1884 and got a job tending bar in a saloon. He whipped the best poker players the town could throw at him and proved to be quite handy with his fists. The town's toughs took him on and regretted it. One wintry night, saloon keepers Tom Carson and Andy Royal lured Stout into a poker session, hoping to double up on him. Stout won anyway and Carson shot him in the back as he was leaving. Stout staggered outside and fell into the arms of N. C. Patterson. Patterson said Stout's dying words were, "I went to the saloon tonight on their invitation to have a little game. I thought Tom Carson was the best friend I had. Boys, don't ever put too much confidence in a man, not even a friend." The jury acquitted Carson and Royal. Carson was shot to death by Bill Holman in 1893 while drinking in Weston's Saloon. Holman was shot to death not long afterwards on the streets of Del Rio by Judge James Cornell. Cornell was acquitted. Andy Royal moved to Fort Stockton, was elected sheriff, and was assassinated in 1894 by an unknown gunman.

CHAPTER FOURTEEN

There was a look of sadness in Charlie Bishop's face the other day as he watched a bunch of ranch kids board the school bus to Junction. Thelma asked her husband what was the matter. "There's not a bowlegged boy anywhere on that bus," Charlie said. It was a profound observation.

Cow ponies with men on their backs are getting to be a rare sight in the Texas hill country. Many ranchers nowadays don't even own a horse. The pickup truck and the border collie have just about replaced Old Paint at roundup time. Of course there are exceptions. But most ranchers are seldom in the saddle any more. Charlie's right. Their kids' legs grow straight as sticks.

The last great horsemen in the Texas hill country was Creed Taylor. Creed lived eighty-six years, and in all his adult life he never once rode on wheels. He hated walking, but he would have hot-footed it to hell and back before taking a wagon to heaven.

Ironically, Creed went to his grave in the thing he most hated. It was an oversight on the part of his family and a sight that his old horsemen friends thought they would never see. When the wagon passed bearing Creed to the cemetery, they shook their heads in disbelief. It all seemed like an evil omen. Only a couple of years before Creed kicked the bucket, a mechanic up in Michigan by the name of Henry Ford had driven a horseless carriage at 91.4 miles an hour.

Creed came to Texas from Tennessee in 1824. He came in an ox-drawn cart, but he couldn't help that. He was only four years old. He went to school in Gonzales and boarded at the home of Almon Dickson, who later was killed in the Alamo with Davy Crockett and company.

Creed grew into as tough a man as you were likely to meet in those days. He was a husky five feet nine inches tall, round-shouldered and bowlegged. He wore a bushy, silver-blue beard, liked his coffee "so strong it will float an iron wedge," and sucked cigarettes rolled in old newspaper. He rolled them thick and long as cigars and smoked them so short that his whiskers

87

often caught on fire. You could always tell where Creed had camped by the butts he left on the ground.

He fought in the Texas army during the war for independence and became one of Ranger Capt. Jack Hays's best Indian scouts.

In 1869, Creed moved to Kimble County and hired stonemasons to build him a huge, two-story ranch house on Devil's Creek near Noxville. It was the largest house in the county and was said to be the finest west of San Antonio. Creed never took ranching seriously, but he could afford to live in style on horse race winnings and his Mexican War pension.

Creed was a shrewd judge of men as well as horses.

One time down in Wilson County, Creed watched with amusement as his horse outran another by three lengths. The owner of the other horse was amazed. The night before, he had slipped into Creed's corral and tested Creed's racer on a trial run. Creed's horse had been slow, so he had put all his money on his nag. He figured his jockey was to blame and threatened to kill him. Creed intervened.

"No you don't," he said. "Don't blame the jockey. I knew your tricks. The reason my horse wouldn't run so fast last night was because I had him fixed so he couldn't. I saw it all from a cedar brake. I unfixed him for the race today."

Creed's best money winner was a horse named Monkey Jack. Monkey Jack was a fantail racer that seldom lost when the wind was right. One day Creed rode over to John Joy's place to challenge Joy's bay filly. "John," he said, "Monkey Jack's a-gettin' a little old, but he can still run rings around that bay filly of yours."

Joy spat a missile of tobacco into the flinty hillside. He would take all the personal abuse a man could dish out, but when somebody talked his horses down he got real red around the ears. "Now, Creed," he said, trying to hold his temper, "you think you got about the fastest thing in the country, but I'm thinkin' 'bout runnin' you anyhow."

It was one of Johnson Fork's most famous races. The betting was heavy. Joy was not a rich man and he and Mrs. Joy had to throw in their feather beds to match the confidence Creed showed on his horse.

The bay filly left Monkey Jack two lengths behind and

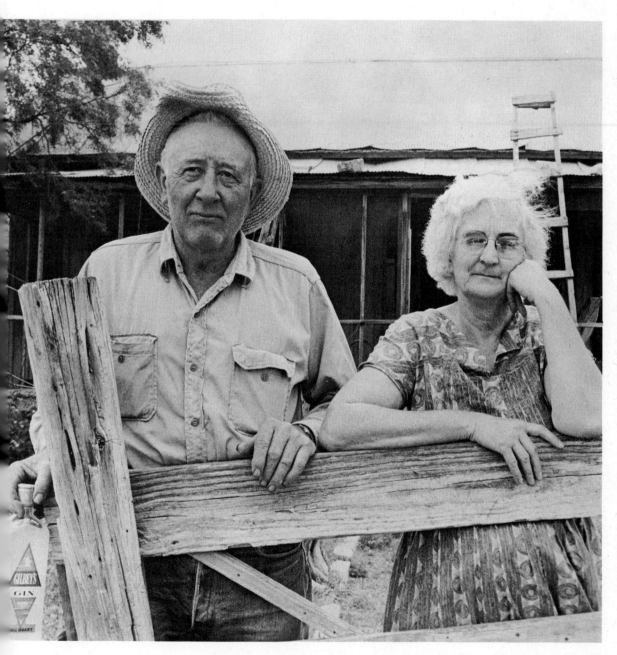

Charlie and Thelma Bishop standing at the front gate in Bois d'Arc.

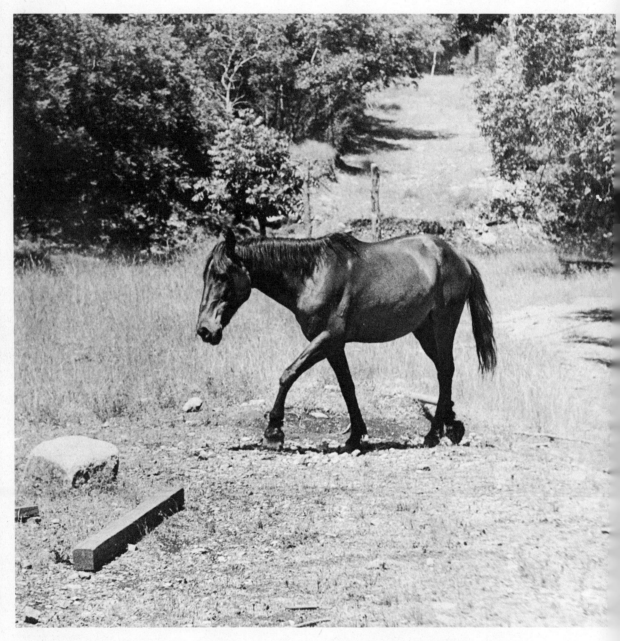

Charlie says everything's changed: "Horses don't get rode by men much any more."

Opposite page
Charlie says the saddle is on the fence more than it's on the horse these days.

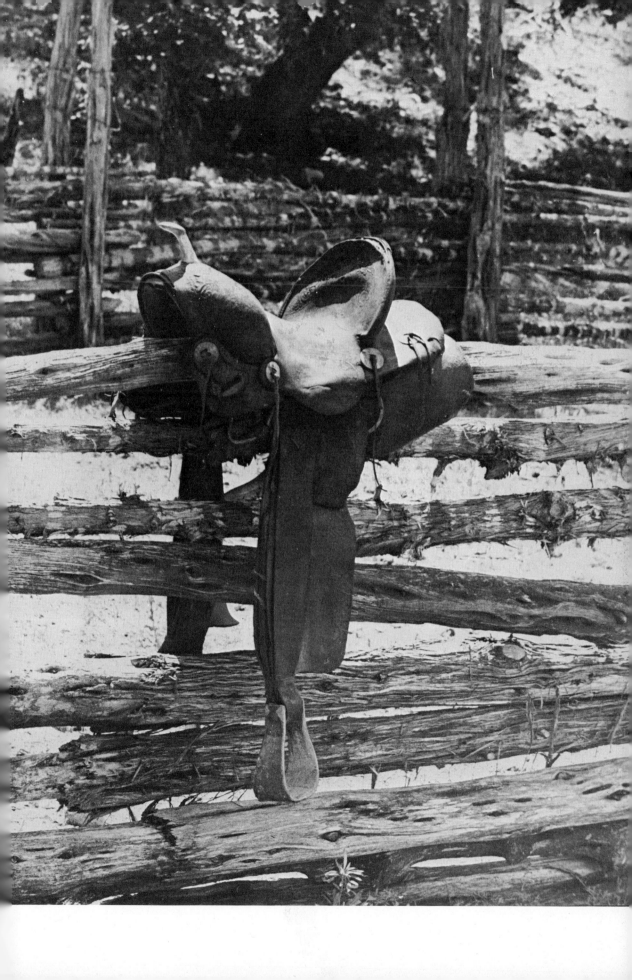

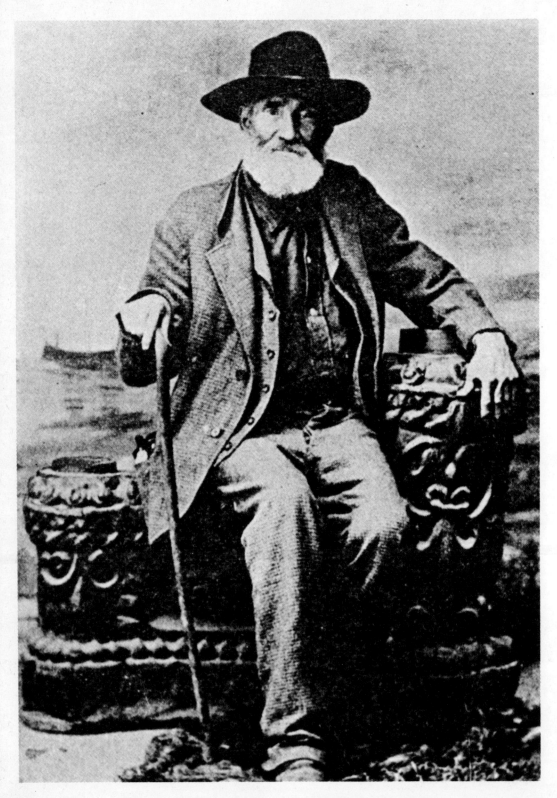

Charlie says Creed Taylor, the greatest horseman in the history of the hill country, wouldn't know the place.

Creed was so mad he almost took a wagon home rather than ride a loser.

One time in 1874, Creed took a lot of ribbing from his neighbors. They accused him of being awfully free with his hospitality. One night Creed had given room and board to a couple of horsemen on their way to Oklahoma. He found out a few days later that his guests were Frank and Jesse James, in flight from a posse after robbing the San Antonio–Austin stage.

One night in 1898, Creed was called to the house of his neighbor, Jess Whitson. The messenger said Whitson was dying and wanted to talk to Creed. Creed wondered why. He and Whitson had been feuding for years, but he wasn't about to fight a man on his deathbed.

"What is it, Jess?" Creed asked suspiciously at the bedside.

"Now, Creed," Jess said, "all I've ever said about you or done to you, I want you to forgive me for if I die. . . ."

Creed said he would.

"All right," Jess said, seemingly relieved. But then he had a second thought. He looked up at Creed and said, "But if I live, by Gatlins, all those things I said still stand good."

JIM BURROWS

1823–1879

Burrows, a bachelor rancher, lived alone on his place with a Negro cowhand, said to be the only Negro in Kimble County at that time. One morning in 1879, Burrows arose to hear his hired hand say sarcastically, "I'd sho like to kill a b'ar fo' my breakfus' dis mawnin'." Burrows thought the cowhand made "b'ar" sound too much like "Burrows." He reached over and got his shotgun and shot the man to death without blinking an eye. After breakfast, he buried the cowpoke, rode into town to tell the sheriff "just for the record," and was home by supper.

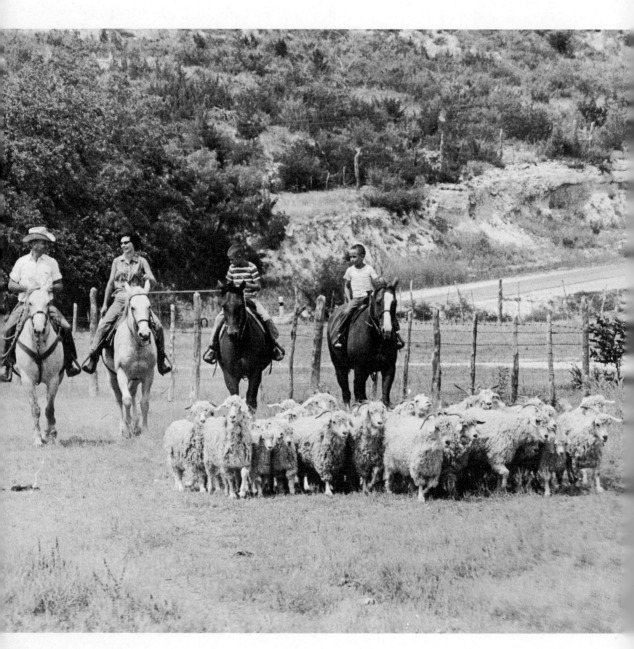

The rising generation, Jack and Rosemary Hoggett and their sons, herding goats on their Kimble County ranch.

CHAPTER FIFTEEN

When Rosemary Patterson of Woodsboro, down in South Texas, married Jack Hoggett of Junction, up in the hill country, Rosemary's friends shook their heads and said it would never work.

All Jack had to offer, they said, was a car, a one-horse trailer, and a rope in his hand.

They had expected Rosemary would marry some bright young banker or businessman who would wrap her in an air-conditioned cocoon and take her off to the big city for a life of wine and roses. She was that beautiful. There was not a single man in all of Refugio County who did not secretly desire her hand. Few had courage to ask.

Jack Hoggett wasn't bashful. When the laconic calf roper from the hills saw Rosemary on the campus at Southwest Texas State College, in San Marcos, he cocked his Stetson over one eye, looped his thumbs over his eighty-eight-pound belt buckle, and went a-courtin'.

After the preacher married them, he plopped her in his car, hitched a horse trailer on behind, and rode off after the rodeos.

That was eleven years ago.

An early, though distant, admirer of Rosemary ran into her husband the other day in a Junction cafe. Jack looked like the same cowpoke of a decade ago, maybe a little heavier with a little less hair under his hat. "Come on out to the ranch tomorrow," he said, "and meet Rosemary and the kids."

When Jack walked out, a rancher asked, "Old friends?"

"Kinda."

"Jack Boy's a goin' Jesse."

"Still a good roper?"

"Good rancher. He's walkin' proof that a young fella just startin' out can make a go of it if he's got a lot of savvy and gets a little help."

"Who helps him?"

"Pierce, his daddy, one of the top ranchers in the country, and other kinfolks. The Hoggetts are in real solid around here."

But how was Rosemary?

The ranch house sat backed up to the South Llano River, seven miles south of Junction. Rosemary came out of the house grinning, her two sons romping ahead. Carleton was ten and Jerry was eight. You could see a little of Jack in them.

Rosemary was more beautiful than ever. She was a woman now, not a girl, and the years had put a strength and character into her face that once was not there.

She wore paint-splattered riding pants. Jack said they had just moved onto the place and Rosemary had been doing two jobs at once—painting the interior walls and making two dozen peach cobbler pies for storing in the freezer. Her parents from Woodsboro and her older sister, Betty, a teacher at Victoria Junior College, were house guests.

Jack sent his sons out behind the house to clean a string of perch they had caught that morning in the Llano. Rosemary fixed dinner while Jack settled into a rocker in the living room.

Their house wasn't new, but it was bigger and better than the one down the road they had been living in. Jack had put in wall-to-wall carpeting and air conditioning.

Jack said he was ranching on about 4000 acres, but that he owned only 274.

"I lease about 2800 acres from my daddy," he said. "The boundary of the 2800 starts a mile east of the house here. Then I lease another 1000 acres, which starts a mile west of the house, from my uncle, C. C. Wright.

"The only way a young man in this country can get ranch land—even to lease it—is from family. The other fella will sell, but at such a high price you can't make enough off the land to afford interest payments on the note. In 1960, I bought a 252-acre tract from my uncle, Jack Turner, for $85 an acre. I should have paid $100 an acre. But that's a family deal. It's the only way somebody starting out can survive. The land I lease costs me about $6600 a year, and that's cheap because it's in the family."

He estimated he had an investment of about $110,000 in ranching. "The secret," he said with a grin, "is to have a good banker."

How did he make the bank notes?

"I buy anything that walks that will make money," he laughed. "You have to be a hustler and a Jack-of-all-trades."

It's true.

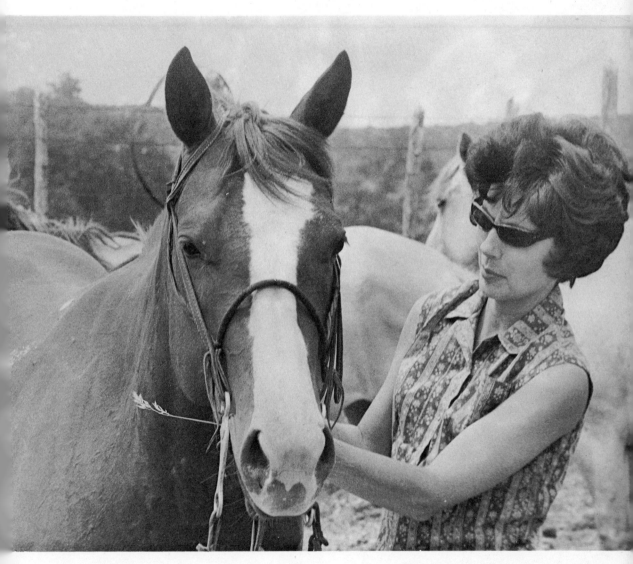

Rosemary Hoggett, a modern ranch wife, with her favorite horse.

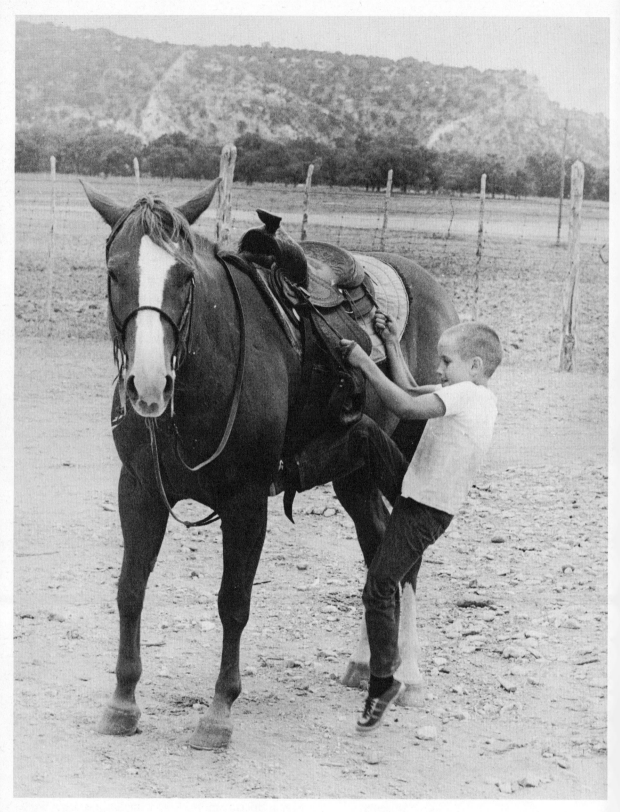

In the hill country, boys and horses go together. Jerry Hoggett saddles up.

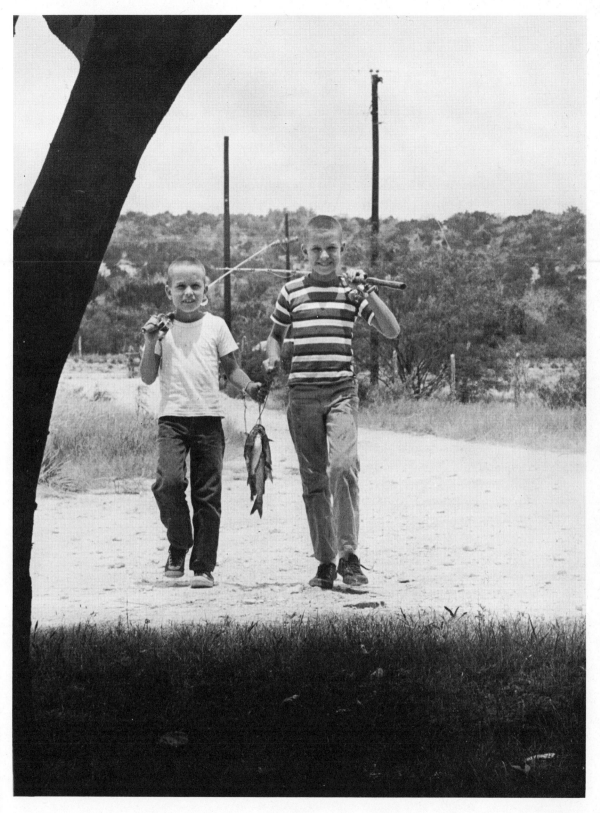

Jerry and Carleton Hoggett come home with their catch of perch from the South Llano River.

Jack runs twelve hundred goats, which he shears twice a year. They graze on grass which looks skimpy, but it must be mineral-rich because he said he doesn't feed his goats a bite all winter. He runs about five hundred sheep and shears them twice a year. He has about a hundred head of range cattle.

Jack employs two full-time hands who do nothing but farm year round. They keep about 200 acres in cultivation, raise oats in the fall and Sudan in the summer. The grain he doesn't sell is fed to the cattle, sheep, and his prize stud goats.

The stock Jack runs on the range doesn't require a lot of looking after, so he and Rosemary tend the ranching chores themselves. They keep one Jersey milk cow, one pet hen, and no hogs. Rosemary has a vegetable garden.

He said there are other ways to make or stretch a dollar if you are enterprising.

The trees on his property along the South Llano bear about a hundred thousand pounds of pecans a year and Jack sells the nuts. He leases a lot of his land to year-round hunters. Rosemary's deep freeze is full of venison.

Jack trades horses for profit, and they keep about a dozen for riding and fall roundups. Rosemary, who hadn't been on a horse before she met Jack, has five of her own. "I wouldn't take five hundred dollars for our sorriest riding horse," he said. "They are a pleasure to have around."

During the fall, Jack gets up at 5 A.M. and milks the Jersey. Then—here comes the kicker—he drives to Junction Junior High School, where he is a full-time mathematics teacher and football coach.

"It interferes with ranching," he admitted. "But the salary makes it worth it. We live on what I make teaching and put what we make ranching into savings and on debts. The ranching profit is never constant. One year I might make two thousand dollars and the next year twenty thousand.

"My daddy will retire in a couple of years. By then, we hope to be in a position to take over his ranches. Then I can quit teaching and become a real rancher."

Rosemary called everyone to dinner. Jerry, after some prodding by his daddy, said grace. Rosemary, who couldn't cook when she met Jack, had laid out quite a banquet—baked ham, garden-fresh green beans, squash and tomatoes, homemade bread, and peach cobbler pie!

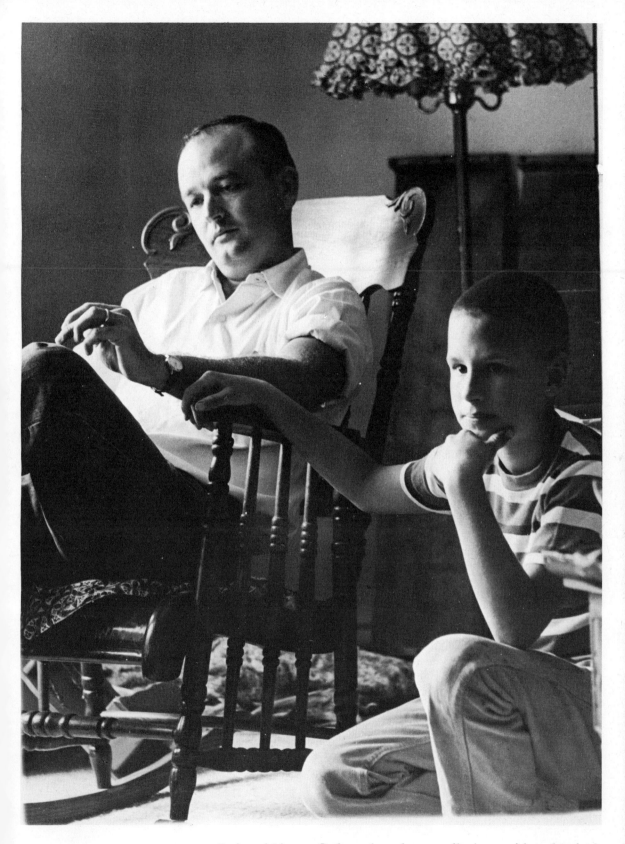

Jack and his son Carleton have lots to talk about with each other.

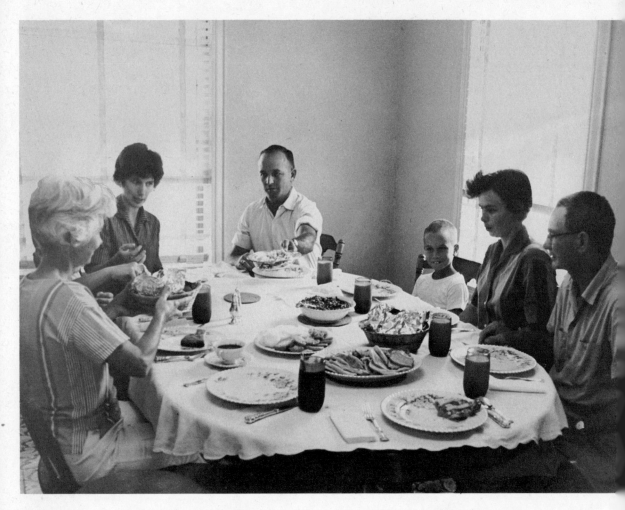

Dinner is family style at the Hoggetts' and includes Rosemary's mother, father, and sister.

They talked and laughed and ate. Rosemary, who is a Cub Scout den mother, said she was taking the pack swimming the next day. Carleton had to play baseball in town. Jack said the mares were about ready for breeding. Rosemary's electric churn was broken. Could Jack take a look at it? Jack thought he might rope a little in the Kerrville rodeo. Maybe they could all go down. That suited the boys just fine.

HEINRICH GROBE

1805–1862

Indians shot eleven arrows into his chest as he worked on a rock fence in the Crabapple community of Gillespie County. His wife, Caroline, wrapped his body in linen and carted him to Fredericksburg for burial. She raised his eight children to maturity.

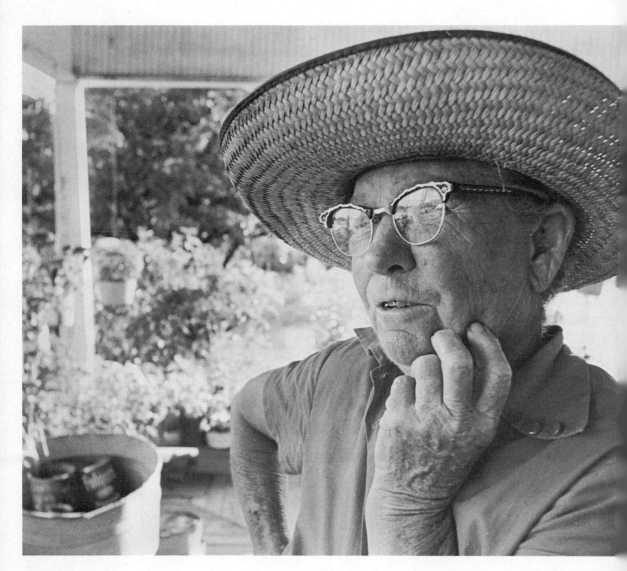

The Widow Schubert built herself a new house but she still prefers to live in her old one.

CHAPTER SIXTEEN

When Widow Schubert's new house began to take shape north-west of Canyon City, in Comal County, the folks in town drove out and looked it over and decided what they had long suspected was surely true. The widow, who every evening came to town to pick up free slop from the cafes for her chickens, certainly had more money than she pretended. The new house was a dream compared to her old house. It was low and modern and had an all-electric kitchen, wall-to-wall carpets, and central air conditioning.

One day a moving van from San Antonio pulled up in front of the new house and the driver and his helper unloaded some of the finest furniture ever seen in Comal County. When the last chair was in place, Widow Schubert took a look around her palace, locked all the doors, and went back to her old house.

That was two years ago, and Widow Schubert still hasn't moved into the new place. It is worrying the dickens out of the folks in Canyon City.

"I can tell you how to get to her place," the man at the real estate office said, "but I don't know if she'll talk. She just might run you off."

Widow Schubert was out in the yard of her old house, chopping weeds in the flower bed that ran around the porch. Two dogs came growling from the shade of a lean-to. The widow yelled at them and they slunk back to their burrows in the sand. She drew back her hoe, took one last chop at a weed, pushed back her straw hat, and said, "Come on inside vhere it is cool. I vas about to quit anyhow."

She served big tins of ice water and talked for an hour. She seemed glad to have someone around.

Pauline Pape Schubert was born sixty-eight years ago, come February, on a farm just six miles from her present place. When she was seventeen, she met Hugo Schubert at a dance at her aunt's house. "Vit my aunt, Hugo vas neighbors," she explained. Hugo was a good dancer. He said he liked Pauline's red hair. Her head was not easily turned. Pauline was not the sentimental sort. She took a hard look at Hugo. He was too skinny to be handsome and he didn't have money. Life with a sharecropper would be hard. But this didn't scare her. She could already pick five hundred pounds of cotton a day. Hugo was honest, hard-working, and, after sundown, a pleasant beau. He owned a hundred-and-ten-dollar mare and an eighty-five-dollar rubber tire buggy, which he parked at Pauline's gate at least two nights a week. Pauline's girl friends were envious. "A vonderful time ve had," she recalled. It took her two years to make up her mind to marry him.

The wedding was at her mama and papa's house. About sixty-five neighbors and kinfolks came to eat and dance and sing. Pauline spent the next day cleaning her mama's house. Then she and Hugo went off to his place, a rented house on a rented farm. "Our first night alone, already, I milk fife cows." The cows were her dowry from Papa.

They raised cotton. Every fourth bale went to the landowner. That first year, they made eight bales. Someday, Hugo promised her, they would have their own house, their own land. Goot, she said, and watched their pennies. She was a good manager.

They moved onto Hugo Halm's place, still renting. Viola was born in 1916. Boy came three years later. When Viola started to Sorrel Creek School, Hugo bought her a donkey for $10 and a Sears, Roebuck saddle for $27.50. When Boy was school age, Pauline managed to get him a donkey and a saddle from a Mexican for $2.50. His $1.25 donkey could trot faster than Viola's $10 donkey.

Hugo wanted to farm in the valley, so they rented Carl Pantermuehe's place. One day Hugo went to New Braunfels with a ten-gallon can of cream to sell. He passed a boy on the road and the boy said, "Mister, will you take me with you? I don't have any folks." Hugo brought him home.

"Ve raised him like a son und paid him fifty cents a day to vork," Pauline recalled. "His name vas Roland Haas, und he died of the cancer six years ago und left a vife und fife kids. He vas a goot boy."

In 1933, Pauline and Hugo had saved enough money to buy her papa's 478-acre farm. They paid four thousand dollars cash and moved into the old home. The house had been built in

1906, but it was sturdy and full of memories for Pauline. At last, she had a home of her own. That same year, Hugo learned he had cancer. "Schnooks," he said to her, "vat for shall I vork when I gonna die pretty soon anyhow?"

He lived for fourteen years, time enough to see Viola and Boy marry. After the funeral, Viola and Boy went back to their families and Pauline went back to the farm. The house was full of ghosts, but they were comforting ones. She knew every nook and cranny and scent and creak of every board. She liked the way the porch ran around the house and the familiar faces in the patterns of the wallpaper. In every piece of furniture was a story, a memory of Hugo, the children, her mama and papa.

But Pauline did not let herself sit and dream of the past. She was never the sentimental sort. The medical bills for Hugo's long illness had left her without money in the bank. And the farm could not run itself.

She started over again, raising sheep and goats and cattle, growing her own vegetables, selling milk and butter and eggs. She was still a good manager. She replaced the coal oil lamps with butane and then electricity. It was a sign of prosperity.

One leads gently into talking about the new house, which sits a few hundred yards away.

The impulse that built it is easy to understand. A woman who has toiled away her life around old farmhouses is not foolish simply because she decides she wants a fine new house to die in. She put into it all the fine things she had never had.

It was not a change of mind, but a change of heart, that keeps her in the old, familiar house. She does not say it. Her explanation is hard and logical.

"All day I vork in da sun und sveat. Den I valk inta dat house und goose bumps I get and maybe pneumonia. It's dat air conditioning. Da old house here is airy und I can run around vit no clothes on to keep cool. Vat do I care? Just me und da dogs are here."

And the ghosts.

But she was never the sentimental sort.

WILLIAM D. (SECO) SMITH

1836–1926

Seco, an Indian-fighting cowpoke who used to swap
yarns with Bigfoot Wallace, was asked by historian
J. Marvin Hunter how he got his name. Seco wrote:
"In 1860, I located on the Seco, about 40 miles from
the town of Bandera, and that is how people came
to call me 'Seco' Smith. There were three different
Smiths in that region. W. L. Smith lived on the
Frio; he was known as 'Frio' Smith. Rube Smith
lived on the Hondo; he was called 'Hondo' Smith.
I lived on the Seco, and ever since I went there
people have called me 'Seco.' These are all Spanish
names. In that language, 'frio' means cold, 'hondo'
means deep, and 'seco' means dry. I don't know
which is most distressing, to be cold, deep or dry."

Opposite page
When she runs out of flowerpots, Pauline Schubert uses old purses for
her front-porch plants.

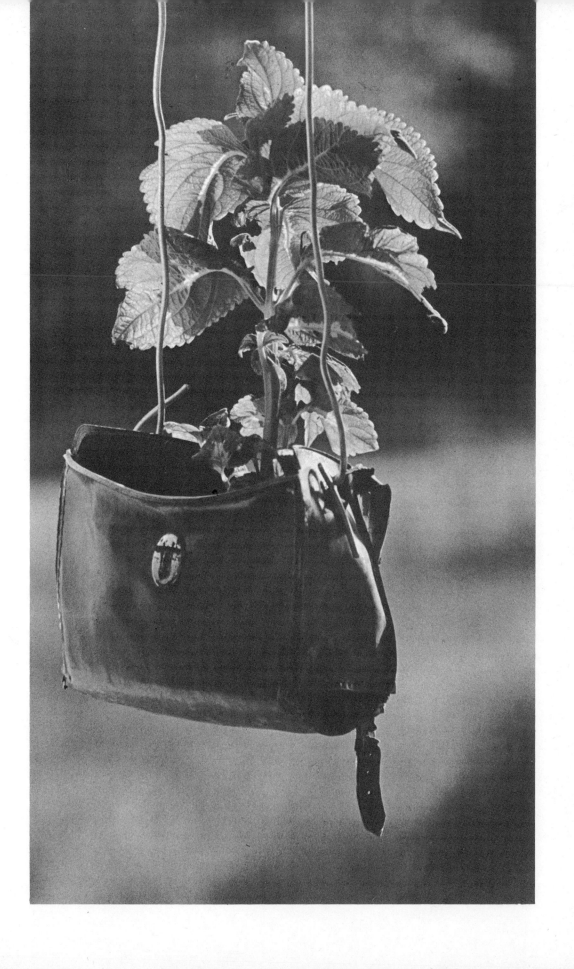

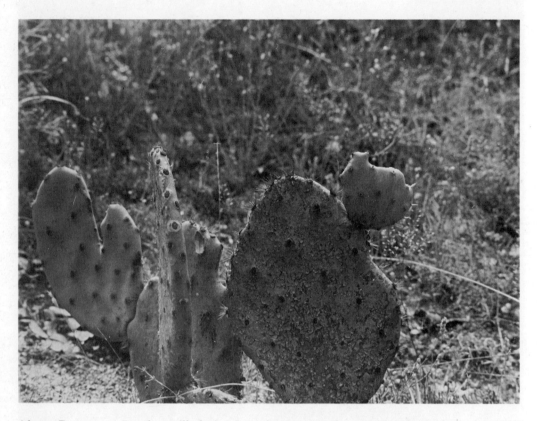

Along Purgatory Road you'll find a luxuriant crop of cactus and prickly pear.

CHAPTER SEVENTEEN

Elmo Jonas stood in his wilting corn patch and watched two Mexican men, strangers in the country, plod past like zombies in the direction of Devil's Backbone.

It was a noonday sun fit for mad dogs and Englishmen. The tar on Purgatory Road ran like lava, scalding grasshoppers. A buzzard, too greedy feeding on a rabbit to get out of the way of a car, lay crumpled on the pavement beside his victim. Ants swarmed out of his eye sockets, and above him his brothers patiently circled.

Somewhere along the roadside, beneath a brown bed of buffalo grass, lay the bones of a baby girl, buried on a searing summer day sixty years before. Vera Gertrude Tausch was nine months and five days old. Did she ever feel on her face the wetness of rain? No, not in this drouthy land, where lizards fry on flintstones and even plastic funeral flowers fade in the malevolent sun.

"Hell could not be hotter," Susie Danforth complained. She stood in an outdoor telephone booth in the little settlement of Wimberley, coaxing coins from the cashbox. Susie is eighty-eight and still collecting for the telephone company. A car loaded with kids clad in bathing suits sped past. "They're going to Jacob's Well to cool off," Susie said wistfully. "If I wasn't so old and dutiful I'd join them."

The road wiggled west like a feverish snake, up rock-ribbed hills and down into canyons choked with cedar and cactus. The creek beds were bone-dry and cows cried for water.

A horseman rested his gelding in the shade of a tree on the road to Johnson City. He wore a sign on his back which read "Nashville or Bust." He said his name was Shel Price and that he was headed for Tennessee and fame and fortune on the Grand Ole Opry.

"I left San Antone three days ago," he said. "I got 56 days and 993 miles to go."

Where was his guitar?

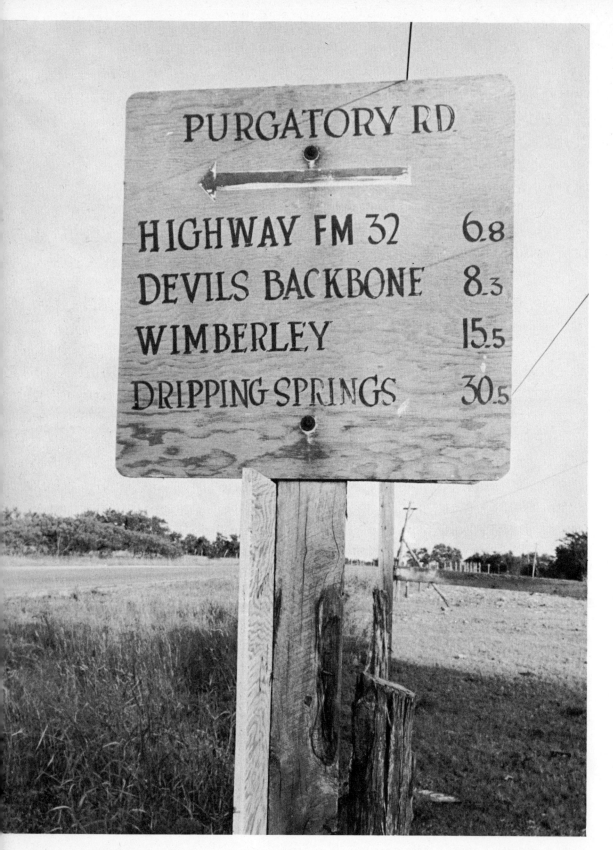

Hill country road signs have a meaning all their own. Here's a highway junction.

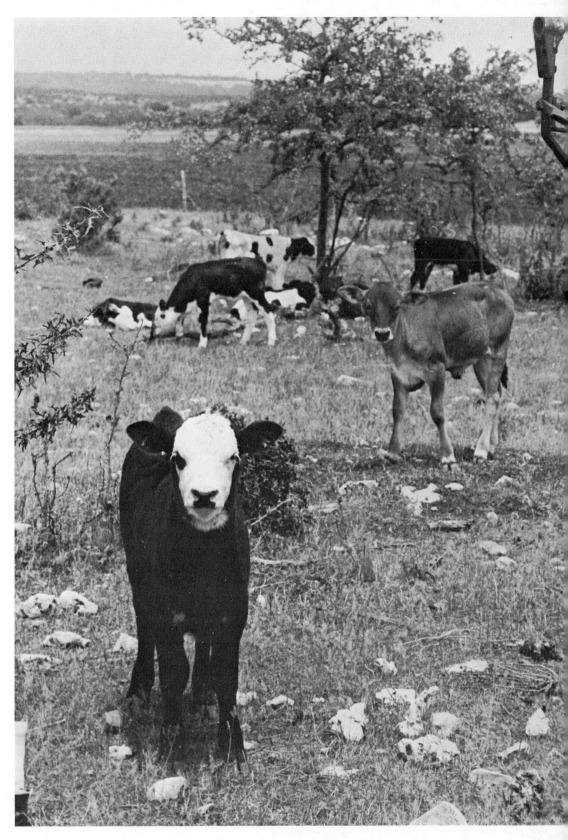

There's no prettier landscape in Texas than a pasture full of baby calves.

"My wife's got it in the car. She's up ahead about ten miles a-waitin' on me and Black Jack. We'll catch her by evenin' and bed down for the night."

She was up ahead all right, sitting in a 1956 Dodge reading a Western novel. This horseback ride to Nashville was a do-or-die deal for her and Shel. He'd been playing the guitar since he was eleven and had never made it big. If this stunt wouldn't get his new recording some attention, nothing would.

The Pedernales ran low. Up on Boggy Mountain, Helmuth Fuchs stomped his boot heel into the ground. "Looky here," he said. "It's so dry it's crackin' and hard as petrified wood. A man could wear out his knees prayin' for rain."

RUBE BOYCE

1854–1934

Two weeks after his marriage in 1877, Boyce shot and killed his wife's brother in a quarrel over cattle. Boyce was acquitted. Two years later, he and three other Kimble County renegades were arrested and charged with the Peg-Leg stage line holdups. They broke out of jail in Austin and fled to Mexico. They were later acquitted. One time Lou Walton asked Boyce why he never learned to read or write. "It takes all my time to dodge bullets," Boyce replied.

CHAPTER EIGHTEEN

Cedar hackers are a strange, clannish people. I get along with them as an employer, but I don't understand them. Never have.

A man from Fort Worth once asked me, "Are cedar cutters happy people?" and I told him, "I don't know. Their idea of happiness is a heck of a lot different from our idea of it. Happiness to them might mean spending their last five bucks on soda pop and wine and marble machines. I've seen 'em work like fiends all day in the hot cedar brakes, then goof off all the money they've made before they get home for supper."

I don't think they know what they want. I've never seen one satisfied. I know they don't want responsibility. They only work when they feel like it.

Things that bother you and me don't faze them. Being always broke, they've got the poorest equipment of any workin' people I've ever seen. They'll load up one of their old trucks with cedar posts and have four or five flat tires before they get to the cedar yard. We would blow our lid. They take it in stride. Guess they're used to it. I don't know. I don't try to explain them. I just work them.

—AL EHRLICH
last of the big-time Texas cedar growers

"Is that true, Oscar, about your people not knowing what they want?"

Do any migratory people know what they want?

The subtlety of his reply surprises. He squats there beside the house (hunkered down, they call it) scratching the ear of a mangy mongrel with his grotesque left hand. He is twenty-six years old, a cedar cutter, an ex-convict, and a cripple with a sixth-grade education. His right arm is off at the shoulder and his left arm is withered. The hand is frozen forever in a claw-like grip.

When he was nineteen, he got tangled in a hot high-line wire, spent eighteen months in a Dallas charity hospital. His wife left him before he got up, saying she couldn't bear to see him crippled. She took their two daughters. He doesn't talk about it. He lives with his seventy-seven-year-old daddy and two dogs in a tiny clapboard house on the edge of a cedar brake outside Johnson City.

Are you sure you want to talk to me? I've got an unsavory reputation.

He has been refused service at a couple of beer joints since he got out of the state penitentiary last April.

He served seven months on a burglary conviction. He was arrested with two other men after deputies found several cases of beer in his car stolen from a tavern on the highway to Marble Falls.

He claims he was a victim of circumstance; that he was in a drunken stupor in the back seat of the car and knew nothing of the burglary until his arrest. Those who know him are inclined to believe him. He is intelligent, loyal to those he trusts, but a quick-tempered battler (six beer joint brawls) when he thinks he is being pushed around. He has an abiding distrust of deputy sheriffs:

I can smell one a mile away.

Prison records show he was an exceptionally well-behaved inmate, scored high on intelligence tests.

His name is Oscar Carter. There is more good in him than even he admits.

His old daddy, John Oscar, has been dozing on a dirty, bare mattress inside the house. He awakes and comes outside and sits in a chair and crosses his long legs. The dog leaves Oscar and goes over and nuzzles the old man. He pets it and listens to his boy.

I was born in a little old town name of Gugan, between Winters and Abilene. Daddy was pickin' cotton at the time. . . .

"I was as good a renter as Williams County had," the old man said. "But the Depression came and I wound up in town hirin' out at first one thang and then another.

"Then me and my brothers got to playin' music for a livin'. I could play anythang with strangs on it. Not braggin', but we could play all right."

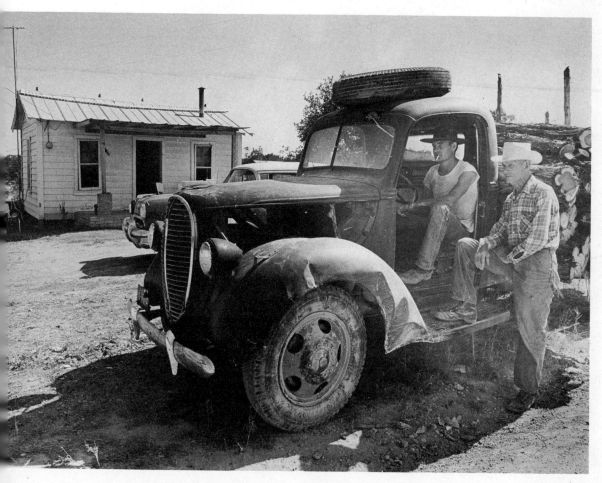

Oscar Carter and his father, John Oscar, are cedar hackers, a clannish breed of men.

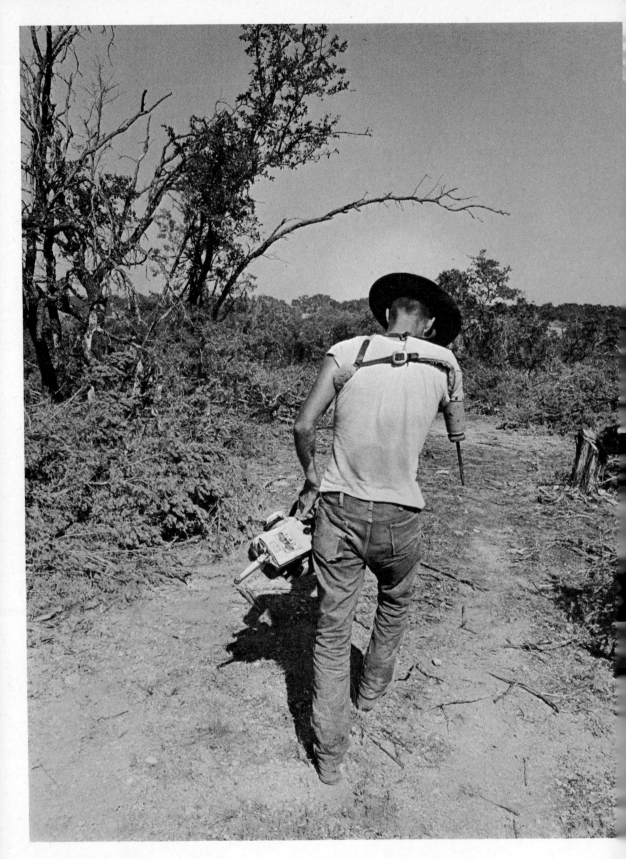

Oscar Carter, with his tools, walking into a cedar brake to begin work.

They sure could. Y'all were known as the Carter Boys, weren't you, Daddy? Didn't y'all play on KNOW radio in Austin?

"Somethin' like that."

Daddy started cuttin' cedar before I was born. I started workin' in the cedar brakes when I was eight. I used a double-bit ax with a short handle.

The old man went and got an ax to show.

Awww, Daddy. Ever'body's seen an ax.

I quit school in the sixth grade to work full time in the brakes.

"I never went to school," the old man said.

Daddy can't write his name, but he used to keep us clean. We coulda gone to school all the way but we were just hardheaded. There was thirteen of us. I got one full sister, seven half brothers and four half sisters.

We used to live in tents in the cedar brakes with about fifteen other families. After work, we'd build a big campfire and sit around and talk and sang songs you never heard.

"We don't stay in the woods no more," the old man said. "Hardly any cedar cutters live thataway now."

The cedar's about gone, I mean the big cedar forests, and there's probably not a hundred choppers left in the hills. Used to be maybe a thousand.

I wished we lived like we used to. It's hard to say in words how I feel about the way it was. It was a free life, I guess you'd say.

"Nobody bossed you," the old man said. "You worked when you took a notion to."

That's right. You cut cedar where you pleased and hauled it where you wanted to. If the contractor talked rough to you, you gave him the finger and went somewheres else.

"And you got paid when you delivered the cedar at the end of the day," the old man said. "You didn't have to wait around no month for your money. You was paid in cash. No taxes."

It was what some people might call a trashy way to live. The kids in the camp ran around hungry and dirty and half naked. That was just the way it was and there wasn't any use in tryin' to change it. The women went around camp bare-

footed and half dressed and at night we used to get them in the truck beds.

I've worked for Al Ehrlich. What he said about cedar hackers is true. He's got us down pretty good. But I wouldn't trade places with him. I really wouldn't. He oughta understand, though, that the reason we have such sorry equipment is because men like him pay sorry wages. We just have to make do with what we've got. One day I blew out ever tire on my truck. I just took off the rubber and drove a load in on the rims. That night, I took a woman to a dance in the truck. It sounded like a tank rollin' down the highway. She didn't care.

I never seen nobody who cut cedar who ever amounted to anythang. It seems almost mandatory. I guess we're what you call a low class of people. I remember when Mama died. Daddy went to the lumber office and asked for a loan of eighty-five dollars to bury her. It was against company policy to lend money to us. Hell, I don't blame them for makin' a rule like that. A cedar cutter's not goin' to pay you what he owes you. He may intend to, but he'll never get around to it. Anyway, Daddy got the loan, and that was surprisin'. And he paid it back and that was kind of surprisin' too. But he's always been proud thataway.

I worked at a lot of jobs but I've always gone back to the cedar brakes. It gets in your blood. One time me and Daddy went to Arizona to look for work. But we got homesick. Daddy said he could just see the cedar trees a-growin' in the hills.

Before I got crippled, I could cut more cedar than most men without half tryin'. Now I strap on my hook, pick up my saw, and go into the brakes knowin' I have to stay with it and fight it when the others are restin'. I still cut more'n the average man. I average about twelve dollars a day—that's about seventy-five posts. I've cut up to fifty-six dollars a day and could average thirty dollars if there was more cedar.

It was getting late. Their voices grew softer as darkness set in. Sounds seem to carry better in the twilight. An old man coughed in the doorway of a trailer house next door. An almost-woman Mexican girl walked down the dirt road in front of the house. Her hair was long and straight and her bare feet made soft explosions in the dust. Oscar watched her and lit a cigarette. His old daddy excused himself and went to bed.

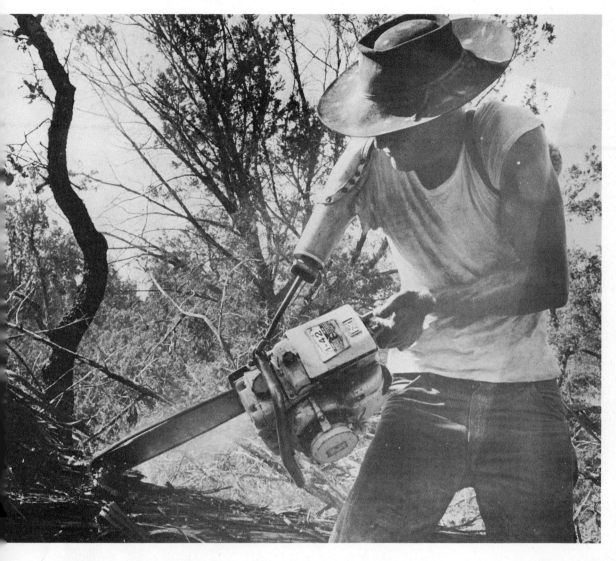

Oscar Carter can handle a chain saw better than most men who have two arms.

Oscar went down to the Maverick Tavern back of town and drank nine beers and smoked a package of cigarettes. And then he went back home and fell into bed with his clothes on.

Before sunup, he heard his old man groaning.

"What's the matter, Daddy?"

"Rheumatism, I reckon. Guess I better get up and take a couple'a bales of hay."

He swallowed two alfalfa pills and was just getting into sleep again when the roosters all over town began crowing. The sun came out with arson in its heart.

THADDEUS E. CAGE

1857–1922

This Blanco merchant was kicked in the mouth by a horse one day in 1890 and could not talk for two days. He lost seven teeth.

CHAPTER NINETEEN

Ⅰt has not rained for two months.

But now, hours before the President of the United States is to speak to the graduating seniors, thunderheads form over Shovel Mountain north of town.

James Ealy Johnson, the President's cousin, turns on his stool at Red's Place and gives the sky a once-over. "Ole Lyndon just might bring us some rain," he says. "Wouldn't that be somethin'?"

In the Johnson City barbershop, Pancho Althaus and his wife Pat are having a run on haircuts. Pat skins heads faster than Pancho, who yaks away like the horse trader he is. A sheepman watches with admiration as Pat makes the hair fly from the head of his boy. "Now wouldn't she be a dilly of a hand for the fall shearing?"

Yesterday the town dozed in the summer sun. Now it is awake, busy with a controlled excitement. New faces are on the streets. Cars with strange license plates line the square. Crider's Motel on Main displays a no vacancy sign.

Deputy sheriffs gather on the courthouse lawn. The cowboys in Red's Place watch them with amusement. The sky is cloud-sopped, but the men behind the stars wear broad-brimmed hats and sunshades. They ride up on mechanical steeds with sofa saddles and pedal stirrups, which naturally fit high-heeled boots. They move about the lawn with a lazy strut, like pompous roosters in a hen house.

In the I.G.A. store, a stranger asks for Amphora pipe tobacco. The clerk shakes her head. "Will Prince Albert do?" Never know who'll turn up here, she tells a customer. A man came in a few weeks ago and asked for cowboy boots. She sent him down the street. She saw his picture in the paper later. It was Dean Rusk.

John Moursund, the principal, and Kittie Leonard, the superintendent, huddle with protocol officers at the high school. It is all so different from the time Lyndon spoke here as vice-president. It had been fairly informal. Lyndon spent most of his time busily brushing June bugs off the necks of the valedictorian and salutatorian.

Mrs. Leonard wonders how she will introduce Lyndon. It has been in her mind for a week. There's so much she would like to say. She and the President grew up together . . . were in the same graduating class . . . got their diplomas here forty years ago, almost to the night. . . . The protocol men are firm. She is simply to say, "Ladies and gentlemen, the President of the United States."

Radio and television crews are busy in the auditorium, setting up platforms for their cameras and equipment. The Washington press corps is arriving.

The rain comes the way they hoped it would; not hard like a gulley washer, but soft and steady, gently soaking the thin skin of the parched hills.

Down on Flat Creek, Jesse Smitherman runs to the barn with two kid goats under his arms, Tippy at his heels. Jesse gets wet, but there's a big grin on his face.

The auditorium fills with people from all over the county. The women fluff their hairdos and look expectantly toward the stage for the President's entrance. Their menfolk watch with great curiosity as the radio and television technicians test a clutter of electronic gadgets. A hush falls over the auditorium. John Moursund, the principal, is at the microphone, asking if there is a doctor in the house. Is something wrong with Lyndon?

Piano chords strike up "Hail to the Chief" and the whispers stop. The President strides on stage and stands a moment before taking a seat. All eyes are upon him, all hands clapping in a standing ovation. He smiles at the audience and nods his head. He seems very tall and robust, almost handsome. His suit is a silky black. His face is deeply tanned and his dark hair, though thinning at the top, is full and graying at the temples.

The piano is out of tune. Rebecca Wolf walks woodenly into the auditorium from a hallway, followed by twenty-nine classmates. The President watches them from the stage. He wears a sentimental expression. Kittie Leonard sits on his left. John Moursund sits beside her and at his left is Lady Bird Johnson. The members of the school board sit behind them. The seniors take seats on stage at the right of the President.

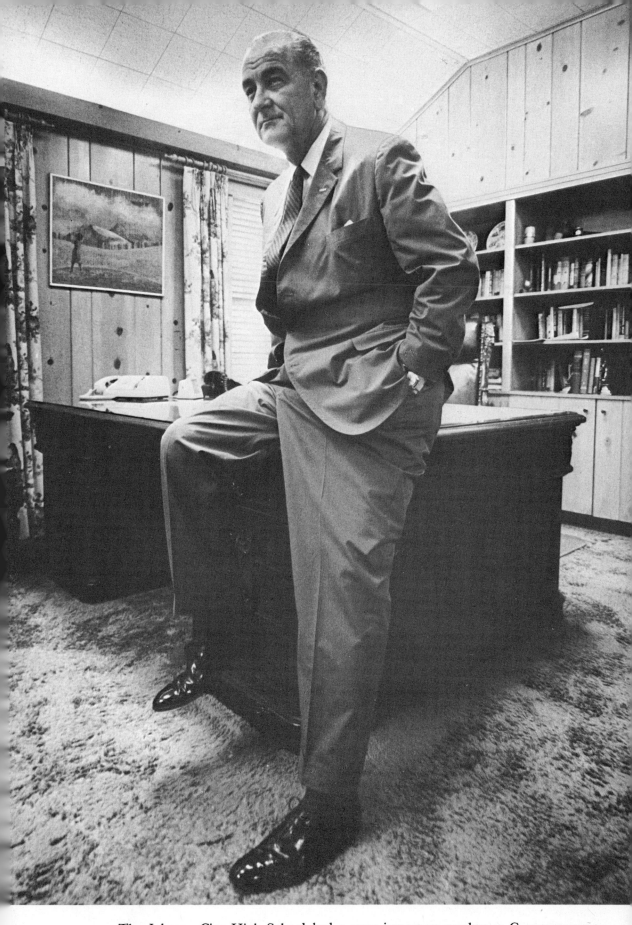

The Johnson City High School had a very important speaker at Commencement.

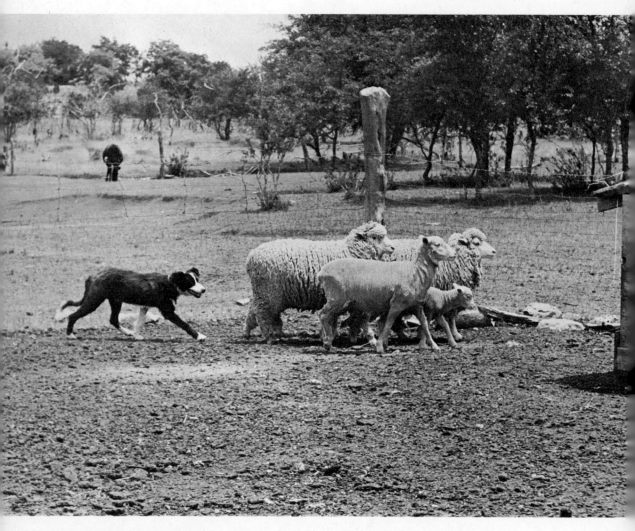

A border collie working sheep.

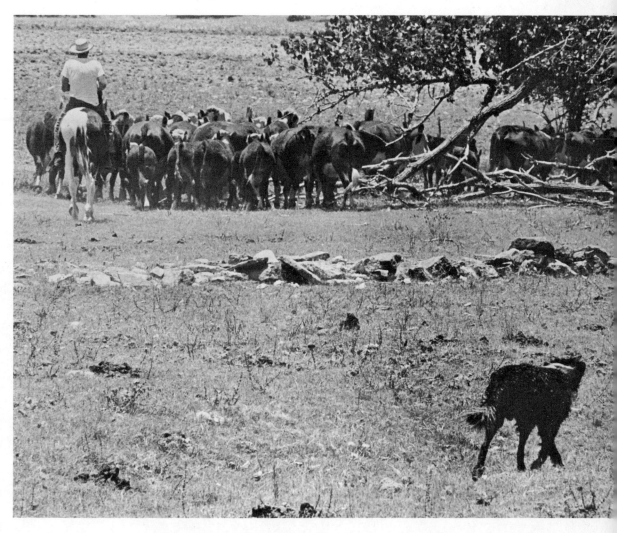

The work goes on on the ranches even when there are big doin's in town.

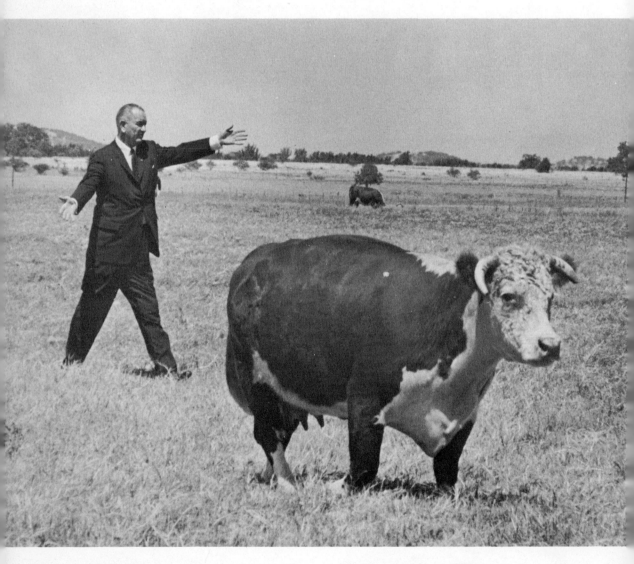

When Lyndon Johnson gets home he continues to display executive ability.

Little Mona Hobbs reads a prayer—perhaps she recites it—
and everyone stands up and pledges allegiance to the flag.

Donna Friedrich delivers the salutatory. She declares, in the
clear, confident voice of youth, "We have been reading lessons
from books, but after tonight, we will make our own history."
The President nods approvingly. Is he remembering what he
said in his graduation speech on this campus forty years ago?

Sherry Latham gives a rundown on the class history, and
then Pat Evans, Becky Wolf, Laura Haynes, and Donna Penick,
all done up in starched white dresses, harmonize on "Commencement Day."

Cathy, the bright, lovely Sibley girl, delivers the valedictory.
She enlarges on the class motto—"Not Finished, Just Begun"
—but sometimes it is hard to hear her. She speaks clearly, but
the radio and television crews are unwittingly rude as they fuss
over their equipment. Parents in the audience frown at them.
The President complains about the glare of the lights from the
camera platform, but they remain on.

John Moursund introduces the seniors. Then David Foster,
the school board president, presents diplomas. Sandra Kay
Crofts recites an acceptance speech. Moursund gets up again to
give out special student awards. The Sibley girl is not only the
prettiest and smartest in the class—but also the most industri-
ous. She takes most of the awards. Foster and Moursund team
to dedicate the high school in the name of the President.

At last, Mrs. Leonard gets up and says, "Ladies and gentlemen, the President of the United States."

He does not talk very long, but he talks with feeling about
the world that awaits a youngster fresh out of Lyndon B.
Johnson High School. He tells them the world of 1964 is really
not much different from the world of 1924, the year he left
the hills to seek "fame and fortune in the West." He tells them
he came back home with "empty hands and empty pockets,"
realizing that the place to begin was the place he had been all
the time.

He tells them he cannot predict their future any more than
he could have predicted his own. Certainly he had no idea he
would one day stand here as President.

But he tells them what America can be if they dream deep
enough and hope and work hard enough. It can be a place, he

says, where they will raise their families free from the dark shadow of war and suspicion among nations.

He tells them it can be a place where their children, and every child, will grow up knowing that success in life depends only on ability and not on the color of skin or the circumstances or region of birth.

Pretty Nina Gutierrez looks at the President with unabashed adulation. She sits on the front row of the class, third from the left.

He ends his little talk by saying he will always be honored to claim that he too came from Johnson City.

As the seniors march out, the President tries to shake hands with each of them. But they have been drilled to robot precision and will not break step, even to shake hands with the Chief. He pumps the hand of about half of them.

That ends the ceremony.

The President comes to the microphone and wonders aloud if any of the other four members of his high school graduating class are in the audience. Kittie Leonard, of course, is already on stage.

"Louise?" he asks, "Are you out there? Georgia?"

Louise Casparis Edwards, Red's oldest sister, and Georgia Cammock Edgeworth stand. They are portly, gray-haired women now. The President calls them on stage to pose for photographers. A thought occurs to him and he strides back to the microphone.

"John Dollahite? Are you there?" he calls.

John doesn't answer.

"John was always shy of the girls," the President jokes. "There were just two of us boys, so I always took his part. I guess John heard the girls were here tonight and didn't come. Thank you."

John Dollahite had trouble all day. The rain came and he rushed out in his field with a combine to harvest the hay before it got wet. The combine broke down and he and his boy had a time until after dark. He was a little sore at the world anyway. He mistakenly thought written invitations had been sent out for the President's commencement address—and he had not received one.

The sun goes down in the usual way over rock-ribbed Devil's Backbone.

SANTA ANNA CRUZE
1845–1920

One day in 1857, Santa Anna came home from
Professor Bristlehead Johnson's Institute for Young
Men, which was on Bear Creek a few miles from
the Cruzes' Hays County ranch, to find his daddy,
Bill, and their faithful scout, Chief Gray Eagle,
murdered by rustlers. One of the horse thieves lay
dead in the corral. Capt. Ferg Kyle buried Bill
Cruze, who was six feet five, beside the Indian. Then
he looped a lariat around the dead rustler's neck and
dragged him off into the bushes and burned him.
Bristlehead Johnson's school closed for good in 1861
when all the students rode off to fight in the Civil
War. Santa Anna, sixteen, was pretty good at calling
hounds with a cow horn and he wanted to be a
bugler for the 33d Texas Cavalry, C.S.A. The
company captain was skeptical. But an old French
soldier of fortune, Paganel, took Santa Anna in hand
and taught him to blow a bugle which Paganel's
father had carried in the Napoleonic Wars. Santa
Anna became the company bugler. After the war,
Santa Anna returned to Lone Man Creek, married,
and bought a ranch. Paganel went off to join
Maximilian in Mexico. Four years passed. One day
Santa Anna rode in off the range to find a vaquero
waiting with a gift. It was Paganel's bugle, wrapped
in burlap. Paganel was dead. From then on, until he
died, Santa Anna Cruze woke the chickens with
reveille and put them to bed with taps.

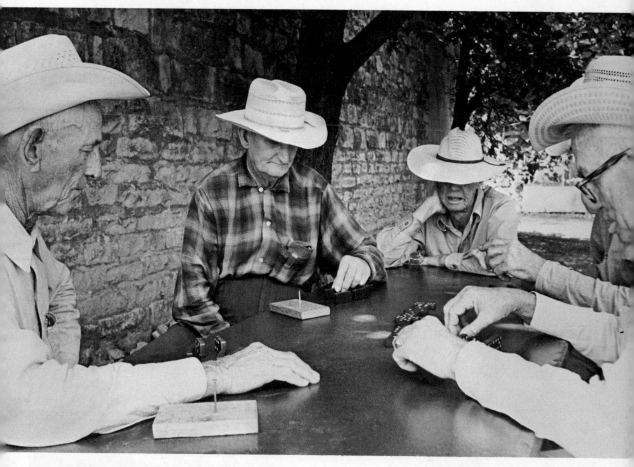

When Johnson City gets back to normal people settle down to important business.

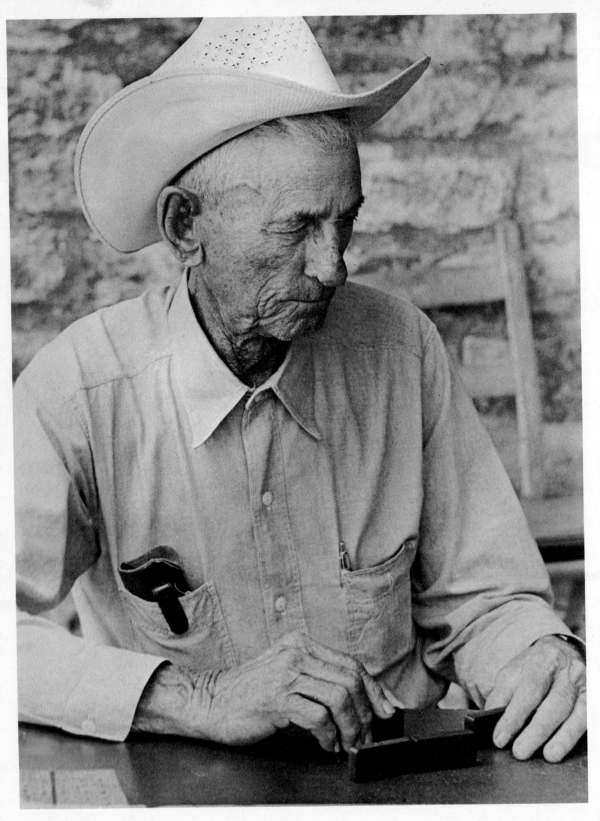

Austin Casparis studies the board before he settles on future strategy.

CHAPTER TWENTY

The town was back to normal the next day as if nothing unusual had happened. Red was behind the bar and his cousin, Ted, who still limps from World War II wounds, was waiting on his favorite stool for James Ealy Johnson.

Zeke Felps and the other domino players were gathering under the mulberry tree beside Casparis' Cafe. Zeke asked Otho Summy, "Didja hear Lyndon last night?"

"Huh-unh," Otho grunted. "Oh," he said, "I was gonna go, but I got to feelin' bad and just didn't."

In his talk Lyndon Johnson had touched on an adventure he had had with Otho, Payne Roundtree, and Otto and Tom Crider when they were boys. Steinbeck could have written the script.

One July day in 1924, just after Lyndon got out of high school, they cranked up a canvas-topped Model T and hit the high road to California, seeking, as Johnson put it, "fame and fortune in the West." Lyndon was the youngest at sixteen, and his mother didn't like his hightailing it a bit. She wanted him in college. But his daddy understood and gave tacit approval.

They chugged westward, stopping twice a day to gulp down fat back and corn bread garnished with molasses. At night, they buried their little sack of money, spread homemade quilts over the treasured spot, and dozed fitfully under the stars.

When their stake was gone, they managed to pick up a little traveling money picking fruit and washing dishes in greasy spoon cafes. By the time they reached the promised land they were ready to leave the wretched place for the hills of home.

Now, forty years later, one of them is President of the United States. Tom Crider is a shop inspector for an oil tool company in Houston. Otto is in the real estate business in Cloverdale, California, and Payne Roundtree is a retired mechanic in Austin.

And Otho? Well, when he's not looking after his cows you can usually find him at the domino table under the mulberry tree beside Casparis' Cafe. Steinbeck couldn't have written a better ending.

Lyndon Johnson told the high school seniors that the Johnson City they would be leaving really isn't much different from the one he knew as a boy. He was talking about values rather than appearances, although the look of things hasn't changed a whole lot either. The same old hot high hills rise above the same sleepy settlements. The sun still blisters. The cedar and cypress and cactus still fight for a foothold in the stingy, shallow soil, and men still wish for rain. But it would be silly to say that time stands still here. Forces are at work changing the character of the people and the country.

The narrow roads that used to bump through the little towns now are superhighways that speed past, and the village squares grow ghosts and weeds. The old-timers who stay, the Otho Summys and the Zeke Felpses, inevitably face the dreaded day when they must wave good-by to their children. Once they dreamed their sons would bury them and take up where they left off on a thousand rocky ranches nestled in a hundred harsh and hallowed hills. Now they sell out to soft strangers in starched blue jeans white at the knees.

The lament of Percy Brigham, the Blanco banker, has a ring of prophecy:

> These playboys are willing to pay high prices for the land. Prices so high that the little rancher has little choice but to sell. Their kids don't want to stay here in these rocky hills and fight drouth to make a livin', so the old folks put their places on the market and retire on the take. . . .

> . . . It'll be getting worse. They'll put more dams down here. More resort property buyers will come in and there'll come a time when there won't be a legitimate rancher left. . . ."

Drive off the main highway and take a lost road through the yucca and mesquite flats and count the empty hulls of houses with rotting corrals out back. You muse and remember George

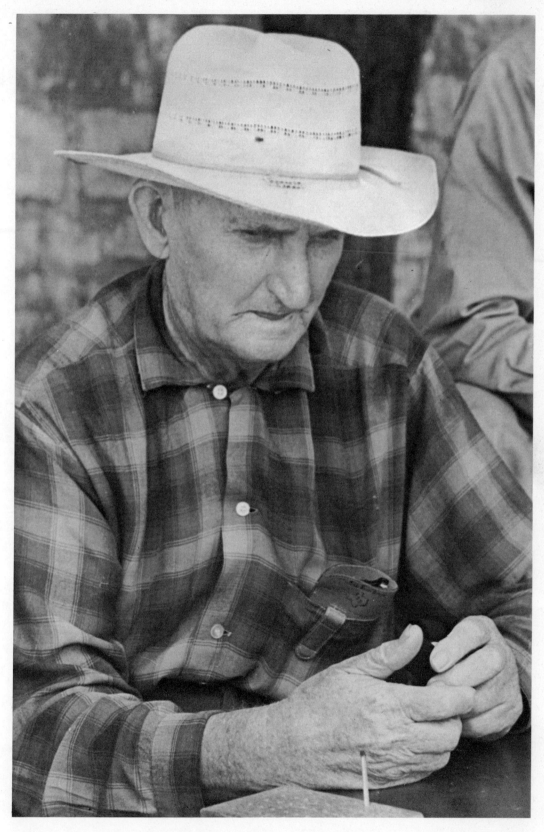

Zeke Felps makes a rough mental calculation about what Lee Green has in his hand.

137

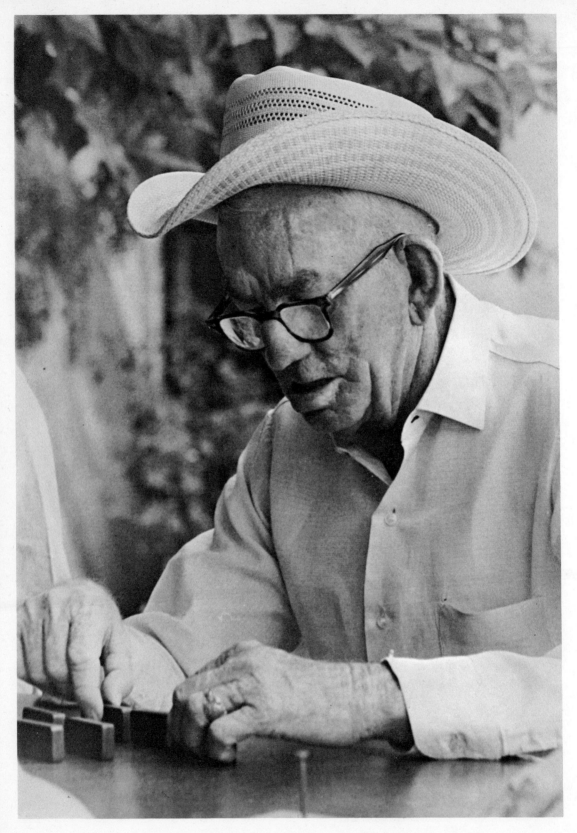

Lee Green ponders whether to play the double five now or to hold it for later.

Sessions Perry finding this message carved on the walls of a West Texas dugout:

> 20 miles to water
> 10 miles to wood
> 6 inches to hell.
> > Gone back East to wife's family.
> > Make yourself at home.

Get back on the asphalt and head for the misty highlands where lakes and rivers have been dammed and count the real estate offices and the swank resort homes with boat basins out back.

This rock-ribbed, lonesome land, this cow-pocked cradle of the cult of rugged and ragged individualism, is being purchased, plotted, and subdivided, irrigated, manicured, and sold off to a generation of Texans tame in the saddle but bold with the ballyhoo of tomorrow.

They make family airplanes in Kerrville now instead of wagon wheels.

Artesian spring waters, which once gurgled pure and sweet for thirsty settlers, are now mixed with mash and brewed and bottled by beer barons.

Every summer, the hills and draws are overrun by city folk seeking a sort of communal solitude in the summer camps and dude ranches. Even communities for artists and convalescents are cropping up.

The old-timers whine, but the progressive businessman isn't bitching. He has moved his store off the square and onto the superhighway under a neon sign. He and his neighbors live in air-conditioned homes and send their children off to college.

The number of ranches dwindles each year, replaced by beef- and mutton-growing syndicates owned by silk-suited city slickers with plenty of money and savvy.

Creed Taylor from Kimble County wouldn't like his hill country now. But Creed could see no farther than his horse could take him. That very man he distrusted, Henry Ford, built the contraption that took five young men from Johnson City to California in 1924. That they failed to find what they were seeking in the West isn't important. What is important is that one of them, perhaps four of them, saw farther than that Model T took them.

139

JOHN K. BACKUES

1838–1874

Backues was just another pioneer settler, now long
forgotten. He took part in a battle against Indians at
the head of Cypress Creek, and was credited with
killing one brave. The Llano County tax roll of
1859 listed his total property as being one horse
valued at fifty dollars. Even in those days, that was
a pretty sorry horse.

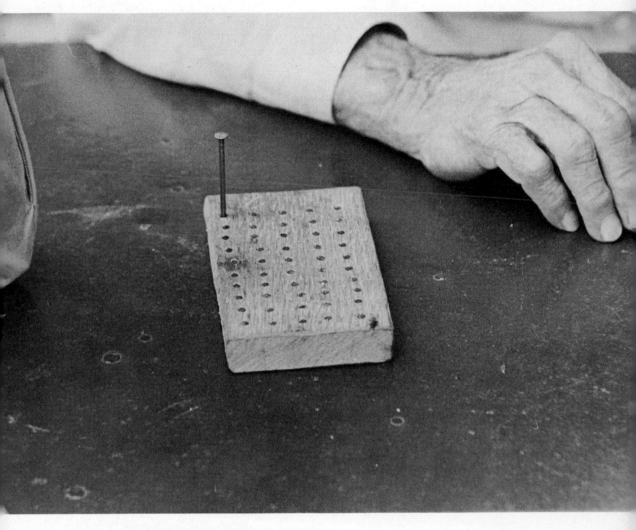

The scoring device preceded IBM machines by many long years in Johnson City, Texas.